Tidy's Physiotherapy

Dedication

To all the physiotherapy students, who have taught me so much.
I thank them for the encouragement and support they have given me over the years.

Also by this author

The Anatomy Workbook (2002)
Butterworth–Heinemann
ISBN 0750 654554

Tidy's Physiotherapy

Thirteenth Edition

Edited by

Stuart B. Porter BSc(Hons) Grad Dip Phys MCSP SRP CertMHS

Lecturer in Physiotherapy
School of Health Care Professions
University of Salford
Manchester
UK

Honorary Research Fellow
Wrightington Wigan and Leigh NHS Trust
Wigan
Lancashire
UK

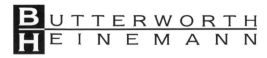

BUTTERWORTH
HEINEMANN

EDINBURGH   LONDON   NEW YORK   OXFORD   PHILADELPHIA   ST LOUIS   SYDNEY   TORONTO   2003

BUTTERWORTH-HEINEMANN
An imprint of Elsevier Limited

First published 2003
 Reprinted 2005, 2006

ISBN 0 7506 3211 9

British Library Cataloguing in Publication Data
A catalogue record for this book is available from the British Library

Library of Congress Cataloging in Publication Data
A catalog record for this book is available from the Library of Congress

Notice
Medical knowledge is constantly changing. Standard safety precautions must be followed,
but as new research and clinical experience broaden our knowledge, changes in treatment
and drug therapy may become necessary or appropriate. Readers are advised to check
the most current product information provided by the manufacturer of each drug to be
administered to verify the recommended dose, the method and duration of administration,
and contraindications. It is the responsibility of the practitioner, relying on experience and
knowledge of the patient, to determine dosages and the best treatment for each individual
patient. Neither the Publisher nor the editors/contributor assumes any liability for any
injury and/or damage to persons or property arising from this publication.

The Publisher

The
Publisher's
policy is to use
**paper manufactured
from sustainable forests**

Printed in The Netherlands by Krips BV

Contents

Contributors

The Responsibilities of Being a Physiotherapist
Judy Mead MCSP
Head of Clinical Effectiveness,
Research and Clinical Effectiveness Unit,
Chartered Society of Physiotherapy,
London, UK

Musculoskeletal Assessment
Lynne Gaskell Grad Dip Phys PGD(Res)
Lecturer, School of Health Care Professions,
University of Salford,
Salford, UK

An Introduction to Fractures
Stuart B. Porter BSc (Hons) Grad Dip Phys MCSP
    SRP CertMHS
Lecturer, School of Health Care Professions,
University of Salford,
Salford, UK

The Intervertebral Disc in Health and Disease: An Introduction to Back Pain
Stuart B. Porter BSc(Hons) Grad Dip Phys MCSP
    SRP CertMHS
Lecturer, School of Health Care Professions,
University of Salford,
Salford, UK

Management of Burns and Plastic Surgery
Sally Dean Grad Dip Phys MCSP
Clinical Specialist, Hand Therapy,
Burns and Plastics Unit,
Whiston Hospital,
St Helens and Knowsley Hospital Services NHS Trust,
Prescot,
Merseyside, UK

Biomechanics
Jim Richards BEng MSc PhD
Senior Lecturer in Biomechanics,
School of Health Care Professions,
University of Salford, Salford, UK

Physiotherapy in Women's Health
Gill Brook MCSP SRP
Eileen Brayshaw MSc MCSP SRP FETC

Yvonne Coldron MSc MCSP MMACP
Susan Davies MCSP SRP
Georgina Evans MCSP SRP
Ruth Hawkes MCSP SRP
Alison Lewis Grad Dip Phy MCSP SRP
Pauline M. Mills MSc MCSP Dip TP
Daphne Sidney Dip Phys
Ros Thomas MCSP SRP
Jacquelyne Todd MCSP SRP PGCE
Kathleen Vits MCSP SRP
Pauline Walsh MCSP SRP

Principles of Paediatric Physiotherapy
Alison Carter MCSP SRP
Superintendent Paediatric Physiotherapist,
Guys & St Thomas NHS Trust,
London, UK

Osteoarthritis
Stuart B. Porter BSC(Hons) Grad Dip Phys MCSP
    SRP Cert MHS
Lecturer,
School of Health Care Professions,
University of Salford,
Salford, UK

Common Chronic Inflammatory Polyarthropathies
J. A. Goodacre MD PhD FRCP
Director of Clinical Research, and Honorary
    Consultant in Rheumatology,
Lancashire Postgraduate School of Medicine and
    Health,
University of Central Lancashire,
Preston, Lancashire, UK

I. Stewart MB CHB FRCP(Edinburgh)
Consultant in Rheumatology,
Blackpool Victoria Hospital,
Blackpool,
Merseyside, UK

Osteoporosis
Kirsty Carne RGN
Osteoporosis Nurse,
National Osteoporosis Society,
Camerton,
Bath, UK

Physiotherapy in Rheumatology
Rachel Lewis MCSP SRP HT
Physiotherapy Department,
Avon Orthopaedic Centre,
Southmead Hospital,
Bristol, UK

Physiotherapy Management of Ankylosing Spondylitis
Juliette O'Hea MCSP MSc PG Dip (Rheum)
Rheumatology Practioner,
Salisbury District Hospital,
Odstock Road,
Salisbury,
Wiltshire, UK

Management of Respiratory Diseases
Stephanie Enright PhD MPhil MSc PG Cert MSCP
Senior Lecturer,
School of Health Care Professions,
University of Salford,
Salford, UK

Cardiac Disease
J. P. Moore PhD
Academic Unit of Cardiovascular Medicine,
University of Leeds, UK

Physiotherapy in Thoracic Surgery
Anne Dyson Grad Dip Phys MCSP SRP
Senior Physiotherapist,
Cardio Thoracic Centre,
NHS Trust,
Liverpool, UK

The Research Process
Lynne Goodacre PhD SROT
Postdoctoral Research Associate,
Lancashire Postgraduate School of Medicine and
    Health,
University of Central Lancashire,
Preston,
Lancashire, UK

Upper and Lower Joint Arthroplasty
Ann Birch BA (OU) MCSP SRP
Senior Physiotherapist,
Wrightington Hospital,
Hand and Upper Limb Surgery Unit,
Wigan,
Lancashire, UK

Ann Price Dip TP Cert Ed MCSP
Superintendent Physiotherapist,
Wrightington Hospital,
Wigan,
Lancashire, UK

Tissue Inflammation and Repair
Elaine Court PhD
Department of Biological Sciences,
University of Central Lancashire,
Preston,
Lancashire, UK

Robert W. Lea PhD
Department of Biological Sciences,
University of Central Lancashire,
Preston,
Lancashire, UK

Neurological Physiotherapy
Alison Chambers Med MCSP SRP
Project Director,
Allied Health Project Developments,
University of Central Lancashire,
Preston,
Lancashire, UK

Christine Smith MSc Grad Dip Phys Cert Ed
Lecturer/Course Leader,
University of Salford,
Salford, UK

Concepts in Exercise Rehabilitation
Duncan Mason Bsc (Hons) SRP
Lecturer Practitioner,
Royal Bolton Infirmary,
Greater Manchester, and University of Salford
    School of Health Care Professions,
University of Salford,
Salford, UK

Sean Kilmurray MSc Grad Dip Phys
Lecturer in Physiotherapy,
The University of Central Lancashire,
Preston,
Lancashire, UK

Physiotherapy for Amputees
Alison Chambers Med MCSP SRP
Project Director Allied Health Project
    Developments,
University of Central Lancashire,
Preston,
Lancashire, UK

Preface to the Thirteenth Edition

This is an exciting time to become a physiotherapist. If you are training or if you are about to commence training as an undergraduate, you are entering one of the most stimulating, varied and rewarding careers possible. The new millennium holds endless possibilities for physiotherapists.

The first edition of *Tidy's Physiotherapy* was published in the 1930s, and the fact that it endures as a bestseller amongst student physiotherapists confirms that students want a clear reference guide to help them through their studies.

This thirteenth edition has been extensively redesigned. Experts from a wide range of clinical and academic backgrounds have rewritten each chapter, to reflect current clinical practice and theory. Previously existing chapters have been updated, and there are new chapters covering a diverse cross-section of the topics to which student physiotherapists need to be introduced.

Physiotherapy as a profession underwent spectacular changes in the second half of the twentieth century. *Tidy's Physiotherapy* now reflects those changes and will evolve as our profession evolves. This new edition covers some key areas and developments in the field of physiotherapy in the early twenty-first century, and the book will look as different in ten years as this edition differs from its predecessor.

Physiotherapy students need a solid foundation upon which to build their knowledge base, and we must not lose sight of this reality. This new edition reflects current trends and innovations whilst acknowledging that just occasionally it is good to have a clearly laid out reference guide for students, for whom the learning curve is especially steep.

Physiotherapy qualifying programmes must prepare students to function effectively in the changing world of healthcare – to be analytical problem-solvers who are autonomous practitioners in their own right. I wonder, though, how many graduates still recall how difficult it was to reflect, hypothesise, reason, analyse and integrate vast amounts of new information when we were new to the profession.

The journey to become a physiotherapist is not an easy one, and we should facilitate the learning process for students, the physiotherapists of the future, in every way possible. Albert Einstein said 'Make everything as simple as possible, but not simpler.' The team of authors in this volume have tried to give student physiotherapists a simple – but accurate and relevant – guide which is grounded in the clinical world and presented in a clear format. I hope that we have succeeded in our aim.

2003   Stuart Porter

Acknowledgements

When I was asked to act as Editor, it soon became clear to me that to accomplish a successful project would involve a team effort involving a diverse group of people who already had extremely busy lives. I have been moved by the willingness and dedication of the contributing authors to devote the time to their chapters, and the grace with which they have accepted my periodic nagging. It is greatly appreciated.

I would also like to thank Heidi Allen, Robert Edwards and Judy Elias at Butterworth–Heinemann for their support and faith in me in entrusting me with the task of editing this book. I would like to thank Richard Cook at Keyword Publishing Services also.

The following people have been an invaluable source of opinions and comments: Marc Hudson, Joanne Fawcett, Hannah Cushion, Laura McLeod, Eleanor Ford, Robert Hodgkiss, Kezia Purdie, David Wilkes, James Baldwin, Vicky Platt, Jamie Murphy, Paul Sparrow, Mark Eales, Steve Morris, Candice Olliver, Amy Glasgow, Chris Hodson, Laura Hay, Natalie Price, Elaine Byrne, undergraduate physiotherapy students who formed the focus group; Patricia Lambert-Zazulak DCR(T) BA PhD, research associate at the Mummy Tissue Bank, Egyptology Department, Manchester Museum for her advice on ancient diseases and trauma; my great friend of 35 years Mark Hothersall for some of the digital image manipulation; Paula-Jayne McDowell, Guidelines Initiative Officer at the Royal College of General Practitioners; Nick Goudge, Kate Slingsby, Kay Hack, Simon Crozier, David Dean and Sharon Baines, lecturers at the University of Salford; Judith Chapman, lecturer at the University of Southampton; Sue Barnard, lecturer in physiotherapy at the University of Southampton; Rod Moore, of Medical Dynamics; Pauline Davey, assistant communications manager at the National Osteoporosis Society; Mr R. F. Adam FRCS MChOrth, consultant orthopaedic surgeon; Fiona Cobbold, senior physiotherapist, and Mike Somervell and Julie Butler, senior occupational therapists, at the Southport & Ormskirk Hospital NHS Trust; Reinier van Mierlo, superintendent physiotherapist at the Royal Preston Hospital; Carol Barnes, senior physiotherapist at Stepping Hill Hospital, Stockport; and the medical photography department at Whiston Hospital. Thanks also go to Andrew and Justine Arlow for their encouragement and advice.

I should also like to thank all my colleagues at the University of Salford School of Health Care Professions for their support; the physiotherapy staff at Wrightington and Ormskirk Hospitals; and the unsung heroes of our profession – the physiotherapy assistants with whom I have worked over the years and who have kept me functioning on numerous occasions.

My thanks go to my wife, Sue, for always having picked me up whenever I have fallen down. Finally, thank you to our three little girls Alison, Claire and Jessica for helping me to believe in magic again and never complaining when they were buried under a mountain of paper during the final months of this project!

The Responsibilities of Being a Physiotherapist

Judy Mead

INTRODUCTION

This chapter aims to provide the reader with an insight into what it means to be a professional (in the context of this chapter, a physiotherapist), focusing on the responsibilities, both ethical and practical, that are inherent in claiming to be a professional.

The current status and privilege of physiotherapists as autonomous professionals will be put in the context of the history of the profession, and the impact of autonomy on clinical practice will be explored. The chapter will reflect on the implications for physiotherapists of the increasing expectations of both the general public and the government for health professionals to deliver high-quality health services. Explanations of how physiotherapists can meet these expectations through clinical governance will be provided. Finally, the reader will be offered a look at the possible future of the profession in the light of the changing shape of health services in the UK.

Physiotherapists come into the profession because they have an underlying sense of – and commitment to – helping others and improving their quality of life. Indeed, Koehn (1994) argues that professions can be thought of as being defined by a distinctive commitment to benefit the client. Physiotherapists want to be able to use their acquisition of knowledge, skills and attributes from qualifying programmes to benefit people, in whatever speciality or with whichever patient group they wish to work once qualified – for example elite athletes, elderly people, the general public with sports injuries or back pain, or people with mental health problems. This chapter will help readers understand how they can make benefiting patients a reality in the context of the expectations of society for the provision of high-quality, safe and effective care.

While earlier editions of *Tidy's Physiotherapy* may have been popular for their prescriptive descriptions of what physiotherapists should do in particular situations or for particular conditions, this edition demands more from the reader. For no two patients are quite the same. Each requires the skills of the physiotherapist to carry out a full and accurate assessment, taking account of the individuality of the patient, and then to use clinical reasoning to problem solve and offer appropriate options for treatment, on which the patient will make a decision. A professional is required to have the maturity to take full responsibility for the privilege of autonomy. This will be by maintaining a competence to practise through career-long learning, through self-evaluation as well as through the evaluation of present practice; by keeping up to date with the most effective interventions and by maintaining the trust of patients by doing good. Readers should realise that while this approach is more challenging, it will also be more rewarding.

CHARACTERISTICS OF BEING A PROFESSIONAL

The most frequently cited characteristics of being a professional are (Koehn 1994):

- belonging to an organisation that sets standards and ideals of behaviour, and which disciplines other members for breaching these
- possessing knowledge and skills not shared by others
- exercising autonomy in their work
- licensed by the state
- making a commitment to assisting those in need.

Setting standards, disciplining members and claiming a unique body of knowledge are described in subsequent paragraphs of this chapter in the context of the role of the UK's professional body, the Chartered Society of Physiotherapy (CSP). While the principles of professionalism should be aspired to by physiotherapists anywhere in the world, the existence and/or role of professional bodies and the way these characteristics are manifested may vary, depending on political, social and financial factors.

Belonging to an organisation that sets standards and ideals of behaviour

Rules of Professional Conduct were endorsed at the very first council meeting of the CSP in 1895 (Barclay 1994) and have been revised and updated at intervals since. *Rules* sets out a framework for the ethical, moral and legal basis of the profession, providing statements of the conduct expected of chartered physiotherapists and students. The current *Rules* (CSP 2002a) set out a number of principles, the basis for all of which is to safeguard patients. They include requirements that physiotherapists should:

- respect the dignity and individual sensibilities of every patient
- work safely and competently
- ensure the confidentiality of patient information
- report circumstances that might otherwise put patients at risk
- not exploit patients
- act in a way that reflects credit on the profession and does not cause offence to patients.

Although the CSP has had *Rules of Professional Conduct* since its inception, *Standards of Physiotherapy Practice* was not published until 1990. This provides statements about the practical application of the ethical principles set out in the *Rules*. The third edition (CSP 2000) has evolved to place more emphasis than in earlier editions on practitioners:

- involving patients in decision-making
- being fully abreast of the evidence of effectiveness in order to inform patients and offer the most effective interventions
- evaluating their practice and measuring a patient's health gain as a result of treatment.

This reflects the increasing expectations of the public to be active partners in their healthcare, the expectations of clinical governance to provide more effective care, and the growing demands of funders of services, as well as patients, to be able to demonstrate the benefits or 'added value' of physiotherapy. All these will be discussed later in the chapter.

Standards of Physiotherapy Practice is written in a way that offers a broad statement of intent (the Standard statement), which is followed by a number of measurable statements about expected performance or activity by the physiotherapist, student or assistant (known as 'criteria'). For example, Core Standard 2 states 'Patients are given relevant information about the proposed physiotherapy procedure, taking into account their age, emotional state and cognitive ability, to allow informed consent.' The criteria for this standard include:

- the patient's consent is obtained before starting any examination/treatment
- treatment options, including significant benefits, risks and side-effects, are discussed with the patient
- the patient is given the opportunity to ask questions
- the patient is informed of the right to decline physiotherapy at any stage without that prejudicing future care
- the patient's consent to the treatment plan is documented in the patient's record.

These measurable criteria allow performance to be assessed against them, through clinical audit, described in more detail later.

The content of this standard and accompanying criteria set out the specific actions required in order to conform, in this case, to an aspect of Rule 2 of *Rules of Professional Conduct*: 'Chartered physiotherapists shall respect and uphold the rights, dignity and individual sensibilities of every patient', which includes guidance on informed consent. This is a good example of how the *Standards* and *Rules* complement each other. They should be used together to ensure compliance with the

characteristics and actions required of members of the physiotherapy profession.

Commitment to discipline other members

The CSP does not 'police' the *Rules* or the *Standards*; that is, it does not directly monitor members' conformance. However, it does have a responsibility to protect patients (self-regulation), as well as to protect the reputation of the profession. Should a member of the public or a colleague make a complaint, therefore, the *Society* has a responsibility to deal with this, and has a formal process for doing so. While it is the *Rules* that must be demonstrated to have been breached in order for disciplinary action to be taken, the *Standards of Physiotherapy Practice* will be used as a benchmark of expected performance in determining the application of the *Rules* in a practice setting.

The ultimate sanction the profession can impose is for a member to be struck off the register, no longer having access to the services of the Society and being unable to use the initials 'MCSP' or the title 'chartered physiotherapist'.

Possessing knowledge and skills not shared by others

Any profession possesses a range of specific knowledge and skills that are either unique, or more significantly developed than in other professions. For physiotherapy, the roots of the profession can be found in massage, the founders of the profession having been a group of nurses who carried out massage. The significance of therapeutic touching of patients still sets physiotherapy aside from other professions. Physiotherapists continue to use massage therapeutically as well as a wide range of other manual techniques such as manipulation and reflex therapy. Therapeutic handling underpins many aspects of rehabilitation, requiring the touching of patients to facilitate movement.

The second core skill is exercise, or movement. Cott et al. (1995) discuss the notion of a 'movement continuum theory of physical therapy', arguing that the way in which physiotherapists conceptualise movement is what differentiates the profession from others. They describe movement as a continuum from a micro (molecular, cellular) to a macro (the person in their environment, or in society) level. The authors argue that the theory is a unique approach to movement rehabilitation because it incorporates knowledge of pathology with a holistic view of movement, which includes the influence of physical, social and psychological factors. They argue that the role of physiotherapy is to minimise the difference between a person's current movement capability and his or her preferred movement capability.

The third core element of physiotherapy is defined as the use of electrophysical agencies (CSP 2002a). Cott and colleagues argue that this, too, can be part of the movement continuum, describing how such modalities complement therapeutic movement strategies at a tissue level, for example by reducing pain or swelling.

Another description of the profession's knowledge and skills can be found in the *Curriculum Framework for Qualifying Programmes in Physiotherapy* (CSP 2002b). This sets out the underpinning knowledge and skills required of newly qualifying physiotherapists, setting this in the context of their application in professional practice areas and environments. These are, in turn, underpinned by a set of professional attributes, identity and relationships, such as understanding the scope of practice and active engagement with patient partnership. Finally, the framework sets out the outcomes that graduates should be able to demonstrate, for example 'enable individual patients and groups to optimise their health and social well-being' and 'respond appropriately to changing demands'.

Definition

Physiotherapy is a healthcare profession concerned with human function and movement and maximising potential. It uses physical approaches to promote, maintain and restore physical, psychological and social well-being, taking account of variations in health status. It is science-based, committed to extending, applying, evaluating and reviewing the evidence that underpins and informs its practice and delivery. The exercise of clinical judgement and informed interpretation is at its core (CSP 2002b).

Exercising autonomy

Autonomy, or 'personal freedom' (*Concise Oxford Dictionary*, 7th edn), is a key characteristic of being a professional. It allows independence, but is mirrored by a responsibility and accountability for action. Central to the practice of professional autonomy is clinical reasoning, described as the 'thinking and decision-making processes associated with clinical practice' (Higgs and Jones 2000). Clinical reasoning requires the ability to think critically about practice, to learn from experience and apply that learning to future situations. It is the relationship between the physiotherapist's knowledge, his or her ability to collect, analyse and synthesise relevant information (cognition), and personal awareness, self-monitoring and reflective processes, or metacognition (Jones et al. 2000).

Autonomy has, however, to be balanced with the autonomy patients have, to make their own decisions. Patient-centred decisions require a partnership between patient and professional, sharing information, with patients' values and experience being treated as equally important as clinical knowledge and scientific facts (Ersser and Atkins 2000). Higgs and Titchen (2001) describe the notion of the professional's role as a 'skilled companion'. The professional is characterised as a person with specialised knowledge which can be shared with the patient in a reciprocal 'working with' rather than 'doing to' relationship, and as someone who 'accompanies the patient on their journey towards health, adjustment, coping or death'. This patient-centred model facilitates the sharing of power and responsibility between professional and patient.

A history of how the physiotherapy profession's autonomy evolved in the UK can be found later in this chapter.

Licensed by the state

Physiotherapists in the United Kingdom have to be registered with the Health Professions Council (HPC) in order to work in the National Health Service (NHS). In the near future this will be a requirement in order to use the title *physiotherapist*, and therefore work in any setting in the UK. This is a government measure to protect patients from unqualified or inadequately skilled healthcare providers.

Within the next few years, the HPC will put in place a system requiring re-registration at intervals of, perhaps, five years, based on a demonstration of an individual's continued competence to practise, probably through the submission of evidence of the outcomes of continuing professional development (CPD). Re-registration is in response to a decrease in public confidence in the NHS following, for example, the report into children's heart surgery in Bristol (Bristol Royal Infirmary Inquiry 2001). Equally disturbing were the revelations about the murders of so many patients by Harold Shipman, a man who had been a previously trusted general practitioner, where health systems failed to detect an unusually high number of deaths.

This has led the government to take a number of measures, including the requirement for all health professionals to re-register at specified intervals, to be seen to be protecting the public through a more explicit and independent process. It will aim to identify poor performers who may be putting the public at risk, as well as providing an incentive for professionals to keep up to date, maintaining and further developing their scope of, and competence to, practise. Disciplinary processes are in place to, ultimately, remove an individual from the register. The means by which individuals can maintain their competence are discussed later in the chapter.

Making a commitment to assist those in need

As stated earlier, one of the characteristics of a professional is to want to 'do good'. This is reflected in the ethical principles of the physiotherapy profession, where there is a 'duty of care' incumbent on the individual towards the patient, to ensure that the therapeutic intervention is intended to be of benefit, as set out in Rule 1 (CSP 2002a). This is a common-law duty, a breach of which (negligence) could lead to a civil claim for damages.

More generally, professionals are perceived to have moral authority, or trustworthiness, if they (Koehn 1994):

- use their skills in the context of the client's best interests, and 'doing good'
- are willing to act as long as it takes for assistance to achieve what it set out to achieve, or for a decision to be made that nothing more can be done to help the client
- have a highly developed internalised sense of responsibility to monitor personal behaviour, for example by not taking advantage of vulnerable patients
- demand from the client the responsibility to provide, for example, sufficient information to allow decisions to be made (compliance)
- are allowed to exercise discretion (judgement) to do the best for the client, within limits.

Koehn argues that trustworthiness is what stands out as a particularly unique characteristic of being a professional – to do good, to have the patient's best interests at heart and to have high ethical standards. Physiotherapists not prepared to maintain such ethics, even in difficult and stressful situations, run the risk of losing the respect as well as the trust of their patients and the public.

RESPONSIBILITIES OF BEING A PROFESSIONAL

Physiotherapists in the UK are granted the right to make their own decisions, in partnership with patients, about meeting needs. Being a professional is a privilege – in particular the trust that is bestowed by the public, which underpins the patient's ability to benefit from treatment. However, this brings with it weighty responsibilities.

Doing only those things you are competent to do

Every physiotherapist has her or his own personal 'scope of practice' (CSP 2002a) – that is, a range (or scope) of professional knowledge and skills that can be applied competently within specific practice settings or populations.

When a person is newly qualified, this scope will be based on the content of the pre-qualifying Curriculum Framework, but will also be informed by the individual's experience in clinical placements, and the amount of teaching and reflective learning that has been possible as part of those placements.

As a career progresses, and as a result of CPD, some physiotherapists will become competent in highly skilled areas such as intensive care procedures, or splinting for children with cerebral palsy, which are unlikely to have been taught pre-qualifying. Others will extend their skills in areas in which they already had some experience, for example dealing with people with neurological problems. Others will enhance their communication and life skills, as well as refining their physiotherapy skills by, for example, working with elderly people or people with learning difficulties.

It is the responsibility of the professional to understand his or her personal scope of practice as it changes and evolves throughout a career. To practise in areas in which you are not competent puts patients at risk and is a breach of the CSP's *Rules of Professional Conduct*.

Maintaining competence to practise

So an individual's scope of practice and competence are constantly evolving, based on professional and life experiences, learning from reading, from evaluating practice, from reflecting on practice, or more formal ways of learning. It includes undertaking programmes of structured CPD. Clinical reasoning skills are continually refined and further developed throughout a career through evaluative and reflective practice, leading to the ability to deal with increasingly complex and unpredictable situations.

Physiotherapists have a duty to keep up to date with new knowledge generated by research, with what their peers are thinking and doing, and by formally evaluating the outcome of their practice. The responsibility for this is reflected in *Standards of Physiotherapy Practice* (CSP 2000). In particular, Core Standards 19–22 are concerned with a requirement that individuals assess their learning needs, then plan, implement and evaluate a programme of CPD based on that assessment.

Responsibility to patients

This chapter has already discussed the importance of the individual physiotherapist as well as the profession as a whole maintaining the attributes of professionals. Trust is perhaps the most essential characteristic with which to develop a sense of partnership with patients that, in turn, will optimise the benefits of intervention. For physiotherapy, many of the other hallmarks for building and securing trust are set out in the profession's *Rules* and *Standards*; for example

- to provide safe and effective interventions (safety of application as well as safe and effective) – Rule 1 and Core Standards 4, 8, 16
- to treat patients with dignity and respect – Rule 2 and Core Standard 1
- to provide patients with information about their options for treatment/interventions – Rule 2 and Core Standard 2
- to involve patients in decisions about their treatment (informed consent) – Rule 2 and Core Standard 2.

Responsibility to those who pay for services

Physiotherapists have an ethical responsibility to payers of services, whether these are commissioners of healthcare, taxpayers or individual patients, to provide efficiently delivered, clinically and cost-effective interventions and services, in order to provide value in an era when resources for healthcare are limited.

Responsibility to colleagues and the profession

A profession has legitimate expectations of its members to conduct themselves in a way that does not bring the profession into disrepute, but rather enhances public perceptions. Physiotherapists have a duty to inform themselves of what is expected of them. Indeed, *Rules of Professional Conduct* states that knowledge and adherence to the *Rules* are part of the contract of membership of the CSP. *Standards of Physiotherapy Practice* makes it clear there is an expectation that all physiotherapists should be able to achieve all the core standards (CSP 2000). Where they do not, programmes of professional development should be put in place to facilitate full compliance, as part of the individual's professional responsibility.

Physiotherapists should not be critical of each other except in extreme circumstances. However, they do have a duty to report circumstances that could put patients at risk. In the NHS, there are procedures and a nominated officer within each trust from whom advice can be sought. Outside the NHS, advice can be sought from the CSP. Physiotherapists are encouraged to be proactive in supporting each others' professional development and in promoting the value of the profession in local workplace settings, in policy-making forums and in the media.

BECOMING AN AUTONOMOUS PROFESSION

The Chartered Society of Physiotherapy was founded in 1894, under the name of the Society of Trained Masseuses. This section will not attempt to relate the history of the profession except in the context of developing autonomy. However, more about the early days of the profession can be found in Dr Jean Barclay's fascinating book *In Good Hands* (Butterworth–Heinemann, 1994).

For many years, doctors governed the profession. One of the first rules of professional conduct stated 'no massage to be undertaken except under medical direction' (Barclay 1994). Even in the 1960s doctors were asserting that they must take full responsibility for patients in their charge and 'professional and technical staff have no right to challenge his views; only he is equipped to decide how best to get the patients fit again' (Barclay 1994). It is hard to believe now that it took more than 80 years to escape the paternalism of doctors, to whom physiotherapists were dependent for referrals. The first breakthrough came in the early 1970s, when a report by the Remedial Professions Committee, chaired by Professor Sir Ronald Tunbridge, included a statement that while the doctor should retain responsibility for prescribing treatment, more scope in application and duration should be given to therapists.

The McMillan report (DHSS 1973) went further, by recommending that therapists should be allowed to decide the nature and duration of treatment, although doctors would remain responsible for the patient's welfare. There was recognition that doctors who referred patients would not be skilled in the detailed application of particular techniques, and that the therapist would therefore be able to operate more effectively if given greater responsibility and freedom.

Eventually, a Health Circular called *Relationship between the Medical and Remedial Professions* was issued (DHSS 1977). This acknowledged the therapist's competence and responsibility for deciding on the nature of the treatment to be given. It recognised the ability of the physiotherapist to determine the most appropriate intervention for a patient, based on knowledge over and above that which it would be reasonable to expect a doctor to possess. It also recognised the close relationship between therapist and patient, and the importance of the therapist interpreting and adjusting treatment according to immediate patient responses.

Autonomy was only achieved by being able to demonstrate competence to make appropriate decisions, building up the trust of doctors and those paying for physiotherapy services. The need to acquire skills of assessment and analysis became a key component of student programmes from the 1970s. Today, qualifying programmes stress even further the development of skills, knowledge and attributes required for autonomous practice.

CLINICAL GOVERNANCE

So far, this chapter has explored the responsibilities of being a physiotherapist from a professional perspective. The focus has been on the individual's personal responsibility as a professional. This section will put all that in the context of a professional's responsibilities to their employer organisation, whether it be in the public or independent sector.

In the NHS, responsibility for the clinical safety of patients and the quality and effectiveness of services is through a system of clinical governance. It seems probable this will apply equally to the independent sector in the near future. But even though clinical governance is the responsibility of NHS trusts, its foundation is based on 'the principle that health professionals must be responsible and accountable for their own practice' (Secretary of State for Health 1998). So the individual's professional responsibility is still paramount.

What is clinical governance?

Definition
Clinical governance is a framework through which NHS organisations are accountable for continuously improving the quality of their services and safeguarding high standards of care by creating an environment in which excellence in clinical care will flourish (Secretary of State for Health 1998). While this definition has been used in England, similar interpretations of the term have been made in Scotland, Wales and Northern Ireland.

A number of key themes were introduced as part of clinical governance.

The accountability of chief executives for quality

Although some chief executives of NHS trusts claim they were always responsible for quality, this had not been a statutory responsibility in the way it was for a trust's finances. Chief executives now have a statutory responsibility for quality.

The introduction of a philosophy of continuous improvement

One-off improvements are not enough – the NHS has to move to a culture of continuous improvement to achieve excellence. In addition, the emphasis has shifted from improving a particular aspect of care in isolation, to examining the whole system of care, crossing professions, departments, organisations and sectors, to ensure the whole process meets the needs of patients through an integrated approach to healthcare.

An aspiration to achieve consistency of services across the NHS

This is founded on two principles:

- If one trust can provide excellence in a service, why can't all trusts?
- Local services should, where possible, be based on national standards, for example National Service Frameworks, or nationally developed clinical guidelines.

There is some evidence to suggest that nationally developed standards or clinical guidelines are likely to be more robustly developed (Sudlow and Thomson 1997) and that their universal implementation locally will ensure consistency and effectiveness.

An emphasis on continuing professional development and life-long learning (LLL)

Clinical governance acknowledges the importance of CPD/LLL for all healthcare workers, in order to keep up to date and deliver high-quality services.

Is clinical governance something new?

Yes and no. Its component parts are all familiar activities, but there is also an underpinning philosophy in clinical governance, to reduce risks for patients, a new and more focused emphasis that was not previously articulated. It can be argued that clinical governance is, at least in part, a response to a loss of public confidence in the NHS discussed earlier, which has undermined public perceptions of the NHS as an organisation they can rely on to 'do good' and of government to protect the public. In addition, the public has become more litigious, suing doctors and trusts more readily for mistakes, drawing money away from front-line clinical services. So clinical governance is about re-building the public's confidence in health services, providing high-quality and effective care and, above all, reducing the risk of harm through negligence, poor performance or system failures.

The components of clinical governance

Although clinical governance should be seen as a package of measures that together ensure excellence and a reduction in risk, it can also be viewed as a number of component parts, some of which have been in place for a number of years and are already familiar (Figure 1.1). They include:

- evidence-based practice and clinical effectiveness
- applying national standards and guidelines locally
- evaluating the effectiveness and quality of services
- continuing professional development/life-long learning
- having the right workforce and using it appropriately.

The following sections deal with these aspects.

EVIDENCE-BASED PRACTICE

At the beginning of this chapter, it was asserted that people who want to become physiotherapists have an inherent desire to 'do good'. But how do we know what works – what interventions have been shown to be effective? It is hard to comprehend that health professionals have not always sought evidence for the

effectiveness of the treatments they use. Perhaps they did – but until the early 1990s this 'evidence' was based on personal experience, opinions derived from that experience, together with the experience of colleagues, or those perceived to be experts and opinion leaders. Is that good enough?

In 1991, Sir Michael Peckham, then Director of Research & Development for the Department of Health, noted that 'strongly held views based on belief rather than sound information still exert too much influence in healthcare. In some instances the relevant knowledge is available but is not being used, in other situations additional knowledge needs to be generated from reliable sources' (Department of Health 1991). At about the same time, a relatively small group of doctors began to write about evidence-based medicine.

Definition
An early definition of evidence-based medicine stated that it is the conscientious, explicit and judicious use of current best evidence in making decisions about the care of individual patients (Sackett et al. 1996).

What do we mean by evidence? Is research the only form of evidence? Certainly for some questions such as the efficacy of particular drugs, or a particular modality such as exercise programmes for the management of back pain, research studies which compare one intervention with another or a placebo (randomised controlled trials) can provide reliable information about the degree to which an intervention is effective. But other forms of evidence are also important (Figure 1.2). What patients tell us about their condition, which treatments they find effective, the degree to which

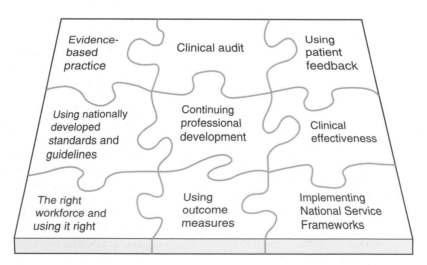

Figure 1.1   Components of clinical governance.

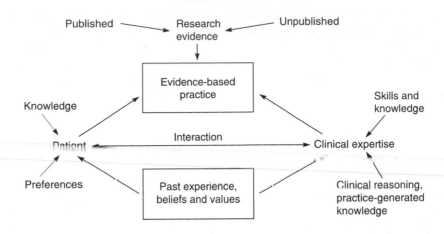

Figure 1.2   What do we mean by 'evidence'? (Adapted from Bury and Mead 1998, with permission.)

interventions improve their ability to get on with their lives, also provides important evidence. The physiotherapist also contributes evidence in the form of clinical expertise, derived from clinical reasoning experience. Thinking and reflecting on what you are doing as a practitioner during or after a clinical encounter will develop such expertise (Jones et al. 2000). Knowledge which arises from and within practice (practice-based and practice-generated knowledge) will become part, along with research evidence, of your rationale for practice (Higgs and Titchen 2001). This was also reflected by Sackett and colleagues, who went on to conclude their definition 'integrating clinical expertise with best available external clinical evidence from systematic research' (Sackett et al. 1996).

A hierarchy of evidence is often described or used in the literature. This ranges from (1) systematic reviews, in which evidence on a topic has been systematically identified, appraised and summarised according to predetermined criteria (usually limited to randomised controlled trials) – said to be the strongest evidence (the most reliable estimate of effectiveness) to (2) expert opinion, perceived as the least reliable. An example is shown in Table 1.1.

However, such a hierarchy fails to recognise that different research methods are needed to answer different types of questions and that, while a qualitative study may be the best research method for a particular question, it still receives a low rating. The hierarchy also fails to recognise the importance of expertise derived from clinical reasoning experience, discussed above. Physiotherapists need to contribute to an ongoing debate to develop a hierarchy that reflects more appropriately a patient-centred approach to practice.

So what does evidence-based practice mean for physiotherapists? Core Standard 4 (CSP 2000) states

that: 'In order to deliver effective care, information relating to treatment options is identified, based on the best available evidence.' A range of sources of information the physiotherapist may need to draw on, including research evidence, patient organisations and clinical guidelines is listed. What practical steps need to be taken to identify and use research evidence?

- Think about the clinical question you are trying to answer in your information search. Identify the population (e.g. people with multiple sclerosis with symptoms of urinary incontinence), the intervention you are looking for (e.g. neuromuscular

Table 1.1 A hierarchy of evidence.

Level	Type of evidence
Ia	Evidence obtained from a systematic review or meta-analysis of randomised controlled trials
Ib	Evidence obtained from at least one randomised controlled trial
IIa	Evidence obtained from at least one well-designed controlled study without randomisation
IIb	Evidence obtained from at least one other type of well-designed quasi-experimental study
III	Evidence obtained from well-designed non-experimental descriptive studies, such as comparative studies, correlation studies and case studies
IV	Evidence obtained from expert committee reports or opinions and/or clinical experience of respected authorities

Adapted from National Institute for Clinical Excellence (2001).

electrical stimulation) and the outcome (e.g. a reduction in symptoms) and use this information to formulate a search strategy.

- Work in partnership with an information scientist to get the best results from a literature search (their information skills and knowledge combined with your clinical skills and knowledge).
- Look first for evidence that has already been synthesised – systematic reviews, nationally developed clinical guidelines or standards. This saves a lot of effort looking for individual studies. If it is a high-quality synthesis, it will also provide a more reliable estimate of effectiveness.
- Know your databases well enough to know which will have the most relevant information for any particular topic.
- Check the titles and abstracts for relevance.
- Critically appraise any relevant papers you have found to assure yourself of their quality, and of the reliability of their conclusions (a list of appraisal instruments can be found at the end of this chapter).
- When you find the 'best available evidence', think about it in relation to your patient and your past experience – is it appropriate for that patient, will you be able to quantify for the patient the degree of likely benefits and harms (if any)?
- Discuss the evidence with the patient and agree together the preferred intervention(s).
- Implement the preferred intervention(s).
- Evaluate the effect of the intervention(s) and act accordingly.

More information about evidence-based practice can be found in Bury and Mead (1998), or at http://www.nettingtheevidence.org.uk/, a catalogue of useful electronic learning resources and links to organisations, which facilitate evidence-based healthcare. See also the section 'Sources of Critical Appraisal Tools' towards the end of this chapter.

CLINICAL EFFECTIVENESS

Clinical effectiveness as defined by the Department of Health sounds very much like evidence-based practice – doing things you know will be effective for a particular patient or group of patients. But the fact that an intervention has been proved to work in research studies, in a relatively controlled environment, does not necessarily mean that it will work for a particular patient. Both patients and practitioners are unique beings, and there are many additional factors, practical and behavioural, that need to be considered to ensure the patient gets the maximum benefit from an intervention.

Definition
Clinical effectiveness was defined by the Department of Health in 1996 as 'the extent to which specific clinical interventions, when deployed in the field for a particular patient or population, do what they are intended to do – that is, maintain and improve health and secure the greatest possible health gain from the available resources' (NHS Executive 1996).

- Is the practitioner sufficiently skilled to apply the intervention safely and effectively?
- Was the practitioner an effective communicator?
- Did the practitioner give the patient an opportunity to fully describe the symptoms and the impact of the problem on the person's life, and to ask questions?
- Did the patient have enough information to be able to give informed consent?
- Were other options discussed, that may have been more acceptable to the patient, even if less effective?
- Would treatment in a hospital setting mean a long, exhausting and expensive journey for the patient?
- Would the patient feel intimidated by a hospital environment?
- Would treatment have been more effective if it had been provided closer to home, for example in the GP's surgery or health centre?
- Would treatment have been more relevant if it had been given in a patient's own home, to be able to develop a programme tailored to the person's lifestyle and environmental needs?
- Wherever treated, did the patient have adequate privacy, warmth and comfort?
- How long did the patient have to wait for treatment – will delay affect the effectiveness of the interventions?

The answer to each of these questions can have an impact on the patient's ability to benefit from an intervention, however effective the research evidence might suggest an intervention is. This also illustrates the complexity of the clinical reasoning process, where highly skilled judgements have to be made based on a consideration of the whole person, physically, emotionally and within society, as well as the environment, practitioner skills and resources available, in order to provide truly effective treatment.

So while evidence-based practice is a key component of clinical effectiveness, clinical effectiveness also takes account of a range of other influences that could affect the patient's ability to benefit from an intervention based on high-quality research evidence.

APPLYING NATIONAL STANDARDS AND GUIDELINES LOCALLY

Standards

One of the tenets of clinical governance is consistency – for the public, being confident that they will experience the same quality of care and have access to the most effective interventions, regardless of where they live. There should be no postcode lottery, where some treatments might be available in some parts of the country and not others; raising the quality of the average and worst services to that of the best. So where there are high-quality national standards, these should be used locally. Two examples of these are set out below.

Nationally developed standards

The CSP's *Standards of Physiotherapy Practice* provides a universal framework for the delivery of services throughout the UK, to which it is expected all physiotherapists will conform. So, for physiotherapy, patients can expect similar values and processes within a healthcare experience.

National Service Frameworks (NSFs)

This government initiative aims to provide the NHS with explicit standards and principles for the pattern and level of services required for a specific service or care group. The NSFs aim to address the 'whole system of care' and each will set out where care is best provided and the standard of care that patients should be offered in each setting. They provide 'a clear set of priorities against which local action can be framed' and seek to ensure that patients will get greater consistency in the availability and quality of services, right across the NHS (Secretary of State for Health 1998).

NSFs have so far been developed for coronary heart disease (including cardiac rehabilitation), mental health, older people (including falls, osteoporosis and stroke) and diabetes. They provide broad statements of expected services; for example in the older-people NSF: 'Older people who have fallen receive effective treatment and rehabilitation and, with their carers, receive advice on prevention through a specialised falls service.' Physiotherapists will therefore need to address the implementation of this standard in any services they provide to older people. Implementation will also provide opportunities to promote the value of physiotherapy to this patient population and highlight the

contribution physiotherapists can make to a trust's compliance with this particular standard.

Clinical Guidelines

> **Definition**
> Clinical guidelines are 'systematically developed statements to assist practitioner and patient decisions about appropriate healthcare for specific circumstances' (Field and Lohr 1992).

The key factors in the development of clinical guidelines are the systematic process for identifying and quality-assessing research evidence, and the systematic and transparent process used for the interpretation of the evidence in the context of clinical practice, in order to formulate reliable recommendations for practice.

National Institute for Clinical Excellence (NICE)

NICE is a Special Health Authority for England and Wales, established by the government in 1999 to provide health professionals and the public with authoritative information about the clinical and cost effectiveness of healthcare. One of its work programmes is to develop clinical guidelines, which is carried out by a series of collaborating centres. NICE has been given a remit by the Department of Health and the Assembly for Wales for developing 'robust and authoritative' clinical guidelines, taking into account clinical and cost effectiveness. More information about the key principles that underpin the way NICE approaches clinical guideline development can be found on its website (www.nice.org.uk).

Scottish Intercollegiate Guidelines Network (SIGN)

SIGN was formed in 1993. Its objective is to improve the quality of healthcare for patients in Scotland by reducing variation in practice and outcome, through the development and dissemination of national clinical guidelines containing recommendations for effective practice based on current evidence. Further information can be found at its website (www.show.scot.nhs.uk/sign).

Professionally led clinical guidelines

The CSP has established a process for the endorsement of clinical guidelines. The criteria for assessing whether the quality of a guideline warrants endorsement can be found in an appraisal instrument developed by a European consortium, known as the AGREE instrument (the AGREE Collaboration: www.agreecollaboration.org). For users of clinical guidelines, CSP-endorsed clinical guidelines can be considered of high quality and should be implemented locally. Further information about the process for the development of clinical guidelines in physiotherapy is available from the CSP (2002e).

EVALUATING SERVICES

How do you know whether you are being effective? Knowing whether you are or not is part of your professional responsibility as a physiotherapist. Rule 1 of *Rules of Professional Conduct* (CSP 2002a) describes the responsibility a physiotherapist has to ensure that any intervention offered to a patient is intended to be of benefit. Several of the CSP's standards of physiotherapy practice include criteria that relate to evaluation, including:

- As part of the assessment process, physiotherapists consider and critically evaluate information about effective interventions relating to the patient's condition (Core Standard 4.1).
- A published, standardised, valid, reliable and responsive outcome measure is used to evaluate the change in the patient's health status (Core Standard 6).
- All physiotherapists participate in a regular and systematic programme of clinical audit (Service Standard 3.2).
- Physiotherapists use the results of audit to assess their learning needs (Core Standard 19.1) and/or as a means to achieve their personal learning objectives (Core Standard 20.3h).

All evaluation is about learning which leads to improvements in the quality and effectiveness of practice. It should be carried out, and the results used, in the context of CPD and reflective practice, to improve an individual practitioner's personal practice and/or the delivery of a whole service. Set out below are four means by which physiotherapists can evaluate their practice. They are not mutually exclusive.

Evaluating the process of care (clinical audit)

In order to evaluate the *process* of care, it is necessary to have a reliable benchmark with which to compare your practice. Earlier, the importance of the local implementation of nationally developed standards and evidence-based clinical guidelines was discussed. These provide such a reliable benchmark. Clinical audit is a tool with

which to measure your own performance (or more often, the performance of the service) against standards or criteria based on the 'best available evidence' of effectiveness. This will identify the extent to which you adhere to those standards or criteria, from which recommendations can be put in place to improve adherance, if necessary.

> **Definition**
> Clinical audit is a cyclical process involving the identification of a topic, setting standards, comparing practice with the standards, implementing changes, and monitoring the effect of those changes (CSP 2000). Further information about clinical audit can be found in an information paper published by the CSP (2002f) and in *Principles for Best Practice in Clinical Audit* published by NICE (2001).

Evaluating the outcomes of care

This will determine the *impact* of the process of care on the patient's life by using specific measures before and after treatment. The use of a test, scale or questionnaire which records what it aims to record (*is valid and responsive*) and is sufficiently well described to ensure that everyone who uses it does so in the same way (*is reliable*) will help to give physiotherapists the chance to see whether the aims of their intervention have had the impact intended.

A database of outcome measures can be found on the CSP website (www.csp.org.uk). This will facilitate the selection of the most appropriate measures for a specific patient or patient group. More information on using measures can be found in a CSP information paper (2001a).

As well as patients themselves having an interest in an objective assessment of their improvement, it is increasingly important for managers and team leaders to present such information to commissioners of healthcare, to demonstrate the benefits of physiotherapy services and their value for money.

Using patient feedback

Another mechanism for evaluating practice is to ask the patient for feedback. This could be through the use of a validated patient assessed outcome measure to provide information about the patient's perception of health gain, or through the use of a structured questionnaire to determine the patient's perception of the quality of the treatment. The CSP's *Standards of Physiotherapy Practice* pack includes a ready-made

Patient Feedback Questionnaire, designed to measure criteria in the core standards, for which only patients can judge compliance. Patients are asked to respond to statements that mirror the criteria (Figure 1.3).

Responses from the feedback questionnaires can be used by individuals or services to reflect on the extent to which the criteria are being met, and to introduce new processes or development opportunities to secure greater conformance, if necessary.

Another valuable source of patient feedback is patients' complaints. These should be considered positively as opportunities to address the issues contained within them, in order to introduce a service improvement. Any issue that becomes a problem for a patient is a problem for the service, which should be analysed. The involvement of the patient making the complaint in this process, if willing, will facilitate the finding of a solution that can then be embedded into systems and processes.

Peer review

Peer review provides an opportunity to evaluate the clinical reasoning behind your decision-making with a trusted peer. It can be applied most effectively to the assessment, treatment planning and evaluative components of physiotherapy practice, where the reasoning behind the information recorded in the patient documentation can be explored. Guidance on peer review can be found in the clinical audit tools document contained in the *Standards of Physiotherapy Practice* pack (CSP 2000).

CONTINUING PROFESSIONAL DEVELOPMENT AND LIFE-LONG LEARNING

Definition

Continuing professional development (CPD) is the range of learning activities in which physiotherapists engage throughout their careers to maintain and develop their capacity to practise safely and competently within their evolving scope of practice (CSP 2002b).

Definition

Life-long learning (LLL) is a theme the government promulgates across all sectors of the population, in order to ensure the workforce is equipped to do the jobs that will contribute to high-quality public services and promote prosperity in the UK.

In healthcare, the connection between CPD/LLL and the quality of services is at the centre of the government's view of a new, modernised NHS. Physiotherapists have always had a strong commitment to CPD, evidenced by the clear statement in Rule 1 of *Rules of Professional Conduct*: 'Chartered physiotherapists shall only practice to the extent that they have … maintained … their

Criteria	Patient feedback questionnaire	Response options
Core Standard 5.3: *The findings of the clinical assessment are explained to the patient*	By the end of your first visit, were the results of the assessment explained?	Yes, no, don't know
Core Standard 8.1: *Physiotherapists ensure that the patient is fully involved in any decision-making process during treatment planning*	I felt involved in deciding about my treatment plan	Strongly disagree, disagree, uncertain, agree, strongly agree
Core Standard 12.3: *All communication, written and verbal, is clear, unambiguous and easily understood by the recipient*	The physiotherapists used words I didn't understand	Strongly disagree, disagree, uncertain, agree, strongly agree

Figure 1.3   Extract from a patient feedback questionnaire (CSP 2000).

ability to work safely and competently …'. The *Core Standards of Physiotherapy Practice*, with which all physiotherapists should conform, include standards for the assessment, planning, implementation and evaluation of a CPD programme. Service Standards 6 and 7 require that all physiotherapy services should have a programme of CPD/in-service training for staff.

The requirement for re-registration of physiotherapists and other healthcare professionals, discussed earlier, will also make CPD an essential component of professional life. The introduction of a philosophy of LLL and individual responsibility for this will be starting in qualifying programmes, equipping students for a lifetime of learning in order to maintain and continually improve their competence to practise. Written evidence of learning and development, and its impact on improving practice, is now an essential requirement. Every physiotherapist must establish a portfolio containing such evidence, which will need to be maintained throughout a career. Guidance on this can be found in *Developing a Portfolio: a Guide for CSP Members* (CSP 2001b).

> ### Some key characteristics of CPD (CSP 2001c)
> • It should comprise a broad range of learning activities (courses, in-service education, reading, supervision, research, audit, reflections on experience, peer review – this is not an exhaustive list).
> • It should demonstrate a clear link between learning and practice.
> • It is about personal development, but also the fulfilling of organisational and service objectives, and enhancing patient care.
> • It should recognise the outcomes of CPD.

The emphasis on the importance of CPD/LLL within clinical governance is a welcome recognition. The challenges for physiotherapists of keeping up to date are huge, with the fast pace of change in healthcare – in particular the rapid increase in the volume of information that has to be evaluated and incorporated into practice. It is hoped that protected time for CPD, including time in the workplace, will become a reality in the NHS, as recommended by the Kennedy Report (Bristol Royal Infirmary Inquiry 2001).

Another form of professional development is reflective practice, a process in which practitioners think critically about their practice and as a result may modify their action or behaviour. 'Reflection enables learning at a sub-conscious level to be brought to a level where it is articulated and shared with others'

(CSP 2001b). Learning from experience requires the development of skills such as self-awareness, open-mindedness and critical analysis.

> ### Definition
> Reflective practice is the process of reviewing an episode of practice to describe, analyse, evaluate and inform professional learning; in such a way, new learning modifies previous perceptions, assumptions and understanding, and the application of this learning to practice influences treatment approaches and outcomes (CSP 2002b).

HAVING THE RIGHT WORKFORCE (and using it appropriately)

Physiotherapists have a professional responsibility to use their skills appropriately. This reflects Rule 1 of *Rules of Professional Conduct*, which states that physiotherapists should 'only practice to the extent that they have established, maintained and developed their ability to work safely and competently'. But there is also a professional responsibility to use resources (human as well as financial) appropriately in delivering healthcare. This means giving consideration to whether you need to refer a patient on, either because the patient requires a higher level of skills than you possess, or requires a specialist in a different clinical area. Equally, consideration should be given to whether there are elements of the treatment programme that can be delegated to a physiotherapy assistant or other support worker (the word 'assistant' is used in the following section to mean both).

The decision about whether to delegate, and which tasks or activities to delegate, is entirely the responsibility of the physiotherapist making that decision. The physiotherapist also takes full responsibility for the application of the tasks or activities carried out by the person who has been delegated. So choosing tasks to be undertaken by an assistant is a complex element of professional activity, which depends on an informed professional opinion.

• *What to delegate?* Physiotherapists need to use their own skills and knowledge to carry out an assessment of a patient in order to formulate a clinical diagnosis and a programme of treatment derived from those findings. This process requires skills of analysis and clinical reasoning, key professional attributes. However, an appropriately trained assistant may well have the attributes required to be able to carry out some or all elements of the treatment programme, based on existing knowledge and skills.

This would include the monitoring of the patient's condition and progress with the plan, and advising the physiotherapist of any variations in either of these. As there are no hard and fast rules about what to delegate, the physiotherapist should consider carefully the scope and nature of the task and ensure this is clearly defined and communicated to the assistant.

- *Who to delegate to?* The factors to be considered here are the competence of the assistant and the nature of the task. The competence of the assistant will be affected by the person's length of service, prior experience and training received, coupled with judgements by the physiotherapist about the assistant's ability to deal with that particular patient in those particular circumstances.

The decision about what to delegate and who to delegate to is one that, while ultimately the responsibility of the physiotherapist, also requires the active involvement of the person to whom the task is being delegated. The assistant, therefore, must be allowed to make an assessment of his or her own competence in relation to the particular task. If either the physiotherapist *or* assistant are concerned about the assistant's competence, the task should *not* be delegated. The physiotherapist will then need to decide whether training is required.

Newly qualified physiotherapists should recognise and value the skills and knowledge many assistants possess, particularly those who have long service within the profession, so that effective partnerships between physiotherapists and assistants can contribute to the efficient and effective delivery of physiotherapy services. Physiotherapy assistant members of the CSP have a *Code of Conduct* (CSP 2002d) to which they are expected to adhere in the same way physiotherapists are to the *Rules*. Users of physiotherapy services have a right to expect those who deliver them to be competent to do so. The physiotherapist has the ultimate responsibility to the patient for ensuring this is the case, but also needs to consider competence in the context of effective resource use, in terms of both finance and skills.

MONITORING CLINICAL GOVERNANCE

NHS physiotherapy managers are responsible for devising, implementing and reporting a departmental clinical governance programme, which should reflect all the aspects of clinical governance discussed in this chapter. Physiotherapists should play an active part in contributing to physiotherapy clinical governance programmes and also participate in relevant multi-professional clinical governance activities such as clinical audit or local protocol/clinical pathway design.

The Commission for Health Improvement (CHI; www.chi.nhs.uk), soon to be renamed the Commission for Healthcare Audit and Inspection (CHAI), is an independent statutory body established to raise standards throughout England and Wales. In Scotland, there are proposals to establish a similar function to CHI, through a new National Quality and Standards Board for Health in Scotland. CHI is tasked with assessing the implementation of clinical governance in every NHS trust and making its findings public. Teams of trained reviewers visit trusts every 3–5 years (and can be called in at any time should concerns be raised) to review trust information and data, talk to staff and patients, and consider the trust's performance in specified categories. The new CHAI, subject to government legislation in 2003, will add to its existing responsibilities those for inspecting hospitals and care homes in the private sector and carrying out value-for-money studies and performance management within the NHS.

Examples of a physiotherapy manager's responsibilities within a clinical governance programme

- Check staff are currently on the state register.
- Deal with and learn from complaints.
- Carry out programmes for quality improvement, including clinical audit and evaluation, and report how these have led to improvements for patients.
- Ensure that nationally produced, high-quality standards and clinical guidelines are implemented locally.
- Have an appropriate skill mix and staffing level to ensure the safety of patients, making appropriate use of human and financial resources, in order to provide effective care.
- Have a process for identifying and supporting staff members whose competence is in question.
- Provide an in-service training programme and time for individual CPD activities.
- Ensure appropriate participation in multi-professional clinical audit and quality improvement activities.

So, being a competent physiotherapist who displays the essential characteristics of a professional in the current climate is a complex and demanding process. Figure 1.4 attempts to summarise the elements of professionalism described in this chapter.

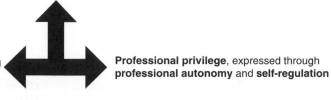

Patient-focused practice, underpinned by sound **clinical reasoning** and professional judgement, ongoing **reflection**, and critical application of the **evidence base**

Professional responsibility, manifested in adherence to a **professional code of conduct/standards of practice**, undertaking structured, evaluated **CPD** to meet identified learning needs, and engagement with the full implications of **clinical effectiveness**

Professional privilege, expressed through **professional autonomy** and **self-regulation**

Figure 1.4   Elements of professionalism.

THE FUTURE

It could be argued that there has never been a better time for the profession. There is the promise of huge injections of cash into the health service (7.5% increase per year in real terms, until 2008) and the number of training places for physiotherapists is set to expand by 60% between 2002 and 2008. This suggests there is a confidence among policy-makers about the value of the profession. Many of the government priority health programmes will be dependent for their success on the provision of effective rehabilitation in order to ensure people can continue to lead independent lives, including services for older people, children and people with long-term conditions. Physiotherapists also have a key contribution to make keeping people fit for work through, for example, the effective management of musculoskeletal problems, or the delivery of cardiac rehabilitation programmes. Ensuring ergonomically safe environments in the workplace and offering a rapid work-based response when treatment is needed provides another example of the value of the profession.

Structural changes

But the extra investment will bring with it an increase in the expectations of the public whose money is being used, and challenges from the government and the public about the need to change and modernise the way in which healthcare is delivered. Services will need to be more responsive to patients' needs, provided in settings closer to patients' own environments, delivered more speedily to maximise health benefits, and utilise available resources more effectively.

Many more physiotherapy services will be provided in primary care and community settings. Primary Care Trusts (PCTs) will hold 60% of the total budget for healthcare in their local area, and local people will have a much stronger voice in the decision-making process about how those funds are used. In addition, the gov-

ernment is committed to increasing integration between health and social care, through Care Trusts, where budgets are pooled in order that they can be used more flexibly to meet the needs of the local population.

More services delivered in primary care and community settings

Physiotherapy already has a track record of delivering responsive and effective services in primary care and community settings. The success of domiciliary and community-based physiotherapy services in avoiding hospital admissions and allowing speedier discharges will be further reinforced through the introduction of intermediate care. The musculoskeletal physiotherapy services delivered in GP practices and health centres, where trust is already established between general practitioners and physiotherapists, has facilitated more direct access to patients and better referrals, making services more efficient as well as effective.

The challenges, however, will lie with greater team working and delegation of tasks, with physiotherapists having to be prepared to be more flexible, often taking on teaching roles in order to allow other staff such as rehabilitation assistants to deliver services. There will be a need to take on some non-physiotherapeutic roles, such as key worker or case manager in order to deliver a more consistent approach to care to vulnerable people living in the community.

Another challenge will be the experience of working in more isolated settings, with less easy access to peer support, supervision or shared CPD with colleagues. At a time when clinical governance, the requirement for re-registration and the need for systems to assure patients about practitioners' competence and safety are to the fore, physiotherapists will need to work hard to create systems to support their ongoing learning, while also ensuring their managers accept their responsibilities too. Networking with colleagues with similar interests and case mix at a local and national level will become more important. Where face-to-face contact is not possible, the use of electronic networks for communication and accessing learning resources will need to be embraced.

Delivering clinically and cost effective services

The profession can thrive only if it can clearly demonstrate the 'added value' it offers to patients through increasing their independence, shorter hospital stays, fewer work days lost and so on. In order to achieve this, the profession needs a two-pronged approach. First, it needs to increase its knowledge base about the effectiveness of specific interventions, through research. Second, it needs to use information from the evaluation of practice to demonstrate the benefit to patients of those interventions. The profession urgently requires high-quality researchers who can access NHS and other funding in order to increase the knowledge base of the profession. Challenges from commissioners of services, to provide evidence for the effectiveness of physiotherapy for particular patient or diagnostic groups, will not go away and physiotherapy services are in increasing jeopardy without it.

The profession must be brave enough to look critically at the outcomes of interventions. Where research evidence shows that particular interventions are ineffective, these should stop being provided. Where patient outcomes are used as a determinant and demonstrate little or no effect, consideration should be given to possible alternative strategies for securing benefit to those patients, which may lie outside physiotherapy. For physiotherapists to continue to provide services in areas where there is little benefit weakens the image of the profession to the public and to colleagues from other professions.

There is a growing emphasis in the NHS on working smarter, looking at systems of care from a patient's perspective, breaking down what are perceived as tribal boundaries between professions, redesigning patient-centred delivery systems rather than 'doing things that way because we always have'. Physiotherapists will need to embrace new ways of working without feeling defensive or appearing to be protectionist. Opportunities will emerge from redesign for physiotherapists to adopt new and highly skilled roles in just the same way as the successful creation of extended-scope practitioner and physiotherapy consultant roles.

Influencing the agenda

To make any of this work, physiotherapists need to be confident about their roles and able to articulate to others the value of physiotherapeutic interventions or approaches from a science-based as well as a holistic point of view. Physiotherapists must adopt a political astuteness that makes them aware of the wider national and local drivers for change in order that opportunities for the profession and for services can be identified and seized positively. They need to be seen to be engaged with and responsive to current agendas through contacts with patient and public representatives as well as senior managers and local politicians.

Characteristics of the profession required to maximise the opportunities being presented

One thing is certain. The delivery of healthcare within organisations, whether state or privately funded, will continue to be highly complex, ever-changing and resource challenged. Qualifying programmes are tasked with equipping physiotherapy students 'with the attitude, aptitude and capacity to cope with change, uncertainty and unpredictability and with a commitment to the concept of quality improvement' (CSP 2002b). Qualifying physiotherapists of today will therefore be better equipped than ever to cope. The NHS is increasingly looking for leaders who are innovative, clear, lateral thinkers and problem solvers. Physiotherapists are well placed to adopt such roles and should be proactive in looking for opportunities to do so. The skill is to turn challenges and pressures into opportunities to demonstrate the 'value added' of physiotherapy which in turn will provide job satisfaction, recognition and benefit for patients and the profession.

Acknowledgements

I am grateful to a number of colleagues who commented on an earlier draft of this chapter and whose thoughts have improved its content, in particular Sally Gosling (who also created Figure 1.4), Ruth ten Hove, Rachel King, Sue Skewis, Ralph Hammond and Pen Robinson.

SOURCES OF CRITICAL APPRAISAL TOOLS

Critical Appraisal Skills Programme

qualitative research:
    www.phru.org.uk/~casp/resources/qualitative.pdf
randomised controlled trials:
    www.phru.org.uk/~casp/resources/rct.pdf
systematic review:
    www.phru.org.uk/~casp/resources/reviews.pdf

Scottish Intercollegiate Guidelines Network

case-control study:
www.show.scot.nhs.uk/sign/guidelines/fulltext/50/checklist4.html

cohort study:
www.show.scot.nhs.uk/sign/guidelines/fulltext/50/checklist3.html

diagnostic study:
www.show.scot.nhs.uk/sign/guidelines/fulltext/50/checklist5.html

randomised controlled trial:
www.show.scot.nhs.uk/sign/guidelines/fulltext/50/checklist2.html

systematic review:
www.show.scot.nhs.uk/sign/guidelines/fulltext/50/checklist1.html

Users' guide series

Guyatt GH, Sackett DL, Cook DJ 1993 Users' guides to the medical literature. II: How to use an article about therapy or prevention, pt A. JAMA 270(21): 2598–601

Oxman AD, Cook DJ, Guyatt GH 1994 Users' guides to the medical literature. VI: How to use an overview. JAMA 272(17): 1367–71

Guyatt GH, Sackett DL, Cook DJ 1994 Users' guides to the medical literature. II. How to use an article about therapy or prevention, pt B. JAMA 271(1): 59–63

Books

Bury T, Mead J (eds) 1998 Evidence-Based Healthcare: a Practical Guide for Therapists. Butterworth–Heinemann: Oxford

Greenhalgh T 2000. How to Read a Paper: the Basics of Evidence-Based Medicine. BMJ Books: London

Clinical guidelines

Appraisal of guidelines for research and evaluation (AGREE) instrument:
www.agreecollaboration.org

REFERENCES

Barclay J 1994 In Good Hands. Butterworth–Heinemann: Oxford

Bristol Royal Infirmary Inquiry 2001 The Report of the Public Inquiry into Children's Heart Surgery at the Bristol Royal Infirmary 1984–1995. Stationery Office: London

Bury T 1998 Evidence-based healthcare explained. In: Bury T, Mead J (eds) Evidence-Based Healthcare – a Practical Guide for Therapists. Butterworth–Heinemann: Oxford

Bury T, Mead J 1998 Evidence-Based Healthcare: a Practical Guide for Therapists. Butterworth–Heinemann: Oxford

Cott CA, Finch E, Gasner D et al. 1995 The movement continuum theory of physical therapy. Physiother Can 47(2): 87–95

CSP (Chartered Society of Physiotherapy) 2000 Standards of Physiotherapy Practice. CSP: London

CSP (Chartered Society of Physiotherapy) 2001a Outcome Measures. CSP: London

CSP (Chartered Society of Physiotherapy) 2001b Developing a Portfolio: a Guide for CSP Members. CSP: London

CSP (Chartered Society of Physiotherapy) 2001c Continuing Professional Development and Life Long Learning. CSP: London

CSP (Chartered Society of Physiotherapy) 2002a Rules of Professional Conduct. CSP: London

CSP (Chartered Society of Physiotherapy) 2002b Curriculum Framework for Qualifying Programmes in Physiotherapy. CSP: London

CSP (Chartered Society of Physiotherapy) 2002c Delegation of Tasks to Assistants: a Guide for Qualified Members and Assistants. CSP: London

CSP (Chartered Society of Physiotherapy) 2002d Physiotherapy Assistants Code of Conduct. CSP: London

CSP (Chartered Society of Physiotherapy) 2002e Guidelines for Developing Clinical Guidelines. CSP: London

CSP (Chartered Society of Physiotherapy) 2002f Clinical Audit. CSP: London

DHSS (Department of Health and Social Security) 1973 McMillan Report: The Remedial Professions (report by a working party set up in March 1973 by the Secretary of State for Social Services). HMSO: London

DHSS (Department of Health and Social Security) 1977 Health Services Development: Relationship between the Medical and Remedial Professions [HC(77)33]. DHSS: London

Department of Health 1991 Research for Health: a R&D Strategy for the NHS. DoH, London

Ersser SJ and Atkins S 2000 Clincial reasoning and patient-centred care. In: Higgs J and Jones M (eds) Clinical Reasoning in the Health Professions. Butterworth–Heinemann: Oxford

Field MJ, Lohr KN (eds) 1992 Guidelines for Clinical Practice: From Development to Use. National Academy Press: Washington, DC

Higgs J and Jones M (eds) 1995 Clinical Reasoning in the Health Professions. Butterworth–Heinemann: Oxford

Higgs J and Titchen A 2001 Rethinking the practice–knowledge interface in an uncertain world: a model for practice development. Br J Occup Ther 64(11): 526–33

Jones M, Jensen G, Edwards I 2000 Clinical reasoning in physiotherapy. In: Higgs J, Jones M (eds) Clinical Reasoning in the Health Professions. Butterworth–Heinemann: Oxford

Koehn D 1994 The Ground of Professional Ethics. Routledge: London

NICE (National Institute for Clinical Excellence) 2001 The Guideline Development Process. Information for National Collaborating Centres and Guideline Development Groups. NICE: London

NHS Executive 1996 Promoting Clinical Effectiveness. Department of Health: London

Royal College of Nursing, University of Leicester, National Institute for Clinical Excellence 2002 Principles of Best Practice in Clinical Audit. Radcliffe Medical Press

Sackett DL, Rosenberg WMC, Gray JAM et al. 1996 Evidence-based medicine: what it is and what it isn't. BMJ 312: 71–2

Secretary of State for Health 1998 A First Class Service: Quality in the New NHS. Department of Health: London

Sudlow M and Thomson R 1997 Clinical guidelines: quantity without quality (editorial). Qual Health Care 6: 60–1

Musculoskeletal Assessment

2

Lynne Gaskell

INTRODUCTION

Students are often in awe of qualified clinicians who assess and make complex clinical reasoning decisions in real time with apparently little effort. Becoming competent in patient assessment, like most things in life, takes practice, refinement and reflection, and it looks easy when performed by an expert. The ability to effectively examine and assess patients is an essential skill for physiotherapists to possess. This chapter introduces some important principles of musculoskeletal assessment. It provides an illustrated guide to many of the important techniques and tests that are valuable tools in the arsenal of the chartered physiotherapist. Furthermore it provides some assessment templates for specific joints of the body. The objectives of this chapter are:

- to identify the appropriate questions to include in a subjective musculoskeletal assessment
- to discuss the use of regional and special questions for particular joints
- to explain the use of appropriate subjective and objective markers
- to explain the use of specific and regional tests at particular joints
- to recognise the need for continuous reassessment.

This chapter includes templates for assessment of the lumbar spine (including a biopsychosocial assessment), the cervical spine, the shoulder, the hip, the knee, the ankle and the foot.

GENERAL ISSUES

Since 1977, chartered physiotherapists in the United Kingdom have been able to work as autonomous practitioners, making treatment decisions independently of other medical professionals. This professional autonomy makes the profession stimulating and exciting but with it comes a great deal of responsibility. Upon qualifying, physiotherapists are legally responsible for their actions and treatments. Increasing numbers of physiotherapists now work in the primary care setting and this trend is likely to continue. Allowing patients direct access to physiotherapists could relieve other medical practitioners of considerable workload.

Recent years have seen the introduction of extended-scope practitioners, clinical specialist and consultant physiotherapy posts. Physiotherapists in these roles are assessing patients usually referred by general practitioners who would otherwise have been examined by a consultant orthopaedic surgeon. These practitioners are required to possess excellent assessment skills, a wide experience of different clinical conditions and pathologies, and to be able to recognise the appropriate course of

action for that particular patient. Audits of these interventions have been encouraging; Gardiner and Turner (2002) found that the extended-scope practitioners showed more consistency between clinical diagnosis and arthroscopic findings in the knee than did their medical counterparts. In the present climate these posts, along with the newly established consultant physiotherapist role, are likely to expand and in doing so will deservedly raise the profile of the physiotherapy profession.

When should physiotherapists assess patients?

- On first patient contact, it is essential to perform an initial assessment to determine the patient's problems and to establish a treatment plan.
- During the treatment, this is particularly appropriate whilst performing treatments such as mobilisations and exercises when the patient's signs and symptoms may vary quite rapidly. Be aware of any improvement or deterioration in the patients' condition as and when it occurs.
- Following each treatment, the patient should be reassessed using subjective and objective markers in order to judge the efficacy of the physiotherapy intervention. Assessment is the keystone of effective treatment without which successes and failures lose all of their value as learning experiences. Subjective and objective markers are explained later in this chapter.
- At the beginning of each new treatment, to determine the lasting effects of treatment or the effects that other activities may have had on the patient's signs and symptoms. In reassessing the effect of a treatment, it is essential to evaluate progress from the perspective of the patient as well as from the physical findings.

Format of the assessment

Listen – history and background
Look – observation
Test – individual structures (range of movement, strength)
Record – an accurate account of findings
Assess – and remember to involve the patient.

Aims of the subjective assessment

To gather all relevant information about the site, nature, behaviour and onset of symptoms, and past treatments. Review the patient's general health, any investigations, medication and social history. This should lead to a formulation of the next step of physical tests.

Symptoms and signs

Symptoms are what the person complains of (e.g. 'my knee hurts'). Signs are what can be measured or tested (e.g. the patient has a positive patellar tap test).

Aims of the objective assessment

The objective assessment aims to seek abnormalities of function, using active, passive, resisted, neurological and special tests of all the tissues involved. This may be guided by the history. However it is important to conduct all tests objectively and equally and not attempt to bias the findings in an attempt to make the hypothesis fit.

Objective examination is concerned with performing and recording objective signs. It aims to:

- reproduce all or parts of the patient's symptoms
- determine the pattern, quality, range, resistance and pain response for each movement
- identify factors that have predisposed or arisen from the disorder
- obtain signs on which to reassess the effectiveness of treatment, by producing reassessment 'asterisks' or 'markers' (Jull, 1994).

SUBJECTIVE ASSESSMENT

Initial questioning

Subjective assessment needs to include the name, address and telephone number of the patient, and the patient's hospital number if appropriate. Both the age and the date of birth of the patient should be recorded. The medical referrer's name and practice should also be recorded for correspondence, discharge letters and so on.

It is also essential for the physiotherapist to obtain sufficient details of the patient's employment. Is the patient currently working? If not, determine the reasons for this. Is it because the person is unable to cope with the physical demands of the job? Do heavy lifting, repetitive movements or inappropriate sustained postures increase the symptoms? These factors may be precursors of poor posture and muscle imbalance, which may accentuate degenerative disease and increase symptoms. However, it is equally important to recognise that withdrawing from normal activities of daily life can result in deconditioning of musculoskeletal structures that may lead to degenerative disease and an increase in symptoms (Waddell 1992; Frost et al. 1998).

Identify the patient's hobbies or interests. Is she able to participate in a sport if desired? If not, determine the reasons. Identify the length of time the patient has been off work or has been unable to participate in physical activities. Evaluate the progression of symptoms. If the person has not been participating in physical activities, and if no improvement has occurred it may be appropriate to advise a return to light training in order to prevent devitalisation of tissues and fear avoidance issues.

Present condition
Area of the symptoms

It is useful to record the area of the pain by using a body chart, because this affords a quick visual reference (Maitland, 2001). The patient may complain of more than one symptom, so the symptoms may be recorded or referred to individually as P1 and P2 and so on. Areas of anaesthesia or paraesthesia may be recorded differently on the pain chart – they may be represented as areas of dots, in order to distinguish them from areas of pain (Figure 2.1).

Severity of the symptoms

The severity of the pain may be measured on a visual analogue scale (Figure 2.2), or on a numerical scale of 0–10 to quantify the pain, where 0 stands for no pain at all and 10 is perceived by the patient as the worst pain imaginable. The mark on a VAS can then be measured and recorded for future comparisons using a ruler. Although these measures are not wholly objective they do allow changes to be monitored as the treatment progresses.

Duration of the symptoms

Establish whether the pain and symptoms are intermittent or constant. Is the pain present all of the time or does it come and go depending on activities or time of day?

Aggravating and easing factors
Positional factors

Most musculoskeletal pain is mechanical in origin and is therefore made better or worse by adopting particular positions or postures that either stretch or compress the structure that is giving rise to the pain. Moreover, aggravating and easing movements may provide the physiotherapist with a clue as to the structure that is causing the pain. Various body or limb positions place different structures on stretch or compression and the resultant deformation produces an increase in severity of the pain. The aggravating and easing factors can be recorded on the pain chart, as in Figure 2.1. It is also necessary to record the length of time that engaging in aggravating activities produces an increase in symptoms or alternatively takes to settle down. This indicates the irritability of the patient's condition.

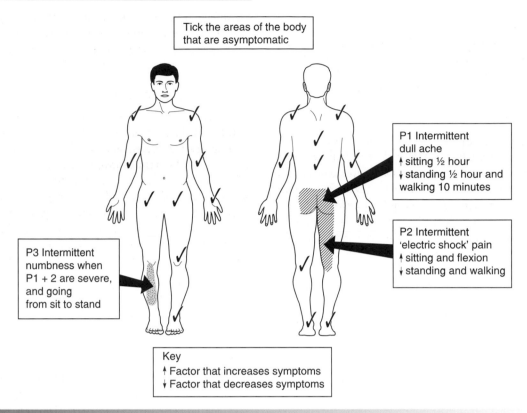

Tick the areas of the body
that are asymptomatic

P1 Intermittent
dull ache
↑ sitting ½ hour
↓ standing ½ hour and
walking 10 minutes

P2 Intermittent
'electric shock' pain
↑ sitting and flexion
↓ standing and walking

P3 Intermittent
numbness when
P1 + 2 are severe,
and going
from sit to stand

Key
↑ Factor that increases symptoms
↓ Factor that decreases symptoms

Figure 2.1   Typical body chart. In this example the patient's details have been recorded.

Time factors

It is useful to record the behaviour of signs and symptoms over a 24-hour period – the diurnal pattern. Do the symptoms keep the patient awake, or awaken the person regularly during the night? Is this due to a particular sleeping posture or to other unrelated factors? On arising, how are the symptoms for the first hour or so of the day, and moreover, do the symptoms vary from the morning to the afternoon and into the evening? Does this follow a particular pattern? This information can be included on the body chart.

Be careful not to confuse time of day with the performance of particular activities that the patient may undertake at that time. Certain pathologies tend to be more painful at characteristic times of the day. For example chronic osteoarthritic changes are characteristically painful and stiff initially on arising from sleep, intervertebral disc related pain is often more painful on arising owing to the disc imbibing water during sleep and thus exerting pressure on pain-sensitive structures. Prolonged morning pain and stiffness, which improves only minimally with movement, suggests an inflammatory process (Magee 1992).

Determining the SIN factors

Once the severity of the symptoms and the aggravating and easing factors have been noted, it is then possible to determine the SIN factor of the condition: severity/irritability/nature. SIN factors are used to guide the length and firmness of the objective assessment and subsequent treatment.

Please mark on this line with a cross how you would rate your pain

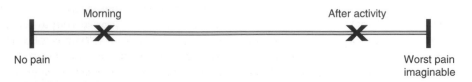

Morning   After activity

No pain   Worst pain
                                     imaginable

Figure 2.2   The visual analogue scale (VAS).

Severity

This can be quantified by the visual analogue scale, numerical scale or other valid pain questionnaire. It can be recorded as high (pain score of around 7–10), moderate (score around 4–6) or low (score around 1–3).

Irritability

This is the time that the person has to perform the activity to increase the pain, and conversely how long it takes before the pain settles to its former intensity. It can be measured as either high (the aggravating factor causes the pain to increase very quickly or instantly and then the pain takes a long time to settle back), moderate (the aggravating factor takes longer to increase the symptom) or low (the aggravating factor can be performed for a long time before exacerbating the patient's symptoms and then on stopping the activity the symptoms subside rapidly). An example of the latter would be that the knee pain is aggravated after jogging for 1 hour and then subsides after 1 minute of rest.

Nature

It is possible to hypothesise the nature of the condition following the subjective history – that is, whether the patient's condition has a predominantly inflammatory, traumatic, degenerative or mechanical cause.

History of the present condition

Insidious onset

Insidious onset means that the patient's symptoms appear without any obvious cause. An example of this would be a degenerative condition such as osteoarthritis. These types of conditions often begin with a small amount of stiffness and pain, which is characterised by exacerbation and remission but is nonetheless progressive.

Traumatic onset

Can the onset of symptoms be related to a particular injury? Identify if there was a definite cause for the patient's symptoms. The mechanism of injury may be indicative of the structures damaged. For example a valgus strain of the knee may stretch the medial collateral ligament of the knee, whereas forced rotation of the knee joint when in a semi-flexed weight-bearing position may tear the menisci.

Progression of the condition

Are the patient's symptoms getting better or worse? Acute soft-tissue injuries normally undergo a period of inflammation and repair and symptoms may subside rapidly within a few days or weeks. However, progressive arthritic diseases may have a history of exacerbation and remissions with a general increase in the severity or frequency of their symptoms, as the disease progresses.

Progression of the condition may indicate how quickly the patient's symptoms will subside.

Chronicity or age of the condition

How long has the patient experienced the symptoms? Is the condition acute or chronic? If the injury is chronic or has not resolved completely, it may indicate a number of different causes, such as mechanical instability from a ligament disruption, functional instability due to weakened muscles, loss of proprioception (and therefore the loss of an inherently protective reflex mechanism at the joint), or malalignment. Furthermore, it may be developing into a degenerative condition. The physiotherapist should identify:

1. Is this the first episode?
2. Is it recurrent?
3. Is it getting better or worse?

Previous treatments

Has the patient received any treatment for this condition in the past, and if so was it effective? Was the improvement partial or total, and did it provide permanent or temporary relief? If the treatment has been effective in the past it may well help again. Be careful not to repeat unsuccessful interventions, as they are unlikely to be therapeutic.

Investigations

Record the results of any investigations that the patient has undergone. Case notes, radiographic films and reports can be ordered and read, as patients may not always be a reliable source of the results of their investigations.

X-rays, MRI scans, CAT scans and bone scans

Scans are now commonly used to aid the diagnosis of musculoskeletal disorders. X-rays are useful in that they show the degree or extent of arthritis present at a joint. They are also useful in determining the extent of osteomyelitis (bone infection) and some malignancies and osteoporosis. Moreover, they are valuable following trauma to identify fractures or dislocations. Be aware, however, that there is a poor correlation between X-rays and spinal symptoms, for non-specific low back and neck pain. What is identified as pathological on these tests may not always be the structure responsible for the patient's signs and symptoms. Routine X-rays are not helpful in non-specific degenerative spinal disease (CSAG, 1994).

CAT (computerised axial tomography) may be used to identify the precise level and extent of disc prolapse and subsequent nerve impingement prior to discectomy. MRI (magnetic resonance imaging) may be used to identify ligamentous and muscular injuries, particularly in athletes, as well as discogenic prolapse. Bone scans are sensitive to 'hot spots' or areas of inflammation present in bone and may detect malignancy or diseases such as ankylosing spondylitis, some fractures and infection sites.

Blood tests

These are used extensively for the confirmation of the diagnosis of particular diseases, such as rheumatoid arthritis, ankylosing spondylitis, osteomyelitis and malignancy.

Other investigations

The patient may be undergoing investigations for other pathologies that could possibly relate to the musculoskeletal condition. These should be noted and recorded.

Past medical history

Determine whether or not the patient is suffering or has suffered any major operations or illnesses. These might affect the vitality of the tissues and be a contraindication to particular treatments. Examples are respiratory or cardiac disease, diabetes, rheumatoid arthritis and epilepsy.

The prolonged use of oral steroid medication should be noted, since this affects bone density and produces a tendency towards bruising. This is commonly found in patients suffering with chronic respiratory diseases, inflammatory bowel diseases or rheumatoid arthritis. Always identify cases of unexplained weight loss and general debility.

Red flag Indicators

Unexplained weight loss, general debility or the patient looking generally unwell – unremitting pain that is unrelieved by changing position or medication – may suggest a non-mechanical basis for the pain. Feeling unwell or tired is common in neoplastic disease affecting the spine (O'Conner and Curner 1992). In these cases, malignant disease should be suspected and the patient should be referred back to the referring general practitioner or consultant immediately with a full report of your findings. Physiotherapy management may well be contraindicated in this situation and may be wasting valuable time for the patient.

Medication

Record the type and dosage of medication prescribed for or taken by the patient. Commonly prescribed drugs for use in musculoskeletal conditions are:

- analgesics (painkillers) such as paracetamol and co-codamol
- non-steroidal anti-inflammatory drugs (NSAIDs) such as ibuprofen
- skeletal muscle relaxants such as diazepam and baclofen.

Medications being taken should alert you to pathologies that the patient may have forgotten to inform you about. For example a person may tell you that she has no significant medical history, but then later in the assessment say that she is currently taking anticoagulation therapy for a recent deep vein thrombosis!

OBJECTIVE ASSESSMENT

Following the subjective assessment it is important to highlight the main findings and determine the SIN factor. A hypothesis may be reached as to the cause of the patient's symptoms and the testing procedures are performed in order to support or refute the physiotherapist's hypothesis.

General observation

Observe the person's gait and general demeanour on entering the department.

Local observation

Note any localised swelling at the joint. This may be measured with a tape measure around the joint or limb circumference. Note any asymmetry of joint contours, redness of the overlying skin suggesting local inflammation, atrophy and asymmetry of musculature, deformity, and malalignment of the joint or joints. Compare one joint closely with the other side whenever possible.

Posture

Observe any asymmetry of posture in standing, walking and sitting. Poor posture is frequently a precursor to muscle imbalance, selective tightness and weakness through over- or underuse of specific muscles. The result of prolonged poor postural habits may lead to an acceleration of certain pathologies such as adhesive capsulitis, shoulder impingement syndrome, spinal pain and arthritis. Poor posture is frequently the cause of aches and pains and may be correctable in the early stages, and improved in later stages. Correction may prevent recurrence or acceleration of specific pathologies.

Palpation

Palpate for the following:

- tenderness
- heat (use the back of your hand which is more sensitive to heat changes)
- swelling
- muscle spasm.

Assessment of movement

Active movements

These are movements performed by the patient's voluntary muscular effort.

Passive movements

These are movements performed by an external source, such as the physiotherapist or a pulley system. There are two types of passive movements.

- Physiological passive movements are movements that can be performed actively by the patient (e.g. flexion or abduction of the shoulder joint).
- Accessory movements cannot be performed actively by the patient (e.g. they incorporate glide, roll or spin movements that occur in combination as part of normal physiological movements). An example of an accessory movement is an anterior–posterior glide at the knee joint.

Resisted movements

These are performed against the resistance of the physiotherapist or weights by the patient's own effort.

Take note

Passive, active and resisted movements are used in the assessment and in the treatment of musculoskeletal disorders, and specific examples of these are included later in the individual joint assessments formats.

Assessment of range of movement

Measurement of joint range using a goniometer

Active movement may be assessed by the use of a goniometer (Figure 2.3) or alternatively by visual estimation. It is measured in degrees. It is useful to practice using the goniometer by measuring the hip, knee and ankle joints in various positions. Either the 360-degree or 180-degree universal goniometers

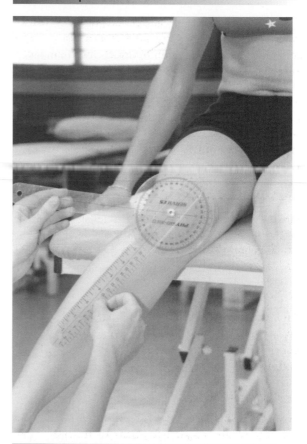

Figure 2.3   Using the goniometer to measure hip joint medial rotation with the hip in 90 degrees of flexion.

may be used. Ensure adequate stabilisation of adjacent joints prior to taking the measurements and locate the appropriate anatomical landmarks as accurately as possible. For details on specific joint measurements using the goniometer, refer to the appropriate joint assessment. Physiological and accessory passive movements are measured respectively in terms of the above and by the end-feel.

Differentiation tests

If a lesion is situated within a non-contractile structure such as ligament, then both the active and passive movements will be painful and/or restricted in the same direction. For example both the active and passive movement of inversion will produce pain in the case of a sprained lateral ankle ligament. However, if a lesion is within a contractile tissue such as a muscle, then the active and passive movements will be painful and/or restricted in opposite directions (Cyriax 1982). For example a ruptured quadriceps muscle will be painful on passive knee flexion (stretch) and resisted knee extension (contraction).

Clinical note

Remember that it is insufficient to measure only the range of movement occurring. The quality of movement should also be observed along with limiting factors to the movement. Is it the pain, muscle spasm, weakness or stiffness that is limiting the movement? This is determined by noting the differences between active, passive and resisted movements.

End-feel

During passive movements, the end-feel is noted. Different joints and different pathologies have different end-feels. The quality of the resistance felt at the end of range has been categorised by Cyriax (1982). For example:

- Bony block to movement or a hard feel is characteristic of arthritic joints.
- An empty feel, or no resistance offered at the end of range, may be due to severe pain associated with infection, active inflammation or a tumour.
- A springy block is characterised by a rebound feel at the end of range and is associated with a torn meniscus blocking knee extension.
- Spasm is experienced as a sudden, relatively hard feel associated with muscle guarding.
- A capsular feel shows a hardish arrest of movement.

Assessment of muscle strength

Symptoms arising from resisted contractions

The Oxford scale is relatively quick and easy to use and is used widely in clinical practice. However, it is not very objective, functional or sensitive to change since the movements resisted are concentric contractions and the spaces between the grades are not linear. Nevertheless it provides a guide to muscle strength and is somewhat sensitive to change.

The Oxford classification

0 = no contraction at all
1 = flicker of contraction only, movement of the joint does not occur
2 = movement is possible only with gravity counterbalanced
3 = movement against gravity is possible
4 = movement against resistance is possible
5 = normal functional movement is possible.

Measurements using isokinetic machines

Objective measurements of strength throughout different joint angles and at different velocities are made more accurately using isokinetic machines such as Cybex or Kin-Kom. These machines are particularly valuable in rehabilitative regimens such as anterior cruciate rehabilitation programmes and can determine the strength ratio of the quadriceps to the hamstrings or the ratios of the operated versus the non-operated leg. Objective markers such as percentages of strength ratios or ratios of operated versus non-operated leg may be used in setting discharge protocols. Isokinetic machines have been found to be reliable and valid in measuring muscle torque, muscle velocity and the angular position of joints (Mayhew et al. 1994). However, they are limited in their use, and Wojtys et al. (1996) suggest that agility and functional exercises may be more beneficial than isokinetic machines in the strengthening of muscle.

Structural differentiation tests

Tests of specific structures are performed in order to reproduce the patient's symptoms or signs, i.e. to reproduce the comparable sign. Differentiation tests are useful to distinguish between two or more structures that are suspected to be the source of the symptoms.

Differentiation tests of muscles and tendons

These are contractile structures and are therefore tested by performing a contraction against resistance. A pain response and/or apparent weakness may indicate a strain of the muscle at any particular point of the range of movement. Full range should be checked since the muscle may be weak only at a particular point in the range. Muscle length may also be tested, particularly those muscles that are prone to become tight and then lose their extensibility. Muscles that pass over two joints and have mobiliser characteristics are particularly prone to tightness. Examples of these are the hamstrings, rectus femoris, gastrocnemius and psoas major. The length of the muscle is tested by passively moving the appropriate joints. The stretch is compared to the other side to determine reproduction of pain and/or restriction of movement.

Passive insufficiency of muscles

This occurs with muscles that act over two joints (Figure 2.4a). The muscle cannot stretch maximally across both joints at the same time. For example, the

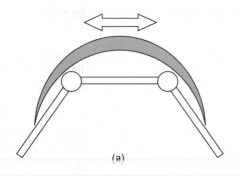

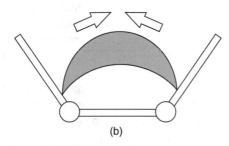

(a)

(b)

Figure 2.4 (a) Passive insufficiency: the muscle cannot simultaneously stretch maximally across two joints. (b) Active insufficiency. The muscle cannot simultaneously contract maximally across two joints.

hamstrings, may limit the flexion of the hip when the knee joint is in extension since they are maximally stretched in this position. However, if the knee is flexed passively, then the hip will be able to flex further since the stretch on the hamstrings has been reduced.

Active insufficiency of muscles

This, too, occurs with muscles that act over two joints (Figure 2.4b). The muscle cannot contract maximally across both joints at the same time. An example is the finger flexors. If you are to make a strong fist, you may notice that the wrist is in a neutral or an extended position when you do this action. Now, if you attempt to actively flex your wrist joint whilst keeping your fingers flexed, you will find that the strength of the grip is greatly diminished. This is because the wrist and finger flexors are unable to shorten any further and so the fingers begin to extend or lose grip strength.

Differentiation tests of ligaments

Ligaments are non-contractile structures and are tested by putting the structure on stretch. Examples are a valgus strain of the knee, to stretch the medial collateral ligament of the knee; or passive inversion of the subtalar joint, to stretch the lateral ligament of the ankle. A positive test would be a pain response or observation or feel of any excessive movement of the joint when compared to the other side.

Differentiation tests of bursae

Bursae are sacs of synovial fluid. Inflammation of these (bursitis) results in tenderness and/or heat on palpation. The tenderness is often very localised to the site of the inflamed bursa.

Differentiation tests of menisci

The history and mechanism of injury, combined with anterior joint tenderness and inability to passively hyperextend the knee, are useful diagnostic markers of meniscal injury. Rotation on a semi-flexed weight-bearing knee is a common cause of injury.

A history of locking, whereby the joint momentarily locks and is unable to actively or passively release itself from the position, is also common. Objectively, the knee joint is unable to fully flex/hyperextend passively.

Characteristics of degenerative joint disease

Signs and symptoms may include:

- pain that increases on weight-bearing activities (standing and walking, walking downstairs particularly)
- insidious onset of symptoms followed by progressive periods of relapses and remissions
- pain and stiffness in the morning
- stiffness following periods of inactivity
- pain and stiffness that arise after unaccustomed periods of activity
- bony deformity (e.g. characteristic varus deformity may follow from collapse of the medial compartmental joint space)
- reduction of the joint space observed on X-ray, with bony outgrowths or osteophytes.

Writing up the assessment

It is imperative to record the assessment immediately following the physical testing. Patient notes should be completed on the day of the assessment for legal reasons.

Ensure that your assessment findings are clear and concise and that they highlight the main points (it may be useful to include one subjective and one objective marker). Formulate a problem list, in agreement with the patient. Agree and record SMART goals (specific, measurable, achievable, realistic, timed) with the patient. Use the problem-orientated medical records (POMR) system.

Remember, if you have insufficient time to conduct a full and thorough assessment, you can always continue with this when the patient attends for his or her subsequent appointment.

SPINAL ASSESSMENTS

THE LUMBAR SPINE

Posture

Normal alignment

Posteriorly, the shoulders, waist creases, posterior superior iliac spines, gluteal creases and knee creases should be horizontal (Figure 2.5). The spine should appear to be vertical. There should be no rotation, side flexion, scoliosis (lateral curvature) or shift (lateral deviation). Laterally, you should observe a normal lordosis in the lumbar spine. *Anteriorly*, the anterior superior iliac spines should be horizontal.

Common deviations from normal posture (Refer to Figure 2.6)

- *Creases* in the posterior aspect of the trunk and particularly adjacent to the spine may indicate areas of hypermobility or instability of that motion segment.
- *Sway back* comprises hyperextension of the hips, an anterior pelvic tilt and anterior displacement of the pelvis.

- *Flat back* consists of a posterior pelvic tilt and a flattening of the lumbar lordosis, extension of the hip joints, flexion of the upper thoracic spine and straightening of the lower thoracic spine.
- *Kypholordosis* consists of a forward-poking chin posture, elevation and protraction of the shoulders, rotation and abduction of the scapulae, an increased thoracic kyphosis, anterior rotation of the pelvis and an increased lumbar lordosis.
- *Shifted posture* (lateral shift) commonly arises from disc herniation, or acute irritation of a facet joint. The shift is thought to result from the body finding a position of ease, whereby the shoulders are displaced laterally in relation to the pelvis. Most commonly the shift occurs away from the painful side (Figure 2.7).

Movements

Assess not only the range of movement occurring, and the pain response, but also localised areas of give and restriction occurring at specific motion segments.

Active movements

Flexion

Flexion should result in a smooth curve. Segmental areas of give or restriction appear as hinging (seg-

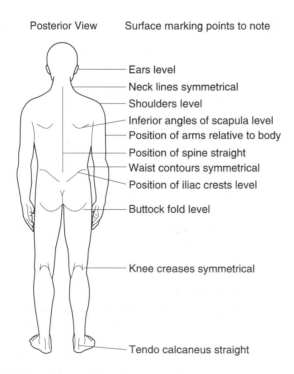

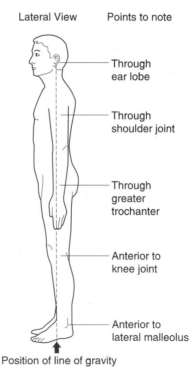

Posterior View	Surface marking points to note
	Ears level
	Neck lines symmetrical
	Shoulders level
	Inferior angles of scapula level
	Position of arms relative to body
	Position of spine straight
	Waist contours symmetrical
	Position of iliac crests level
	Buttock fold level
	Knee creases symmetrical
	Tendo calcaneus straight

Lateral View	Points to note
	Through ear lobe
	Through shoulder joint
	Through greater trochanter
	Anterior to knee joint
	Anterior to lateral malleolus

Position of line of gravity

Figure 2.5   Examination of the spine.

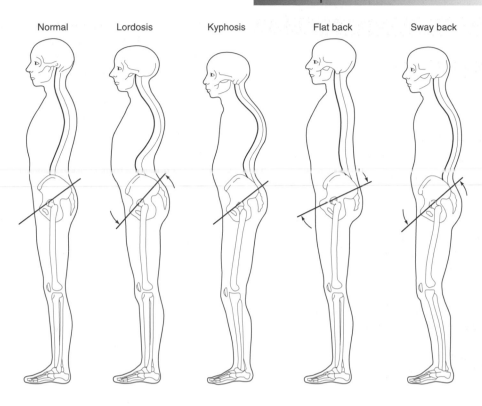

| Normal | Lordosis | Kyphosis | Flat back | Sway back |

Figure 2.6   Abnormal postural curves of the spine.

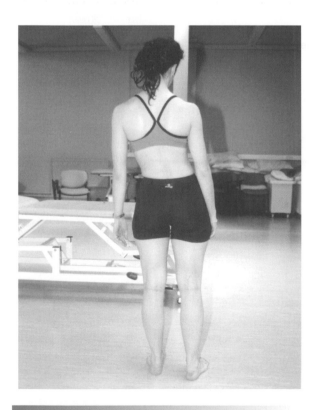

Figure 2.7   Lateral shift.

mental hypermobility). Lack of movement in lumbar spine may be compensated by flexion at the hips or thoracic spine flexion. The gross movement may be measured as fingertip to floor distance with a tape measure. Note any limitation of movement lateral deviation and pain response (Figure 2.8).

Extension

Observe extension in relation to areas of give or restriction. Observe for hinging at specific motion segments indicating areas of hypermobility. This may appear as horizontal lines appearing across the hypermobile segment. Note any limitation of movement and pain response.

Side flexion (Figure 2.9)

Normal movement should be observed as a smooth curve. Areas of give or restriction will be observed as hinging (segments of hypermobility) or plane lines (areas of hypomobility). Compare with the other side for symmetry. Note any 'coupling' of movements, i.e. the trunk may flex or rotate to compensate for restriction of side flexion.

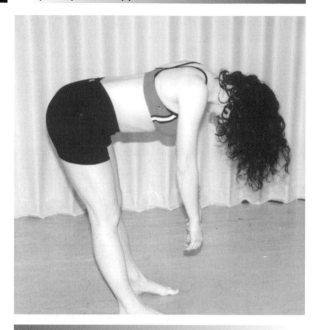

Figure 2.8   A faulty lumbar flexion pattern. All movements occur at the hip joint while the lumbar spine remains in an extended position.

Passive physiological intervertebral movements (PPIVMs)

These can be used to confirm any restriction of motion seen on active movement tests, to detect restriction of movement not discovered by the active movement tests. PPIVMs also detect segmental hypermobility (Magarey 1988; Maitland 2001).

Overpressure

If the plane movements have full range and are pain-free, then overpressure applied slowly and with care can be administered. At the end of the available range the physiotherapist may apply a small oscillatory movement to assess the quality and end-feel of the movement. Also the range of further movement should be noted, as well as the pain response.

Repeated movements

Repeating movements several times may alter the quality and range of the movement and may give rise to latent pain. McKenzie (1981) advocates the use of

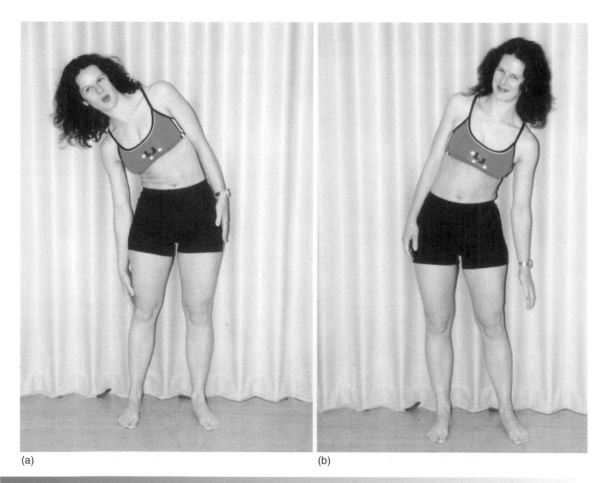

(a)   (b)

Figure 2.9   Side flexion (a) to the right, and (b) to the left. Note the difference, and the pain response.

repeating flexion and extension in both standing and lying to determine the movement that may centralise patient's symptoms (Figure 2.10). According to Palmer and Epler (1998), progressive worsening of pain on repeated movements indicates a disc derangement, the pain either becoming more intense or spreading more distally. Centralisation of symptoms means that the referred pain becomes more proximal, i.e. pain experienced at the medial aspect of the shin may centralise to the buttock. Thus, the exercise is believed to be reducing the patient's symptoms and the disc derangement.

Combined movements

According to Edwards (1992): 'Although the use of combining movements is not always necessary – adequate results being obtained by standard examination procedures – there are times when they are helpful. Often, with the more difficult mechanical problems, their use is essential.'

For example lumbar spine extension may be performed and, whilst maintaining that extension, side flexion may be added. Symptoms are likely to vary with the addition of a second movement and this may indicate whether or not there is a regular or irregular stretch component to the signs and symptoms. For example if a disc prolapse is aggravated by flexion, it would be reasonable to hypothesise that the addition of contralateral side flexion would also further increase the symptoms, because both of the movements are stretching the pos-

terior component of the disc and posterior longitudinal ligament. Combining ipsilateral side flexion to flexion would be expected to lead to a reduction in the patient's symptoms, since the ipsilateral side flexion is reducing the stretch component.

Differentiation between the hip and lumbar spine as a source of symptoms

The hip joint may give rise to pain in the buttock or groin, and in order to differentiate between pain arising as a result of spinal or hip pathology it is important that the therapist discounts the hip joint as a possible source of symptoms. With the patient supine, full flexion, medial and lateral rotation is performed actively and passively at the hip joint. These are the movements commonly painful or restricted by degenerative joint conditions such as osteoarthritis. If these movements are pain-free and full range, then it is unlikely that the hip is a source of symptoms. Compare both sides.

Assessing the sacroiliac joint

Sitting flexion (Piedello's sign)

The seated patient is asked to flex forwards. The physiotherapist palpates the sacral dimples bilaterally. Both sacral dimples should move equally in a *cephalad direction* (i.e. towards the head). (This tests the movement of the sacrum on the ilium.) Excessive rising of one side indicates hypomobility at that sacroiliac joint.

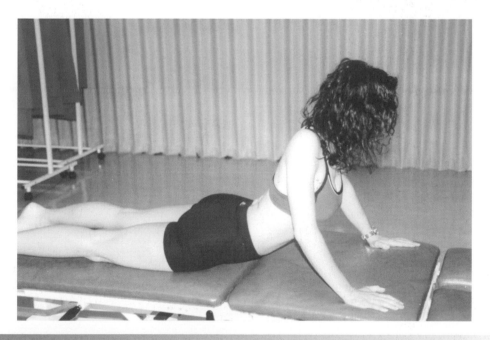

Figure 2.10   Repeated extension in prone.

Standing flexion (stork test)

With the patient standing, the physiotherapist locates the sacral dimples (level of S2) and places the other hand centrally at the sacrum. The patient is instructed to stand on one leg whilst flexing the non-weight-bearing hip and knee. The sacral dimple on the non-weight-bearing side should appear to move *caudally* (towards the floor) by approximately 1 cm as the ilium rotates posteriorly. Hypomobility is observed if the dimple does not move distally in relation to the sacrum.

Compression tests

Posterior ligaments

These test the integrity of the *posterior* sacroiliac ligaments. The patient lies supine and the hip is passively flexed towards the ipsilateral shoulder (Figure 2.11). A downward thrust is applied along the line of the femur. Observe for pain response, clunk and difference in end-feel between both sides. The test is repeated for (oblique) hip flexion towards the contralateral shoulder, and (transverse) hip flexion towards the contralateral hip.

Anterior ligaments – Fabers test

Flexion plus abduction plus external rotation (the 'faber' test) tests the integrity of the anterior sacroiliac ligaments. The test is also described as the 'four test' because of the position of the patient's limb, a combination of flexion, abduction and external rotation. The physiotherapist pushes the leg downward, just proximal to the

knee joint whilst stabilising the oposite hip with the other hand. A normal finding would be to lower the leg to the level of the opposite leg. Observe for pain response or limitation of movement (Figure 2.12).

Neurological Testing

Compression or traction of spinal nerve roots by disc trespass and/or osteophytes may give rise to referred pain, paraesthesia and anaesthesia and also give positive neurological signs. Neurological signs should be carefully monitored as deterioration may indicate worsening pathology.

Dermatomes

A dermatome is an area of skin supplied by a particular spinal nerve. Dermatomes may exhibit sensory changes for light touch and pin prick. Test each dermatome individually, on the unaffected and then the affected side. The Appendix lists dermatomes of upper and lower limbs.

Myotomes

A myotome is a muscle supplied by a particular nerve root level (see the Appendix). These are assessed by performing isometric resisted tests of the myotomes L1 to S1 in middle range, held for approximately 3 seconds. Test the unaffected side, then the affected: LI–L2 for the hip flexors (see Figure 2.15) L3–L4 for knee extensors, (see Figure 2.16), L4 for foot dorsiflex-

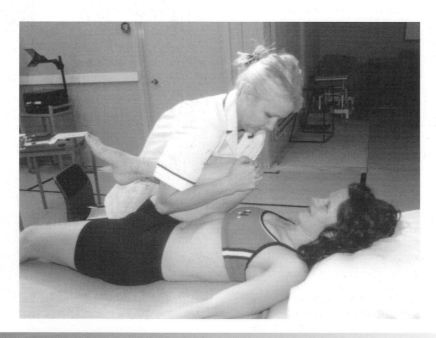

Figure 2.11 Compression testing of the posterior sacroiliac ligaments.

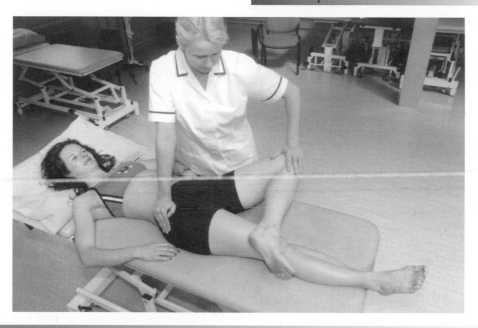

Figure 2.12   The faber or four-test. Normal range of movement.

ors and invertors, L5 for extension of the big toe, S1 for plantarflexion (see Figure 2.17) and knee flexion, S2 for knee flexion and toe standing, S3–S4 for muscles of the pelvic floor and the bladder.

Reflexes

- Test the non-affected first then affected side second. Note dull reflexes may indicate lower motor neurone dysfunction. Brisk reflexes may indicate an upper motor neurone dysfunction.
- L3 corresponds to the quadriceps. The patient sits with the knee flexed and the therapist hits the patellar tendon just below the patella (Figure 2.13).
- S1 corresponds to the plantarflexors. Dorsiflex the ankle and strike the Achilles tendon. Observe and feel for plantarflexion at the ankle (Figure 2.14).

The Babinski reflex

The Babinski reflex (or plantar response) is an abnormal response and occurs when a blunt object is drawn up the lateral aspect of the sole of the foot. Normally the great toe (big toe) flexes. Abnormally the great toe extends indicating upper motor neurone damage. Note that this primitive reflex is seen in the newborn but disappears with time.

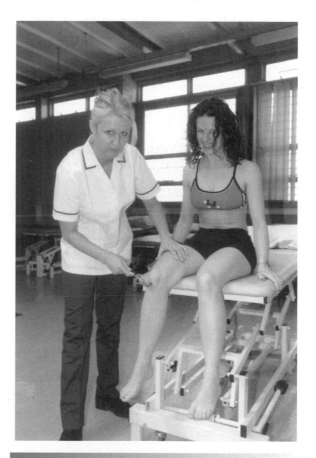

Figure 2.13   The quadriceps reflex (L2, L3, L4).

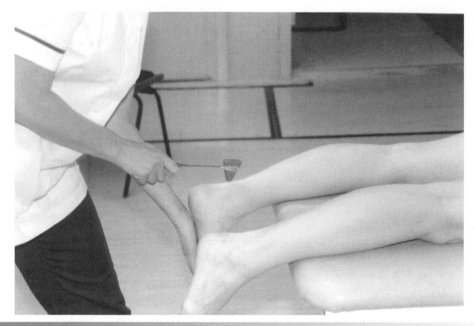

Figure 2.14   The Achilles tendon reflex (S1, S2).

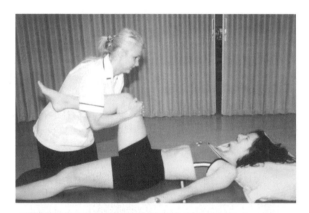

Figure 2.15   Resisted hip flexion to test myotome L1–L2.

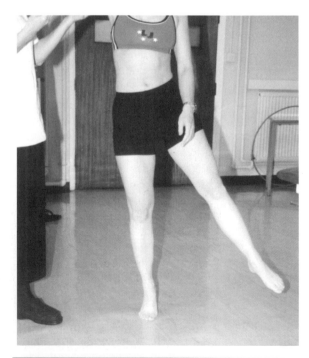

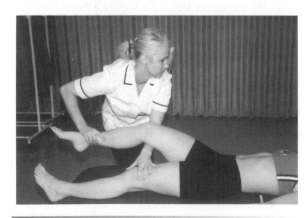

Figure 2.16   Resisted knee extension to test myotome L3.

Figure 2.17   Toe standing (plantar flexion) to test myotome S1.

Adverse mechanical tension

Passive neck flexion

The patient is supine. The physiotherapist passively flexes the patient's neck. Observe for any low back pain response, which may suggest disc pathology.

Straight leg raise (SLR)

This is also known as Lasegue's test. The patient is supine. The physiotherapist lifts the patient's leg whilst maintaining extension of the knee (Figure 2.18). An abnormal finding is back pain or sciatic pain. The sciatic nerve is on full stretch at approximately 70 degrees of flexion, so a positive sign of sciatic nerve involvement occurs before this point (Palmer and Epler 1998). Any pain response and range of movement is noted and comparison made with the other side. Factors such as hip adduction and medial rotation further sensitise the sciatic nerve; dorsiflexion of the ankle will sensitise the tibial portion of the sciatic nerve; plantarflexion and inversion will sensitise the peroneal portion of the nerve.

Prone knee bend (femoral nerve stretch)

The patient lies prone and the physiotherapist flexes the person's knee and then extends the hip (Figure 2.19). Pain in the back or distribution of the femoral nerve indicates femoral nerve irritation or reduced mobility. Comparison is made with the other side.

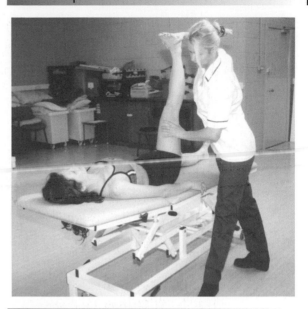

Figure 2.18   SLR test adding dorsiflexion of the ankle joint.

Slump test

This tests the mobility of the dura mater. The patient sits with thighs fully supported with hands clasped behind the back. The patient is instructed to slump the shoulders towards the groin (Figure 2.20). The physiotherapist applies gentle overpressure to this trunk flexion. The patient adds cervical flexion, which is maintained by the therapist. The patient then performs unilateral active knee extension and active ankle dorsi-

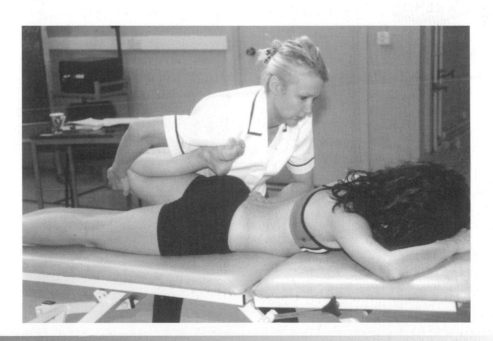

Figure 2.19   Femoral nerve test.

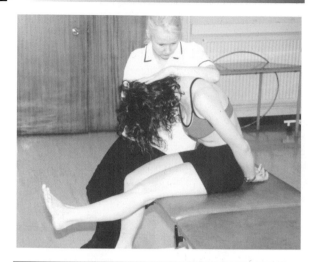

Figure 2.20   Slump test with single knee extension.

flexion. The physiotherapist should not force the movement. The non-affected side should be assessed first.

Any symptoms are noted at the particular part in range. If the dura mater is tethered, symptoms will increase as each component is added to the slump test. The patient is instructed to extend the head – a reduction in symptoms on cervical extension is a positive finding, indicating abnormal neurodynamics.

Testing for lumbopelvic stability

Stability of the lumbar spine is necessary to protect the lumbopelvic region from the everyday demands of posture and load changes (Panjabi 1992a). It is essential for pain-free normal activity (Jull et al. 1993) and should always be assessed.

With the patient in crook lying with the hips at 45 degrees flexion, he or she is instructed to maintain a neutral spine (it may be useful to tell the patient to maintain such a lordosis that an army of ants could just crawl through!). The person then performs an abdominal in-drawing by contracting the transversus abdominis muscle whilst attempting to maintain the spine in neutral. To challenge the transversus abdominis and multifidus stabilising muscles (and consequently the spinal position), the patient adds the leg load by alternately lifting the heels from the floor and sliding out the leg whilst maintaining a neutral spine position. The maintenance of a neutral spine posture can be assessed by using a biofeedback device. An inability to maintain the spine in neutral will result in the lumbar spine extending as the leg is lifted. The intra-abdominal pressure mechanism is controlled primarily by the diaphragm and transversus abdominis which provides a stiffening effect on the lumbar spine (Hodges and Richardson 1997).

Palpation

Soft-tissue thickening over the articular pillar at one or more spinal levels is a common finding in cases of degenerative disease of the lumbar spine, as is hard bony thickening and prominence over the apophyseal joints. Note any general tightness, or localised thickening of muscular tissue or ligamentous tissue. In general,

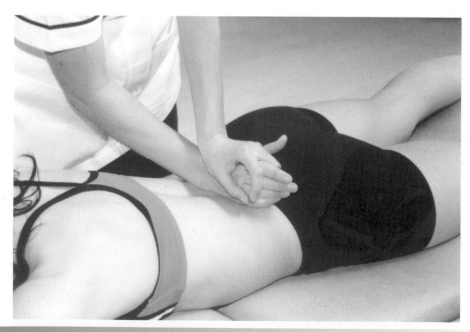

Figure 2.21   Unilateral pressures applied to the lumbar spine over the articular pillar. Note the pressure is applied through the physiotherapist's pisiform bone.

the older the soft-tissue changes, the tougher they are; the more recent, the softer they are. However, a thickened or stiff area is not necessarily painful or the source of a patient's symptoms (Maitland 2001).

Accessory spinal movements

The physiotherapist applies central PA (postero-anterior) pressures on the spinous processes, and unilateral (one-sided) pressure over the articular pillar (Figure 2.21), noting areas of hyper- and hypomobility. Record any pain experienced by the patient, and the corresponding spinal level.

Case Study: Lumbar Spine

A 30-year-old labourer was referred for physiotherapy following a lifting injury at work. He complained of left-sided low back and medial shin pain and intermittent paraesthesia affecting his left great toe. The pain was aggravated by flexion and eased by standing and walking. On examination he had a marked shift to the right. Flexion was reduced to fingertips to knees and his left SLR was reduced to 50 degrees.

Owing to the rapid onset of symptoms associated with a lifting injury in a flexed posture, and the pain being aggravated by flexion and eased by extension activities, the injury was hypothesised to be discogenic. Clinical trials suggest that the most usual sources of low back pain are the intervertebral disc, the zygapophyseal (facet) joint and the sacroiliac joint (Maitland 2001).

The patient was treated by rotations to the right (as demonstrated on another patient in Figure 2.22), which centralised his pain. His shift was manually corrected on the first visit. He was prescribed repeated extension exercises in prone, as advocated by McKenzie (1985), to do at home every 2 hours. By the third visit

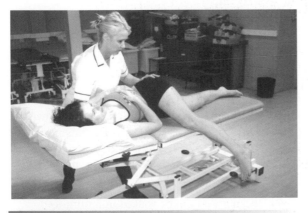

Figure 2.22   Right-sided lumbar rotation, used to treat left-sided back and leg pain.

his pain had centralised to left low back pain, and his SLR was 80 degrees. He was then treated by unilateral mobilisations on the left at grade 4. This alleviated his symptoms and he regained full range of all movements.

Prior to discharge, he was given a programme of abdominal and multifidus exercises. He was also given postural and ergonomic advice prior to his return to work. The multifidus and the transverse abdominus muscles have been found to be primarily responsible for imparting local stability to the lumbar spine in the joint's neutral zone (Wilke et al. 1995; Gocl et al. 1993; Panjabi 1992; Hodges and Richardson 1996).

Biopsychosocial Assessment (Lumbar Spine)

Although historically there has been no change in the pathology or prevalence of low back pain (LBP), disability due to non-specific LBP has increased dramatically in modern western societies. Medical interventions for chronic LBP using a limited biomedical approach have been relatively unsuccessful and the cost to NHS physiotherapy services was estimated to be £151 million per annum (Maniadakis and Gray 2000). Low back pain has been described as a twentieth-century healthcare disaster (Wadell 1992). In 80% of cases of LBP no significant pathology is ever found despite considerable disability. Recent guidelines based on systematic reviews of contemporary literature have recommended a biopsychosocial approach in the assessment and treatment of LBP (CSAG 1994; RCGP 1999).

Fundamental differences between acute and chronic pain

It is not satisfactory to view chronic pain simply as acute pain that has persisted for a long period. Acute and chronic pain are different clinical entities. We now acknowledge that there are many different mechanisms and processes involved in the genesis of chronic pain states which are not relevant in acute pain. The diversity of these elements has led to the use of a biopsychosocial approach to indicate that there are biological, social and psychological factors relevant within an individual that can be either causing or maintaining the chronic pain state

Acute pain is basically a protective mechanism to reduce the possibility of increasing the injury. It is usually self-limiting, and lasts until the tissues are healed. It is usually associated with an increased sympathetic nervous activity. This may be associated with feelings of anxiety, panic; nausea etc. and may be observed during traumatic injuries to the bones and soft tissues.

Chronic pain is detrimental because it lasts long after the injury has healed. Tonic self-sustaining neural loops are set up to perpetuate the pain. Decrease in sympathetic activity may cause depression and apathy. Chronic pain outlasts the normal time of healing, and has no recognisable end-point (Grichnik and Ferrante 1991).

Predictors of chronic incapacity

Can disability from low back pain be predicted? Psychosocial researchers in the last decade have found common psychosocial and social traits in people who have developed chronic disability due to LBP. Many subjects with chronic LBP have been reported to have a psychological profile that predisposes them to develop chronic pain (Burton et al. 1995; Carrageen 2001). Additionally, people aged between 50 and 60 years are more likely to become disabled due to LBP (Burton et al. 1995).

Further major predictors are listed here.

- people who have unrealistic beliefs about their pain and the nature of their disease (Waddell 1992)
- people whose occupation involves heavy manual work and sustained postures
- people with a previous history of sickness absence
- people who seek multiple investigations and treatments (Waddell 1992; Harding and Watson 2000)
- people with low educational achievement or low-status occupations (Cats-Baril and Frymoyer 1991; Frymoyer 1992)
- people who have pending compensation issues (Tait and Chibnall 2001)
- people with fear-avoidance beliefs – i.e. that a fear of activity may be more disabling than the original injury (Vlaeyen 1995; Fritz et al. 2001)
- people who exhibit 'illness behaviour', which may include attention seeking, grimacing, catastrophising about their problems or LBP, inappropriate coping strategies, excessive use of splints, braces, walking aids, over-reliance on the NHS, and passive rather than active treatment modalities.

In view of the above factors, it is necessary to screen patients with LBP in order to attempt to reduce the likelihood of chronic disability. It is important to note that a patient's general physical fitness may be a poor predictor of chronic incapacity (Deyo et al. 2001). The identification of the patients at risk of progression to chronicity (failure to respond to treatment) is by means of psychosocial questionnaires, because clinical variables contribute practically nothing to our predictive ability (Burton 1997). The psychosocial traits concerned (coping strategies, depressive tendencies, inappropriate beliefs about pain and activity) are present in the acute phase – they are not just the result of persistent symptoms (Burton 1997).

Management guidelines for LBP (CSAG 1994; RCGP 1999)

In the early management of acute LBP, analgesia with non-steroidal anti-inflammatory drugs (NSAIDs) should be administered immediately following an acute onset. Manipulative therapy is advised in the early stages, and active exercise and physical activity should be encouraged. Bedrest is ineffective as treatment for back pain, but is acceptable in moderation in the acute situation for 1–2 days.

Encourage physical activity and an early return to work and sport whenever possible. Practice psychosocial management: educate the patient of the importance of good postural habits and activities of daily living. Challenge the patient who has unrealistic beliefs about the LBP condition and prognosis.

Biopsychosocial assessment

The biopsychosocial assessment differs from the physical assessment in that it incorporates psychological and social issues in more depth. This gives the physiotherapist a good overview of the patient's circumstances, his or her overall mood state, beliefs, attributes and thoughts about the problem, about therapy and about the future.

Psychological factors

A previous history of anxiety and depression, general attitudes and expectations is noted. The patient's perceived level of control over the pain is also assessed with particular regard to the use of active or passive coping strategies (these are often referred to as 'internalised' or 'externalised' locus of control).

Social factors

Identify social areas, including work issues, pending compensation, a history of injury, sickness benefits, and daily functioning, because these may effect the outcome.

Physical examination

A body chart and physical examination may or may not be conducted, as the physiotherapist deems necessary. However, if red flags are noted then a neurological examination is indicated. Assessments may include functional tests such as:

- the distance that can be walked in 5 minutes
- the number of times the person can stand from sitting in 1 minute

Flags

'Yellow flags' are psychosocial factors including a previous history of anxiety and depression, impending compensation, absence from work, sickness benefit, invalidity benefit, passivity and high levels of dependency and poor coping skills. 'Red flags' are clinical features that should alert the therapist to the possibility of severe pathology. They include bladder and bowel malfunction, saddle anaesthesia, bilateral paraesthesia, neurological signs, unexplained weight loss, a past history of carcinoma, general debility and fever.

- the number of times the person can step up and down in 1 minute.

Outcome measures questionnaires

The following questionnaires and tools are validated, reliable and sensitive. They can be used prior to and following intervention to determine efficacy.

- the Oswestry Disability Index (Fairbank et al. 1980)
- the visual analogue scale
- the Present Pain Index
- the short-form McGill Pain Questionnaire (Melzack 1987)
- the Hospital Anxiety and Depression Questionnaire (Zigmond and Snaith 1983)
- the locus of control questionnaire (FABQ).

Treatment of biopsychosocial aspects of LBP disability

Many studies have reported decreases in pain levels and disability following intensive back rehabilitation programmes combining exercise and cognitive therapy (e.g. Frost et al. 1998; Guzman et al. 2001). The aims of chronic spinal rehabilitation programmes are to:

- reduce the patient's pain if possible, or enable the patient to cope more effectively with the pain
- reduce the patient's disability
- encourage when possible a return to work and hobbies to promote better physical functioning (by challenging the unhelpful belief that pain always equates to harm)
- encourage an active patient-centred approach to LBP management.

Van Korff and Saunders (1996), in a survey of LBP sufferers in the USA, found that patients wanted to understand the following four things:

1. the likely course of their back problem
2. how to manage the pain
3. how to return to normal activities of daily living
4. how to minimise recurrences of back pain.

Example of the content of a back rehabilitation programme

- Pre-intervention questionnaire and physical tests for outcome measures.
- Circuit training, including aerobic and strengthening regimes, with emphasis on postural control, spinal stability, back extensors and deep abdominal musculature.
- Patient-centred discussions, seminars on anatomy, pathology, medication, self help measures, posture and exercise, etc.
- Relaxation workshops.
- Post-programme questionnaire and physical tests.
- Follow-up questionnaires at 1 and 12 months to determine how they are managing their LBP.

THE CERVICAL SPINE

Following on from the subjective assessment, the physiotherapist should highlight the main findings and formulate a hypothesis regarding the clinical diagnosis. The SIN factors will determine the vigour of the examination. The physiotherapist will attempt to find the patient's comparable sign by means of movement or palpation.

Special questions

Patients presenting with disorders of the cervical spine may also complain of headaches, dizziness, nausea and vertigo. Record this in your assessment. These may be symptoms of vertebrobasilar insufficiency (VBI).

Posture

Note the symmetry of the head on the neck, and the neck relative to the thorax. The chin should be at 90 degrees to the anterior aspect of the neck. There should be no obvious horizontal skin creases posteriorly. A plumbline from the tragus of the ear should fall behind the clavicle.

Assess the cervical lordosis. A decreased lordosis predisposes the vertebral bodies and discs to bear more weight. An increased lordosis increases the compressive loads on the zygapophyseal (facet) joints and posterior elements. Observe for muscle hypertrophy, hypotrophy, spasm, tightness or general asymmetry.

An acute wry neck (torticollis) presents as a combination of flexion and rotation or side flexion away from the painful side. Patients with chronic pathology often have a poking chin posture which consists of excessive upper and middle cervical extension and lower cervical/cervicothoracic flexion. This results from a weakness of the deep cervical flexors and overactivity of sternocleidomastoid and levator scapulae muscles (Figure 2.23).

Note that cervical posture is influenced by lumbar posture, and hence the poking chin posture is exaggerated by lumbar and thoracic flexion (Figure 2.23). Cervical and shoulder posture should therefore be viewed in both the sitting and standing postures.

The shoulders should ideally be level, but this is often not the case because of handedness. For example in a right-handed person the right shoulder is often held slightly lower than the left.

Movements

It is important to not only assess the range of movement occurring in the cervical region but also the quality of that movement. Particularly note the motion segments where the movement is occurring. Hinging may be observed which indicates areas of hypermobility or instability. Conversely, areas of hypomobility or stiffness are observed as areas of plane or straight lines.

Key points

For consistency and reliability of re-assessment, the same order of active movements should be carried out each time.

Active movements

Flexion

The movement should be performed to either the patient's pain or the limit of movement. During flexion the cervical lordosis should be obliterated, and the spine appears to be flexed or neutral. The spinous

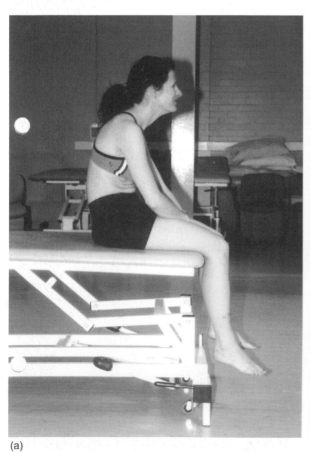

(a)

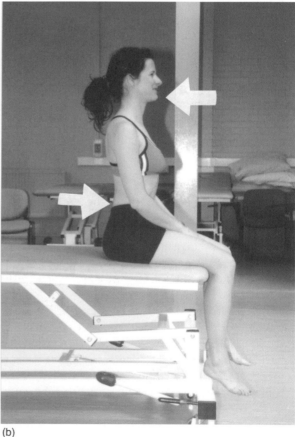

(b)

Figure 2.23   (a) Poking-chin posture, exaggerated by thoracic and lumbar flexion. (b) Correction of cervical posture by maintaining the lumbar spine in a neutral position.

process of C7 should be the most prominent, C6 and T1 less so. The chin should approximate the chest. Common faulty patterns are the upper cervical spine remaining in extension or chin poke. Loss of range, areas of give and restriction should be noted, as well as the pain response, muscle spasm and crepitus.

Extension

The entire cervical spine should extend, and the face should be almost parallel to the ceiling. A vertical line should be observed from the chin to sternum. Common faulty movement patterns include a loss of lower cervical extension and the head does not move posteriorly to the shoulders. Furthermore, excessive hyperextension of the upper and mid cervical spine may occur earlier on in the movement and the chin pokes forward.

Side flexion

Often this movement is the most restricted in degenerative spinal pathologies. Tightness in the contralateral sternocleidomastoid and trapezius may be observed. Common faulty patterns include coupling with rotation due to tightness in anterior flexor musculature. Observe range, pain response and areas of give or restriction. Compare the sides for symmetry.

Right and left rotation

Observe the range of movement available and the patient's pain response, muscle spasm and crepitus. Common faulty patterns include coupled movements with side flexion and the eyes not moving in a purely horizontal plane (Figure 2.24). Compare the right and the left sides.

Overpressures repeated and combined movements

If the plane movements are full range and pain-free, then overpressure may be applied. At the end of the available range the physiotherapist may apply a small oscillatory movement to feel the quality and end-feel of the movement, and the range of further movement. The pain response is also noted. Combined movements may be examined in an attempt to reproduce the patient's pain or restriction of movement. The patient should if possible perform repeated movements, since this may alter the quality and range of the movement and may give rise to latent pain (McKenzie 1990).

The shoulder complex

Observe full shoulder elevation through flexion and abduction for the shoulders bilaterally, because

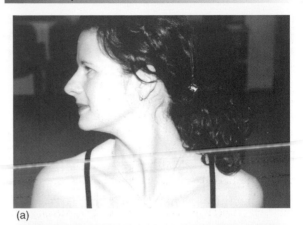
(a)

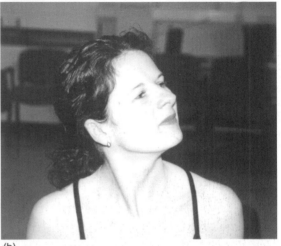
(b)

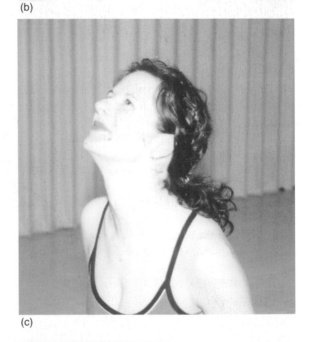
(c)

Figure 2.24   (a) Normal right cervical rotation. (b) Faulty position: right side flexion limited and completed with contralateral rotation. (c) Faulty position: extension with chin poke, upper cervical extension, lower cervical spine remaining flexed.

during the last few degrees of elevation the thoracic spine extends to allow for full shoulder elevation. A stiff kyphotic thoracic spine will limit shoulder elevation.

Passive physiological intervertebral movements (PPIVMs)

PPIVMs may be used to confirm any restriction of motion seen on active movement and to detect restriction of movement not discovered by the active movements. They are also used to detect segmental hypermobility (Magarey 1988; Maitland 2001).

Vertebral Artery Testing

> **Key point**
> Vertebrobasilar insufficiency (VBI) is a contraindication to cervical manipulation and high-grade mobilisations, particularly rotations, extensions or longitudinal distractions and traction.

Differentiation test to determine between vestibular and VBI symptoms

The patient stands and rotates the cervical spine to the right and left. Note is taken of symptoms such as dizziness or nausea. Either vertebrobasilar artery insufficiency or the vestibular apparatus could cause symptoms produced as a result of this manoeuvre. In order to differentiate between these two structures, the physiotherapist fixes the patient's head and the patient keeps the feet static and facing forwards. The patient then rotates his or her body to the right and to the left whilst maintaining the head in a static position (Figure 2.25).

If symptoms such as dizziness or light-headedness are produced with this manoeuvre then they are due to vertebrobasilar pathology, because the head remains still (and the vestibular apparatus will be unaffected) and the cervical spine is rotating effecting the artery.

Vertebrobasilar testing (Maitland 2001)

This test is performed in both sitting and supine positions.

1. Sustained rotation for 10 seconds is performed to each side. Note any symptoms.
2. Sustained extension for 10 seconds is performed. If the patient is asymptomatic then:

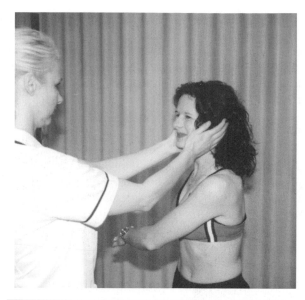

Figure 2.25 Differentiation test to determine between vestibular and VBI symptoms.

3. Combined rotation and extension to each side is sustained for 10 seconds. Note any symptoms. A positive test would be to induce feelings of dizziness and nausea.

> **Key point**
> If the patient has grossly restricted range of movement then the test for vertebrobasilar insufficiency is not valid.

Neurological Testing

Dermatomes

Test for normal sensation, the cutaneous area supplied by a single posterior root of each spinal segment, light touch with the dorsal aspect of the hand or cotton wool and pinprick sensation for each dermatome, C1 to T1. Refer to the Appendix for dermatome illustrations.

Myotomes

Isometric testing of the muscles supplied by a spinal segment in mid range for a few seconds is performed at each level from C1 to T1 (Figure 2.26). Weakness may indicate a lower motor lesion from a prolapsed disc, or another space-occupying lesion. Refer to the Appendix for myotomes.

Reflexes

Test for normal reflexes: biceps (C5–C6), triceps and brachioradialis (C7). Compare one side with the other.

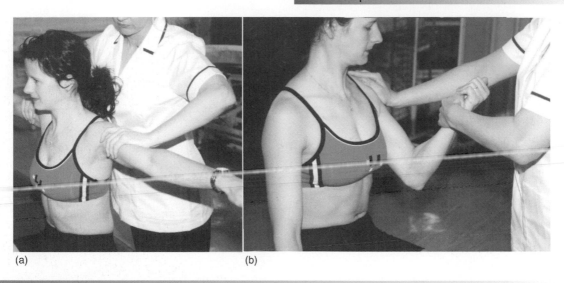

(a)   (b)

Figure 2.26   (a) Resisted shoulder abduction (C5) myotome. (b) Assessment of C6 myotome in resisted biceps.

Note brisk reflexes which may be indicative of an upper motor neurone lesion, and dull reflexes which may be indicative of a lower motor neurone lesion.

- C5–C6 corresponds to biceps brachii. The person's arm should be semi-flexed at the elbow with the forearm pronated. Place your thumb or finger firmly on the biceps tendon and hit your finger with the hammer (Figure 2.27).
- C6 to C8 correspond to triceps. Support the person's upper arm and let the forearm hang free. Hit the triceps tendon above the elbow (Figure 2.28).

Mechanical tension tests

The upper limb tension test (ULTT) is referred to as the SLR test of the cervical spine. This test mobilises the brachial plexus and particularly biases the median nerve to determine the degree to which neural tissue is responsible for producing the patient's symptoms. Certain movements of the arm, shoulder, elbow, wrist and hand, and similarly the neck and the lower limb, can cause neural movement in the cervical spine. These tests are so important that all physiotherapists should know and use them (Butler 1991).

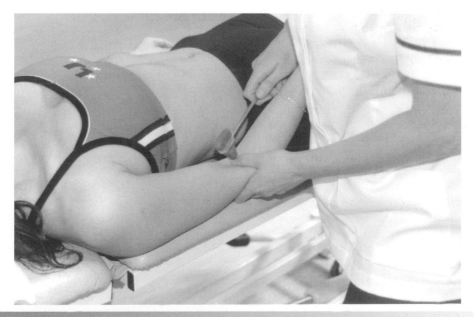

Figure 2.27   The biceps reflex (C5, C6).

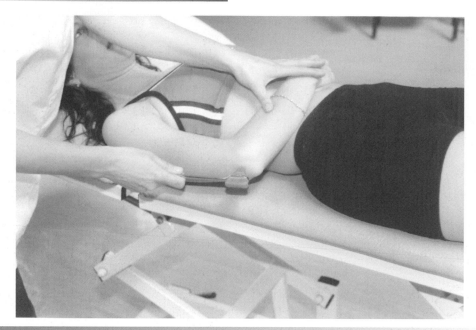

Figure 2.28   The triceps reflex (C6, C7).

The physiotherapist depresses the patient's shoulder, then adds in 90° abduction, 90° lateral rotation of the shoulder, elbow extension, forearm supination and wrist and finger extension to the supine patient (Figure 2.29a). Sensitising manoeuvres such as ipsilateral (same side) or contralateral (opposite side) cervical rotation and side flexion are added (Figure 2.29b). Symptoms of pain, paraesthesia and restriction are noted, and compared with the other side. Common findings will be reduced range or the reproduction of symptoms on the affected side.

Palpation

Palpate the soft tissues, noting the positions of vertebrae and myofascial trigger points (localised irritable spots within skeletal muscle). These trigger points produce local pain in a referred pattern and often accompany chronic musculoskeletal disorders. Palpation of a hypersensitive nodule of muscle fibres of harder than normal consistency is the physical finding typically associated with trigger points (Alvarez and Rockwell 2002).

Observe for local or referred pain, thickening of structures or stiffness. Remember that anomalies of the bifid spinous processes of the cervical vertebrae and differences in their spacing are not uncommon and may not be clinically significant (Maitland 2001).

Soft-tissue changes including sub-occipital thickening and shortening in the extensors and prominence and thickening of the articular pillar of C2–C3 facet joints are common in degenerative disorders. Soft-tissue changes around the cervicothoracic junction

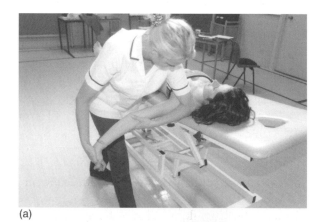

(a)

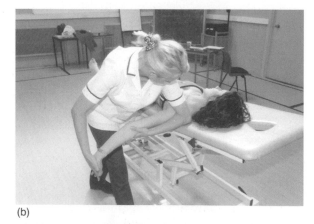

(b)

Figure 2.29   (a) Upper limb tension test (ULTT). (b) ULTT with contralateral right side flexion of the cervical spine.

are also commonly found, and may be referred to as a Dowager's hump.

Bony anomalies

Osteophytes may be palpable at the C2–C3 facet joints, in patients with pre-existing spinal pathology (Maitland 2001). Approximation of the spinous processes of C6–C7 is also a common feature.

Accessory spinal movements

With the patient prone, central pressure on the spinous processes C2 to T6 and unilateral pressures on the articular pillars C2 to T6 is applied by the physiotherapist, noting levels of stiffness, pain response, muscle spasm and areas of hypermobility (Figure 2.30).

Case Study: Cervical Spine

A 50-year-old woman with a 2-year history of central neck and occasionally bilateral shoulder pain (4 on the visual analogue scale) was referred for physiotherapy. On examination she had a marked protracted cervical spine (poking chin posture) which could, however, be corrected by the patient on demand. Her cervical range of movement was approximately two-thirds on all movements. Neurological testing was normal. Palpation revealed stiffness at levels C5 and C6 to central posterio-anterior pressures over the spinous processes.

The patient was treated with grade III postero-anterior (PA) central pressures (as in Figure 2.30) and was given postural correction exercises. Priority one cervical neutral shin slides against a wall. Following three treatment sessions her pain was reduced to 1 on the VAS and her range of movement was almost full. She was given deep flexor exercises on the fourth visit along with exercises for normal range of movement. On the fifth visit she was asymptomatic, and was discharged to continue with the exercises at home.

Both manipulations and mobilisations aim to reduce pain and increase the joint range of motion for spinal conditions (Johnson and Rogers 2000; Maitland 2001). Studies have shown that cervical mobilisation produces a hypoalgesic (pain-relieving) effect and can decrease visual analogue scores (Sterling et al. 2001). The majority of studies conclude that spinal mobilisations have a positive short-term effect on pain (Bronfort et al. 2001; Coulter 1996). Koes et al. (1992) observed an improvement in physical functioning when compared to other physiotherapy modalities, placebo or general practitioner involvement. It could be argued that by improving pain in the short term the patient will return to normal activities more quickly

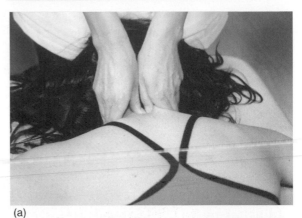

(a)

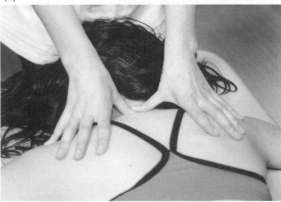

(b)

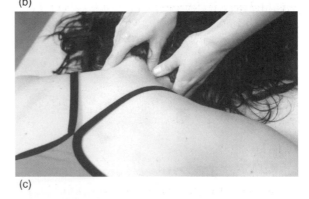

(c)

Figure 2.30   Accessory movements: (a) central PA pressure on spinous process; (b) central PA with thumbs superimposed; (c) unilateral pressure on the left articular pillar.

and thus avoid the potential for deconditioning and chronicity.

Muscle imbalance procedures were instituted into the woman's programme to improve the patient's postural awareness, to increase the strength of the deep cervical flexors, and to stretch out the tight sub-occipital extensors. According to Heimeyer et al. (1990) it is important for the therapist to differentiate between people who have protracted chin posture but who can voluntarily correct it, and those who cannot. For the person in this case study, the posture was correctable, so the role of the physiotherapist as adviser was paramount. Repeated sessions of electrotherapy for example would have been inappropriate or would have provided a short-term solution to the pain only. Treatment should be geared towards behaviour modifications – the change of bad postural habits. In this case the combination of manipulative therapy, corrective exercises and advice was employed with success.

PERIPHERAL JOINT ASSESSMENTS

THE SHOULDER JOINT

Key point
The patient should be suitably undressed to view the cervical spine, thoracic spine, shoulder girdles, shoulders and both arms.

Posture

It is important to assess the posture of the cervical and thoracic spine because a scoliosis, kyphosis or poking chin posture will affect the mechanics of the shoulder, by altering the plane of the glenohumeral joint. The spinal and shoulder complex postures should be observed with the patient in both sitting and standing.

Posterior alignment

The shoulders should ideally be level, but for a right-handed person the right shoulder is often held lower than the left, and vice versa. Elevation of the shoulder girdle may be due to tightness or overactivity in the levator scapulae or the upper fibres of trapezius, and lengthening or weakness in the lower fibres of trapezius.

Observe the symmetry of the scapulae. They should lie flat against the thoracic wall and the medial borders lie approximately 50–75 mm lateral to the spine. Winging of the scapulae is observed when the whole length of the medial border of the scapula is displaced laterally and posteriorly from the wall of the thorax. This may result from weakness in the serratus anterior muscle or a lesion of the long thoracic nerve. Pseudo-winging of the scapulae occurs when the inferior angle of the scapula is displaced from the thoracic wall.

Observe the soft-tissue contours of the shoulder for symmetry, and areas of atrophy and hypertrophy. The acromion processes should be horizontal to, or slightly higher than, the point at the root of the scapula. If the root of the scapula is higher this indicates tightness or overactivity of the levator scapulae and rhomboid musculature, which causes a downward rotation of the glenoid fossa. This may be a precursor to impingement syndromes and rotator cuff pathologies. Moreover, the levator scapulae may cause anterior shear on the cervical spine and give rise to cervical and scapula pain.

Anterior alignment

Note any irregularities of the clavicle, sternoclavicular and acromioclavicular joints resulting from previous fractures or dislocations. Note the soft-tissue contours regarding symmetry atrophy and hypertrophy, particularly in the deltoid, upper trapezius and sternocleidomastoid muscles.

Lateral alignment

Note the relative positions of the humeral head: no more than one-third of the humeral head should lie anteriorly to the acromion process. Excessive forward translation may result from tightness in the pectoral muscles and elongation of the posterior shoulder capsule. The patient's arms should lie comfortably at the side with the thumbs facing almost forwards. Excessive medial rotation of the shoulders will result in the thumbs facing inwards towards the body. Excessive protraction of the shoulders with an increased thoracic kyphosis and tightness in the pectoral muscles is a common faulty posture.

Palpation

Palpate the local skin temperature, noting any increase suggestive of underlying inflammation. Palpate the acromioclavicular and sternoclavicular joints, observing for pain or tenderness. Palpate the supraspinatus and infraspinatus tendons for tenderness associated with tendonitis, calcification and strain. Palpate the upper trapezius and levator scapulae for tenderness and trigger points. These hyperirritable areas within the muscle and connective tissue are thought to be due to a secondary tissue response to disc or joint disorders (Hubbard and Berkhoff 1993). They are painful to compression and may cause referred pain.

Muscle length tests
Levator scapulae

With the patient supine, flex and lateral flex the cervical spine away to resistance and add ipsilateral rotation (rotation to the same side as side flexion). Depress the shoulder girdle and compare range and pain response on both sides.

Pectoralis minor

With the patient supine, the lateral border of the spine of the scapula should be within 25 mm of the plinth. If pectoralis minor is shortened, the lateral border of the spine of the scapula is more than 25 mm from the plinth since the shoulder girdle is protracted

Movements

Differentiation tests
Since the cervical and thoracic spines may refer pain to the shoulder and scapula areas, full active movements and accessory movements of these areas should be assessed. Note any increase or referral of pain around the shoulder or scapula areas. Overpressure may be used if the movements are pain-free. Furthermore, the upper limb tension test (ULTT) may be performed to rule out referral of pain from neural structures. Refer to the objective assessment of the cervical spine for descriptions of these techniques.

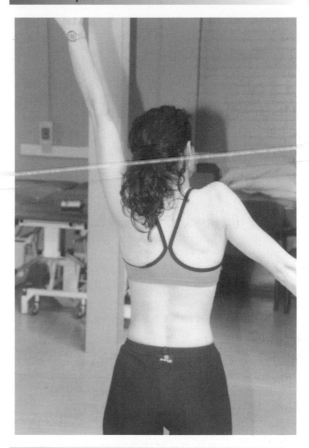

Figure 2.31   Reversed scapulohumeral rhythm of the right shoulder.

Active movements

Full active movements of the shoulder girdle and joint are performed, noting any restriction, asymmetry and pain response. Note the capsular pattern for the glenohumeral joint is limitation of lateral rotation, abduction and medial rotation (Cyriax 1982).

Shoulder girdle movements

Assess shoulder girdle elevation, depression, protraction and retraction, observing for pain asymmetry and crepitus.

Shoulder joint flexion

Observe flexion through to elevation and return of movement, assessing the scapulohumeral rhythm. Normal should be in the ratio of 2:1 (humerus: scapula). Reversed scapulohumeral rhythm occurs in conditions causing restriction of the glenohumeral joint, such as adhesive capsulitis ('frozen shoulder').

Shoulder joint abduction

Observe abduction through to elevation and return (Fgure 2.31), again noting the scapulohumeral rhythm.

Key point
A painful arc of movement is observed in patients suffering from impingement syndromes, whereby the superior aspects of the rotator cuff, biceps tendon and bursae are impinged by repetitive overarm activities. Pain is experienced between 90 and 130 degrees of abduction.

Impingement may be caused by loss of scapular stability. Faulty patterns of scapula motion include early rotation and elevation of the scapula (reversed scapulohumeral rhythm). This may implicate weakness in the stabilisers (e.g. lower fibres of trapezius, rhomboids and serratus anterior), or shortness and overactivity in the upper trapezius and levator scapulae.

Impingement may also be caused by weakness or inhibition of the rotator cuff muscles that produces a superior translation of the humeral head (i.e. subscapularis, teres minor and lower infraspinatus). There may also be late timing of lateral rotation during abduction which may cause impingement.

Tightness of pectoralis minor can cause increased protraction of the scapula which decreases the sub-acromial space.

Repetition of the movement may induce an element of fatigue, and abnormal movements may derive from that. A juddering movement of the scapula on return from elevation implicates poor eccentric control.

Differentiation. If abduction reproduces the person's pain, then differentiation between the glenohumeral and subacromial structures may be required.

1. If the movement is repeated and compression applied to the glenohumeral joint causes an increase in symptoms, then the glenohumeral joint is implicated.
2. If the movement is repeated and a longitudinal force in a cephalad direction is applied (increasing compression on the subacromial structures), with an increase in pain, the subacromial structures are implicated.

Failure to initiate or maintain abduction when placed passively into abduction is a sign of rotator cuff rupture, and the patient should be referred to a consultant for a repair/further investigations.

Shoulder joint rotation

Test medial and lateral rotations, both beside the trunk and at 90 degrees of abduction. Note pain response and limitation of movement.

Shoulder joint horizontal flexion and extension (Scarf-test)

Pain on these movements implicates the acromio-clavicular joints as the source of pain or restriction.

Shoulder joint extension

Compare both sides for range and pain response.

Shoulder functional movements

Functional movements such as hand behind the back (HBB), and the hand behind the neck (HBN), should also be assessed. These movements are grossly restricted in patients with adhesive capsulitis.

Other shoulder joint abnormalities

Sporting activities that give rise to symptoms, such as the late cocking stage of throwing a ball overhead, should also be assessed to determine faulty mechanics.

Passive movements

All movements performed actively can be repeated passively, noting the differences in range. Observe the differences in end-feel and compare these with the unaffected side.

Key point
Note that the capsular pattern for the glenohumeral joint is limitation of lateral rotation, abduction and medial rotation (Cyriax 1982).

Accessory movements

Acromioclavicular and sternoclavicular joints

Test anteroposterior (AP) and posteroanterior (PA) draw, and caudal glide.

Glenohumeral joint

Test anteroposterior (AP) and posteroanterior (PA) draw, caudal and cephalad glide, and lateral distraction (Figure 2.32).

Further tests (Maitland 2001)

The following tests should be performed only in shoulders of low irritability, and when no comparable sign has been found. They stress a number of different structures around the shoulder and are therefore not diagnostic:

- locking test of the shoulder
- quadrant test of the shoulder (Figure 2.33)

Resisted muscle testing

This provides a guide of strength ratios and pain response. Test: abduction and flexion at around 30–60 degrees; internal and external rotation beside the trunk and at 90 degrees of elevation in the plane of the scapula; and resisted muscle testing in positions of function and/or pain.

Muscle length tests

It may be useful to test the length of muscles that are prone to shortness – latissimus dorsi, pectoralis major and minor, upper fibres of trapezius, levator scapulae and sternocleido-mastoid.

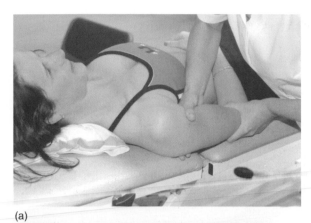

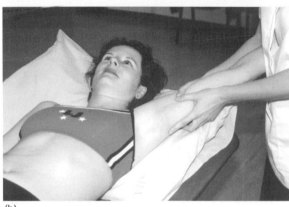

(a)

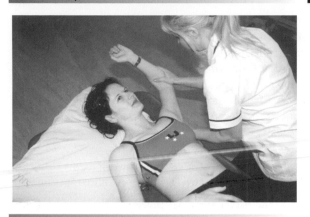

Figure 2.33   Quadrant test of the shoulder.

(b)

Figure 2.32   (a) Lateral glide of the glenohumeral joint. (b) Caudal glide of the shoulder in elevation.

Acromioclavicular joint compression and distraction

End-of-range overpressure into horizontal flexion compresses the acromioclavicular joint and may give rise to pain arising from this joint. Acromioclavicular distraction tests the instability of the acromioclavicular joint, by applying a downward traction on the arm whilst palpating the joint line. Reproduction of pain or palpable separation of the joint line is a positive test.

Tests for Shoulder Instability

Anterior draw/translation (Lachmann's of the shoulder)

This is performed in supine with the patient's arm at around 30 degrees of abduction, 45 degrees of lateral

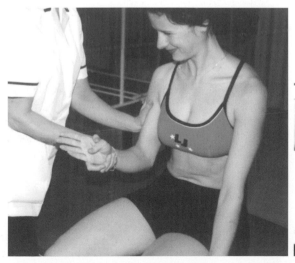

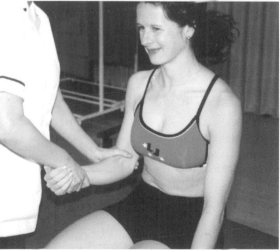

Figure 2.34   (a) Resisted lateral rotation at the shoulder. (b) Resisted medial rotation at the shoulder.

rotation and slight flexion. The physiotherapist grasps the humeral head with one hand, and the medial hand is used to stabilise the shoulder girdle. The lateral hand applies the anterior translation force in the same way as the anterior draw test of the knee. Laxity of the joint (excessive anterior translation) is a positive sign (Figure 2.35).

Posterior draw test

This is performed in supine with the patient's gleno-humeral joint at the edge of the examination couch in abduction not exceeding 90 degrees. Posterior pressure is applied on the anterior aspect of the humeral head. Excessive movement compared with the other side is a positive sign.

Inferior draw (sulcus) test

This is performed in sitting or supine, arm by the side. The physiotherapist exerts a strong downward traction force on the arm, grasping the head of the humerus with both hands, to the limit of movement, pain or apprehension, whilst monitoring the superior contour of the shoulder joint. Excessive inferior glide or a significant depression or sulcus distal to the acromion is a positive sign.

Impingement Test

Supraspinatus (empty-can test)

This is performed in sitting or standing with 90 degrees of abduction bilaterally, full available medial rotation, and 30 degrees of horizontal flexion (Figure 2.36). Supraspinatus is the main support for the suspended arm in this position. The physiotherapist resists abduction of the shoulder. Pain on resistance is a positive test for a lesion of the supraspinatus muscle or tendon. Following the objective assessment record your findings clearly and asterisk objective findings.

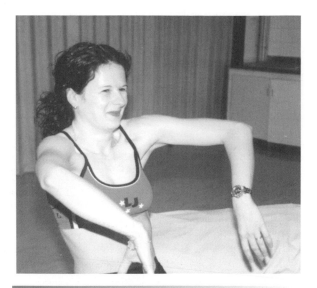

Figure 2.36   The empty-can test position. Resistance to abduction is applied by the therapist.

Test Yourself

Match these five scenarios to the likely pathology:

1. reduced range of movement particularly on active and passive rotations and abduction
2. painful arc of movement between 90 and 120 degrees
3. inability to actively abduct the arm away from the body and maintain the position when the arm is placed there passively
4. pain and weakness on resisted elbow and shoulder flexion
5. excessive movement on passive anterior, posterior and sulcus draw tests of the shoulder.

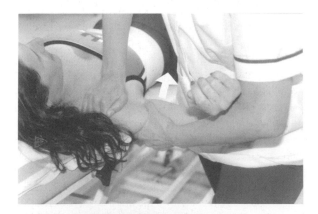

Figure 2.35   Anterior draw of the glenohumeral joint in abduction with stabilisation of the shoulder girdle.

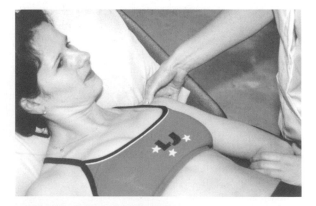

Figure 2.37   Palpation of the supraspinatus tendon. The patient's hand is behind the back.

Answers

(1) Frozen shoulder (adhesive capsulitis). (2) Impingement of supraspinatus under the acromion. (3) Rupture of the rotator cuff musculature. (4) Ruptured biceps brachii muscle. (5) Global instability.

THE HIP JOINT

Key point
The patient should be suitably undressed to view the hip, pelvis and spine. Note that the hip joint is too deep to observe an effusion or palpate the joint line.

Gait

Observe the person's gait from the front, back and side. Assess the patient with and without a walking aid as deemed appropriate. Ask the patient to walk forwards and backwards, whilst observing:

- stride length symmetry
- the time spent on the single leg support phase on each leg
- corresponding factors of pain, stiffness and/or weakness during the cycle.

Posture

Standing

With the patient standing, view from the front, rear and sides. Note:

1. pelvic tilting: a line joining the two anterior sacroiliac joints should be horizontal (the same applies posteriorly)
2. the relative levels of the PSIS to the ipsilateral ASIS viewed from the side: differences may be suggestive of sacroiliac rotatory asymmetry
3. rotational deformity of the hips: may be observed as in-toeing or out-toeing
4. leg length discrepancy: this may be observed by the differences in the horizontal levels of the gluteal and knee creases
5. scoliosis of the lumbar spine: this may be structural or a compensation for a leg length discrepancy
6. inequality of weight distribution: the patient may reduce the amount of weight borne on the painful side
7. increased lumbar lordosis: this may suggest a fixed flexion deformity of the hip(s)

8. bruising in the abdominal or groin area: suggestive of a sportsman's hernia
9. muscle wasting: particularly of the quadriceps and gluteal muscles is common and may appear as hollowing posteriorly or laterally at the buttocks.

Supine

With the patient supine, note the following:

1. leg rotation, through observing the relative positions of the patella and/or the feet
2. pelvic rotation
3. leg length discrepancy, through observing the relative position of the medial malleoli or heels.

Leg length discrepancy

Apparent leg length discrepancy is measured from the xiphoid of the sternum to the tip of the medial malleolus using a tape measure (compare with the other leg). *True* leg length discrepancy is measured, using a tape measure, from the ASIS to the tip of the medial malleolus. A difference in leg length of up to 1–2 cm is considered normal by some clinicians. If there is a leg length difference, measure the length of the individual bones – i.e. thigh and leg.

Key point
From the movement of supine to sitting, one leg may appear to be longer in supine and shorter in sitting. This is caused by anterior rotation of the innominate bone on the affected side and is an SI joint dysfunction.

Muscle length assessments

The Thomas test

This test determines the presence of a fixed flexion deformity at the hip. With the patient supine, the hip is fully passively flexed, and the lumbar lordosis is obliterated. If the contralateral (opposite) hip rises off the bed, this indicates a fixed flexion deformity of that hip. This may be due to tightness or restriction in the capsule, iliopsoas or rectus femoris.

To differentiate between the iliopsoas and rectus femoris as the source of restriction, the patient's knee is passively extended (Figure 2.8). If this results in the patient's hip dropping down into less flexion, then the restriction is in the rectus femoris muscle because by extending the knee an element of stretch has been removed. If the hip is unaffected and remains, in the same degree of flexion, independently of the knee

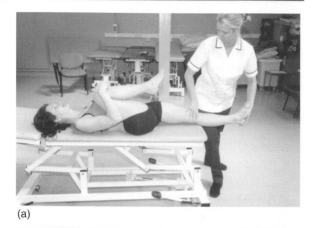

(a)

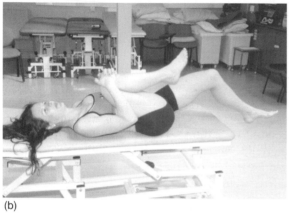

(b)

Figure 2.38   The Thomas test: (a) normal; (b) abnormal.

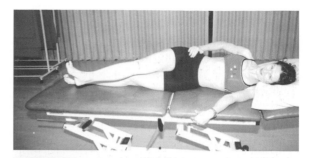

Figure 2.39   Modified Obers test.

extension, then the restriction is in the iliopsoas muscle. This is measured and recorded.

The length of the following muscles may be tested since they are prone to shortening: quadratus lumborum, tensor fascia lata and the hamstrings.

Modified Ober's test (iliotibial band)

With the patient in side-lying and the uppermost hip fully laterally rotated, the knee joint in unlocked extension, the uppermost leg should drop (adduct) to the plinth (Figure 2.39). A tight iliotibial band would result in the leg not being able to adduct to the plinth.

Piriformis test

With the patient supine, or side-lying, with hip at 90 degrees flexion, adduct maximally to resistance and externally rotate. (Note piriformis is a medial rotator in flexion.) Pain in the buttock or in the distribution of the sciatic nerve may signify compression of the sciatic nerve by the piriformis muscle (Figure 2.40).

Hamstrings

With the patient sitting, spine in neutral, the hip at 90 degrees, the person should be able to extend the knee to within 10 degrees of full extension (Figure 2.41).

Quadratus lumborum

Test side flexion against a wall without associated flexion or rotations. Compare the two sides. A shortened quadratus lumborum will result in limitation of contralateral side flexion.

Movements

Allow the patient to functionally demonstrate his or her aggravating movement in order to determine the likely structures implicated in producing the symptoms.

Lumbar spine differentiation

The lumbar spine may give rise to referred pain in the region of the hip or groin, so it is important to exclude the lumbar spine as a possible cause of symptoms arising at the hip joint. Flexion, extension and bilateral side flexion should be observed actively in standing. Loss of range of motion and pain

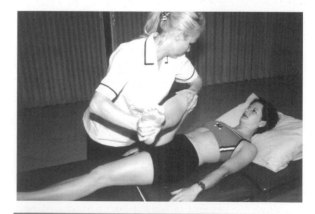

Figure 2.40   Piriformis stretch. Note that, in the flexed position, piriformis becomes a hip medial rotator.

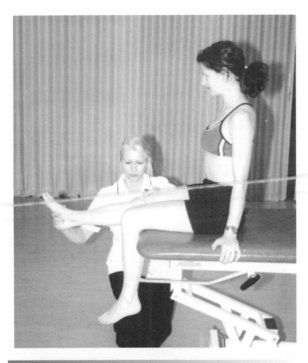

Figure 2.41   Assessment of hamstring length. Note that the lumbar spine remains in neutral. This picture shows normal hamstring length.

- Palpate the psoas major and adductor longus tendons to localise strains and contractures of these structures.
- Palpate the greater trochanter of the femur for tenderness associated with bursitis. Palpate the ischial tuberosity for suspected hamstring strains.
- Tenderness located over the ASIS may indicate a strain of the sartorius muscle or contusion of the spine following contact sports. This is referred to as a 'hip-pointer'
- Palpate the lower abdominal musculature for suspected inguinal or sports hernias.

Active movements

> **Key point**
>
> Note pain, crepitus and/or limitation of movement. Apply overpressure to the movement if it is pain-free to see whether this reproduces the symptoms not elicited on other movements. Measure both the normal and affected hip for comparison.

Hip flexion/extension

The patient is supine or side lying. The axis of the goniometer is placed directly over the greater trochanter of the femur. The static arm should be parallel to the patient's trunk. The dynamic arm should be placed parallel to the femur. Note loss of range or pain response.

Hip abduction/adduction

The patient is supine. The axis of the goniometer is placed over the ASIS. The static arm should be in line between the left and right ASIS. The dynamic arm should be parallel to the long axis of the femur. Note loss of range or pain response.

Hip rotation

Hip rotation can be easily measured with the patient sitting. Note that the hip joints are approximately 90° flexed (Figure 2.3). The axis of the goniometer is placed at the mid-point of the patella. The static arm is perpendicular to the floor. The dynamic arm should be parallel to the anterior midline of patella. If active movements are full range and pain free then gentle overpressure can be applied noting any reproduction of symptoms.

The normal ranges of movement at the hip joint should be approximately:

response should be noted, particularly if these movements reproduce the patient's hip pain or the patient's comparable sign. If the movements are pain-free and full range, then overpressure may be applied to observe whether this reproduces the patient's symptoms. Accessory movements of the lumbar spine, femoral nerve stretch and SLR should also be screened.

Trendelenberg test

A positive Trendelenburg test demonstrates that the hip abductors are not functioning owing to weakness or pain inhibition and are unable to perform their role of stabilising the pelvis on the weight-bearing leg. To perform the test the patient stands on the unaffected leg and flexes the other knee to a right-angle. The pelvis should remain level or tilt up slightly on the NWB side. The patient then stands on the affected leg and flexes the knee of the other leg. If the pelvis drops on the NWB side this signifies a positive Trendelenberg test (Figures 2.42 and 2.43).

Palpation

- Palpate the head of the femur lateral to the femoral artery.
- Rotate the hip passively to elicit crepitus or tenderness at the joint.

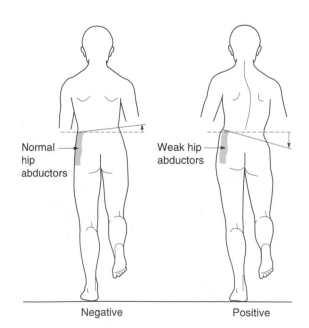

(a)   (b)

Figure 2.42   Trendelenburg test of right hip abductors: (a) normal; (b) abnormal or positive sign.

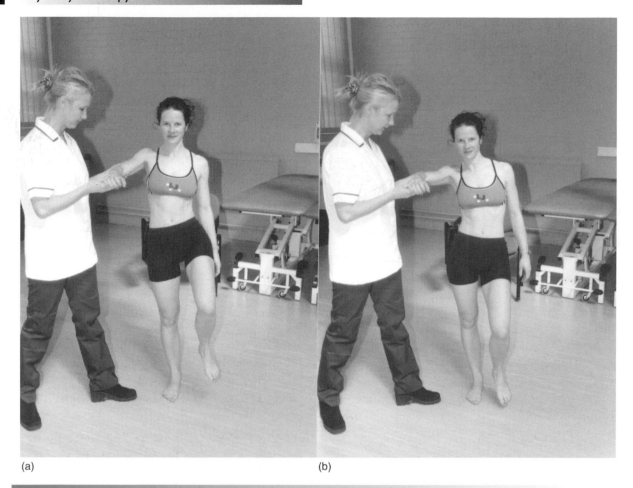

Normal
hip
abductors

Weak hip
abductors

Negative   Positive

Figure 2.43   Schematic of Trendelburg's sign.

- 0–120 degrees for unilateral flexion, 0–150 for bilateral flexion
- 10–15 degrees for extension
- 0–40 degrees for abduction
- 0–25 degrees for adduction
- 0–35 degrees for medial rotation
- 0–45 degrees for lateral rotation (Figure 2.44).

Key point
The capsular pattern for the hip joint is in order of greatest loss: flexion, abduction and medial rotation, slight limitation of extension and full range of lateral rotation (Cyriax 1982).

Passive movements

Flexion, extension, abduction, adduction, internal and external rotation should be performed passively by the

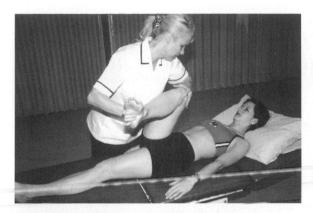

Figure 2.44   Resisted lateral rotation of the hip in flexion.

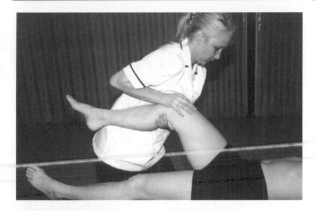

Figure 2.46   Compression applied through the hip joint.

therapist (Figure 2.45). Note any differences between active and passive ranges and identify reasons for this.

Muscle strength testing

Test the muscles both isometrically and isotonically through range to detect weakness at any particular point in the range. Compare with the opposite side. Pain inhibits muscle contraction and it is therefore important to differentiate between true weakness and pain-induced inhibition.

With the patient side-lying, test the strength of the hip abductors and adductors (weakness of adductors is a common finding in recurrent groin strains). With the patient supine, test the strength of the hip adductors, flexors and medial/lateral rotators (Figure 2.44).

Accessory movements

Test:

- cephalad longitudinal accessory movement (Figure 2.46)
- caudad longitudinal accessory movement
- lateral transverse (joint distraction).

Flexion/adduction combination and the hip quadrant test may be performed on non-irritable hips when all plane movements are clear with overpressure (Figure 2.47; Maitland 2001).

Neural tests

Neural tests may be performed if the symptoms produced at the hip appear to be originating from neural or spinal structures:

- femoral nerve stretch test (prone knee bend)
- sciatic nerve stretch test (straight leg raise)
- slump test.

For descriptions of these tests refer to the objective assessment of the lumbar spine.

Functional tests

Observe the patient performing activities that reproduce their pain. If appropriate assessment activities such as hop, squats, walking forwards, backwards, sideways, etc.

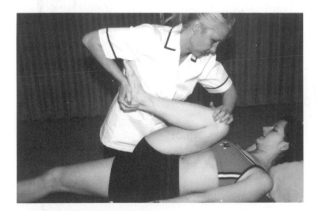

Figure 2.45   Passive hip and knee flexion.

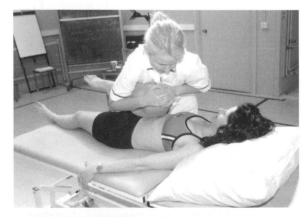

Figure 2.47   Quadrant test of the hip (flexion and adduction).

Key point

On completion of the assessment, specific objective signs that reproduce the patient's symptoms should be marked with an asterisk * or highlighted. This is commonly referred to as a 'comparable sign' and needs to be reassessed at each treatment, to determine the effectiveness of the physiotherapy intervention. Record your findings clearly.

Differentiation tests

The hip joint may refer pain to the knee. To differentiate between the hip and knee joints as a source of symptoms, the hip joint is tested by observing full flexion of the hip joint and then medial and lateral rotation in 90-degree flexion passively. Observe for any pain response or limitation of movement compared with the other side. If the movements are full range and pain-free, it is unlikely that the hip joint is the source of pain (Figure 2.44).

Test Yourself

Match these five scenarios to the likely pathology:

1. local tenderness at the ischial tuberosity and pain on resisted knee flexion
2. pain in the groin on coughing, resisted adduction sit-ups and weightbearing
3. a 3-year history of pain and stiffness particularly on medial rotation
4. local tenderness and heat palpated in the area of the greater trochanter having an insidious onset
5. increased or exaggerated lumbar lordosis and a positive Thomas test.

Answers

(1) Hamstring strain. (2) Sportsman's hernia. (3) Osteoarthritic (OA) hip. (4) Trochanteric bursitis. (5) Tightness in the hip flexors (iliopsoas.)

THE KNEE JOINT

Key point

The patient should be suitably undressed to view the hip, knee and ankle joints.

Gait

Observe the person's gait as they walk forwards and backwards. Make particular note of the equality of stride length, dwell time on each leg, reluctance to bear weight, and any pain responses.

Knee Examination

Posture with patient standing

Observe any deformities such as genu varum, genu valgus or genu recurvatum (Figure 2.48). Note any evidence of muscle atrophy, particularly evident in the vastus medialis muscle. Observe the relative positions and size of the patellae. 'Patella alta' is the term used to describe a small high riding patella.

Note any foot, ankle or subtalar deformity, such as foot pronation which will cause medial rotation of the tibia and hence affect the mechanics of the knee joint.

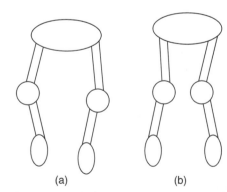

(a)   (b)   (c)

Figure 2.48   Leg posture deformities: genu varum (bow legs); (b) genu valgus (knock-knees); (c) genu recurvatum (hyperextending knees).

Swelling and discoloration

Swelling that extends beyond the joint capsule may suggest an infection or a major ligamentous injury, and the suprapatellar pouch will appear distended.

The Q angle

On your patient, draw a straight line across the middle of the patella. From the centre of this, draw a straight line going downwards through the centre of the tibial tuberosity, and another going upwards towards the ASIS (Figure 2.49). Normal values are approximately 12 degrees for males and 15 degrees for females. An increase in the Q angle is a predisposing factor in anterior knee pain and lateral dislocation of the patella.

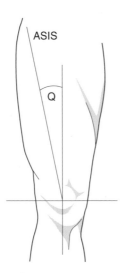

†Figure 2.49   Measuring the Q angle.

Bruising may suggest trauma to superficial tissues or ligaments. Redness of the skin suggests an underlying inflammation. Palpate the temperature around the knee joint with the back of the hand: heat is indicative of an underlying inflammatory disorder.

Observe scar tissue that may be indicative of previous surgery or trauma.

Effusions

An effusion (swelling confined within the joint capsule) will appear to obliterate the natural hollows at the sides of the patella. The synovial membrane of the knee is expansive, and extends the width of 3–4 fingers above the superior aspect of the patella.

Loss of muscle bulk

Observe loss of bulk in the quadriceps muscles, particularly in the vastus medialis which atrophies earlier than vastus lateralis following trauma, degenerative diseases and pain episodes. Measure the circumference of both thighs at 5, 8, 15 and 23 cm above the upper pole of the patella with a tape measure to obtain an objective marker (Magee 1992).

Ask the patient to perform a static quadriceps contraction. Palpate the tone, compare left with right sides of the musculature. Inability to actively extend the knee may result from rupture of the quadriceps tendon or quadriceps weakness, patella fractures, rupture of the patellar ligament, or avulsion of the tibial tubercle. Note any loss of tone in the anterior and posterior tibial muscles and again measure if appropriate at specific recorded distances below the patella.

Patellar tap

Patellar tap is a simple test to determine the presence of an effusion at the knee joint. It is performed with the patient supine. Any excess fluid is squeezed out of the suprapatellar pouch by sliding the index finger and thumb from 15 cm above the knee to the level of the upper border of the patella (Figure 2.50). Then place the tips of the thumb and three fingers of the free hand squarely on the patella and jerk it quickly downwards. A 'click' sound indicates the presence of effusion. The test will, however, be negative if the effusion is gross and tense, such as with a haemarthrosis of the knee (blood within the joint) following an anterior cruciate rupture.

Fluid displacement test

This is performed as above, by squeezing excess fluid out of the suprapatellar pouch and then stroking the medial side of the knee joint to displace any excess fluid in the main joint cavity to the lateral side of the joint. Repeat this procedure by stroking the lateral side of the

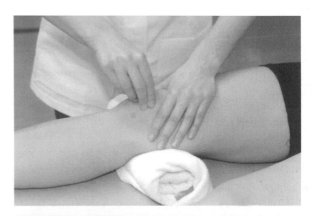

Figure 2.50   Patellar tap test.

joint. Any excess fluid will be seen to move across the joint and distend the medial side of the knee.

Tenderness at the knee (tibiofemoral joint)

Identify the joint line clearly by flexing the knee and observing for hollows at the sides of the patella ligament – these lie over the joint line.

1. Tenderness at the joint line is common in meniscal and fat pad injuries.
2. Tenderness along the line of the collateral ligaments of the knee joint is common at the site of a lesion following a tear, particularly at the upper and lower attachments and at the ligament's midpoint. Associated bruising and oedema may also be a feature of acute injuries.
3. Tenderness at the tibial tubercle – in children and adolescents, tenderness and hypertrophy of the tibial tubercle prominence – is associated with Osgood Schlatter's disease. Tenderness is also found following acute avulsion injuries of the patella ligament and its tibial attachment.
4. Tenderness and swelling in the popliteal fossa may indicate the presence of a Baker's cyst. This condition is associated with degenerative changes or rheumatoid arthritis involving the knee joint.
5. Tenderness at the adductor tubercle may indicate strain in the adductor magnus muscle.
6. Femoral condyle tenderness may indicate the presence of osteochondritis dessicans.

Patellofemoral joint assessment

A knee assessment should include assessment of both the tibiofemoral and patellofemoral joint. Observe the position of the patella and compare both sides.

- Determination of a high or small patella (patella alta) is made by calculating the ratio of the length of the patellar tendon to the longest diagonal length of the patella. The normal value for this ratio is 1.02 plus or minus 20% (Simmons and Cameron 1992). Patella alta is a predisposing factor in anterior knee pain and recurrent dislocation of the patella.
- Observe any tilting, lateral glide and rotation of the patella during a quadriceps contraction. Compare this with the other side.
- McConnell (1996) described a 'critical test' for the patellofemoral joint. Resisted inner-range quadriceps contraction is performed with the patient sitting at various degrees of knee flexion to determine whether this reproduces the patient's symptoms. Compare both sides (Figure 2.51).

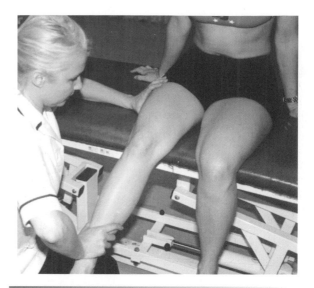

Figure 2.51   Critical test for patellofemoral pain. The test works because of the different contact areas of the patella against the femoral condyles in varying degrees of knee flexion.

- The McConnell critical test may be repeated with the patella taped in the corrected position. This will determine whether the taping is effective and should be incorporated into the treatment programme. Taping is believed to enhance activation and earlier timing of vastus medialis in quadriceps contractions and thus restore patellar tracking to normal.
- Observe any excessive pronation of the feet which may increase the Q angle (Figure 2.49).
- Test for tightness in the following structures: lateral retinaculum, iliotibial band, hamstrings and calves. Tightness of the above structures will increase dorsiflexion, and therefore pronation of the foot and ankle during the gait cycle. All of this will increase the Q angle (Olerud and Berg 1984).
- Perform passive accessory movements to test the mobility and pain response of the patella in all directions. Observe pain, laxity, or muscle spasm.
- Perform Clarke's test. The patient is asked to contract the quadriceps whilst the patella is pressed firmly down against the femur. Pain is produced in conditions such as chondromalacia or osteoarthritis affecting the patellofemoral joint.

Movements

Active movements

The patient is in half lying. Measure the active range of flexion and extension on each leg. The normal range of movement at the knee joint is approximately *minus* 5 degrees to 135 degrees of flexion. Note limitations of pain, stiffness or spasm. Overpressure the movement if full active movement is pain-free.

The axis of the goniometer should be positioned over the lateral femoral condyle. The static arm should be parallel with the long axis of the femur towards the greater trochanter. The dynamic arm should be positioned parallel to the long axis of the fibula and lateral malleolus (Figure 2.52). Hyperextension is present if the knee extends beyond 0 degrees (i.e. when the tibia and femur are in line).

Failure to hyperextend or lock out the knee fully may be a sign of a meniscal tear, which is blocking the movement of the joint. Moreover, a springy end-feel may be indicative of a bucket-handle tear of the meniscus. A rigid block to extension is common in arthritic conditions effecting the knee.

Passive movements

Check the range of extension and flexion passively. If there is a difference in active and passive range determine reasons for this.

Valgus stress test (medial collateral ligament of the knee)

With the patient supine, the physiotherapist applies a valgus force to the knee joint (i.e. the femur is pushed medially, and the leg pulled laterally) whilst the joint is held in extension (Figure 2.53a). A positive sign is observed as excessive opening up on the medial side of the joint. With the knee held in extension, a positive sign suggests major ligamentous injury involving the medial collateral, posterior cruciate and potentially the anterior cruciate. The test is performed again with the knee in 20–30 degrees of flexion.

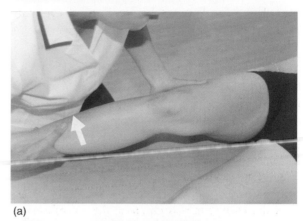

(a)

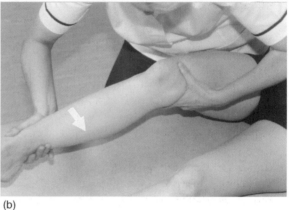

(b)

Figure 2.53   Stress tests: (a) valgus; (b) varus.

Varus stress test (lateral collateral ligament of the knee)

With the patient supine, the physiotherapist applies a varus force to the knee joint (i.e. the femur is pushed laterally, and the leg pulled medially) whilst the joint is held in extension (Figure 2.53b). A positive sign is observed as excessive opening up on the lateral side of the joint. As with the valgus stress test, with the knee held in extension a positive sign suggests major ligamentous injury involving the lateral collateral, posterior cruciate and potentially the anterior cruciate. The test is performed again with the knee in 20–30 degrees of flexion.

Anterior draw test (anterior cruciate ligament)

With the patient crook lying, the physiotherapist sits on the patient's foot to stabilise the leg and grasps around the proximal tibia and tibial tuberosity and pulls the tibia forwards (Figure 2.54a). A positive sign is elicited by excessive translation of the tibia anteriorly

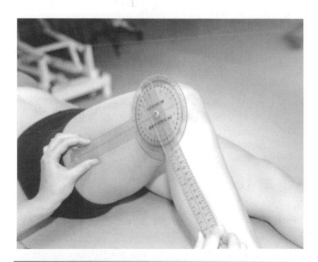

Figure 2.52   Measuring knee flexion using a 360-degree goniometer.

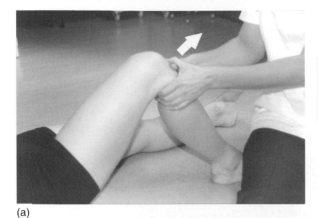

(a)

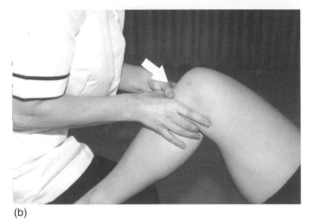

(b)

Figure 2.54   Draw tests: (a) anterior; (b) posterior.

(the normal translation is approximately 6 mm). Translation of 15 mm confirms rupture. Compare this with the other side. This test also stresses the posterior joint capsule, the medial collateral ligament and the iliotibial band (Magee 1992).

Rupture of the anterior cruciate ligament

Figure 2.55 illustrates the positive PA draw following rupture of the ACL.

Posterior draw test (posterior cruciate ligament)

With the patient crook lying, the physiotherapist sits on the patient's foot to stabilise the leg and grasps around the anterior aspect of the proximal tibia, and pushes the tibia backwards (Figure 2.54b). A positive sign is elicited by excessive translation of the tibia posteriorly. Compare this with the other side. This test also stresses the arcuate-popliteus complex,

posterior oblique ligament and anterior cruciate ligament (Magee 1992).

Sag sign

A 'sag sign' is observed with the patient in crook-lying, whereby the tibia is posteriorly displaced in relation to the femur. (Posterior displacement may give the false impression that the patient has a rupture of the anterior cruciate ligament since when an anterior draw test is performed a considerable amount of movement is noted. This is due to the tibia returning to its normal position however.

Lachman's test (modified anterior draw test)

The patient is supine with the knee resting over the physiotherapist's thigh at around 20–30 degrees of flexion (Figure 2.56). The physiotherapist grasps around the medial proximal aspect of the tibia with the right hand. The lateral aspect of the patient's femur is stabilised by the therapists left hand. Anterior and posterior translation of the tibia is produced by the physiotherapist's right hand. This tests the anterior cruciate, the posterior oblique ligament and the arcuate-popliteus complex (Magee 1992). The Lachman test has been shown to be sensitive for the diagnosis of anterior cruciate injury (Kim and Kim 1995).

The pivot shift test

This is a test for anterolateral instability of the knee joint. With the foot in medial rotation and the knee in 30 degrees of flexion, a valgus stress is applied to the knee whilst simultaneously extending it. A 'clunk' indicates a positive test and suggests anterior cruciate ligament pathology (McRae 1999).

Key point

Peripheral tears of the menisci can now be sutured arthroscopically. Many authorities believe that McMurray's tests described below may be of limited value (Evans et al. 1993).

McMurray's medial and lateral meniscus tests

The physiotherapist palpates the medial aspect of the joint line, and passively flexes and then laterally rotates the tibia, so that the posterior part of the medial

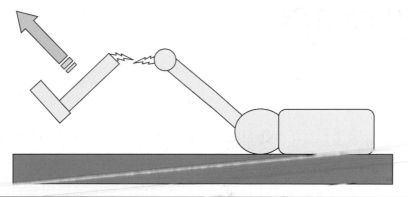

Figure 2.55   Schematic of positive PA draw following rupture of the ACL.

meniscus is rotated with the tibia. The joint is then moved back from a fully flexed position to 90 degrees of flexion, to test for the posterior part of the meniscus. A positive test occurs if pain is elicited, or a snap or click of the joint will occur if the meniscus is torn. The test is then repeated for the lateral meniscus by medially rotating the tibia.

Note that the examiner may be able to detect clicking or snapping sounds when performing this test, since there are various structures in the knee joint that can produce these signs. It is thus easy for this test to produce a false positive result (Palmer and Epler 1998).

Apley's compression/distraction test (for differentiation between meniscus and ligament)

The patient is prone with the knee flexed at right-angles. The physiotherapist medially and laterally rotates the tibia whilst applying a distraction force through the knee joint. The test is repeated by applying a compressive force through the knee joint. If the patient's symptoms are worse on compression then the symptoms are likely to be arising from a meniscal injury. Conversely, if they are worse on distraction then they are likely to be arising from a ligamentous injury.

Proprioception

Proprioception is tested with the patient standing on the unaffected leg and then on the affected leg whilst maintaining balance. Progressive adaptations may include standing on one leg with the eyes closed, standing on a wobble board, catching and throwing a ball etc.

Accessory movements
Patellofemoral joint

- Medial, lateral, cephalad and caudad glides.
- Medial and lateral rotation.
- Compression and distraction.

Superior tibiofibular joint

- Anteroposterior and posteroanterior glides.
- Compression.

Tibiofemoral joint

- Anteroposterior and posteroanterior glides.
- Medial and transverse glides.

Quadrant tests

These are performed on non-irritable knees when plane movements are pain-free.

- flexion/adduction quadrant
- flexion/abduction quadrant
- extension/adduction quadrant
- extension/abduction quadrant.

Following the objective assessment record your findings clearly and asterisk objective markers.

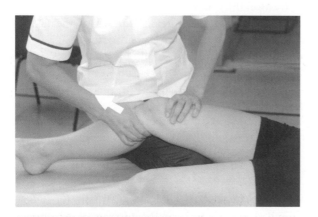

Figure 2.56   Lachman's test.

Test Yourself

Match these five scenarios to the likely pathology:

1. The knee is stiff and painful for about half an hour in the morning, aches at the end of the day, and has been like that for a long time.
2. The knee locks and has to be jiggled around to unlock it.
3. Since a tackle last week the knee keeps giving way and becomes very swollen.
4. The knee is very red and swollen. The person also feels feverish and generally unwell.
5. When the person walks downstairs he feels pain behind his kneecap.
6. There is pain on the inside of the knee and it hurts doing sideways movements.

Answers

(1) Osteoarthritis. (2) Torn meniscus. (3) Ruptured anterior cruciate. (4) Infective arthritis. (5) Chondromalacia patella. (6) Torn medial collateral ligament.

THE ANKLE AND FOOT

Key point
The patient should be suitably undressed to view the legs, ankles and feet.

Gait

Observe the patient's gait both barefoot and with shoes. Ask the patient to walk backwards and forwards. Assess the normal heel to toe pattern and stride length, rhythm, the posture of the longitudinal arch and weight-bearing on both feet. Note any pain, stiffness and weakness. Inspect the patient's footwear for areas of uneven or greatest wear.

Foot and Ankle Examination

Pulses (leg circulation)

Palpate the posterior tibial and dorsalis pedis pulses, to establish the state of the distal circulation. Circulation is often poor in patients suffering from peripheral vascular disease or diabetes. Compare both sides.

Oedema

Note any oedema, suggesting a systemic rather than a local cause for the patient's symptoms. This may indicate heart failure or excessive water retention. Bruising is suggestive of muscle or ligament injury. This is commonly situated on the lateral aspect of the foot beneath the lateral malleolus, following lateral ligament tears.

General Condition

Note the skin texture, colour and nail condition, which identifies the state of the peripheral circulation.

Temperature

Feel for any increase in temperature around the joint and compare with the opposite foot. A foot with impaired arterial circulation is colder than normal and may appear cyanosed (blue); conversely a warm foot may be indicative of an inflammatory response, for example following an injury or associated with conditions such as rheumatoid arthritis.

Tenderness

- Tenderness localised over and just proximal to the malleoli often occurs following a fracture.
- Tenderness and pain in the area distal and inferior to the lateral ligaments is common following inversion sprains. The anterior talofibular ligament (ATF) is the most commonly injured since the ligament is most often torn in the combined position of inversion and plantarflexion. This is the loose packed position and one in which the anterior band of the lateral ligament is particularly placed on stretch.
- Tenderness along the line of the long flexor tendons and/or the peroneal tendons may indicate the presence of tenosynovitis. This may be accompanied by local thickening.
- Tenderness at the articular surface of the talus is common in osteoarthritic conditions.
- Tenderness at the heel is found in conditions such as calcaneal exostosis (bony spurs), tendocalcaneal bursitis and plantar fasciitis.
- Diffuse tenderness under the metatarsal heads may be a sign of Morton's neuroma. This is a condition characterised by inflammation and pain around 3rd and 4th digital nerves. Pain is reproduced on squeezing the medial and lateral sides of the forefoot together.
- Diffuse tenderness and swelling on both the plantar and dorsal surfaces of the forefoot is a common finding in rheumatoid arthritis.

- Tenderness on the mid posterior aspect of the calcaneus may be a sign of a calcaneus bursitis.
- Tenderness along the Achilles tendon may be a sign of a sprain or tendonitis in the Achilles tendon.

Alignments

Observe the posture of the heel relative to the leg. The heel and lower leg should be parallel and the calcaneus should rest squarely on the ground. Note any postural misalignment such as excessive supination or pronation.

> ### Foot pronation and supination
>
> A *pronated* foot has the appearance of rolling in on the medial side with bulging of the navicular bone medially. Additionally, the longitudinal arch appears flattened. A *supinated* foot has the appearance of rolling outwards with the inner border raised.

Excessive pronation may cause posteromedial shin splints, plantar fasciitis, hallux valgus or Achilles tendonitis. Excessive supination may cause anterolateral shin splints, dropped first ray (metatarsal) or plantar fasciitis.

Note whether the heel is inverted or everted. Posteriorly the Achilles tendon and the calcaneus should be vertically aligned. *Calcaneal varus* is observed as the calcaneus being inverted relative to the leg; *calcaneal valgus* is observed if the calcaneus is everted relative to the leg.

Is the foot splayed or flattened? This may be due to weakness of the intrinsic muscles and subsequent flat-tening of the longitudinal arch. Observe the posture of the medial arch and assess its height in comparison with the other.

Note any wastage of the calf musculature. Compare both sides. Measure the circumference of the leg with a tape measure at specified points below the patella.

The leg and hindfoot

With the patient prone, the physiotherapist bisects the calcaneus by drawing a vertical line through the posterior aspect of the calcaneus, then bisects the lower leg by drawing a vertical line on the posterior aspect of the lower third, and places the subtalar joint in a neutral position. If the lines are parallel there is correct alignment of the leg and hindfoot (Figure 2.57a). *Rear foot varus* is observed as the calcaneus appearing to invert relative to the leg (Figure 2.57b); *rear foot valgus* is observed as the calcaneus appearing to evert relative to the leg.

The hindfoot and forefoot

As above, observe the position of the whole foot. Correct alignment is observed if the hindfoot and forefoot are in line and perpendicular to the floor. *Forefoot varus* is observed if the first toe is superior to the lateral toes. *Forefoot valgus* is observed if the fifth toe is superior to the medial toes.

> ### Key point
>
> Complex foot misalignments may require referral to a podiatrist.

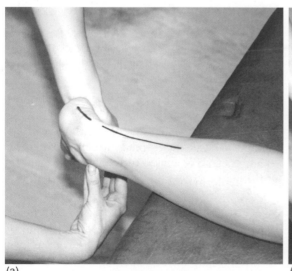
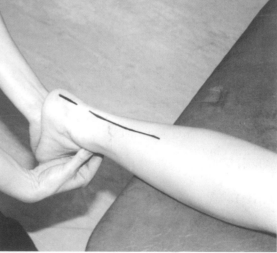

(a)   (b)

Figure 2.57   Alignment of the right leg and hindfoot: (a) calcaneal varus); (b) normal.

The toes

Look for:

- clawing (hyperextension of the metatarsophalangeal joints and flexion of the other phalanges)
- mallet toe (flexion of the distal interphalangeal joints)
- hammer toe (hyperextension of the metatarsophalangeal and flexion of the proximal interphalangeal joints)
- hallux valgus (lateral deviation of the first interphalangeal joint)
- hallux rigidus (stiffness of the first interphalangeal joint).

Functional activities

Assess the patient's ability to stand on heels, toes and the inner and outer borders of the feet. Test the patient's proprioception. This may be performed with the patient standing on one leg or on a wobble board, with the eyes open and then closed. To make this more difficult the patient can catch and throw a ball whilst trying to maintain balance. Balance on the unaffected leg is assessed and then compared with the affected side. Also, when appropriate, test the patient's ability to hop, squat and jump, noting any stiffness or pain response.

Movements

Active movements

Ankle joint

The patient is in supine or sitting. Measure plantar and dorsiflexion. Movement occurring at the tarsal joints is easily mistaken for movement at the ankle, and vice versa. Note pain or stiffness compared with the other side. Overpressure the movement if it is full range and pain-free.

The axis of the goniometer is placed 15 mm inferior to the lateral malleolus. The static arm should be parallel to the fibula. The dynamic arm should be parallel to the long axis of the fifth metatarsal (Figure 2.58).

- Normal range of plantarflexion is approximately 50–55 degrees.
- Normal range of dorsiflexion is approximately 10–15 degrees.

Note that the knee needs to be in slight flexion if full dorsiflexion is to be achieved. This takes the stretch off gastrocnemius.

Subtalar and midtarsal joints

In the normal foot, 80% inversion and eversion occurs at the subtalar joint. Most of the remainder occurs at

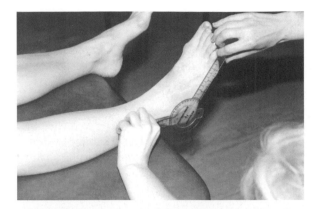

Figure 2.58 Measurement of ankle plantarflexion/dorsiflexion.

the midtarsal joints, with a little at the tarsometatarsal joints. Determine the range by percentage of the abnormal to the normal. Test:

- combined inversion and adduction (supination)
- combined eversion and abduction (pronation).

Inversion and eversion

Inversion is the movement whereby the soles of the feet face inwards towards one another. Eversion is the movement whereby they face outwards.

Toe movements

Observe flexion and extension at all the toes and compare with the opposite side.

Passive movements

All the movements measured actively can be measured and tested passively. Note any difference between active and passive ranges and identify possible reasons for discrepancies.

Muscle strength

The dorsiflexors, plantarflexors, invertors and evertors are tested by isometric and isotonic resisted movements. Assess any weakness or pain elicited at any part of the range.

Ligament tests

Lateral ligament stress test. The patient lies supine and the physiotherapist grasps the heel and passively inverts the foot, feeling for any opening at the lateral side of the foot (Figure 2.59). A positive test may reveal increased inversion movement, a sulcus dimple on the lateral side of the foot, or a pain response.

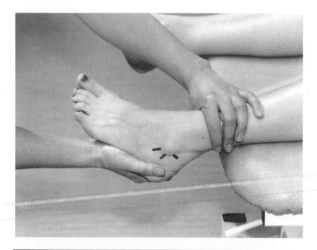

Figure 2.59   Passive inversion of the plantarflexed foot to test the anterior talofibular ligament.

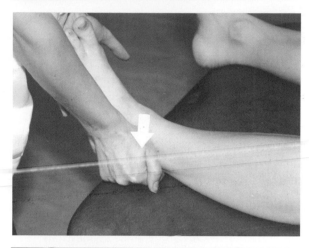

Figure 2.60   AP glide at the inferior tibiofibular joint.

To differentiate between the three bands of the lateral ligaments, the test should be performed in:

- plantarflexion and inversion to strain the anterior band
- inversion only to strain the calcaneofibular band
- a combination of dorsiflexion and inversion to strain the posterior band.

Medial ligament stress test. The patient lies supine and the physiotherapist grasps the heel and passively everts the foot. A positive test may reveal increased movement of eversion compared with the other side and/or may elicit a pain response.

Anterior draw test at the ankle. This detects the integrity and stability of the anterior talofibular and calcaneofibular components of the lateral ankle ligaments. The patient lies supine. The physiotherapist stabilises the distal leg, grasps around the talus and pulls it forwards. A positive test reveals an anterior displacement of the talus in the mortise of the lower end of the tibia and fibula and suggests major lateral ligament disruption. Observe for laxity, an audible 'clunk', or the presence of a lateral suction dimple.

Accessory movements (Maitland 2001)
Inferior tibiofibular joint

Perform posteroanterior and anteroposterior glides (Figure 2.60).

Ankle joint
Perform:

- posteroanterior and anteroposterior glides
- longitudinal movement cephalad and caudad
- medial and lateral rotation.

Subtalar joint
Perform medial and lateral glides.

Metatarsophalangeal and interphalangeal joints
Perform:

- posteroanterior and anteroposterior glides
- rotations and distractions.

Thompson's squeeze test

This tests the integrity of the gastrocnemius/soleus Achilles tendon complex. With the patient prone, the physiotherapist squeezes the calf firmly just distal to its maximum circumference (Figure 2.61). If the tendon is intact, the foot will plantarflex. A positive test will occur if the tendon or muscle is ruptured and the ankle will not plantarflex. A palpable gap in the tendon or muscle belly may sometimes be observed if the tendon is ruptured. Following on from the objective assessment write up your findings clearly and asterisk an objective marker.

Test Yourself
Match these five scenarios to the likely pathology:

1. One ankle keeps giving way and feels unstable. There is poor proprioception on one leg.
2. There is pain in the plantar aspect of the heel on weight-bearing, or toe extension.
3. There is pain under the medial malleolus, increasing on resisted inversion.
4. There is longstanding, insidious pain and stiffness in the ankle, increasing on weight-bearing.

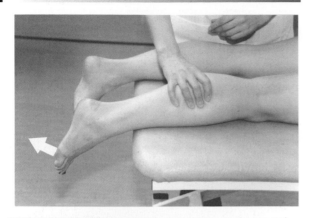

Figure 2.61   Thompson's test of the right calf. Slight plantarflexion of the ankle suggests an intact Achilles tendon.

5. The patient has a history of an inversion strain combined with swelling and bruising under the lateral malleolus.

Answers

(1) Lengthened lateral ligaments. (2) Plantar fasciitis. (3) Tendonitis of tibialis posterior. (4) Osteoarthritis of the ankle. (5) Lateral ligament sprain.

REFERENCES

Alvarez DJ, Rockwell PG 2002 Trigger points: diagnosis and management. Am Fam Phys 65(4): 653–60

Bronfort G, Evans R, Nelson B et al. 2001 A randomized clinical trial of exercise and spinal manipulation for patients with chronic neck pain. Spine 26(7): 788–99

Burton K, Tillotson M, Main C, Hollis S 1995 Psychological predictors of outcome in acute and chronic low back trouble. Spine 20(6): 722–8

Butler DS 1991 Mobilisation of the Nervous System. Churchill Livingstone: Edinburgh

Carrageen EJ 2001 Psychological and functional profiles in select subjects with low back pain. Spine 1(3): 198–204

Cats-Baril W, Frymoyer J 1991 Identifying patients at risk of becoming disabled because of low back pain: the Vermont Rehabilitation Engineering Centre Predictive Model. Spine 16:(6): 605–7

Coulter I 1996 Manipulation and mobilization of the cervical spine: results of a literature survey and consensus panel. J Musculoskel Pain 4(4): 113–23

CSAG (Clinical Standards Advisory Group) 1994 Back Pain Management Guidelines. HMSO: London

Cyriax J 1982 Textbook of Orthopaedic Medicine: Diagnosis of Soft Tissue Lesions, 8th edn. Ballière Tindall: London

Deyo RA, Weinstein JN 2001 Low back pain. N Engl J Med 344: 363–70

Edwards BE 1992 Manual of Combined Movements. Churchill Livingstone: Edinburgh

Evans PJ, Bell GD, Frank C 1993 Prospective evaluation of the McMurray test. Am J Sports Med 21(4): 604–8

Fairbank J, Davies J, Coupar J, O'Brian JP 1980 Oswestry Low Back Pain Disability questionnaire. Physiotherapy 66: 271–3

Frost H, Lamb S, Klaber E et al. 1998 A fitness programme for patients with chronic low back pain: 2-year follow-up of a randomised controlled trial. Pain 75: 273–9

Fritz JM, George SZ, Delitto A 2001 The role of fear-avoidance beliefs in acute low back pain: relationships with current and future disability and work status. Pain 94(5): 7–15

Frymoyer JW 1992 Predicting disability from low back pain. Clin Orthopaed Rel Res 221: 101–9

Gardiner J, Turner P 2002 Accuracy of clinical diagnosis of internal derangement of the knee by extended scope physiotherapists and orthopaedic doctors: retrospective audit. Physiotherapy 88(3): 153–7

Goel VK, Kong W, Hans JS, Weinstein JN, Gilbertson LG 1993 A combined finite element and optimisation investigation of the lumbar spine with and without muscles. Spine 18: 1531–41

Grichnik KP, Ferrante FM 1991 The difference between acute and chronic pain. Mt Sinai J Med 58(3): 217–20

Guzman J, Esmail R, Karjalainen K et al. 2001 Multidisciplinary rehabilitation for chronic low back pain: systematic review. BMJ 322: 1511–16

Harding V, Watson P 2000 Increasing activity and improving function in chronic pain management. Physiotherapy 86(12): 619–30

Heimeyer K, Lutz R, Menninger H 1990 Dependence of tender points upon posture: a key to the understanding of fibromyalgia syndrome. J Man Med 5: 169–74

Hides JA, Richardson CA, Jull GA 1996 Multifidus recovery is not automatic after resolution of acute, first episode low back pain. Spine 21(23): 2763–9

Hodges PW, Richardson CA 1996 Inefficient muscular stabilisation of the lumbar spine associated with low back pain: a motor control evaluation of transverse abdominus. Spine 21(22): 2640–50

Hodges PW, Richardson CA 1997 Contraction of the abdominal muscles associated with movement of the lower limb. Phys Ther 77: 132–44

Hubbard DR, Berkhoff GM 1993 Myofascial trigger points show spontaneous needle EMG activity. Spine 18: 1803–7

Johnson D, Rogers M 2000 Spinal manipulation. Phys Ther 80(8): 820–3

Jull JA, Richardson CA, Topperberg R, Comerford M, Biu B 1993 Towards a measurement of active muscle control for lumbar stabilisation. Aust J Physiother 39: 187–93

Jull GA 1994 Examination of the articular system. In: Grieve's Modern Manual Therapy, 2nd edn, p. 511. Churchill Livingstone: Edinburgh

Kim SJ, Kim HK 1995 Reliability of the anterior drawer test, the pivot shift test, and the Lachman test. Clin Orthop 317: 237–42

Koes BW, Bouter LM, Van Maeren H et al. 1992 A blinded randomised clinical trial of manual therapy and physiotherapy for chronic back and neck complaints: physical outcome measures. J Manip Physiol Therap 15(1): 16–23

Magarey ME 1988 Examination of the cervical and thoracic spine. In: Grant R (ed.) Physical Therapy of the Cervical and Thoracic Spine, pp. 81–109. Churchill Livingstone: New York

Magee DJ 1992 Orthopaedic Physical Assessment, 2nd edn. WB Saunders: Philadelphia

Maitland G 2001 Maitland's Vertebral Manipulation, 6th edn. Butterworth–Heinemann: Oxford

Maniadakis N, Gray A 2000 The economic burden of back pain in the UK. Pain 84: 95–103

Mayhew TP, Rothstein JM, Finucane SD, Lamb RL 1994 Performance characteristics of the Kin–Com dynamometer. Phys Therap 74(11): 56–63

McConnell 1996 Management of patellofemoral problems. Man Therap 1: 60–6

McKenzie RA 1981 The Lumbar Spine: Mechanical Diagnosis and Therapy. Spinal Publications: New Zealand

McKenzie RA 1985 Treat Your Own Back. Spinal Publications, New Zealand

McKenzie R A 1990 The Cervical and Thoracic Spine: Mechanical Diagnosis and Therapy. Spinal Publications, New Zealand

McRae R 1999 Pocketbook of Orthopaedics and Fractures. Churchill Livingstone: Edinburgh

Melzack R 1987 The short-form McGill Pain Questionnaire. Pain 30(2): 191–7

O'Conner MI, Curner BL 1992 Metastatic diseases of the spine. Orthopaedics 15: 611–20

Olerud C, Berg P 1984 The variation of the Q angle with different positions of the foot. Clin Orthop 191: 162–5

Palmer ML, Epler M E 1998 Fundamentals of Musculoskeletal Techniques, 2nd edn. Lippincott: Philadelphia

Panjabi MM 1992a The stabilising system of the spine. 1: Function, dysfunction, adaptation and enhancement. J Spinal Dis 5(4): 383–5

Panjabi MM 1992b The stabilising system of the spine. 2: Neutral zone and instability hypothesis. J Spinal Dis 5(4): 383–9

RCGP (Royal College of General Practitioners) 1999 Clinical Guidelines for the Management of Low Back Pain. RCGP: London

Simmons E, Cameron JC 1992 Patella alta and recurrent dislocation of the patella. Clin Orthop 274: 265–9

Sterling M, Jull G, Wright A 2001 Cervical mobilisation: concurrent effects on pain, sympathetic nervous system activity and motor activity. Man Therap 6(2): 72–81

Tait RC, Chibnall JT 2001 Work injury management of refractory low back pain: relations with ethnicity, legal representation and diagnosis. Pain 91(1/2): 47–56

Vlaeyen JW, Kole Snijders AM, Boeren RG, van Eek H 1995 Fear of movement/(re)injury in chronic low back pain and its relation to behavioral performance. Pain 62(3): 363–72

Von Korff M, Saunders K 1996 The course of back pain in primary care. Spine 21: 2833–7; discussion 2838–9

Wojtys EM, Huston LJ, Taylor PD 1996 Neuromuscular adaptations in isokinetic, isotonic and agility training programmes. Am J Sports Med 24: 187–92

Waddell G 1992 Biopsychosocial analysis of low back pain. Baillière's Clinical Rheumatology 6(3): 523–55

Wilke HJ, Wolf S, Claes LE, Arand M, Weisand A 1995 Stability increase of the lumbar spine with different muscle groups: a biomechanical in-vitro study. Spine 20: 192–8

Zigmond AS, Snaith RP 1983 The Hospital Anxiety and Depression Scale. Acta Psychiatr Scand 67(6): 361–70.

An Introduction to Fractures

Stuart B. Porter

This chapter looks at some basic facts and concepts about fractures but should not be seen as a definitive guide to fracture management. Suggested further reading is included at the end of the chapter.

DEFINITION AND CLASSIFICATIONS

> ### Definition of a fracture
> A fracture is an interruption in the continuity of bone. The terms fracture and break mean the same thing in medicine. The symbol # (hash) represents a fracture.

Classification of Fractures

Fractures may be *open* or *closed* (Figure 3.1). With closed fractures there is no communication between the fracture and the outside environment; with open fractures there is such a communication. An open fracture is the same as a *compound* fracture.

Open types of fracture occur when the bone end or some other object has pierced the skin. These fractures are an additional cause for concern because of the possibility of the introduction of micro-organisms leading to bone infection (osteomyelitis).

Twisting injuries commonly give rise to spiral fractures (Figure 3.2). A direct blow could give a transverse

or oblique fracture depending on the angle of the force and whether the limb is fixed or moving at the time of the trauma. Longitudinal forces tend to result in compression or crush fractures. In some cases there are a number of fragments of bone and this is termed a 'comminuted' fracture (not to be confused with 'compound'). Loose fragments of bone are known as 'butterfly fragments'.

The type of fracture sustained may also relate to age or disease. In young children the bones are still relatively malleable and so fractures are more likely to present as an incomplete fracture – a greenstick fracture. The analogy is attempting to break a green twig, which will bend and split but not snap. The elderly often have decreased bone mineral density (osteoporosis) and fractures may occur with relatively little force applied.

Although it is helpful to categorise common fracture types and mechanisms, any bone may break in a variety of ways, so no two fractures will be exactly alike.

THE CAUSES OF FRACTURES

Trauma

Most fractures are due to some form of injury. This might be a direct blow, a fall from a height, or a weight falling onto a part of the body. Other fractures may be caused by indirect trauma such as falling on an outstretched hand, leading to the transmission of force up the arm causing a fracture of the clavicle. Twisting forces may result in fractures of the tibia and fibula, for example during soccer or skiing when the weight of the body rotates on a fixed foot. Stress or fatigue fractures are caused by repeated minor trauma, which can occur after walking or running long distances, and often affect the foot metatarsals. These are commonly seen in athletes.

Pathological Fractures

These occur as the result of a disease that affects the composition of the bone itself, making it liable to fracture as the result of a relatively trivial injury. There are a number of such diseases but those most commonly seen clinically are osteoporosis, Paget's disease, carcinoma, osteomyelitis, or osteogenesis imperfecta (brittle bone disease).

CLINICAL FEATURES OF FRACTURES

Clinical features vary depending on the cause and nature of the injury, and range from unconsciousness, to the patient being able to use the limb although com-

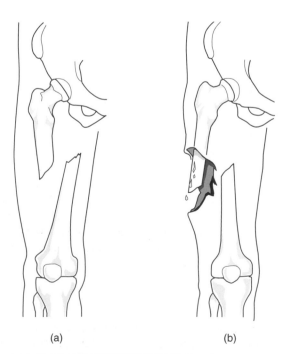

Figure 3.1 (a) Closed fracture. (b) Open or compound fracture. (Adapted from Dandy and Edwards 1998, with permission.)

(a)   (b)

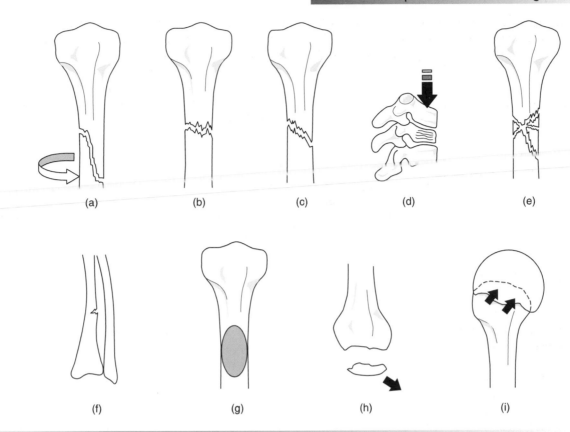

Figure 3.2 Classification: (a) spiral; (b) transverse; (c) oblique; (d) compression; (e) comminuted; (f) greenstick; (g) pathological; (h) avulsion; (i) impacted.

plaining of pain – such as following fatigue fractures and some impacted or crack fractures. It is a myth that a person with a broken bone will not be able to move the limb, although that is of course sometimes the case. Some will have their fracture diagnosed only days or weeks after the event; for example fracture of the scaphoid bone is often not detected upon initial X-ray and can be misdiagnosed as wrist sprain. The clinical features of fractures are summarised below.

Pain

This may be immediate from the local inflammatory reaction and trauma, but the cause may not be obvious in some cases. There will be marked tenderness around the site of the fracture. Once reduced, a fracture is remarkably painless.

Deformity

This is noticeable when there is displacement of the bone fragments. Some fractures exhibit classical deformities – for example the 'dinner fork' deformity which occurs following a Colles fracture of the distal radius, caused by displacement of the distal fragment.

Oedema

This is localised immediately after the injury and becomes more extensive with time. It may be necessary to apply a temporary cast or splint and then reapply the plaster as soon as the swelling has subsided. Oedema may be apparent below the level of the plaster and it is often necessary to elevate the limb, exercise the fingers or toes not encased in plaster and perform isometric contractions of the muscles within the cast in an attempt to encourage muscle pump activity (Sheriff and Van Bibber 1998; Tschakovsky et al. 1996). Once the plaster has been removed, atrophied muscles may not provide an adequate muscle pump on the veins, in which case swelling may reappear especially after activity or non-elevation.

Muscle spasm

Muscle spasm is an attempt by the body to stop things from moving. It often affects powerful muscle groups such as the quadriceps and may cause displacement or overriding of the bone ends. Traction may be needed to counteract this.

Abnormal movement/crepitus

There may be grating between the broken ends of the bone. Do not deliberately attempt to elicit this, though, because that might result in further damage.

Loss of function

This may be complete following severe fractures but some activity may be possible when the injury is less severe, such as a stress, impacted or crack fractures. Sometimes normal function can be regained very quickly with appropriate assessment, advice and treatment, whereas in other cases there are a number of problems for which more intensive treatment may be required. Modern orthopaedics is now geared towards early mobilisation with minimal surgical trauma, and physiotherapy needs to complement this.

Shock

Hypovolaemic shock is a possibility following fractures. A fractured shaft of femur may haemorrhage as much as 3 pints (1.7 L).

Limitation of joint movement

Joint mobility can be affected by many factors: adhesion formation, pain, spasm, fear, mechanical obstruction, or swelling. Movement may also be limited because of weak muscles, in which case it will be possible to move the joint passively through total range. The physiotherapist's role is to identify the cause of the problem and to select the appropriate procedure to alleviate or eliminate the cause of the loss of movement – 'the right tool for the right job'. For example there is little point in using accessory joint mobilisations if muscle spasm is the limiting factor, and a hot pack would not be appropriate if there were a bony block to movement. If the fracture involves the articular surface of the joint this may also cause limitation of movement and future cartilage degeneration. For this reason certain fractures are now treated aggressively with almost immediate movement (aggressive in this context meaning soon, not rough!). For example a patient with a fractured tibial plateau may be placed on a CPM unit immediately to maintain synovial sweep and joint nutrition. (CPM is discussed later in this chapter.)

Muscle atrophy

There will be a loss of strength in disused muscle groups. Assessment of each individual will dictate the rehabilitation programme – there is no standard 'recipe' for the treatment of fractures. Any exercises given to a person must be realistic, attainable, adaptable, functional and memorable since patients often become confused about their exercises.

FRACTURE HEALING

Healing of Compact Bone

Bone has the incredible ability to replace itself with new bone, not scar tissue. Healing starts within seconds of a fracture being sustained and is still ongoing years later – this makes ascribing a healing timescale difficult.

Wolff's law states that bone responds to the stresses that are imposed upon it by rearranging its internal architecture to best withstand the stresses. In other words bone is laid down where it is needed and absorbed where it is not. It is important to understand this concept when dealing with people who have sustained fractures. Bone is a living tissue, not the brittle, chalky specimens that students may be familiar with. It is continually in a dynamic equilibrium of growth and reabsorption. Figure 3.3 shows the process of fracture healing in compact bone taken through five stages.

Haematoma

As a result of the tearing of blood vessels within seconds of the injury, a haematoma forms at the fracture site. Very small portions of bone immediately adjacent to the fracture die, and are gradually absorbed.

Periosteal and endosteal proliferation

There is a proliferation of cells from the deep surface of the periosteum adjacent to the fracture site. These cells are precursors of the osteoblasts and form around each fragment of bone. At the same time cells proliferate from the endosteum in each fragment and this tissue gradually forms a bridge between the bone ends. During this stage the haematoma is gradually reabsorbed.

Callus formation

The proliferating cells mature as osteoblasts or in some instances as chondroblasts. The chondroblasts form cartilage and are found in varying amounts at a fracture site. Osteoblasts lay down an intercellular matrix of collagen and polysaccharide which then becomes impregnated with calcium salts, forming the immature bone called callus or woven bone. This is visible on X-ray and gives evidence that healing is taking place.

Consolidation

Osteoblastic activity results in the change of primary callus to bone, which has a lamellar structure, and at the end of this stage union is complete. New bone

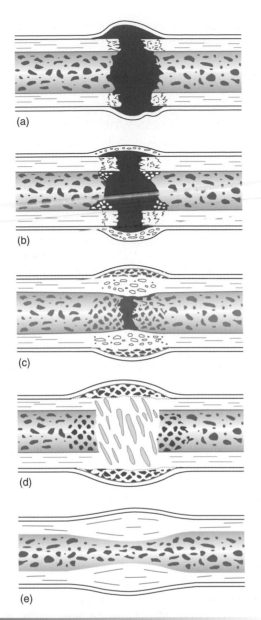

Figure 3.3   Fracture healing: (a) haematoma; (b) periosteal and endosteal proliferation; (c) callus formation; (d) consolidation; (e) remodelling.

forms a thickened mass at the fracture site and obliterates the medullary cavity. The amount of this new bone varies for a number of reasons. It tends to be more extensive if there has been a large haematoma or it has been impossible to obtain exact apposition of the bone fragments.

Remodelling

The lamellar structure is changed and the bone adapts by strengthening along the lines of stress imposed upon it. The surplus bone formed during healing is gradually removed and eventually the bone structure appears very similar to the original. In children, healing is usually very good and it is difficult to see the fracture site on a radiograph. In adults there may be a permanent area of thickening, which might be felt or seen, in a superficial bone.

Healing of Cancellous Bone

This follows a different pattern from that described above. As with compact bone, a haematoma will form, but since there is no medullary cavity, the second stage differs. Cancellous bone has a greater area of contact between the fragments of bone, and penetration of the bone-forming tissue is facilitated by the open arrangement of trabeculae as it grows out from both fragments. Osteogenic cells lay down intercellular matrix, which calcifies to form woven bone. The process of remodelling then continues to form the cancellous bone.

When is a Fracture Healed?

One of the most common questions asked by patients is 'When will my fracture be healed?' Unfortunately the answer to this question is not always straightforward and depends upon many factors, including the type of bone fractured, the type of fracture sustained, the age of the person, the treatment undergone, and the nutritional status of the person.

The current mainstay for evaluating when a fracture is healed is still based upon a combination of clinical judgement, X-ray evaluation and historical knowledge on specific fracture behaviours. A fracture is considered to be clinically healed based upon the combination of physical findings and symptoms over time.

The following suggest complete healing:

- absence of pain on weight bearing, lifting or movement
- no tenderness on palpation at the fracture site
- blurring or disappearance of the fracture line on X-ray
- full or near full functional ability (Hoppenfeld and Urthy 1999).

Time for a Fracture to Unite

This depends on a number of factors.

- *Type of bone.* Cancellous bone heals more quickly than compact bone. Healing of long bones depends on their size so that bones of the upper limb unite earlier (3–12 weeks) than do those of the lower limb (12–18 weeks).
- *Revascularisation* of devitalised bone and soft tissues adjacent to the fracture site.

- The *mechanical environment* of the fracture (Marsh and Li 1999).
- *Classification of the fracture.* It is easier to obtain good apposition of bone ends with some fractures than with others. This may depend on the initial position of the fragments before reduction and the effect of muscle pull on the fragments.
- *Blood supply.* Adequate blood supply is essential for normal healing to take place. Certain fractures can be notoriously slow to heal (e.g. fractures of the lower third of tibia). This part of the bone has a poor blood supply due to the fact that under normal circumstances it does not require one as there is little muscle bulk here, therefore little demand for nutrients and oxygen.
- *Fixation.* Adequate fixation prevents impairment of the blood supply which may be caused by movement of the fragments. It also maintains the reduction thus preventing deformity and consequent loss of function. Interestingly if a fracture is rigidly immobilised, the stimulus for callus to form is lost, so a small amount of movement at a fracture site actually encourages fracture healing.
- *Age.* Union of a fracture is quicker in children and consolidation may occur at between 4 and 6 weeks. Age makes little difference to union in adults unless there is accompanying pathology.
- Certain *drugs* such as non-steroidal anti-inflammatory drugs may interfere with fracture healing as they have an impact upon the inflammatory process.
- *Smoking.* There are increased rates of delayed union and non-union in people who smoke who have sustained open tibial fractures (Adams et al. 2001).
- *Ultrasound.* Recent work has suggested that low-intensity ultrasound may accelerate fracture healing (Azuma et al. 2001).

COMPLICATIONS OF FRACTURES

Critical blood disorders

Pulmonary embolism and *deep vein thrombosis* are two possible complications of a fracture. *Shock* may be caused by hypovolaemia or loss of blood. Femoral shaft fractures may bleed as much as 3 pints (1.7 L) and pelvic fractures may lose 6 pints (3.4 L). Clinical signs of this are tachycardia (rapid heart rate), pallor from reduced peripheral perfusion, hypoxia (decreased oxygen saturation), confusion, and a state of semi-consciousness.

Infection and *tetanus* are threats, especially following open or compound fractures. Most people are now immunised against tetanus or given booster tetanus injections if they have a large open wound. Osteomyelitis (bone infection) can be stubborn to respond to treatment.

Fat embolism (ARDS – acute respiratory distress syndrome)

If a person sustains multiple fractures of large bones, or crushing injuries, or if large amounts of marrow become exposed, there may be leakage of microscopic fat globules into the circulatory system. These may become trapped in the lungs. Symptoms include respiratory distress, shortness of breath, drowsiness, decrease in saturation of oxygen levels, and petechiae (tiny haemorrhages which appear on the chest). ARDS is potentially fatal.

Skin plaster sores

Reassure the patient that large amounts of dry flaky skin following removal of plaster is normal. Reddened areas or sores caused by plaster or splints must be reported to the relevant team member.

Muscle damage and atrophy

Muscle fibres may be torn, crushed or ruptured as a result of the injury and this will cause additional bleeding and swelling. Tendons may be severed, particularly in the case of open fractures, or sometimes there may be a rupture following a fracture. Surgical intervention is usually necessary to repair a rupture.

Compartment syndrome

If muscles become damaged or inflamed at the time of injury, and intramuscular pressure builds up with no means of release, death (necrosis) of the tissues from ischaemia (lack of blood supply) may result. It is defined as the condition in which high pressure within a closed fascial sheath reduces capillary blood perfusion below the level necessary for tissue viability. Compartment syndrome is seen most commonly in the anterior tibial muscles or forearm muscles.

Clinical signs of a limb with compartment syndrome are the five Ps:

- Pale
- Painful
- Pulseless
- Paraesthesiae
- Paralysed.

Treatment revolves primarily around accurate diagnosis. Check colour, sensation and movement after any injury or surgery, elevate and cool the limb. Surgical decompression (fasciotomy) may be necessary as an emergency procedure.

Avascular necrosis

Bone receives its blood supply by the soft-tissue structures attached to it or by intra-osseous vessels. In certain instances one part of the bone is very dependent on the intra-osseous (within the bone) vessels for its blood supply, and if this is interrupted because of a fracture, avascular necrosis may occur (part of the fractured bone may die). It can occur in fractures of the neck of femur leading to avascular necrosis of the head, and in fractures of the scaphoid bone where the proximal pole may be affected. This may be a cause of non-union of the fracture and as the fragment usually includes an articular surface it can lead to osteoarthritis.

Problems with union

Delayed union may occur if the gap between the bone ends is too big, the blood supply is poor (lower one-third of the tibia), the area is infected, or if internal fixation is used (this sometimes removes the stimulus for callus formation).

There may be distinct pathological changes and radiological evidence of *non-union*. There appears to be no callus formation and the fractured ends of bone become dense and the outline clear-cut. The gap between the bone fragments may be filled with fibrous tissue and form a pseudo-arthrosis. The lower third of the tibia has notoriously poor healing capabilities, even occasionally in the young and healthy.

A fracture may heal in a less than perfect position – *malunion*. Overlapping of the fragments could lead to shortening and this would affect function. Angulation or rotation of the fragments may impair function because of the resulting altered biomechanics.

Growth disturbance

In younger people there may be growth disturbance if the fracture includes the epiphysis (growth plate).

Sudeck's atrophy/reflex sympathetic dystrophy (RSD)/algodystrophy/causalgia

The term *complex regional pain syndrome* is now being used to describe these pathological states. This is a complication where the patient complains of severe pain on movement, or at rest, out of proportion to the initial injury. The limb is swollen. The skin appears shiny and discoloured and feels cold; in extreme cases this may lead to the limb becoming exquisitely tender and discoloured. Osteoporosis and permanent contractures may follow.

Management is difficult. Sympathetic nerve blocks and active physiotherapy management programmes are often employed with varying degrees of success (Viel et al. 1999). Vasodilator drugs such as guanethedine are occasionally successful. It may also respond to nerve blocks , local analgesia, TENS, and other local therapies but recovery is slow and may take several months. Fortunately this complication is comparatively rare.

Intra-articular fractures

Fractures involving the articular cartilage predispose the joint to osteoarthrosis in the future (e.g. fractures of the tibial plateau). This is due to the area of roughness that inevitably results after a fracture, and also because the immobilisation of the fracture results in cartilage death (see below). For the latter reason, some fractures are now treated aggressively by physiotherapists from an early stage.

Another problem with intra-articular fractures is that, if callus is attempting to form within a joint cavity, it is constantly being washed away by synovial fluid – for example after a fractured neck of femur.

Visceral injuries

A fractured pelvis may damage the bladder or urethra. A fractured rib may cause a pneumothorax. A skull fracture may cause brain injury. These are just three examples.

Adhesions

These may be within the joint (intra-articular) or around the joint (peri-articular). Adhesions are the price paid for immobilising a fracture. Intra-articular adhesions may occur when the fracture extends into the joint surface and there is a haemarthrosis or bleeding within a joint cavity. If this is not absorbed, fibrous adhesions may form within the synovial membrane. Peri-articular adhesions may occur if oedema is not reduced and is allowed to organise in the surrounding tissues. This leads to adhesion formation between tissues such as the capsule and ligaments and results in joint stiffness, which is less of a problem now that new techniques of fixation allowing early mobilisation have been developed.

Capsular adhesions are common, for example in the capsule of the shoulder joint which possesses dependent folds on its inferior aspect to permit the huge range of motion at this joint. These may stick together after fracture or injury causing limitation of movement.

Injury to large vessels

If a large artery is occluded in such a position as to cut off the blood supply to the limb, this may lead to gangrene; or if there is partial occlusion an ischaemic contracture may develop. These injuries must be dealt with as an emergency by the surgical team.

Thrombosis of veins may occur in the neighbourhood of the fracture. This presents as a sudden development of a cramp-like pain in the part, by an increase of swelling, and by marked tenderness along the line of the vein. Anything that appears to be abnormal in the circulatory system must be reported to the surgeon immediately. Blood vessels may sustain damage; for example, following supracondylar humeral fractures the brachial artery may be damaged.

Nerve injury

Certain fractures (e.g. mid-shaft humerus) may lead to radial nerve palsy; hence the importance of a knowledge of functional anatomy when treating. If a plaster is too tight it may cause nerve damage. The common peroneal nerve is vulnerable to this if a plaster cast is moulded too tightly around the fibular head, resulting in foot drop as the tibialis anterior muscle is affected and unable to perform its function of decelerating the foot upon heel strike, and permitting toe clearance during the swing-through phase of gait.

PRINCIPLES OF FRACTURE MANAGEMENT

Once a fracture has been diagnosed, the most suitable treatment must be decided upon. This should be the minimum possible intervention that will safely and effectively provide the right environment for healing of the fracture. Interestingly, nature has devised a system by which a slight amount of movement at a fracture site is useful in stimulating callus formation, and if a fracture is plated or immobilised in such a way that practically eliminates motion between the bone ends, callus will not form (Figure 3.4; Cornell and Lane 1992).

This is a common dilemma in orthopaedics. In the same way that there is no recipe for the physiotherapy treatment of a fracture, there is no single recipe for the surgical management of fractures. This 'see-saw' will be referred to in the case study later in this chapter.

Reduction

Reduction means to realign into the normal position, or as near to the normal anatomical position as possible (Figure 3.5). Reduction of a fracture may be either open or closed. *Closed reduction* means that no surgical intervention is used, the fracture being manipulated by hand under local or general anaesthesia. *Open reduction* means that the area has been surgically opened and reduced.

Reduction may not always be necessary even when there is some displacement. For example, fractures of the clavicle may heal with a bump which may be a problem only in the cosmetic sense; function is the most important end-point.

However, when there is poor alignment of the fragments or the relative positions of the joints above and below the fracture are lost as a result of angulation or rotation of the bone ends, or if there is loss of leg length, then accurate anatomical reduction is necessary. X-rays are used to ascertain the exact position of the fragments before and after reduction. Real-time X-rays can now be taken using image intensifiers so that the surgeon can more accurately reduce. Improvements in CT and MRI scanning mean that complex fractures can be studied in great detail preoperatively, which assists the planning of surgery.

Immobilisation

The objectives of immobilising a fracture are:

- to maintain the reduction
- to provide the optimal healing environment for the fracture
- to relieve pain.

In some fractures where there is no likelihood of displacement, fixation may not be necessary, or minimal fixation will suffice – for example neighbour strapping for some finger fractures (Figure 3.6).

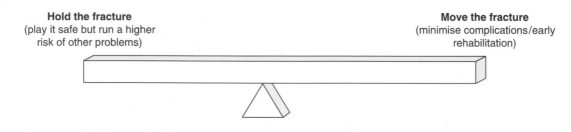

Hold the fracture
(play it safe but run a higher risk of other problems)

Move the fracture
(minimise complications/early rehabilitation)

Figure 3.4   The mobilisation see-saw.

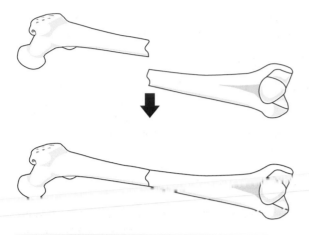

Figure 3.5   Reduction of a fracture.

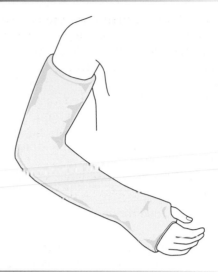

Figure 3.7   Plaster of Paris immobilisation.

Common methods of fracture immobilisation

Plaster of Paris (PoP)

This is a plaster-impregnated bandage which can be moulded to the part when wet, which sets in time. The standard method of external splinting is still plaster of Paris (Figure 3.7).

Synthetic materials are now used for splinting some fractures because of their light weight, and waterproof qualities. Custom-made lightweight thermoplastics can be moulded to the limb and re-moulded if swelling or atrophy cause changes in the limb contour. Some synthetic casting materials, however, are less malleable and cannot be moulded as effectively as plaster of Paris. They can occasionally cause allergies.

A plaster saw is needed to remove a cast. This special tool has an oscillating blade that will cut through the hard cast without damaging the skin.

The advantages and disadvantages of using PoP are listed in Table 3.1.

Medical note

Medical advice should be sought if any of the following occur to a limb that is in plaster of Paris or similar splint:

- pale or blue coloration of the skin on the injured part
- numbness, tingling, or throbbing of the injured part
- inability to move the fingers or toes
- excessive pain in the injured part
- swelling, bulging, or puffiness around the edges of the cast
- a foul smell from under the cast
- if it becomes loose and slides around.

Functional bracing (cast bracing)

It has now been found unnecessary to fix some fractures as rigidly as was thought necessary in the past, and an example of this is cast bracing (functional bracing). Functional braces have hinges to allow movement (see the case study towards the end of the chapter – Figure 3.24).

The soft tissues of the limb squeeze against the inside of the brace and, in conjunction with the use of a heel cup, permit weight to be taken through the substance of the brace. This has reduced many of the problems that were seen as a direct result of prolonged

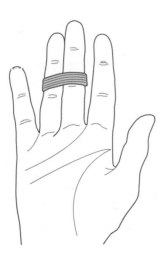

Figure 3.6   Neighbour strapping splint applied to both sound and damaged fingers to assist movement of the latter.

Table 3.1 The advantages and disadvantages of PoP.

Advantages of PoP	Disadvantages of PoP
<ul><li>No surgery or its complications</li><li>No infection risk</li><li>Quick to apply</li><li>Rapid patient discharge</li><li>Cheap, relatively easy to apply with training</li><li>New lightweight casts are an alternative</li><li>Radio translucent (bones can be X-rayed through the cast)</li><li>May absorb fluids or bleeding. The extent of bleeding can be traced on the cast itself and monitored daily</li><li>Can be moulded for several minutes before hardening</li></ul>	<ul><li>It may not be possible to reduce the fracture correctly or maintain reduction</li><li>May require surgery at a later date</li><li>Plaster needs removal/or windowing (removal of a piece of the cast) to inspect the skin</li><li>May need removal in case of increased swelling or reapplication once swelling has subsided</li><li>Smelly if it gets wet</li><li>Heavy</li><li>May crack</li><li>May rub the skin and cause sores</li></ul>

immobilisation. Another benefit of allowing movement of joints, provided that it does not unduly stress the fracture site, is that it may promote union by improving the area's blood supply.

Internal fixation

Surgical intervention by applying a plate and screws to the fracture is known as *open reduction and internal fixation*, often abbreviated to ORIF (Figure 3.8).

Advantages of ORIF

It permits a detailed inspection and accurate surgical assessment of the site of injury and procedure to be undertaken.

Disadvantages of ORIF

- Surgery inevitably causes additional trauma and potential exposure to micro-organisms.
- It can convert a closed fracture into an open fracture.
- It requires surgery with all its sequelae and potential complications. Ironically, rigid fixation may remove the stimulus for callus formation. The implants may be removed 12–18 months in the future or if they start to become a problem. For example, the screws may become an irritant. In the young, they will be removed, as whilst they are in, bone will not grow and respond to stress normally, as some of the stresses will be taken by the implants themselves.

Intramedullary (IM) nailing

Here a hollow metal rod is introduced at one end of a long bone, travels down the medullary canal and may be locked with screws distally and proximally (Figure 3.9). The proximal aspect of the nail is threaded and

this permits a tool to be threaded onto the nail at a later date for its removal.

IM nailing for fractures of long bones has revolutionised management of many fractures, which up

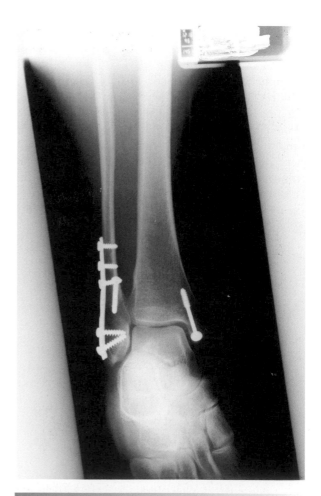

Figure 3.8   Fracture of the tibia/fibula fixed by plate and screws.

paction of bone ends (dynamisation). It allows the bone to once again take its normal stresses and strains and adapt in accordance with Wolff's law. The endosteal proliferation which occurs as part of the normal fracture healing process may be lost with certain types of internal fixation. Fractures of the shaft of tibia and humerus may also be nailed in this way.

External fixation

Figure 3.10 shows fixation of a fractured tibia using an external fixator. Pins or wires are driven into the fragments and held by a piece of apparatus on the outside of the body. Figure 3.11 shows an external fixator for a comminuted intra-articular fracture of the distal radius. Figure 3.12 shows an external fixator for an unstable pelvic fracture.

The advantages and disadvantages of external fixation are listed in Table 3.2.

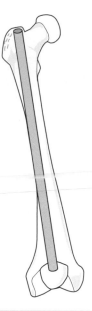

Figure 3.9   Intramedullary nailing.

until a few years ago would have been managed by prolonged bedrest. The trauma is less than with open techniques and results in decreased hospital stay, more rapid patient mobilisation, and rehabilitation with minimal risk of complications associated with immobility. The implant rather than the bone may take stresses and strains and for this reason the surgeon may choose to remove the locking screws at a later stage. This permits the nail to move slightly and cause com-

Ilizarov method

The Ilizarov method of fracture fixation had its origins in Russia in the 1940s. It incorporates an axial system of wires or pins fitted through the bone and connected to a circular ring. It has proved successful in cases of non-union (Schwartsman et al. 1990). This method also incorporates the principle of 'distraction osteogenesis', and can be used in the restoration of large skeletal defects, limb lengthening, and the correction of skeletal deformities (Figure 3.13).

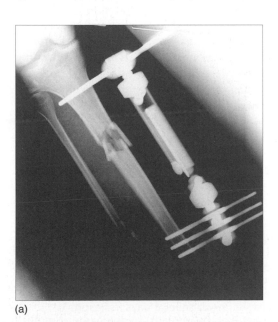

(a)

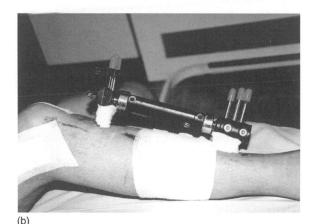

(b)

Figure 3.10   Fixation of a fractured tibia using an external fixator. Pins or wires are driven into the fragments and held by a piece of apparatus on the outside of the body, as shown in the external view. Photo reproduced by kind permission of Mr R.F. Adam.

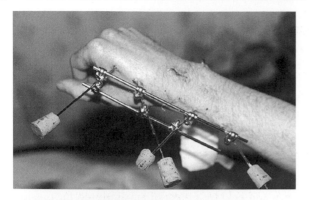

Figure 3.11 Fixation of a comminuted intra-articular fracture of the distal radius. Photo reproduced by kind permission of Ms Fiona Cobbold. ©

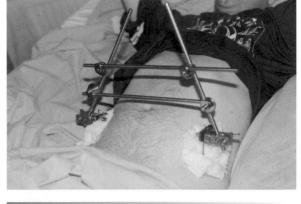

Figure 3.12 External fixator for an unstable pelvic fracture.

Skeletal traction

Figure 3.14 shows an example of skeletal traction. The pin shown is a Steinman pin. This can be inserted through a bone and a weight system attached to allow localised, effective traction. Common sites for this are the tibial plateau or the calcaneum. Pin sites must be kept clean and free of infection. These pins are usually tolerated well and are not as painful as they appear.

Traction

Traction is the application of a pulling force to a part of the body, and it may be either a direct or an indirect pull. Traction is less common on the orthopaedic ward nowadays, although it still has its place. Uses include:

- to restore bone or limb length if it has been reduced by fracture or disease
- to maintain correct limb length, and overcome muscle spasm which may be the cause of limb shortening after a fracture

- to correct deformity in a joint
- to reduce a dislocated joint
- to immobilise a joint
- to relieve pain preoperatively
- to promote rest and healing postoperatively.

PHYSIOTHERAPY AND FRACTURES

General Issues

Before commencing any orthopaedic assessment, consider the points in the accompanying box on page 83.

Most orthopaedic units have in place standardised protocols and postoperative care plans for particular surgical or orthopaedic interventions, and the student must adhere to these. To say that orthopaedics is routine is, however, an oversimplification – nothing that deals with the human body is routine. Providing the best possible treatment to orthopaedic patients will take many years of practice, reflection and fine-tuning of clinical reasoning skills.

Do not let this dishearten you. Clinical reasoning is not an abstract concept, it is often basic common sense

Table 3.2 Advantages and disadvantages of external fixation.

Advantages of external fixation	Disadvantages of external fixation
<ul><li>Minimal disruption to the fracture site</li><li>Enables inspection of the wound and fracture</li><li>Can be adjusted with minimal trauma</li><li>Can be used for limb lengthening procedures</li><li>Can be used to pin multiple fragments (e.g. comminuted fractures)</li><li>Allows preservation of tissues in open or compound fractures, degloving injuries or burns</li></ul>	<ul><li>Infection risk at pin sites</li><li>Needs meticulous wound care</li><li>Cosmetically ugly</li><li>Functional impairment (e.g. adjacent joints may be restricted or soft tissues pierced by fixator)</li><li>Anaesthetic risk and its associated complications</li><li>Patient will need several days in hospital</li><li>Stresses taken by implant, so decreased stimulus for callus formation</li><li>Heavy</li></ul>

Statement	Consequence for the physiotherapist
No two orthopaedic patients are alike	Do not ask for a 'treatment recipe'. Your approach should be flexible and dynamic and will change as a result of many factors
No two assessments are alike	Learn the basic assessment framework but tailor your assessment slightly to each individual
No two treatment courses are alike. Patients do not always do what the textbook says!	Keep an open mind, recognise when a treatment is not working and change or modify it
No single assessment can predict the outcome of the problem	Experienced physiotherapists are able to 'assess as they treat'. This means that the patient is continually receiving the most appropriate attention and the situation is dynamic. Treatment goals may need modification and should not be totally inflexible

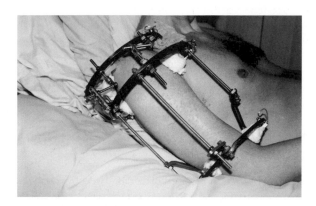

Figure 3.13   Ilizarov fixation for fractured humerus and scapula.

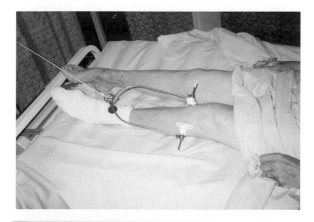

Figure 3.14   A Steinman pin. This woman sustained a fractured shaft of femur and, owing to her general health, surgery was not indicated. She was managed conservatively.

and nobody expects you to get it right immediately. Your knowledge will improve every time you assess a patient and evolve with experience. Clinical reasoning will be honed as you gain experience. In the early undergraduate stages, you will need a framework to begin with, rather like a route map. Each student will eventually lose the map in their own time but by the time they have lost the map it is no longer necessary anyway. With this in mind the following section gives pointers about assessing patients who have sustained fractures.

The problem-oriented medical record system (POMR) is now the appropriate format to use. But within this system, how physiotherapists assess fractures depends very much on the time elapsed since the fracture and the stage or rehabilitation at which they are performing the assessment. For example, students are often dismayed on their clinical placement to find that they are unable to perform a complete assessment of a patient who has just been put into plaster of Paris. Their treatment plan may consist of:

1. Attain safe non-weight-bearing on elbow crutches.
2. Negotiate stairs safely.
3. Plan for safe discharge home.
4. Advise on isometric exercises.

There may be little else that can be done at this stage. The points below therefore assume assessment of a hypothetical patient who has just undergone removal of plaster or discharge from the orthopaedic team.

Patient Assessment

An assessment is essential if you are to plan out a safe and appropriate treatment. Assess a fracture like any other condition, but be aware of any specific instructions or limitations. For example is the patient allowed to fully or partially bear weight? Students often rush into collecting data; instead take time and think about what you are doing. If you omit something, make a note and remember to follow it up next time.

Previous medical history

Are there any warning signs or findings that might affect your treatment options? For example a person with internal fixation in place would not be considered for certain electrotherapy treatments. Or a patient with advanced osteoporosis would not be considered for high-impact gym work.

Social history

Do not underestimate the importance of asking these questions.

- Is the patient living alone?
- Does the person need to go up stairs?
- Is the person losing money through non-employment?
- What are the person's hobbies?
- Does the person care for sick relatives?
- What does that person need to be able to do to be 'normal'?

The most effective physiotherapists are able to listen to what the patient tells them and incorporate this into the treatment plan. Do not ask leading or multiple questions, but keep your questioning on track and relevant and do not lose sight of why you are there. Set long- and short-term goals as you would with any other patient, but be prepared to adapt them if necessary.

Setting Goals for Orthopaedic Patients

Without goals we have nothing to measure our performance against. This simple summary should help you plan goals for patients. When you set goals for any patient (orthopaedic or otherwise) the goals need to be SMART:

- **S**pecific
- **M**easurable
- **A**chievable
- **R**ealistic
- **T**imely

Typical examples of orthopaedic goals possessing all the SMART characteristics are:

1. Goal – Mr X will be able to safely negotiate stairs, partial weight bearing with two elbow crutches in 4 days time.
2. Goal – Mrs Y will have attained 50 degrees of active knee flexion by 1 week from today.

3. Goal – Mrs Z will be able to transfer safely from bed to chair within 2 days.

Test yourself

Each of these goals fails to achieve one or more of the SMART criteria:

1. Mr X will be totally pain free within 1 day of sustaining his fractured femur, tibia and humerus.
2. Mr X will be able to walk in 8 months' time.
3. Mr X will be much better in 1 week.
4. Mr X will mobilise full weight-bearing on the unstable fracture within 1 week.
5. Mr X will have more knee flexion within 1 week.

Answers

(1) Not realistic, it is extremely unlikely that Mr X will be totally pain-free 1 day after three such major fractures. (2) Not timely, the end-point of this goal is too far in the future. (3) Not specific – what does 'much better' mean? (4) Not achievable, the orthopaedic protocol does not permit this. (5) Not measurable and not specific – what does 'more' mean?

The Problem-Oriented Medical Record (POMR)

The POMR system is based on a data collection system that incorporates the acronym SOAP.

- **Subjective.** Any information given to you by the patient: allergies, past medical history, past surgical history, family history, social history (living arrangements, social conditions, employment, medication), review of systems.
- **Objective.** All information obtained through observation or testing; e.g. range of joint movement, muscle strength.
- **Analysis.** A listing of problems based on what you know from a review of subjective and objective data. For patients with multiple problems, number and list each problem consecutively, with the most important listed first.
- **Plan.** As the name implies this refers to the plan of forthcoming treatment.

The Objective Assessment

Basic background information to record

- Occupation
- Drug history

- X-rays/scans/other tests
- Family history
- Date of next clinic appointment
- Specific surgical instructions.

History of present condition

Include the date of onset, mode of onset, course, and treatment to date. Note specific instructions, for example partial weight bearing for the next 3 weeks. If the patient does not know his or her own postoperative instructions, do not guess. Speak to the other team members to establish treatment parameters.

Pain

It is not sufficient to ask merely whether or not the patient has pain. Ask the person about the location, type, duration and radiation of the pain. Is it related to time of day or certain activities, and does it have alleviating or aggravating factors? Visual analogue scales may be used as an attempt to quantify pain (see Chapter 2). Remember that dull aching of the fracture site may be considered normal, especially after activity. This may signify bone remodelling. Sharp pain of a prolonged nature is more cause for concern – hence the need to understand the physiology underlying healing.

Objective examination

See Table 3.3.

Muscle strength

This should be tested surrounding the affected area, above and below the site of injury as necessary. Do not forget that there may be wide-ranging weakness in many muscle groups. For example, a person who has had an arm immobilised in a collar and cuff for 2 weeks after a Colles' fracture may have significant rotator cuff weakness through disuse atrophy. Remember that when recovered, a muscle might need to act as agonist, antagonist, synergist or fixator – you need to understand the functional anatomy of the area.

Specific tests

These may be appropriate, such as leg length, observation of gait and posture. No test is irrelevant if it adds to the substance of your assessment database. If it can be objectively measured and is pertinent to your patient then include it. Students often 'go through the motions' of assessment and ask questions without appreciating why they are asking them. It is valuable therefore to continually ask yourself why are you doing a musculoskeletal test and what does the result tell you? If you are not sure why you are doing a particular test, do not perform it until you have spoken to your supervisor.

Think about your patient as a whole: what does the person need to be able to do in order to return to full function? Ask this important question appropriately and it will reap dividends for the remainder of your treatment sessions. Tailor your assessment to the individual and tailor your treatment to what your assessment is telling you. For example, if Beethoven had been a patient of yours, how would you have assessed his hand function? Ask relevant questions and find out what the patient needs to be able to do. Do not assume that the patient's problems will be straightforward, unchanging, or what the textbook stated! When the assessment is complete, discuss it with the patient, colleagues if necessary – and obtain written consent to treat.

Form a problem list. Keep it simple, but be objective and be specific. Formulate short- and long-term goals; for example, Mr Johnson will be fully weight-bearing in 1 month with a normal gait.

General points

Think about how you will realistically progress your treatment and how you will measure any progression (e.g. grip strength, isokinetic machine, goniometry). Work as part of the multi-disciplinary team (MDT) and think about who else needs to have input into the case – but at the same time do not forget your own role. Be aware of potential complications, reassure and

Table 3.3 Objective examination.

Look	Feel	Move
Swelling	Swelling	Active first
Spasm	Heat	Then passive
Deformity	Sensation	Then overpressure (care – this
Bruising	Tenderness on palpation	may be inadvisable
Oedema	Spasm	depending upon the stage
Atrophy		of fracture healing)
		What is the quality and
		amount of movement and
		what is the end feel?

encourage your patient – who is the most important member of the MDT. Make the patient responsible for his or her own recovery – a partner in fact. Home exercises should be clear, practical and monitored. Reassess progress as necessary. Are you attaining your goals? If not, change or modify your goals or your treatment. Before you discharge the patient remember that a normal limb needs:

- full active movement
- accessory movement
- full strength
- full function
- anything else specific to that patient.

Does the patient need follow-up appointments or domiciliary physiotherapy? The physiotherapist is a member of the multi-disciplinary team. The membership and relative roles of this team change according to the nature of the injury and the stage of treatment but the physiotherapist must liaise and work with the other members throughout the rehabilitation period. Initially if the patient is in hospital the members of the team will include: the patient, medical staff, nurses, occupational therapist, pharmacists, radiographers, district nurse, and corresponding domiciliary staff.

COMMONLY ENCOUNTERED FRACTURES AND SOME PRINCIPLES OF MANAGEMENT

Fractures of the Upper Limb

Fractures of the clavicle and scapula

Scapular fractures are not particularly common and usually occur as a result of direct trauma. The clavicle often fractures following a fall on to the side or as a result of a fall on an outstretched hand. The fracture is usually in the middle or the junction of the outer and middle thirds of the bone. The pull of sternocleidomastoid muscle can cause displacement.

These fractures are usually immobilised by a brace, a sling, or a collar and cuff. Complications include a restricted range of movement in the shoulder girdle or shoulder joint since the two work together, and associated muscle weakness.

Fractures of the proximal humerus

These may be classified using the Neer classification:

- Group 1 – minimal displacement
- Group 2 – anatomical neck fracture with less than 1 cm displacement

- Group 3 – displaced or angulated surgical neck
- Group 4 – displaced fracture of greater tuberosity
- Group 5 – fractures of the lesser tuberosity
- Group 6 – fracture dislocations.

Fractures of the surgical neck of humerus

These usually occur in elderly people as the result of a fall on the outstretched hand. There may or may not be displacement of the fragments, but in a large number of cases the fragments are impacted. This means that one bone fragment has been driven into the other, often stabilising the fracture at the time of injury. Displaced fractures, and particularly those occurring in the elderly, are not usually reduced for a number of reasons:

- Lack of good alignment does not affect union.
- It is preferable to avoid surgery in the elderly unless essential.
- Early movement is important to avoid a stiff shoulder.

Fractures of the shaft of the humerus

These fractures usually occur in the middle third of the bone and may be due to direct or indirect trauma. *Direct trauma* may give rise to transverse or oblique fractures and sometimes presents as a comminuted fracture. Displacement may result due to muscle pull, and if the fracture is below the insertion of deltoid the upper fragment will be abducted. *Indirect trauma* tends to give a rotational force resulting in a spiral fracture.

In stable fractures the fixation can be minimal and consist of a sling alone or with a posterior slab from below the shoulder to the wrist with the elbow at 90°. This allows the weight of the arm to maintain reduction. If the fracture needs sturdier fixation, IM nailing is possible or a complete plaster from the shoulder to the wrist or hand may be applied.

Because the fracture usually occurs in the middle part of the shaft, the radial nerve may be affected as it winds through the radial groove. Since the radial nerve supplies the wrist and forearm extensor muscles, a wrist drop may result. The injury may compress the radial nerve and cause a neuropraxia, or if it is stretched it may result in axonotmesis. Normally these will recover spontaneously although an axonotmesis will take longer as degeneration of the nerve has occurred within the sheath. In an open fracture the radial nerve may be severed resulting in a neurotmesis and this will require surgical suturing.

Delayed union or non-union can be complications but are not very common.

Fractures of the condyles of the humerus

These fractures are common in children following a fall. A supracondylar fracture is the most common type (Figure 3.15). After reduction the arm may be immobilised in one of the following ways depending on the type of fracture:

- plaster with the elbow at approximately 90° or a little more and extending from below the shoulder down to the wrist or hand (the plaster should be cut so that it is possible to feel the radial pulse at the wrist)
- a posterior slab plus a collar and cuff
- a collar and cuff.

Some fractures of the condyles may extend on to the articular surfaces and thereby cause additional problems. One of the most serious complications that can occur is damage to the brachial artery, which could be severed or contused owing to its close proximity to the fracture site. Therefore circulation must be monitored. Impairment of the circulation requires emergency treatment as occlusion can lead to irreversible ischaemic effects within a few hours. If the circulation is not restored, Volkmann's ischaemic contracture may develop. This affects the flexor muscles of the forearm, which are replaced by fibrous tissue which contracts and produces flexion of the wrist and fingers. The skin and nerves will also be affected by the diminished blood supply.

Another problem following elbow fractures is post-traumatic ossification – sometimes known as myositis ossificans. If there is a severe injury, the periosteum may be torn from the bone resulting in bleeding and the formation of a haematoma. Osteoblasts invade this blood clot and new (ectopic) bone forms. This can also occur as the result of forced extension of the elbow. First indications that this is developing may be pain and loss of movement. The elbow should be rested in a sling or collar and cuff for about 3 weeks to allow the haematoma to be absorbed. If this does not occur and bone is formed it may be necessary to remove the bone tissue surgically. If deformity develops at the elbow – such as a cubitus valgus – this may cause a stretch on the ulnar nerve, which may require surgical intervention with a transposition of the nerve from the posterior to the anterior aspect of the elbow. Fractures that extend on to the articular surfaces and cause disruption of the joint may cause a permanently stiff elbow, lead to the development of osteoarthritis, or both.

Fractures of the radial head

Management of these ranges from no immobilisation at all in undisplaced fractures, to screw fixation, excision or replacement arthroplasty.

With fractures of the radius and/or ulna, both bones may be fractured as a result of direct or indirect violence such as a fall on the outstretched hand. The resulting displacement may be difficult to correct and in some instances may require open reduction. Accurate anatomical reduction is very important because loss of the normal relationship between the two bones may result in impairment of pronation and supination – a very important component of hand function. In children the damage may not be so severe and they may sustain a greenstick fracture with minor angulation which normally will heal without any complications. Fracture of the ulna with radial head subluxation is called a *Monteggia fracture*, while fracture of the radius and subluxation of the lower end of ulna is called a *Galeazzi fracture*.

Colles' fractures of the distal radius are very common, particularly in the elderly, as a consequence of osteoporosis. They are usually caused by a fall on the outstretched hand. This may result in the typical dinner-fork deformity due to the backward (towards the dorsum) displacement of the distal fragment (Figure 3.16).

After reduction the Colles wrist may be immobilised with a complete plaster from just below the elbow to the hand, ending just above the proximal crease on the palm, or alternatively a plaster slab. The position of the wrist and whether or not there is a complete plaster will depend on the pattern of the displacement. If there is gross swelling it may be necessary to use a plaster back slab and then a complete plaster when the swelling has reduced. Fixation is usually maintained for 4–6 weeks.

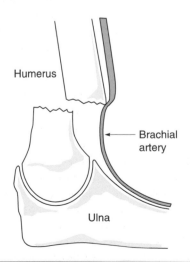

Figure 3.15   Supracondylar fracture of the humerus.

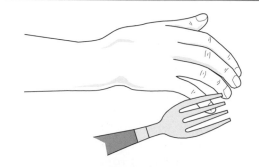

Figure 3.16   Colles' (dinner-fork) fracture.

A less common fracture is the *Smith's fracture* which is similar to a Colles but with volar (towards the palm) as opposed to dorsal displacement of the distal fragment.

Fractures of the proximal radius are less common and tend to occur in younger people following either a direct blow or a fall on the outstretched hand which causes a fracture through the head of the radius. Fractures of the ulna alone are not as common as those of the radius.

There are a number of complications that can occur with fractures of the lower end of the radius, although these are rare considering the numbers of fractures dealt with in fracture clinics. Loss of shoulder movement may occur as it could be injured when the person falls, or be a consequence of wearing a sling or collar and cuff. Rupture of the extensor pollicis longus may be noted, occurring 4–8 weeks after the fracture. A late complication can be that of Sudeck's atrophy. Median nerve neuritis can also be a complication if displacement causes stretching or compression of the nerve.

Fracture of the scaphoid

This fracture tends to occur in young adults as the result of falls on the outstretched hand. It may be overlooked either because the person considers it to be a strain, or the fracture may not be visible on the initial X-ray. Healing is often slow in this fracture and in some instances there may be non-union. In the latter case the arm is usually placed in a so-called 'scaphoid plaster' as a precaution and X-rayed again after a couple of weeks. If these fractures are accurately diagnosed within 1 week followed by plaster immobilisation, non-union could be prevented (Roolker et al. 1999).

If the fracture occurs through the waist of the bone the blood supply to the proximal part of the bone will be impaired and avascular necrosis may develop. Long-term complications include the development of osteoarthrosis.

Fractures of the phalanges or metacarpals

Accurate anatomical reduction and fixation is essential, but it is also important to keep the period of immobilisation as short as possible if a good functional result is to be obtained. The position of the fixation will vary depending on which phalanx or phalanges are fractured and on the subsequent stability of the reduced fracture. This can be very important in relation to regaining function of the hand, and the team has to decide on the priorities in each case.

In certain unstable fractures internal fixation may be the method of choice, but if external fixation is used a rolled gauze bandage may be placed in the palm and the finger placed over this with flexion at the metacarpophalangeal joint and as near extension as possible at the interphalangeal joints. In stable fractures, a garter or neighbour strap splint may be used which fixes the injured finger to the adjacent finger and gives some support while encouraging some movement.

Bennett's fracture

This is a fracture dislocation affecting the carpometacarpal joint of the thumb.

Fractures of the Lower Limb

Fractures of the pelvis

The majority of pelvic fractures are caused by direct violence, falls, or following crushing injuries. Shock sustained by the patient at the time of the injury, or from damage to the internal organs, may be a complications. Common fractures include *pubic ramus* fractures (secondary to osteoporosis) which are managed conservatively with analgesia and gradual mobilisation. These fractures can be very painful as the hip adductors have their origin in this area, so walking is understandably painful.

The skill as a physiotherapist here is to gain the confidence and respect of the patient and gradually mobilise the person to recovery. It also highlights the need for teamwork when co-ordinating analgesia with mobilisation.

The pelvis may be thought of as a ring; like a ring it will often break in two places at once. An isolated fracture is not as a rule serious unless it is complicated by damage to the internal organs. The same is true of double or even multiple fractures provided that there is no fracture or dislocation in the iliac segment. But if there are two or more fractures or dislocations with at least one in each segment, then the displacement may be considerable. It is brought about both by the causative force and by the pull of the muscles passing from the spine to the pelvis or femur.

When the pelvic ring is severely disrupted then rapid reduction and fixation is necessary. If it is possible to reduce the displacement manually then fixation may be by means of a plaster spica, but otherwise another method of external fixation may be used, by placing pins through the iliac bones and fixed to a transverse bar. Skeletal traction may be used for certain pelvic fractures. Complications may include injuries to the bladder or urethra and possibly to other tissues within the pelvis.

Avulsion fractures occasionally occur in the pelvis at the anterior iliac spines, more specifically at the attachment of rectus femoris and sartorius. They are caused by forcible contraction of the muscle, pulling off the tip of the bone.

Fracture of the neck of femur

This is probably the most common and most significant fracture in terms of morbidity, mortality and socio-economic impact in developed countries (Reginster et al. 1999). Mortality after fracture is high: Schurch et al. (1996) found that the 1-year death rate were as high as 23.8% following fractured neck of femur.

The following is Garden's classification of femoral neck fractures:

- Type 1 – inferior cortex is not completely broken.
- Type 2 – cortex is broken but there is no angulation.
- Type 3 – some displacement and rotation of the femoral head.
- Type 4 – complete displacement.

In addition, femoral neck fracture is classified by its location (Figure 3.17):

1. subcapital
2. transcervical
3. basicervical
4. intertrochanteric
5. subtrochanteric.

Femoral neck fractures are extremely common in the elderly, often following falls, and most orthopaedic units will have a number of these fractures at any one time. The bones architecture may have been so weakened that patients state that they 'heard a crack' before they hit the ground. In other words the fracture caused the fall, not the fall the fracture. Osteoporosis is often referred to as the silent epidemic as it may not present any clinical signs until fracture. It is discussed elsewhere in this textbook.

The resulting fracture is usually displaced with lateral rotation of the femoral shaft so that the leg will be laterally rotated in comparison with the other limb.

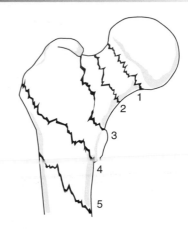

Figure 3.17   Classification of femoral neck fractures: (1) subcapital; (2) transcervical; (3) basicervical; (4) intertrochanteric; (5) subtrochanteric.

Occasionally the fragments are impacted in slight abduction and the patient may be able to get up and walk after the injury. Displaced fractures will need operative fixation (Figure 3.18); the usual method is to excise the head and perform replacement arthroplasty using one of the metal prostheses available (e.g. Thompson's hemiarthroplasty – Figure 3.19). This is the method of choice for displaced fractures because of the dangers of avascular necrosis, and because of the benefits of early mobilisation, which is so important in the frail.

An alternative method of fixation is a compression screw plate called a 'dynamic hip screw' – so called because it permits dynamic movement at the fracture site which stimulates healing. Minimally displaced (e.g. Garden type 1) fractures may be managed by cannulated screw fixation.

Complications

The blood supply to the femoral head is predominantly via a periarticular anastomosis (Palastanga et al. 1998). Avascular necrosis (death of part of the bone owing to lack of blood supply) can occur as the blood supply to the head of the femur may be impaired following a fractured neck of femur (Figure 3.20).

Fractures of the shaft of the femur

These fractures are usually the result of severe violence and may occur at any part of the shaft, and may be of any type – transverse, oblique, spiral – and may be comminuted. Usually there is marked displacement with overlap of the fragments, which could lead to limb shortening if it is not corrected. Angulation may occur depending on the injury and on powerful muscle spasm pulling the fragment in the direction of the attached muscles.

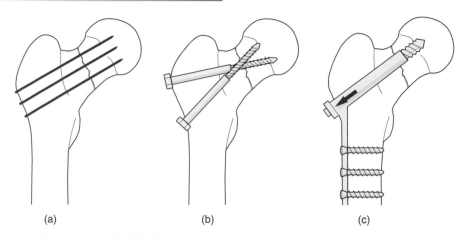

(a)   (b)   (c)

Figure 3.18   Methods of fixation for femoral neck fractures. (Reproduced from Dandy and Edwards 1998, with permission.)

For children under the age of 3 years 'gallows' traction may be used. A modern, more acceptable alternative to traction is the use of an intramedullary (IM) nailing (Figure 3.9) which can be performed by the closed technique. The nail is passed through the greater trochanter and down the medullary canal of a long bone and through the fracture site. This is preferable to the previously favoured method of prolonged traction or open reduction, as there is less risk of infection and the complications of bedrest and immobility.

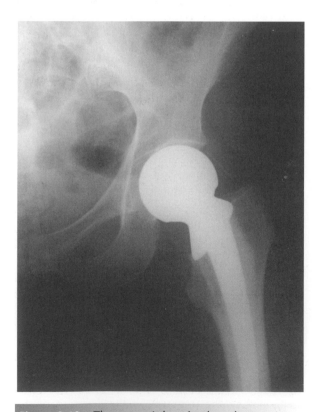

Figure 3.19   Thompson's hemiarthroplasty.

If the fracture is an open fracture there is a risk of infection. Delayed union or non-union is occasionally a complication of this injury, as is malunion. If the overlap of the fragments is not reduced or there is redisplacement, this can occur with consequent shortening of the femur. When the fracture has been fixed internally with an intramedullary nail, mobilisation can occur more rapidly. The patient may be on bedrest for 2–3 days but may be able to undertake active exercises. This will depend on how satisfactorily the nail is in maintaining reduction. Following this the patient will start walking with partial weight bearing and progress to full weight bearing once the surgeon is satisfied that the reduction is satisfactory and that union is progressing normally.

Fractures around the knee

These include fractures of the tibial condyles, the patella and the femoral condyles.

Injury to the tibial condyles may comprise either a comminuted compression or a depressed plateau fracture. In the former, reduction is not usually attempted and early mobilisation is encouraged. Depressed plateau fractures require reduction to try to achieve an anatomically correct articular surface. Constant passive motion (CPM) may be used immediately after the fracture or after surgery to preserve synovial sweep and maintain articular cartilage nutrition.

Fractures of the femoral condyles are not very common but a supracondylar fracture occurs more frequently.

Complications

- Stiff knee could occur as the result of adhesions or because of disruption of the articular surfaces in fractures of the tibial condyles or patella.

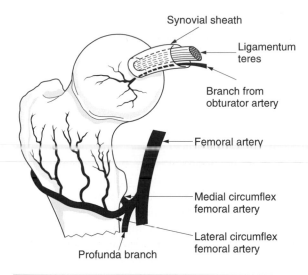

Figure 3.20   Arterial supply to the hip.
(Reproduced from Palastanga et al. 2002, with
permission.)

- Secondary osteoarthritis may occur as a late complication following disruption of the articular surfaces.
- Genu valgum may develop following depression of the lateral tibial condyle.
- Haemarthrosis may be a problem after fractures of the tibial condyles. This may need to be aspirated (drained) and bandaged, but the swelling that occurs as a result of a synovitis will gradually absorb. If other soft-tissue structures are damaged there may be further swelling, in which case the limb should be elevated to assist drainage.

Fracture of the patella

This can be caused by a direct blow on the knee or a sudden violent contraction of the quadriceps resulting in an avulsion fracture. The former tends to cause a crack or comminuted fracture whereas the latter may produce a transverse fracture. Internal fixation may be required if there is separation of the fragments. If the chances of regaining a smooth contour of the articular surfaces are low then the surgeon may decide to excise the patella (patellectomy) as this results in very little loss of function and is preferable to a stiff knee or development of osteoarthritis, particularly in the elderly patient. More severe patellar fractures may require wiring or screw fixation.

Fractures of the tibia and fibula

These fractures are common and occur at all ages, as a result of direct or indirect violence. Often they are open fractures either because of the direct violence or because the anterior tibia is very close to the surface and the fragments may extrude through the skin.

Direct violence, commonly due to road traffic accidents or soccer, is likely to give an oblique or transverse fracture. It may be comminuted and further complicated by soft-tissue damage. Fractures caused by a rotatory force, such as may occur in skiing, are usually spiral and the fractures of the two bones are at different levels.

Fixation will depend on the type of fracture and the amount of soft-tissue damage. In closed fractures or those where the fracture is stable after reduction, the leg may be managed in a long plaster from the thigh to just above the toes, with the knee slightly flexed and the ankle at a right-angle. Later a rocker or plaster boot may be applied so that the patient can walk on the plaster but the time at which this occurs will depend on the fracture. Alternatively a functional brace with a hinge at the ankle may be used and this has the advantage of allowing more movement and a better walking pattern. If there is a lot of soft-tissue damage and consequent swelling, a split plaster may be applied and the leg elevated on a Braun frame. This is replaced with a plaster once the swelling has subsided.

Another method that is used to immobilize this fracture is external fixation. Sometimes internal fixation is used with either an intramedullary nail or plate and screws. Common practice now is to commence active movement in elevation immediately after surgery and delay the application of a plaster until movements are sufficiently regained.

Complications

Fractures of the tibia or fibula alone are not very common. The tibia can be the site of a stress fracture due to repeated minor trauma probably associated with sport. Infection is a possible complication as many of these are open fractures; fortunately the problem is less serious these days with the advent of antibiotics and improved wound care.

Vascular impairment can occur due to damage to a blood vessel or a plaster cast that is too tight. Great care must be taken by all concerned with the management of these patients to monitor for any signs of circulatory deficiency.

Compartment syndrome is common, as is delayed union or non-union. Occasionally these fractures are very slow to heal or there may even be non-union owing to the lower third of the tibia having such a poor blood supply.

Fractures around the ankle

Figure 13.21 shows fractures resulting from an abduction/lateral rotation force or an adduction force. Complications include limitation of movement in the ankle joint and foot resulting from peri-articular and intra-articular adhesions or from disruption of the articular surfaces. The latter may also lead to the later development of secondary osteoarthritis.

For fractures without displacement, a below-knee walking plaster may be applied for 3–6 weeks. When there is displacement it is important for the surgeon to try to ensure that reduction establishes the normal anatomical relationship at the ankle joint. If reduction cannot be attained by manipulation and plaster immobilisation it may be necessary to have an open reduction with internal fixation (ORIF) and use a screw or screws to maintain a good position of the fragments followed by immobilisation in a below-knee plaster. The modern trend is towards immediate postoperative active exercise (with adequate analgesia), then subsequent application of a cast once good movement (particularly dorsiflexion) is attained. Tri-malleolar fractures are generally unstable.

Fractures in the foot

Fractures of the calcaneum usually occur as the result of a fall from a height on to the feet, fracturing the calcaneum in one or sometimes both feet. It may well be accompanied by a fracture of one of the lower thoracic or upper lumbar vertebrae. (Take note if a patient with a fractured calcaneum complains of back pain.) Calcaneal fractures can be extremely painful and carry a poor functional prognosis if inversion and eversion are not regained, since their movements are essential for normal function of the foot in such activities as adapting to uneven surfaces.

The emphasis of physiotherapy management is on the reduction of the oedema and mobilisation. Once the patient is allowed to bear weight it is important to re-educate gait as well as concentrating on strengthening muscles and regaining range of movement in the ankle and foot. It may not be possible to regain any movement at the mid-tarsal joints and the patient will have to learn to adapt to this loss of movement. The arches of the foot may have flattened and this could be the result of weak muscles, deformity of the foot, or both. In the former case the muscles can be strengthened, but if the latter is the case the arches will not

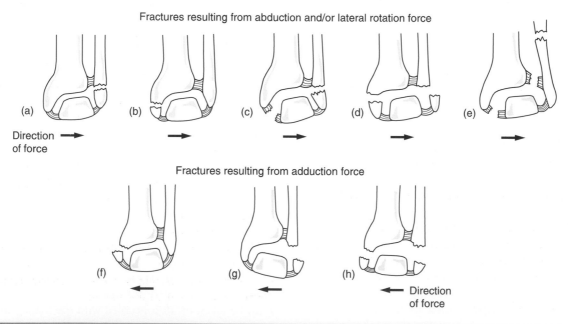

Fractures resulting from abduction and/or lateral rotation force

(a)   (b)   (c)   (d)   (e)

Direction of force

Fractures resulting from adduction force

(f)   (g)   (h)   Direction of force

Figure 3.21   Parts (a)–(e) show fractures resulting from an abduction/lateral rotation force: (a) fracture of lateral malleolus; (b) avulsion fracture of medial malleolus; (c) fracture of lateral malleolus, rupture of medial ligament, and lateral shift of talus; (d) fracture of lateral and medial malleoli and lateral shift of talus; (e) tibio-fibular diastasis – rupture of tibio-fibular and medial ligaments, fracture of shaft of fibula, and lateral shift of talus. Parts (f)–(h) show fractures resulting from an adduction force: (f) fracture of medial malleolus; (g) avulsion fracture of lateral malleolus; (h) fractures of lateral and medial malleoli plus medial shift of talus.

reform: the patient may continue to have persistent pain and tenderness for a long time after the fracture has healed and it is difficult to relieve.

Generally speaking it is advisable to commence early active mobilisation in elevation. Cryotherapy/TENS, flowtron boot, and patient-controlled analgesia (PCA) have all been used with success. In later stages, accessory mobilisations to the affected joints may be appropriate.

The phalanges and metatarsals are most likely to be fractured by a heavy object falling on the foot. This will also cause soft-tissue damage and consequently swelling is likely to be severe. These fractures do not as a rule require reduction or immobilisation. However, a below-knee walking plaster is usually applied for fractures of the metatarsals to relieve pain and enable the patient to walk. If swelling is severe the patient will need to rest in bed with the leg elevated for a few days.

Another type of fracture that occurs in the metatarsals is a stress fracture – often known as a 'March' fracture. It is caused by repeated minor trauma that may arise from prolonged walking particularly on hard surfaces, and usually in someone who is unaccustomed to walking long distances. It is usually a crack fracture affecting the shaft or neck of the second or third metatarsal. No fixation is required but a walking plaster may be applied if the pain is severe

Complications

Complications include stiffness, particularly if there has been disruption of the subtalar joint articular surfaces. Secondary osteoarthritis may develop later as a result of the disruption of the joint surfaces.

Spinal fractures

These are not dealt with in this text.

CONTINUOUS PASSIVE MOTION (CPM)

Use of CPM is now widespread in the orthopaedic setting (Figure 3.22). Like any other modality in medicine, has its place and its limitations. Salter (1993) has made an interesting study of the uses of CPM.

Benefits of CPM

- There is maintenance of synovial sweep and thus hyaline articular cartilage nutrition. This is useful after certain intra-articular fractures (e.g. tibial plateau).
- Regular rhythmical motion can act as an analgesic, can stimulate circulation, and may assist in reduction of swelling.

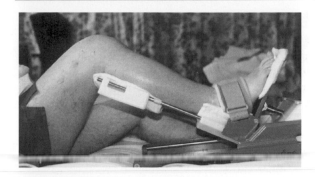

Figure 3.22   A demonstration of CPM.

- CPM has been used following anterior cruciate reconstruction particularly following patellar tendon graft. It is possible that this encourages more rapid revascularisation and therefore strength of the donor graft.
- It is possible to increase the flexion/extension in a controlled manner that is immediately obvious to the patient and can assist in giving the patient a goal to strive for.
- Some units have counters so that the healthcare team can tell exactly for how long the patient has been using the unit.
- CPM units are now available for shoulder, wrist and other joints.
- CPMs may now be used in the patient's home.

Disadvantages of CPM

- It is passive, and therefore by definition will not build muscle strength. Some patients mistakenly neglect active exercises in the belief that they no longer need to undertake them. It is the responsibility of the physiotherapist to ensure that this situation does not occur.
- Some patients are distressed by the appearance of the unit and feel threatened. Most units have a panic button so the patient can stop the unit for rest, meals or toileting.
- The units can be bulky and expensive.
- If incorrectly positioned they can cause pressure problems and be uncomfortable.
- They pose an infection risk if not properly cleaned, and policies for their use followed.

CASE STUDY: FRACTURED SHAFT OF THE FEMUR

Note that the material in this section does *not* represent a recipe for the management of all fractures of the femur.

Background

Ms Jones is a 25-year-old law student who was involved in a road traffic accident. She was driving and as a result of a head-on collision the dashboard was pushed backwards into her knees. She sustained a fractured shaft of the left femur (Figure 3.23a). She was treated by intramedullary fixation (Figure 3.23b). Ms Smith spent 10 days in hospital and has now come to the out-patient physiotherapy department. She did not sustain any other injuries.

On examination

Ms Jones is partial weight-bearing, and is mobilising with two elbow crutches and wearing a functional (cast) brace. She is independently mobile although needs help to remove her training shoe and sock. The brace was custom-made by the occupational therapists (Figure 3.24) and it is unlocked to permit 0–90 degrees of knee flexion. The physiotherapist may unlock the brace by a further 10 degrees each week. The patient must wear the brace when walking but is permitted to remove it to perform knee flexion exercises and to take a shower.

She is extremely anxious about what is going to happen to her and confused about how much or how little she should be doing. The only exercise she can remem-ber is straight leg raise (SLR). She is articulate, co-operative and keen to take advice. She cannot currently attain heel strike and she states that this is because it causes her calf to be painful – although deep vein thrombosis has been excluded. She has been told to keep moving and as a result she is walking long distances every day. Her leg aches badly at bedtime and she is worried that the fracture has 'moved', although X-rays show that it has not displaced since the time of surgery.

Objective examination

There are two incisions; one proximal to the greater trochanter, one lateral to the knee joint. These have healed. The patient has a reddened area over the lateral malleolus, which is due to the brace rubbing her skin.

Knee joint

The range of movement of the knee joint with the brace removed is shown in Table 3.4.

Patello-femoral joint

All accessory movements are reduced by approximately 50% on the left side.

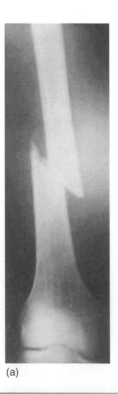

(a)

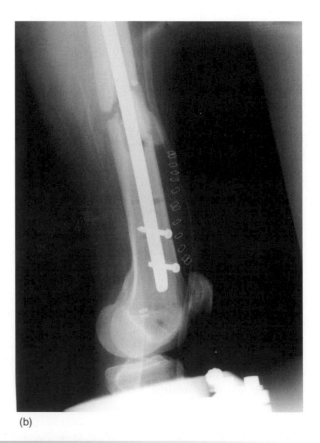

(b)

Figure 3.23   (a) The femoral fracture. Note that spasm in the quadriceps has resulted in overriding of the fracture fragments. (b) Note the locking screws and skin staples visible on X-ray.

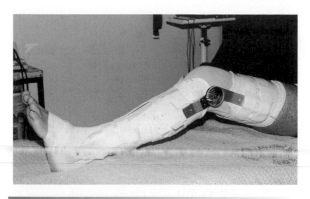

Figure 3.24   The functional brace. The heel cup is essential for correct off-loading of weight from the fracture. Photo courtesy of Mike Somervell and Julie Butler.

Ankles

There is full active range plantar flexion in both ankles. Terminal dorsiflexion of the affected side causes calf 'tightness' when the left knee is in the fully extended position. The range of plantar and dorsiflexion is full, however. Small joints of the foot, intertarsal, and tarso-metatarsal have some loss of accessory movement of the subtalar and intertarsal joints of the affected side. There is some oedema of the ankle. Capillary filling is poor.

Muscle strength (Oxford grade – left:right)

	L	R
Quadriceps	4	5
Hamstrings	4	5
Tibialis anterior	4	5
Gastrocnemius	4	5

Pain

Figure 3.25 shows the pain recorded using a visual analogue scale.

Limb girth

See the chart.

Limb girth	10 cm above palella apex	20 cm above palella apex
Left leg	48 cm	44 cm
Right leg	56 cm	52 cm

Short-term problems

Do not underestimate the impact of apprehension and confusion. If a person is nervous, frightened or confused, whatever you plan to tell, teach or ask of them will be adversely influenced. Do not think only of the fracture, take a holistic approach. Physiotherapists are not technicians, they are also educators. It is perfectly valid to undertake with her a teaching session on fracture healing and to discuss your aims of treatment. This might seem time-consuming but consider your aims of treatment and your role as her physiotherapist. The quality of your communication and subsequent discussion of your management plan will influence her eventual health outcome. There is now strong research evidence suggesting a positive correlation between effective professional–patient communication and improved patient health outcomes.

The sore caused by the brace is a high priority. The physiotherapist needs to refer the patient to the occupational therapist for adjustment of the brace. If the sore develops to the point where she cannot tolerate the brace, your ability to progress her treatment will be adversely affected.

Table 3.4 Features of the patient's knee joint.

	LEFT KNEE			RIGHT KNEE		
	Passive[a]	Active[b]	Over-pressure[c]	Passive	Active	Over-pressure
Flexion	0–60	0–40	–	130	130	–
Extension	Full extension possible but causes posterior knee discomfort			Full 0-degree extension painless		
Lateral rotation	Full			Full		
Internal rotation	Full			Full		

[a]Limited by apprehension. [b]Limited by aching at the fracture site and quadriceps spasm. [c] Not tested in view of fracture status and patient apprehension.
The units are degrees.

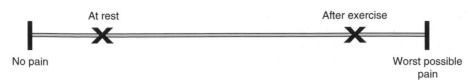

Figure 3.25   The patient's pain scale.

Pain and aching at the end of the day is normal – your goal here is to explain *why* the pain is happening and that it signifies bone healing. Do not assume that your patient will automatically know this. Some patients equate pain with 'no pain no gain' and see it as a positive factor whereas others will be frightened by pain. In this person's case it seems likely that too much walking is being undertaken; she needs advice on smaller, more frequent walks with attainable goals. For example she could be told to walk the length of the home every hour. Knee flexion may be painful, in which case your role as her physiotherapist is to identify the specific cause and minimise or reduce it prior to active exercise. This might consist of asking the patient to take her analgesia one hour before commencing her exercises, or the application of TENS or hydrotherapy as a supplement to exercise.

Her current exercise regimen is unacceptable. Repeated straight leg raising will do nothing to provide functional quadriceps strength and at worst it will cause backache. Straight leg raising is probably one of the most abused exercises in physiotherapy. It will strengthen the hip flexors but little else. She needs functional exercises such as inner range quadriceps, hamstring, gastrocnemius and anterior tibial and hip abductor work within the permitted limits of the fracture rehabilitation. These must be taught and explained clearly, written down if possible and the rationale behind them explained to the patient. Patients often become confused about their exercises, keep them simple and understandable. Patient compliance with exercise is poor in general (Campbell et al. 2001), and the more you can do to make home exercises simple and practical, the more success you will have in educating and rehabilitating your patient.

Loss of knee flexion due to callus may be impeding soft tissue mobility. Pain, fear or muscle spasm might also be causes of limited mobility; since she has more passive than active range, something other than the joint is limiting her movement. Your role is to identify the cause and treat it accordingly. Heat pack or massage may relieve spasm. The brace limits flexion to 90 degrees but there is no reason why you should not aim for 90 degrees at this time.

With regard to the oedema, an inefficient muscle pump is a likely cause. She is not attaining heel strike but is walking great distances; these will both exacerbate dependent oedema. Little and often is the key, with elevation during periods of rest, and a graduated increase of walking distance. Massage might be used to relieve oedema but can be time-consuming.

This person has a loss of limb girth on the affected side. This will be due to disuse atrophy. Decreased limb girth is not so important as muscle function but may be distressing to the patient; reassure her that function will come first, then bulk. Whilst it is not a true reflection of quadriceps girth or strength, and it does give the person something specific to aim for.

Loss of accessory movement needs to be addressed in the treatment plan, for example to the small joints of the foot and mid-tarsal joints. The loss of accessory motion at the patello-femoral joint should also be addressed; the function of this joint cannot and should not be isolated from the function of the knee joint itself. It is relatively easy to identify immediate problems, but unfortunately this alone is insufficient; you also need to be aware of potential or longer-term complications:

Potential and long-term problems: the bigger picture

- Adaptive shortening of the Achilles tendon leading to permanent soft tissue contracture may occur if her gait is not corrected as a consequence of her not attaining heel strike. She currently does not have any soft-tissue contracture since her measurements are full.
- Encourage her to walk shorter distances with a normal gait.
- Check that her pain is being controlled adequately so that she is not afraid to attain heel strike.
- Explain this to the patient so that she can take an active role in her own rehabilitation.
- Make sure that a potential problem does not become a real one.
- Fixed flexion deformity of the knee joint is also a possibility if the importance of attaining full knee extension is not explained to the patient.
- Fibrous adhesions may occur if oedema is allowed to organise.

- Retro-patellar adhesions may form as a result of immobility of the knee's expansive synovial membrane and might become a cause of stiffness. The likelihood of this happening might be reduced by isometric contractions of the quadriceps and articularis genus muscle whose task it is to retract the synovium of the knee joint (Ahmad 1975).
- Degeneration of hyaline articular cartilage occurs if a joint is not subjected to movement. The patient should be encouraged to undertake general mobility and exercise little and often.
- Generalised osteopaenia, or a reduction in bone mineral density, may result if weight is not placed through the limb. The see-saw needs careful consideration here – see earlier in this chapter.

Treatment plan

- The patient must effectively become involved in the management of her condition.
- Commence partial weight-bearing gait and progress within protocol guidelines.
- Re-educate normal gait – i.e. heel strike.
- Mobility of all unaffected joints must be maintained, during the period of immobilisation.
- Regain movement and function to normal. This is person-specific and full function might not be attained until removal of the nail in one or two years' time.
- Draw up a thorough and fully understood home exercise programme which can be monitored and progressed as needed. It is better to teach two exercises well and have the patient thoroughly understand them than teach ten exercises, which are too complex and confusing to the patient.
- Strengthen appropriate muscles dependent upon your assessment findings.
- Progress to full weight-bearing within rehabilitation guidelines; check any protocols and specific guidelines.

Overall progress and discharge

Study the simplified graph in Figure 3.26. If we plot a hypothetical 'improvement versus time' graph, the student might *hope* for this pattern. ('Improvement' may mean different things to different people. For purposes of clarity it has been shown as a single item.) If this were the case, recovery could always be predicted, all patients could use the same treatment regimen, one assessment would be sufficient, a discharge date could be predicted many weeks in advance, and undergraduate training would take about a month! Unfortunately this is not the case.

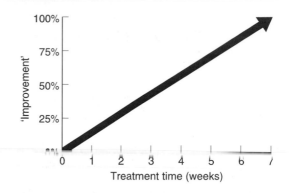

Figure 3.26   A hypothetical improvement chart.

It is more likely that you will see a pattern of peaks, troughs, and plateaux with a general trend towards recovery. The overall shape of the real improvement curve displays the gradual attainment of a plateau in improvement.

This pattern of recovery is common: the patient may gain 10 degrees of knee flexion per week for the first 3 weeks of treatment, then improvements will slow to the point where it takes a further 3 weeks to attain an additional 5 degrees. This presents the physiotherapist with a constantly changeable situation – which is one of the reasons why the profession is so stimulating. It also poses the problem of when to discharge the patient. The final decision must be a mutually agreed decision between physiotherapist and patient, and it is at this point that previously agreed goals are essential. It may be the case that 95% 'improvement' is the maximum possible improvement attainable whilst the IM nail remains in situ. For example there may be some residual discomfort on running or squatting. Experienced physiotherapists will be able to integrate their knowledge of anatomy, physiology and biomechanics and explain to the patient that now is the time for discharge and that the further 5% will occur following implant removal. Without a sound prior assessment and formulation of goals, appropriate patient discharge may be jeopardised, resulting in discharge that is too early or treatments that become repetitive, non-adaptive and inappropriate. The advantage of physiotherapists being autonomous practitioners is that with a little thought and a sound initial assessment one can avoid the situation where the patient is seen 'twice a week for 8 weeks' with no change in treatment or progression. The patient and physiotherapist 'own' the process.

FURTHER READING

Atkinson K, Coutts F, Hassenkamp AM 1999 Physiotherapy in Orthopaedics – A Problem Solving Approach. Churchill Livingstone: Edinburgh

Bruckner P, Bennell K 1997 Stress fractures in female athletes: diagnosis, management and rehabilitation. Sports Med 24(6): 419–29

Duckworth T 1995 Lecture Notes on Orthopaedics and Fractures. Blackwell Science: Oxford

McRae M 1999 Pocketbook of Orthopaedics and Fractures. Churchill Livingstone: Edinburgh

Stewart MA 1995 Effective physician–patient communication and health outcomes: a review. CMAJ 152(9): 1423–33

Tidswell M 1998 Orthopaedic Physiotherapy. Mosby: New York

REFERENCES

Adams CI, Keating JF, Court-Brown CM 2001 Cigarette smoking and open tibial fractures. Injury 32(1): 61–5

Ahmad I 1975 Articular muscle of the knee – articularis genus. Bull Hosp Joint Dis 36(1): 58–60

Azuma Y, Ito M et al. 2001 Low-intensity pulsed ultrasound accelerates rat femoral fracture healing by acting on the various cellular reactions in the fracture callus. J Bone Miner Res 16(4): 671–80

Campbell R, Evans M, Tucker M et al. 2001 Why don't patients do their exercises? Understanding non-compliance with physiotherapy in patients with osteoarthritis of the knee. J Epidemiol Commun Health 55(2): 132–8

Cornell CN, Lane JM 1992 Newest factors in fracture healing. Clin Orthop 277: 293–311

Dandy DJ, Edwards DJ 1998 Essential Orthopaedics and Trauma, 3rd edn, p. 94. Churchill Livingstone: New York

Hoppenfeld S, Urthy VL 1999 Treatment and Rehabilitation of Fractures. Lippincott Williams and Wilkins: Baltimore

Marsh DR, Li G 1999 The biology of fracture healing: optimising outcome. BMJ 55: 856–69

Palastanga N, Field D, Soames R 1998 Anatomy and Human Movement: Structure and Function, 3rd edn. Butterworth–Heinemann: Oxford

Palastanga N, Field D, Soames R 2002 Anatomy and Human Movement, 4th edn, pp. 3, 20. Butterworth–Heinemann: Oxford.

Reginster JY, Gillet P et al. 1999 Direct costs of hip fractures in patients over 60 years of age in Belgium. Pharmacoeconomics 15(5): 507–14

Roolker W, Maas M et al. 1999 Diagnosis and treatment of scaphoid fractures: can non-union be prevented? Arch Orthop Trauma Surg 119(7–8): 428–31

Salter RB 1993 Continuous Passive Motion (CPM) – a Biological Concept for the Healing and Regeneration of Articular Cartilage, Ligaments and Tendons. Williams and Wilkins: Baltimore

Schurch MA, Rizzoli R et al. 1996 A prospective study of socioeconomic aspects of fracture of the proximal femur. J Bone Miner Res 11(12): 1935–42

Schwartsman V, Choi SH, Schwartsman R 1990 Tibial nonunions: treatment tactics with the Ilizarov method. Orthop Clin N Am 21(4): 639–53

Sheriff DD, Van Bibber R 1998 Flow-generating capability of the isolated skeletal muscle pump. Am J Physiol 274(5:2): H1502–8

Tschakovsky ME, Shoemaker JK et al. 1996 Vasodilation and muscle pump contribution to immediate exercise hyperemia. Am J Physiol 271(4:2): H1679–701

Viel E, Ripart J et al. 1999 Management of reflex sympathetic dystrophy. Ann Med Interne (Paris) 150(3): 205–10

4

The Intervertebral Disc in Health and Disease: An Introduction to Back Pain

Stuart B. Porter

The anatomy of the human spine, the pathomechanics of low back pain, and physiotherapy approaches to the management of back pain quite easily justify whole textbooks. This chapter will introduce the student to some general concepts. Suggested further reading is included at the end of the chapter.

This chapter will cover:

- the structure and function of the intervertebral disc
- common pathological processes affecting intervertebral discs
- differential diagnoses of back pain
- an overview of some current research findings relating to the management of acute low back pain.

The chapter should be read in conjunction with Chapter 2 on musculoskeletal assessment, in particular the section on biopsychosocial assessment for low back pain.

THE INTERVERTEBRAL DISC: ITS STRUCTURE AND FUNCTIONS

Mobility and Articulation

Approximately a quarter of the height of the vertebral column is made up not by its bones but by the intervertebral discs (Figure 4.1). These are often described as shock absorbers, allowing load to be transmitted from one vertebra to the next.

An equally important role of a disc is to permit controlled, small-amplitude movements between the vertebrae above and below it (Figure 4.2a). Between two adjoining vertebrae, only small movements are possible. When added together, the result is a column that is extremely mobile without sacrificing stability (Figure 4.2b). The normal spine is self-stabilising, and for

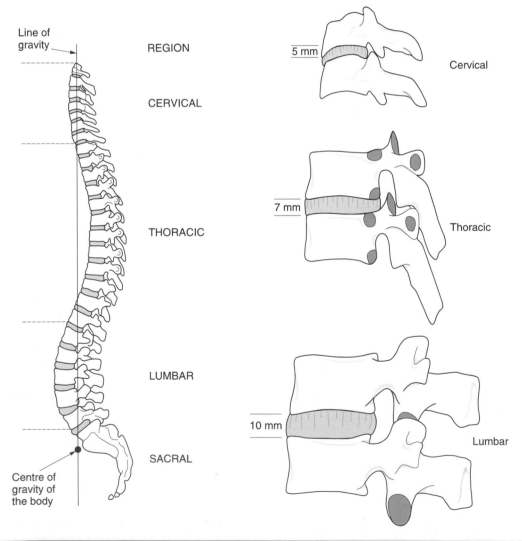

Figure 4.1   Lateral view of the adult vertebral column. (Reproduced from Palastanga et al. 2002, with permission.)

humans to stand erect takes very little muscle action – illustrated by the fact that people who have spent prolonged periods in bed can sit upright with relative ease. A spinal column minus muscles is still able to support itself, but if the spinal ligaments are severed the intrinsic stability of the spinal column is lost (Palastanga et al. 1998).

There are three points of articulation between each pair of vertebrae, forming an articular triad – they are the central intervertebral joint and the two facet joints (Figure 4.3). The motion segment consists of: the space between the vertebrae, the disc and its endplates, anterior/posterior longitudinal ligaments, facet joints and their capsules, ligamentum flavum, the contents of the spinal canal, and supraspinous and interspinous ligaments. Spinal motion is controlled not only by the thickness and shape of the discs, but also by small pairs of synovial joints located at the posterior of each motion segment – known as facet or zygapophyseal joints. Each motion segment possesses two facet joints that control and limit certain torsional or twisting movements in the spine depending on their orientation, and these vary from lumbar to thoracic to cervical regions.

Intervertebral Disc Structure

The disc consists of an outer ring called the annulus fibrosus and a soft gel-like central portion called the nucleus pulposus (Figure 4.4). When considering the disc and its pathology, or describing the structure to patients, it is useful to compare the disc to a jam doughnut, with a contained soft inner part and a hard outer portion. The disc contains fibrocytes and chondrocytes in an elaborate avascular matrix of collagen and proteoglycans (Guiot and Fessler 2000).

Discs are thickest in the lumbar spine, where each is approximately 10 mm deep. They also tend to be

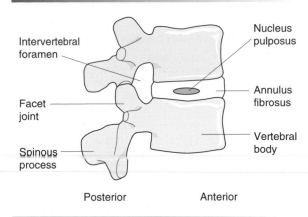

Figure 4.3   The motion segment (simplified).

wedge-shaped, so the combined effect of these multiple wedges is to give the spine its curvatures. The curvatures in the cervical, lumbar and thoracic spine add to the strength of the spine and its remarkable ability to withstand compression. The normal disc is so strong that falls from a height will often cause fracture of the vertebral body rather than damage to the disc.

The annulus fibrosus

The annulus fibrosus is the outer portion of the disc and it provides an envelope, which restrains the nucleus. The annulus is just elastic enough to permit some bulging of the disc, which helps to dissipate stress from one vertebra to the next. It is made up of crisscross sheets or lamellae of collagen bundles – this allows the disc to resist excessive twisting from different directions. The lamellae form incomplete rings and the angle made by their fibres becomes more acute when the disc is loaded.

The outer portion of the annulus possesses nerve endings, which can explain the presence of back pain symptoms which occur even when discs appear normal (Yoshizawa et al. 1980; Bogduk 1991).

The annulus is not the same anteriorly and posteriorly in the lumbar spine. Anteriorly there are about 20 thick lamellae, running between the vertebral rims, weakly anchored to the anterior longitudinal ligament. Posteriorly these lamellae are fewer in number, thinner, and fused with the posterior longitudinal ligament. A previously unknown ligament has recently been described, the superficial annulus fibrosus ligament (SAFL), situated on the anterior part of the L5 disc. (Hanson et al. 2000).

The nucleus pulposus

The nucleus normally sits centrally within the disc (Figure 4.4), except in the lumbar spine where it tends

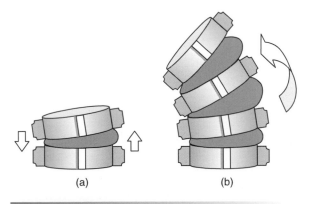

Figure 4.2   The roles of intervertebral discs. (a) Small movements only between adjacent vertebrae. (b) Summation of movements results in great mobility.

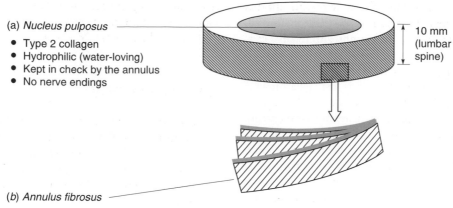

(a) *Nucleus pulposus*

- Type 2 collagen
- Hydrophilic (water-loving)
- Kept in check by the annulus
- No nerve endings

10 mm (lumbar spine)

(b) *Annulus fibrosus*

- Criss-cross arrangement of lamellae or sheets
- Each layer has a slightly different orientation of fibres, making the disc resistant to torsional movements
- Permits a small amount of disc bulging
- Type 1 collagen (typical of tendon) provides the disc with tensile strength
- Type 2 collagen (typical of cartilage) provides the disc with compressive strength
- Annulus consists of outer ligamentous and inner fibrocartilaginous portions
- Nerve endings in outer portion

Figure 4.4   Characteristics of the nucleus pulposus and annulus fibrosus.

to be located towards the back. The nucleus has a high water content and is turgid, as a consequence if a fresh disc is sectioned it immediately bulges. This pressure within the disc has the effect of 'pushing' the vertebra above and below it apart, placing the surrounding ligaments under tension, further enhancing the stability of the spinal column.

The nucleus is ideally suited to withstanding axial loading as it cannot be significantly compressed, and it is held in check by the outer annulus. Tension in the ligamentum flavum is thought to compress the motion segment and pre-stress the disc (Oliver and Middleditch 1991). The nucleus acts hydrostatically during loading (Nachemson and Morris 1964) – 'hydrostatic' refers to the pressure exerted by a fluid (Figure 4.5).

The vertebral endplate

The endplates are found above and below each disc, are approximately 1 mm thick and have several functions. The endplate is thought to permit osmosis of nutrients between the vertebral body and the disc, it restrains the disc, and may also protect the vertebra from pressure. Herniation or bulging of the nucleus into the vertebral body through the endplate may occur but this is often asymptomatic (Giles and Singer 1997).

Pressures within the Disc

Classical experiments by Nachemson and Morris (1964; see also Nachemson 1966) provided insight into the pressures within the disc. The results correlate with the clinical signs and symptoms described by people

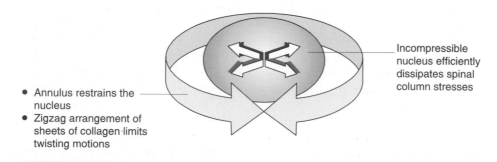

- Annulus restrains the nucleus
- Zigzag arrangement of sheets of collagen limits twisting motions

Incompressible nucleus efficiently dissipates spinal column stresses

Figure 4.5   The disc annulus and nucleus interact to provide a resilient hydrodynamic complex.

with disc disease. For example, people with annular tears often say that their pain is least in lying, worst when sitting, and they are often observed standing in clinic waiting rooms in preference to sitting. Extremely high intra-discal pressures are recorded when a person sits slumped forward in a chair.

Intervertebral discs undergo a daily battle between compressive loading – tending to squeeze water out of the disc – and the tendency of the nucleus to take up water when the load is relieved. This accounts for the fact that people are taller in the morning than in the evening. In the young, this equilibrium is stable, but with increasing age discs tend to lose water more readily and become less able to cope with stresses. Spinal load changes with the angle of the motion segment, and lower discs have to bear more of the weight of the body. The pressure within degenerated discs is less than that found in normal discs (Sato et al. 1999). The explanation for high intra-discal pressure in sitting may be because of the slightly flexed posture and the compressive effect of psoas major on the spine.

SPINAL MUSCLES

The exact roles of all the muscles of the spinal column are still not altogether clear. The abdominal muscles play an important role in trunk rotation and in raising intra-abdominal pressure, thereby stabilising the spinal motion segments (Grakovetsky et al. 1985). The extensor muscles of the spine may be able to control individual vertebral movements, and it seems likely that the erector spinae complex works in complex patterns to resist the tendency of the spine to flex in various postures. The erector spinae complex does not play an important role in rotation of the trunk (Macintosh et al. 1993), but despite many complex biomechanical and computer simulation studies, no single model as yet explains them satisfactorily (Nordin and Frankel 1989). In the past, it was thought that exercising the spinal extensors was of chief importance in preventing back pain.

There are now convincing arguments that this complex of small paraspinal muscles play more of a sensory proprioceptive role rather than having a direct stabilising effect on the spine. It has also been argued that the role of the short spinal muscles (multifidus, rotatores, interspinales and intertransversarii) is to stabilise the motion segment, allowing the longer, more superficial muscles to act efficiently. Recent muscle imbalance theories suggest that a mismatch between the strengths of surrounding muscle groups may be a cause of pain in the spine (Lee et al. 1999). Put simply, muscle imbalance theory suggests that certain muscles become over-active and shorten, whilst their antagonist group becomes lengthened and inhibited. Muscle imbalance

is an interesting concept and may be precipitated by pain, type of activity or ligamentous instability (Oliver and Middleditch 1991). Muscle imbalance is discussed in Chapter 21.

DISC PATHOLOGY

It is important to be aware that disc pathology can take several forms, and that disc pathology is not the only cause of low back pain. In fact the majority of back pain is non-specific (Giles and Singer 1997). Differential diagnoses of back pain are considered later in this chapter.

Throughout life, discs endure various pathological processes, but the naming of these pathologies is still inconsistent. In this chapter, two of the most common pathologies will be considered – *disc protrusion* and *disc degeneration*.

Disc Protrusion (Prolapse)

Discs undergo the ageing process in a similar manner to the changes discussed in Chapter 9 on osteoarthritis (OA). The term 'slipped disc' is misleading, since the disc does not slip. Earlier in this chapter, the disc was compared to a jam doughnut and the analogy continues to be useful when trying to understand a 'slipped disc': imagine a crack in the wall of the doughnut, through which oozes jam under pressure. Protrusions can be classified as shown in Figure 4.6 (American Academy of Orthopedic Surgeons 1987).

The most common age range affected by disc prolapse is 20–55 years. The nucleus dries out with age, making true extrusion less likely in older age groups.

Although all lumbar discs are prone to prolapse, the most common sites are L5–S1 and L4–L5, accounting for 80–90% of all lumbar disc lesions. C5–C6 and C6–C7 are vulnerable sites in the cervical spine, these being the levels at which there is a change from mobility to relative stability in the spine.

Aetiology

Intervertebral disc prolapse is the combined result of repetitive loading, biochemical alterations and degenerative changes (Oliver and Middleditch 1991). Repeated flexion–extension movements lead to cracks in the annulus, which provide an escape route for the normally restrained nucleus (Callaghan and McGill 2001; Kuga and Kawabuchi 2001).

Prolapses may develop as small annular tears accumulate over many months. In such cases the final straw is often something trivial such as sneezing or picking up a pencil from the floor, and these patients can often recall a history of minor episodes of back pain which

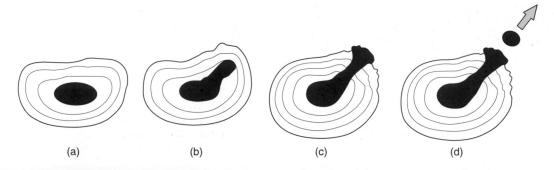

Figure 4.6   Intervertebral disc protrusions. (a) In the normal disc the nucleus is contained within the annulus. (b) With a bulge or protrusion the posterior longitudinal ligament remains intact but the nucleus impinges on the annulus. (c) With an extrusion the nucleus escapes from the annulus but is still contained by the posterior longitudinal ligament. (d) With sequestration a portion of disc escapes and may become loose within the epidural space.

may identify the occurrence of these annular tears. It is also possible for a disc to prolapse suddenly. Both of these mechanisms have been reproduced on cadaver discs (Oliver and Middleditch 1991).

There may also be abnormal movement of the nucleus:

- It may move through the endplate upwards into the vertebral body. This is known as a Schmorl's node (see Figure 4.9). This pathology tends to occur in younger adults and often does not produce symptoms until later degenerative changes occur.
- It may move centrally backwards. This movement is limited by the posterior longitudinal ligament which is narrowest over L4–L5 and L5–S1, and so the nucleus may extrude backwards at these sites.
- It may move posterolaterally. This is very common, since the posterolateral part of the annulus suffers the highest pressures in life (Edwards et al. 2001).

If the spine is forcefully flexed, nuclear fluid bursts through the annulus, which can result in irritation or compression of the nerve roots, dura mater and possibly the posterior longitudinal ligament and ligamentum flavum. Analysis of extruded disc material removed after spinal surgery has found that, in approximately half of the cases, the extruded fragment consisted predominantly of nuclear material, whereas in the other cases it consisted mainly of endplate material (Brock et al. 1992).

Extruded nuclear fluid is replaced by fibrous tissue, which contracts with time. Dehydration of the nucleus may play an important role in the reduction of the lumbar disc herniation (Henmi et al. 2002). This may cause adhesions between the ligaments, nerve root, dura mater and periosteum, or other soft tissues, and results in persistent pain or tethering of neural tissue if no attempt is made to restore mobility of these tissues.

The tendency for adhesion formation is possibly an explanation for the poor long-term postoperative results following spinal surgery and the relative success of micro discectomy which is less invasive and causes less trauma to surrounding tissues.

Osteophytes may form at the margins of the vertebral bodies. The annulus pulls on the periosteal attachment round the vertebral body margin and osteoblasts lay down bone at the traction sites

Clinical features and diagnosis

Intervertebral disc protrusions often go unnoticed because they are not producing any symptoms. Disc lesions are not visible on X-ray, but scans such as magnetic resonance imaging (MRI) and computer-assisted tomography (CAT) will show them (Figure 4.7). Such scans now reveal that disc protrusions are common coincidental findings. Up to 50% of 'normal' 40-year-olds demonstrate abnormal CAT findings such as herniated disc, facet joint degeneration and spinal stenosis (Wiesel et al. 1984).

Symptoms

Unlike a lateral ligament sprain at the ankle, for example, which produces local symptoms at the site of injury, a person with a disc prolapse may exhibit a wide range of signs and symptoms, some of which can be various distances away from the prolapse itself. The clinical presentation of disc lesions thus varies greatly.

Because the nerve root is in close proximity to the disc, a prolapse can cause nerve root irritation, and the person can exhibit a variety of motor and or sensory problems depending on which nerve roots are involved. If extruded nucleus pulposus is exposed to a nerve root, it acts as an irritant and may produce excruciating nerve root pain. There may be no back pain at

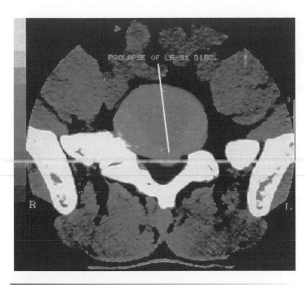

Figure 4.7 CT scan of posterolateral disc prolapse. This shows a horizontal 'slice' of the spine and has the benefit over an X-ray in revealing soft tissues as well as bone.

all but a vague pain in the back of the thigh, for example, which can be misinterpreted as a hamstring injury.

The spinal level involved may be tender on palpation, with local muscle spasm. The muscles themselves will becomes painful if they have been in a state of spasm for a long period. Palpation over the lumbar spine provokes tenderness and when pressure is applied can increase the spasm.

Sharp pain in the back can arise suddenly because of bending, sneezing, twisting or lifting. Classically, the patient is unable to straighten up and is 'stuck' – often having heard or felt something 'go'. The onset may alternatively be gradual following repeated episodes of exercise or unaccustomed activity. In this case it starts as a minor discomfort until gradually the patient becomes very aware of increasingly constant pain. A long car journey, for example, can result in central backache, and the patient cannot straighten up. Pain is worse on coughing and X-rays will not show any abnormality.

In summary, the site of the pain may be:

- central on the back
- diffuse over the lumbosacral area
- poorly localised (the dura mater does not follow any specific dermatomal innervation and so dural pain is in this category)
- referred down one or both legs (this may mimic muscle injury, and disc lesions are occasionally misdiagnosed as torn hamstrings).

Referred pain is pain that is felt at a location away from the site of its origin. It is of two main types.

Referred pain

There are many potential causes of referred pain, including:

- piriformis muscle syndrome (Durrani and Winnie 1991)
- the intervertebral disc (Ohnmeiss et al. 1997)
- lumbar facet joint lesions (Suseki et al. 1997)
- fibrous adhesive entrapment of lumbosacral nerve roots (Ido and Urushidani 2001)

The symptom may be a dull, poorly defined ache over the back, sacroiliac joint, buttock and thigh. This is thought to be due to mechanical pressure from the disc bulge, or chemical irritation. Experiments in which fresh nucleus pulposus tissue is applied to nerve roots results in increased nerve excitability and mechanical hypersensitivity of the nerve (Takebayashi et al. 2001).

The second type of symptom is referred pain down the leg. This is often thought to be due to nerve root irritation, although that is not always the case (Ohnmeiss et al. 1997). Generally the leg pain is aggravated by movements, especially flexion/extension, and eased by lying down. Pins and needles (paraesthesiae) may be felt in a nerve root distribution (dermatome) and numbness may be detected when tested by touch, pinprick or temperature test tubes. There may be a subjective feeling of weakness or that the leg is going to 'give way' – this is usually due to nerve root compression or irritation. Very large or central disc prolapses may give rise to bilateral leg pains. Compression of a nerve root that interrupts impulse transmission results in weakness of the muscles supplied by that nerve. Large bulges may cause long tract signs such as spasticity or bladder/bowel disturbance. These symptoms are referred to as 'red flag' symptoms and should not be ignored.

The quadriceps (L3–L4) and tendo–calcaneal (L5–S1) reflexes are diminished when there is pressure in the corresponding nerve roots. Flexion is limited, erector spinae stands out in spasm, and the movement that can occur usually deviates to one side in an attempt to avoid reproducing the person's pain. Side flexion is generally free to one side with some discomfort, and restricted to the opposite side. Extension is not possible, beyond neutral, especially where there is a protrusion that cannot be compressed.

The spine may be held rigid with or without a scoliosis; this is termed an 'antalgic posture' (*ant* meaning against or away from, *algia* pain) because straightening or correcting the position aggravates the pain in the leg. Most of the body weight is taken on the non-painful leg. The patient does not like to sit equally on both buttocks, leg pain increases following prolonged periods of sitting, and individuals are often seen to raise one buttock off the chair whilst waiting for treatment and might prefer to stand rather than sit. Standing up from sitting takes time and the patient 'walks the hands up the thighs'. This type of pain is usually relieved by a change of position.

Leg pain often worsens at night. The person is stiff on waking and has to struggle to get moving. There may also be a limp because the patient cannot take a normal stance phase on the affected leg. Gait is often slow. Sciatic nerve stretch (straight leg raising with foot dorsiflexion) – known as Lasegue's sign – is an indicator of nerve root tethering. This is often slightly reduced on the unaffected leg and very limited on the affected leg. Passive neck flexion with the person in lying causes movement of the spinal cord in the spinal canal and may cause pain if there is a mechanical tethering of nerve roots. This may aggravate the back pain and may aggravate the leg pain as well.

Coughing and sneezing can also provoke pain. The latter is more painful because it is involuntary whereas the patient can often prepare for a cough. The pain is related to the raised abdominal pressure moving the affected segment and tending to force the nucleus backwards.

Disc Degeneration

Lumbar spondylosis

Pathogenesis

Also known as 'wear and tear of the spine', the main characteristic of lumbar spondylosis is the loss of water from a disc. Other changes include decreased cell viability, decreased proteoglycan synthesis, and an alteration of the distribution of collagen within the disc (Guiot and Fessler 2000). Tears also occur in the nucleus, annulus and endplates.

Nourishment of the adult disc is more precarious than that of an immature disc. The first signs of spondylosis often present clinically at about the age of 30, but 45 is a more common age. The pathological changes that occur are the same regardless of site, but the differences in functional anatomy give rise to different clinical signs and symptoms.

Pathology involves a coarsening of the annulus fibrosis, and collagen fibres separate and cracks appear in the annulus. The nucleus pulposus dehydrates and becomes more fibrous with the disc losing height overall. These changes can be present without causing any signs or symptoms. 'Lipping' of the vertebral bodies occurs, owing to altered disc biomechanics, which causes traction of the periosteum by the attachments of the annulus fibrosis. There can also be decalcification within the vertebral body. The intervertebral ligaments may become contracted and thickened especially at the sites where there are gross changes. The dura mater of the spinal cord, which forms a sleeve round the nerve root, may undergo low-grade, chronic inflammatory changes. This can result in nerve root adhesions with associated neural symptoms.

Facet joint degeneration

Spines that show indications of spondylosis (Figures 4.8 and 4.9) also often show osteoarthritic changes in the corresponding facet joints. In the normal spine, facet joints do bear some load, and this load rises dramatically when disc height is diminished as in spondylosis (Adams and Hutton 1983). Lordotic postures result in increased loading of the facet joints, whereas slightly flexed postures equalise compressive stress across the disc, and unload the facet joints (Dolan and Adams 2001). Osteophytes form at the margins of the articular surfaces of the facets joints and these, together with the capsular thickening, can cause pressure on the nerve root and reduce the lumen of the intervertebral foramen.

Clinical features

Usually pain starts as a niggle and later becomes constant. It is described as a poorly localised aching type pain with stabbing on certain movements. Acute pain may be precipitated by unaccustomed activity, such as a weekend of gardening or lifting. A common site for pain is across the sacrum, between the sacroiliac joints for example, which may radiate down one or both buttocks and to the lateral aspects of one or both hips. Central pain can occur in the L4–L5–S1 region. Unlike with disc prolapse (see above), sitting usually eases the pain, and coughing does not cause an increase in back pain.

Referred pain (see above) tends to follow one or more dermatomes:

- groin – L1
- anterior aspect thigh – L2
- lower third anterior aspect thigh and knee – L3
- medial aspect leg to the big toe – L4
- lateral aspect leg to the middle three toes – L5
- little toe, lateral border foot, lateral side posterior aspect whole leg – S1
- heel, medial side posterior aspect whole leg – S2

(See the Appendix for an illustration of dermatomes.)

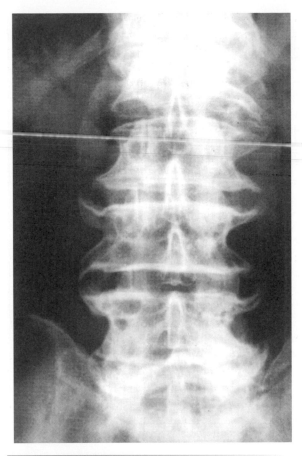

Figure 4.8   Lumbar spondylosis seen on conventional X-ray. (Reproduced from Dandy and Edwards 1998, with permission.)

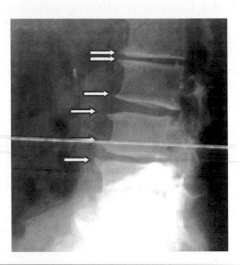

Figure 4.10   Lateral X-ray of the lumbar spine of a 55-year-old male with lumbar spondylosis. Arrows indicate anterior osteophytes.

SUMMARY OF COMMON SPINAL PATHOLOGIES

See Table 4.1.

OTHER CAUSES OF BACK PAIN

There are many possible causes of back pain, including scoliosis (a lateral curvature of the spine), spondylolisthesis (a forward slip of one vertebra on another), spinal stenosis (a decreased diameter of the spinal canal), leg length inequality, joint hypermobility, and other postural abnormalities. Sheuermann's disease (spinal osteochondrosis) is a disorder affecting the

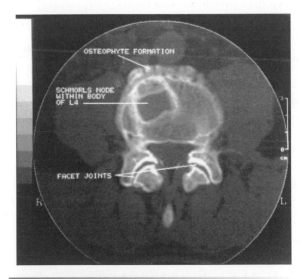

Figure 4.9   CT scan showing lumbar spondylosis at the L4 level, with a large Schmorl's node and degenerative hypertrophy of the facet (zygapophyseal) joints, which appear irregular in contour and sclerotic.

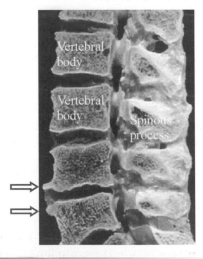

Figure 4.11   Autopsy specimen. Arrows indicate anterior osteophytes.

Table 4.1 Common spinal pathologies.

	Disc herniation	Osteoarthritis	Spinal stenosis	Ankylosing spondylitis	Muscle tear
Common age of onset	25–55	35 onwards	55 onwards	Mid teens onwards; often misdiagnosed in early stages	Any age
Pain pattern	Sudden/acute or insidious with or without nerve root pain Long tract signs result if prolapse is large Pain is worse on sitting, eased by standing Straight leg raise test is positive	Aching after activity Morning stiffness Worse on standing Eased by sitting Straight leg raise usually negative	Pain after activity	Low back and sacroiliac joint pain Worse in mornings or after inactivity Eased by exercise	Sudden onset Stiffness after immobility Eased by local heat
X-ray findings	Negative	Bony changes such as osteophytes and loss of joint space	Difficult to assess CT or MRI may be more helpful	Syndesmophytes and bony ankylosis Squaring of the vertebral bodies	None Spasm may cause vertebral malalignment if it is severe

thoracic spine and involving epiphyses resulting in vertebral 'wedging'.

Fracture of a vertebral body or transverse process and fracture/dislocations may be due to trauma or secondary to tumours or osteoporosis.

Other possible causes of back pain are: osteoporosis, muscle imbalance, pregnancy, renal pathology, gynaecological disease, malignancy, aortic aneurysm, overuse syndromes, myofascial or soft-tissue injury, discitis, and many other medical pathologies.

Ankylosing spondylitis and other inflammatory seronegative arthritides cause spinal pain and are covered elsewhere in this book.

Idiopathic and psychogenic back pain have no known cause; all investigations are normal yet pain persists, which can be distressing for the patient who fears being branded a malingerer.

MANAGEMENT OF LOW BACK PAIN

Some General Issues

Back pain is a tremendous problem in Western society, in terms of the suffering it causes to the individual, the numbers of people affected and the impact upon the economy. This chapter will not debate the merits of the many treatment techniques available to the physiotherapist in the management of low back pain. Instead it presents a summary of research findings in an attempt to clarify some of the misconceptions about back pain which have persisted for so long.

Students entering the physiotherapy profession will soon become aware that techniques, theories and therapies appear, evolve, and are then discredited, supported or modified on a regular basis. Physiotherapists often disagree or give conflicting advice about how to assess, examine and treat the spine. Whilst new ideas and debate are important if physiotherapists are to gain a deeper understanding of back pain, the situation can be confusing to the student and depressing for the person who is suffering from back pain. There was little agreement amongst healthcare professionals for many years, so much of the advice and treatment given to back pain patients was anecdotal and based upon studies which had been of poor methodological quality.

Best practice for the management of back pain has always stimulated great debate amongst physiotherapists (Foster et al. 1999) and no gold standard yet exists. Perhaps we should look at our terminology as a starting point. 'Back pain' is still used as a diagnosis, but 'back pain' is actually a symptom, not a diagnosis, and gives us no more information than a diagnosis of 'headache'. It is therefore not surprising that the management of 'back pain' has stimulated such debate and controversy.

Physiotherapists and other professionals can now take comfort in the fact that the knowledge base has increased rapidly. More consistent research findings are emerging, and more systematic, randomised controlled trials and reviews are being undertaken. The quality of physiotherapy research being undertaken in the twenty-first century is generally of higher quality than it has been in the past.

Techniques of Management

Firstly, a diagnostic triage is essential to differentiate between:

- non-specific low back pain (simple backache)
- nerve root pain
- possible serious pathology (e.g. tumour).

The guidelines discussed in this section relate to simple backache.

The accompanying chart (Table 4.2) is adapted from *Clinical Guidelines for the Management of Acute Low Back Pain*, produced in 1999 by the Royal College of General Practitioners (Waddell et al. 1999). This multiprofessional collaborative document was produced as a collation of some of the research findings in low back pain. Some of the findings are summarised below.

Most back pain is *self-limiting*, but there are still thousands of cases of chronic back pain referred to physiotherapy departments every year. These place considerable stresses upon the healthcare system. They pose a complex set of clinical judgement and management problems to the physiotherapist.

Effectively managing people with chronic back pain requires a combination of approaches, including 'back schools' (Lonn et al. 1999; Hodselmans et al. 2001) and cognitive therapies (Pettinen Rose et al. 1997; van Tulder et al. 2001). Psychosocial factors are now known to be strongly linked to the presentation and prognosis of chronic back pain. It has been shown for example that psychosocial factors and insurance claims are more significant than biomechanical workload when analysing back pain (Nachemson 1992). Management of chronic back pain should be geared towards the reduction of disability, through modification of the environment, and cognitive therapy (van Tulder et al. 2001).

The most effective back pain management programmes are multidisciplinary (Brander et al. 1997), and as with all physiotherapy programmes education is crucial. This is particularly true in the case of chronic back pain, where multidisciplinary therapies such as back schools encourage patients to become partners in the management of their own condition (Holman and Lorig 2000). The social support offered by such approaches is also important, and it is now becoming clear that social and psychological factors cannot be

Table 4.2 Clinical guidelines for the management of acute low back pain.

Exercises	Drugs	Activity	Manipulation
Specific spinal exercises do not seem to be effective in relieving acute low back pain, but back school and rehabilitation programmes are useful in chronic stages.	Paracetamol and non-steroidal anti-inflammatory (NSAID) drugs may help. Muscle relaxants may help if spasm is severe.	Bedrest is ineffective as a treatment for back pain unless the pain is so severe that movement is impossible.	Manipulation may provide short-term benefits in acute low back pain. It gives high levels of patient satisfaction.
Back rehabilitation should be considered for patients who have not managed to recommence activities after 6 weeks.			

Warning. This chart gives general guidelines based upon analysis of results from acceptable research studies. Be aware that there will be individuals who do not respond to the above. A degree of flexibility and clinical judgement is always required.

ignored when considering chronic back pain. Back schools offer a holistic approach, many of which have sessions devoted to ergonomics, strategies for breaking the fear–avoidance cycle, functional restoration programmes, basic anatomy and physiology, and ergonomic advice.

It is important to make use of the most recent research findings to provide the best advice for patients. This is of course the point of clinical research. An example of this might be encouraging people with back pain to stop smoking, since nicotine levels consistent with those seen in persons smoking 30 cigarettes a day have been shown to result in necrosis of the nucleus pulposus, as well as hypertrophy, cracking and detachment of the annulus (Uematsu et al. 2001). Cigarette smoking also affects metabolite and solute exchange within the disc (Holm and Nachemson 1988).

Waddell et al. (1999) identified the risk factors associated with chronicity of back pain, which are:

- a prior history of back pain
- total loss of employment in the past year
- radiating leg pain
- reduced straight leg raise (SLR)
- nerve root irritation symptoms and signs
- decreased abdominal muscle strength
- poor physical fitness
- smoking
- depression
- disproportionate illness behaviour
- low job satisfaction
- social (e.g. marital) problems
- ongoing medico-legal proceedings.

FURTHER READING

Giles LGF, Singer KP 1997 The Clinical Anatomy and Management of Back Pain. Vol. 1: Clinical Anatomy and Management of Low Back Pain. Butterworth–Heinemann: Oxford

Nordin M, Frankel VH 1989 Basic Biomechanics of the Musculoskeletal System, 2nd edn. Lippincott Williams & Wilkins: Baltimore

Palastanga N, Field D, Soames R 1998 Anatomy and Human Movement: Structure and Function. Butterworth–Heinemann: Oxford

Waddell G, McIntosh A, Hutchinson A, Feder M 1999 Low Back Pain Evidence Review. Royal College of General Practitioners: London [available at www.csp.org.uk/effectivepractice/outcomemeasures/publications.cfm]

REFERENCES

Adams MA, Hutton WC 1983 The mechanical function of the lumbar apophyseal joints. Spine 8(3): 327–30

American Academy of Orthopedic Surgeons 1987 A Glossary on Spinal Terminology, pp. 34–5. American Academy of Orthopaedic Surgeons: Chicago

Bogduk N 1991 The lumbar disc and low back pain. Neurosurg Clin N Am 2(4): 791–806

Brander VA, Malhotra S et al. 1997 Outcome of hip and knee arthroplasty in persons aged 80 years and older. Clin Orthop 345: 67–78

Brock M, Patt S et al. 1992 The form and structure of the extruded disc. Spine 17(12): 1457–61

Callaghan JP, McGill SM 2001 Intervertebral disc herniation: studies on a porcine model exposed to highly repetitive flexion/extension motion with compressive force. Clin Biomech (Bristol, Avon) 16(1): 28–37

Dandy DJ, Edwards DJ 1998 Essential Orthopaedics and Trauma, 3rd edn, p. 442. Churchill Livingstone: New York.

Dolan P, Adams MA 2001 Recent advances in lumbar spinal mechanics and their significance for modelling. Clin Biomech (Bristol, Avon) 16 Suppl. 1: s8–s16

Durrani Z, Winnie AP 1991 Piriformis muscle syndrome: an underdiagnosed cause of sciatica. J Pain Symptom Manage 6(6): 374–9

Edwards WT, Ordway NR, Zheng Y et al. 2001 Peak stresses observed in the posterior lateral annulus. Spine 26(16): 1753–9

Foster NE, Thompson KA et al. 1999 Management of non-specific low back pain by physiotherapists in Britain and Ireland: a descriptive questionnaire of current clinical practice. Spine 24(13): 1332-42

Giles LGF, Singer KP 1997 Clinical anatomy and management of low back pain. Butterworth–Heinemann: Oxford

Gracovetsky S, Farfan H, Helleur C 1985 The abdominal mechanism. Spine 10(4): 317–24

Guiot BH, Fessler RG 2000 Molecular biology of degenerative disc disease. Neurosurgery 47(5): 1034–40

Hanson P, Qvortrup K, Magnusson SP 2000 The superficial annulus fibrosus ligament: an incipient description of a separate ligament between the lumbar anterior longitudinal ligament and the intervertebral disc. Cells Tissues Organs 167(4): 259–65

Henmi T, Sairyo K, Nakano S et al. 2002 Natural history of extruded lumbar intervertebral disc herniation. J Med Invest 49(1/2): 40–3

Hodselmans AP, Jaegers SM et al. 2001 Short-term outcomes of a back school program for chronic low back pain. Arch Phys Med Rehabil 82(8): 1099–105

Holm S, Nachemson A 1988 Nutrition of the intervertebral disc: acute effects of cigarette smoking (an experimental animal study). Ups J Med Sci 93(1): 91–9

Holman H, Lorig K 2000 Patients as partners in managing chronic disease: partnership is a prerequisite for effective and efficient health care. BMJ 320(7234): 526–7

Ido K, Urushidani H 2001 Fibrous adhesive entrapment of lumbosacral nerve roots as a cause of sciatica. Spinal Cord 39(5): 269–73

Kuga N, Kawabuchi M 2001 Histology of intervertebral disc protrusion: an experimental study using an aged rat model. Spine 26(17): E379–84

Lee JH, Hoshino Y et al. 1999 Trunk muscle weakness as a risk factor for low back pain: a 5-year prospective study. Spine 24(1): 54–7

Lonn JH, Glomsrod B et al. 1999 Active back school: prophylactic management for low back pain (a randomized, controlled, 1-year follow-up study). Spine 24(9): 865–71

Macintosh JE, Pearcy MJ et al. 1993 The axial torque of the lumbar back muscles: torsion strength of the back muscles. Aust N Z J Surg 63(3): 205–12

Nachemson A 1966 The load on lumbar discs in different positions of the body. Clin Orthop 45: 107

Nachemson AL 1992 Newest knowledge of low back pain: a critical look. Clin Orthop 279: 8–20

Nachemson A, Morris JM 1964 In-vivo measurements of intradiscal pressure. J Bone Jt Surg 46A(5): 1077

Nordin M, Frankel VH 1989 Basic Biomechanics of the Musculoskeletal System. Lippincott Williams & Wilkins: Baltimore

Ohnmeiss DD, Vanharanta H et al. 1997 Degree of disc disruption and lower extremity pain. Spine 22(14): 1600–5

Oliver J, Middleditch A 1991 Functional Anatomy of the Spine. Butterworth–Heinemann: Oxford

Palastanga H, Field D, Soames R 1998 Anatomy and Human Movement: Structure and Function. Butterworth–Heinemann: Oxford

Palastanga N, Field D, Soames R 2002 Anatomy and Human Movement, 4th edn. Butterworth–Heinemann: Oxford.

Pettinen Rose MJ, Reilly JP et al. 1997 Chronic low back pain rehabilitation programs: a study of the optimum duration of treatment and a comparison of group and individual therapy. Spine 22(19): 2246–51; discussion 2252–3

Sato K, Kikuchi S, Yonezawa T 1999 In–vivo intradiscal pressure measurement in healthy individuals and in patients with ongoing back problems. Spine 24 (23) 2468–74

Suseki K, Takahashi Y et al. 1997 Innervation of the lumbar facet joints: origins and functions. Spine 22(5): 477–85

Takebayashi T, Cavanaugh JM et al. 2001 Effect of nucleus pulposus on the neural activity of dorsal root ganglion. Spine 26(8): 940–5

Uematsu T, Matuzaki H et al. 2001 Effects of nicotine on the intervertebral disc: an experimental study in rabbits. J Orthop Sci 6(2): 177–82

van Tulder MW, Ostelo R et al. 2001 Behavioral treatment for chronic low back pain: a systematic review within the framework of the Cochrane Back Review Group. Spine 26(3): 270–81

Waddell G, McIntosh A et al. 1999 Low Back Pain Evidence Review. Royal College of General Practitioners: London

Wiesel SW, Tsourmas N et al. 1984 A study of computer-assisted tomography. I: The incidence of positive CAT scans in an asymptomatic group of patients. Spine 9(6): 549–51

Yoshizawa H, O'Brien JP et al. 1980 The neuropathology of intervertebral discs removed for low-back pain. J Pathol 132(2): 95–104

Management of Burns and Plastic Surgery

Sally Dean

This chapter introduces the reader to current practice and physiotherapy management in the field of burns and plastic surgery. Towards the end of the chapter there is a case study of a person with burns, and a selection of further reading.

INTRODUCTION TO BURNS

An external burn injury comprises damage to the skin, and there can be loss of skin and underlying tissues with impairment of skin functions. The effects of a burn depend on its cause and extent and the site of damage. If serious, a burn injury is thought to be the most severe trauma that is survivable. For a survivor, life is altered in all aspects: in appearance, in physical function and psychologically.

Classification of Burns

Erythema

The skin remains intact, the erythema lasts for a few days, and the patient does not normally seek medical help unless the problem is extensive, as can occur with sunburn.

Superficial

The tissue damage results in seepage of fluid in between the layers of epidermis, causing a blister, which is surrounded by a dark red erythema. Movement of the burned areas can be very painful. Blisters will continue to appear over the first 24 hours after burning.

Partial thickness

1. In a superficial partial-thickness burn the epidermis is destroyed.
2. In a deep dermal burn both the epidermis and part of the dermis are destroyed.

There are blisters, patches of white destroyed tissue, and red areas (Figure 5.1). Sensation varies according to the depth of dermal damage and the sensory nerve endings involved.

Full-thickness

The epidermis, dermis and other underlying tissues are destroyed. The presenting surface may be black, white or yellow. It is inelastic and unable to stretch (the eschar).

If the burn is circumferential (e.g. around the forearm, chest or finger) the damaged skin can perform a tourniquet effect as swelling develops. In these cases the tension must be released by longitudinal incisions through the eschar along its full length (escharotomy; Figure 5.2). This procedure will be performed within the first hours of admission to hospital. The skin is dead, therefore no analgesia is required.

Aetiology of Burns

The most common causes of injury are by fire, by chemicals, by scalding, by electricity and by inhalation.

- *Fire burns.* These occur when the patient is caught by fire. Because the clothes ignite, the burns are often partial- or full-thickness. Flash flames tend to cause partial-thickness burns.

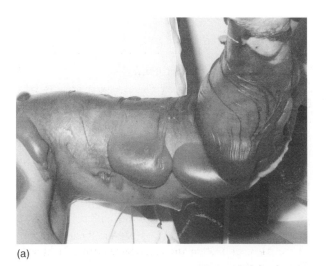

(a)

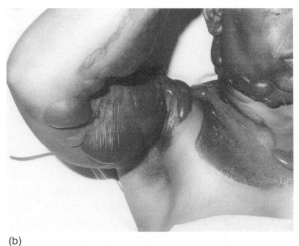

(b)

Figure 5.1   Partial-thickness burns to both upper limbs and neck with extensive blister formation.

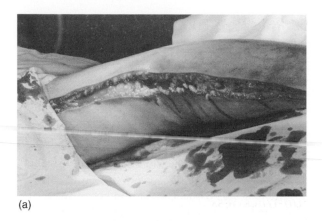

(a)

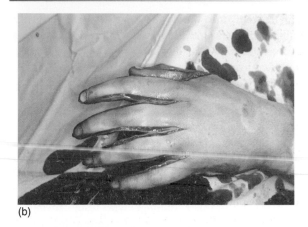

(b)

Figure 5.2   Full-thickness burns: inelastic leather-like skin with escharotomies to (a) lower limb and (b) fingers.

- *Chemical burns.* Caustic substances (e.g. cement) can cause deep burns. The depth of tissue involved can be limited by prompt action.
- *Scalding.* Hot water is the most common cause of scalds. It may be as a hot drink, or by boiling fluid from a pan or kettle. Scalds are common in the elderly, often caused when climbing into a hot bath and being unable to climb out again. These burns will vary in depth relative to the exposure time.
- *Electrical burns.* Burns will appear on the skin where there has been contact with a live wire. There will be a burn at the entry and exit site of the electric current. Neither the depth nor the size of the burn is predictable. There can be extensive damage to deep structures with little external evidence. Often this type of injury is complicated by cardiac and respiratory arrest.
- *Inhalation burns.* Direct thermal injury can be sustained by inhalation of flames, hot gases or steam. This places a major threat to the upper airway, causing oedema of the larynx, pharynx and trachea. Early diagnosis of an inhalation injury is essential. The patient must be intubated before the oedema becomes extensive, as this will prevent the passing of the endotrachael tube.

Prevention of Burns

There have been a number of studies relating to burn prevention, but from these there emerges no clear method for effective prevention (British Burns Association 2001, p. 62). A large number of burns result from domestic accidents in the home, young children and the elderly being particularly vulnerable. It is essential to ensure that:

- kettles and hot pans are out of the reach of children

- electrical sockets have shutters, and electrical cables are secure with the insulation intact
- circuit breakers are in use with external appliances
- matches and cigarette lighters are stored safely
- thermostatic valves are fitted to bathroom taps
- smoke alarms are fitted
- clothes, especially children's, are flameproof.

A number of burns are industrial, caused by chemicals, electrical accidents, molten metals, friction burns or blowbacks. The Health and Safety at Work Act 1974 and other legislation has gone some way to preventing such accidents by enforcing rising standards of safe working practices.

PATHOLOGICAL CHANGES WITH BURNS

Shock

Definition of shock

'The inability of the circulatory system to meet the needs of tissues for oxygen and nutrients and the removal of their metabolites' (Dietzman and Lillehei 1968; cited by Settle 1986).

Shock can last for 2–3 days, and longer in the elderly. Within minutes of the burn being sustained, oedema gathers beneath the damaged areas, a result of increased capillary permeability of the affected tissues. There is loss of protein and electrolytes from the blood. The main changes are:

- reduced plasma volume – hypovolaemia

- increased ratio of red blood cells to plasma in the blood vessels – resulting in increased blood viscosity and slowing of the circulation
- reduction of cardiac output
- increased heart rate.

During this stage the main dangers are from pulmonary oedema, occlusion of arteries, cardiac failure, renal failure, liver failure, and permanent brain and vital organ damage.

Inhalation Injury

Thermal pulmonary damage will result from the inhalation of steam, or from flames igniting a fuel/oxygen gas mixture in the airways. Injury to the alveoli will be caused by the inhalation of corrosive and toxic fumes released as products of combustion. It may be difficult to diagnose such an injury when the patient is first admitted and further investigations are required.

Carboxyhaemoglobin (COHb) levels are raised in patients with smoke inhalation and the level of blood COHb can be used in diagnosis. A level of COHb of over 15% at 3 hours after the incident is strong evidence of smoke inhalation.

Hypoxia can result from alveolar damage, causing ventilatory insufficiency, impairment of the circulation and reduced oxygen transport (COHb). A Pao_2 of less than 10 kPa when inspired oxygen concentration is 50% is suggestive of an inhalation injury.

The airway will have mucosal oedema in the bronchi, carbonaceous sputum and possible bleeding or ulceration of the lining of the bronchial tree. To find diagnostic evidence of these a fibreoptic bronchoscopy can be carried out.

None of the above physiological changes would give rise to alteration of a normal X-ray of the lung fields in the early post-burn period, so X-rays are of no value in the initial diagnosis of an inhalation injury.

Eschar Removal

The burned skin becomes crusted and leathery. If left untreated it begins to separate at 3–4 weeks.

After a superficial burn the skin is healed underneath. Following a deeper burn, tissues are exposed which require skin grafting.

Healing and Reconstruction

After superficial burns, the skin heals and can be normal. Following burns that have destroyed the epidermis, there is scar tissue. Over a number of weeks this tissue can become contracted and bound down or may have excessive growth as in keloid scarring.

Where there is extensive destruction of the skin, the patient undergoes grafting and reconstructive surgery, which may take months. In the case of children there may have to be episodes of surgery for many years.

Complications of Burns

See Table 5.1.

PROGNOSIS OF THE BURNS PATIENT

Age
Burns in people aged over 60 years or under 5 years carry a poor prognosis.

Total burn surface area (TBSA)

The greater the total burn surface area, the poorer the prognosis. A formula for gauging outcome is: percentage chance of survival = [100 – (age in years + percentage TBSA)]. For example, a 60-year-old with 30% TBSA has a 10% chance of survival [100 – (60 + 30)].

Table 5.1 Complications of burns.

- Heart problems
- Inhalation injuries
- Pneumonia
- Adult respiratory distress syndrome – ARDS (shock lung)
- Infection of the wound site
- Infection of the urinary tract
- Septicaemia
- Renal and liver failure
- Joint effusion and periarticular swelling
- Calcification of periarticular tissues
- Contraction of scar tissue causing joint deformity
- Psychological trauma to the patient

A 20-year-old with the same TBSA has a chance of survival of [100 − (20 + 30)], or 50%.

It is interesting to note that if both legs are burnt, 36% TBSA is affected. Therefore, a 50-year-old with such extensive burns has [100 − (50 + 36)] or 14% chance of recovery.

A method for gauging the total body surface area is 'the rule of nines'. This rule divides the body surface into 11 areas, each constituting 9% of the total (Figure 5.3). The perineum is counted as 1%. Other charts may be used (e.g. the Lund and Browder chart).

An experienced doctor should carry out the assessment of the TBSA, as the correct percentage area will determine the correct volume of fluid replacement required for the resuscitation process.

The accuracy and variability of burn size calculations using Lund and Browder charts currently in clinical use and rule-of-nines diagrams have been evaluated. The study showed that variability in estimation increased with burn size initially, plateaued in large burns, and then decreased slightly in extensive burns. The rule-of-nines technique may overestimate the size of the burn, but it is somewhat faster than the Lund and Browder method (Wachtel 2000).

Key point

Patients with poor prognosis must be treated with the same care and attention as any other

Inhalation burns

A high percentage of patients with facial burns develop pneumonia. Where there are inhalation burns as well, the mortality rate is very high.

CLINICAL FEATURES OF BURNS

The following signs and symptoms may be present depending on the extent of the burn.

At the site of the burn

- Redness – erythema.
- Blisters.
- Weeping of plasma – straw-coloured.
- Yellow/white skin – leathery in nature.
- Blackened crispy tissues – exposed blackened structures.

Inhalation injury

- Burnt lips and nose.

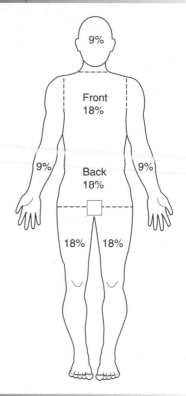

Figure 5.3   Illustrating the 'rule of nines'.

- Soot in the nostrils and mouth.
- Singed nasal and facial hair.
- Hoarseness of the voice.
- Sore throat.

During shock (up to 3 days post-burn)

- Restlessness and disorientation.
- Coldness and paleness of the skin.
- Collapsed veins and rapid pulse.
- Sweating.
- Thirst.
- Hypotension.
- Tachycardia.
- Rapid breathing – later becoming gasping.
- Cyanosis.

Post-shock phase

- Separation of the burned skin (eschar).
- Formation of scar tissue.
- Contraction of scar tissue, causing (a) pain due to traction of the sensory nerve endings; (b) limitation of joint movement; (c) joint deformities; (d) loss of function.

Long-term

The severity of dysfunction and disfigurement depends on the site and extent of burn:

- possible amputation of a limb
- disabling damage to the hands
- possible loss of independence
- loss of employment
- facial damage making rehabilitation of the patient and family very difficult.
- social rejection
- emotional trauma for both the patient and relatives.

MANAGEMENT OF BURNS

First Aid

A friend, relative or stranger may rescue the victim of a serious burn accident. The decisions made and the treatment given at the scene of the accident – especially the quality of the first aid – has often had a profound effect on mortality and morbidity (British Burns Association 2001, p. 17).

Flame burns must be smothered. Cold water applied continuously over the burnt area relieves pain and limits the depth of the burn, because heat is conducted to the deeper tissues for several minutes after the flames have been extinguished.

With *chemical burns*, contaminated clothing must be removed and copious quantities of running water applied to the area. Neutralizing agents need to be identified and applied accordingly.

With *scalds*, thorough and continuous dousing with cold water can limit the extent of the damage and reduce the pain.

With *electrical burns*, the patient may require CPR before attention can be paid to the injury. Unlike heat burns, these injuries do not spread and it is sufficient to cover the area with a clean cloth that has been soaked in clean cold water.

Hospital Referral

Referral guidelines

The determining criterion for admission to a burns unit was traditionally the area of skin injured. Now it is based on the complexity of the injury. Guidelines for burn injury referral have been set (British Burns Association 2001, pp. 68–9).

Minor burns

These are defined as less than 10% surface area in a child or less than 15% in an adult. If the injury is non-complex these injuries are cleaned with chlorhexidine and covered with a bactericidal non-stick dressing. The patient can rest at home and, depending on local circumstances, the dressings are changed every 2–3 days by a district nurse or at the hospital dressings clinic.

Major burns

These are injuries that involve 10% or more of the body surface area in children and 15% or more in an adult. If the injury is complex the patient will be admitted to the burns unit or intensive care unit.

Medical Management

Early hospital management (including the shock phase).

This involves:

- maintenance of a clear airway
- pain relief
- assessment of TBSA
- maintenance of fluid balance (see below)
- removal of adherent clothing and covering of the burns with sterile cotton dressings
- application of neutralizing agents for chemical burns
- reassurance and explanation to the patient
- transfer to a burns unit or admission to an intensive care unit.

Whether the person is sent to the operating theatre for shaving of burns and grafting depends on the depth of the burns, the age of the patient and whether the patient is fit for surgery.

Resuscitation

Fluid replacement is administered over a 36-hour period (from the occurrence of the burn, not the time of arrival at hospital).

The volume of plasma required by the burns patient is related to the TBSA and the size of the patient (Evans et al. 1952; cited by Settle 1986, p. 14). To calculate the volume of fluid required for resuscitation, the following formula is used (Muir and Barclay 1962): mL of plasma $= \frac{1}{2}$ TBSA $\times$ age of patient.

The wound areas

Management of wound areas varies according to the experience of the staff and facilities available. The two main themes are 'open' or 'closed'.

Open method

This method leaves the wound exposed. If exudate is cleaned away regularly, the area dries out. Bacterial growth is inhibited and this method is used for areas that are difficult to dress, such as the face. Healing of the epithelium tends to be slower than with the closed method.

Closed method

The primary layer of dressing is non-adherent, for example petroleum jelly gauze. This is then covered with layers of absorbent cotton gauze or gamgee, held in place by crêpe bandages or net. With bandages securing the dressings the patient may be able to begin to mobilise about the ward with the aid of the physiotherapist (see below).

When a hand is affected, a polythene bag containing chlorhexadine may be placed over the hand and bandaged to the forearm. The patient is able to regularly exercise the hand freely through full range of motion. The bag is changed daily or more frequently if indicated by large amounts of exudate collecting in the bag. The bag is changed to dry dressings at the nurse's discretion. The physiotherapist must be aware of the change and encourage the patient to maintain the range of motion as this becomes more difficult as the wounds begin to dry.

Surgical Management of Full-Thickness Burns

Escharectomy is removal of the dead, burnt skin by a method of excision or shaving. This may be carried out on the day of admission depending on the stability of the patient. A bleeding surface remains which has to be grafted.

Grafting involves covering the open tissues with a layer of split skin (see under plastic surgery below). This may be from an uninjured area on the patient (an autograft) or from another person (allograft). Sometimes pigskin is used where there are extensive areas to be covered. Grafts other than autografts do not give permanent cover but provide protection for 2–3 weeks.

Donor sites take 10–14 days to heal and can be very painful during the first few days. Where there is a shortage of available donor sites on the body owing to the area of the burn, the 'split-skin' that is removed for grafting purposes has to be extremely thin so that the donor area can be used again after 14 days. Unfortunately these very thin grafts have a greater tendency to contract.

Extensive burns require considerable excision and grafting carried out every 1–2 weeks. This is a long and distressful period for the patient who has to have repeated anaesthesia and operations.

Grafts are kept in position with petroleum jelly gauze and bandages, and splints can be applied to immobilise the joints adjacent to the grafts. The dressings are taken down at 24 hours after grafting to look for any formation of haematoma or seroma. The change of dressings can be very painful and the process may be carried out on the ward, under a general anaesthetic or with the use of Entonox.

REHABILITIVE PHYSIOTHERAPY OF A BURNS PATIENT

Introduction

The rehabilitation process commences on the day of admission. The ultimate goal for the burns team is to return the individual to society with unaltered appearance, abilities and potential. This is very often impossible owing to the nature of the burn, but the goal remains the same. The process of rehabilitation involves healthcare professionals, support groups and the individual's family and friends. The burns care team consists of a multidisciplinary team of professionals who specialise in the care of the burns patient. In addition to medical, nursing and therapy staff, a dietitian, psychologist, cosmetologist and plastic surgery prosthetist (to name a few) may be involved in the rehabilitation process.

It is impossible to say exactly what intensity of treatment a burns patient should receive, as this depends on the complexity and extent of the injury. The more complex burns require intensive physiotherapy and need an experienced therapist to assess their needs and develop a treatment plan (CSP Therapy Standards Working Group 2000).

Inpatients may be in a special ward, intensive care unit or a regional burns unit. The latter is most advantageous because the patient receives specialist attention, but difficulties can arise for relatives needing to undertake long journeys to visit. The physiotherapist, and other team members, must recognise the devastating effect a bad case of burning can have on the family. It is important to recognise mood changes – guilt, depression, anger, bewilderment and bitterness – which can arise in the patient and family. The cause of the accident clearly has a bearing on these moods. The physiotherapist has to gauge what is the appropriate reaction – sympathy, cajoling, encouragment or optimism – whilst achieving the aims of treatment.

Aims

The aims of physiotherapy are to:

- achieve a clear airway and so prevent respiratory complications
- maintain joint range of movement, and prevent contractures or deformities
- maintain soft-tissue length
- maintain muscle strength
- regain maximum function
- minimise scarring
- help the patient to gain independence and return to an active lifestyle.

Respiratory Care

Shaking, clapping, postural drainage, coughing and suction can be used to clear secretions. If it is very uncomfortable for the patient to have hand pressure applied to a chest burn, then a piece of foam may be used under the hands. Tipping is contraindicated if there is facial oedema but the patient may lie supine or on either side. A ventilated patient usually requires suction and humidification. A little treatment, often, is the most effective. Humidification may be necessary for the non-ventilated patient especially when there has been inhalation of smoke or fumes. Breathing (expansion) exercises are also important to maintain ventilation of all lung areas. The physiotherapist must not be afraid to treat with the vigour required to achieve these aims even when the chest skin is burnt.

Intensive respiratory care is required in the following situations:

- for the elderly patient
- for burns affecting face, mouth and respiratory passages
- for immobile patients
- where there is a history of a chronic respiratory condition
- pre- and postoperatively
- for patients with a full-thickness burn to the chest to keep the eschar mobile.

Joint Range of Movement

Positioning, splinting and exercise are used for maintaining and improving joint range.

Positioning

The position of comfort for the patient is usually that of joint flexion. Unfortunately this allows scar tissue to contract and cause deformities. Therefore, it is essential that joints be held in the correct position during recovery. The correct positions to be maintained are described below.

Head and neck

A small roll (towel) behind the neck and/or a pillow under the shoulders will help to maintain extension of the cervical spine. The patient may be in lying (chest and leg burns) or in half-lying with facial burns (because of facial oedema).

Upper limbs

The upper limbs should be elevated on pillows with the shoulder in abduction and slight flexion, the elbows and wrists in extension, and the hands with metacarpophalangeal joints in flexion, interphalangeal joints in extension, and thumb in palmar abduction. The joints of the hand are held in position by static splints.

Lower limbs

The lower limbs are rested with the hip joints in extension and slight abduction, knees in extension and ankles in 90-degree dorsiflexion (in a foot drop splint). Elevation is obtained by raising the end of the bed, not by placing pillows under the legs, which would put the hips into flexion.

Splinting

Splints may be static or dynamic.

Static splints

Static splints are used when it is essential to maintain a certain joint position until movement can start or to maintain a satisfactory resting position between exercises. These are designed and made to individual requirements using thermoplastics and modified as the patient recovers, such as after passive stretching. Splinting may be required at night only to prevent soft-tissue tightening whilst the patient is asleep. Nearly all patients will require hand-resting splints and foot-drop splints.

Dynamic splints

Dynamic splints can permit controlled movement of various joints. For example, an MCP extension splint to all four fingers allows some flexion of the fingers, thus allowing damaged extensor tendons to move in a limited range but not to be overstretched.

With a dynamic finger MCP joint flexion and thumb abduction splint (Figure 5.4), wrist extension is maintained and leather loops are positioned over the proximal phalanges of each finger and pulled volarly by elastic traction. The thumb is pulled into abduction to widen the first web space.

With a flexor glove wrist extension is maintained, and straps pass from the fingers to the volar aspect of

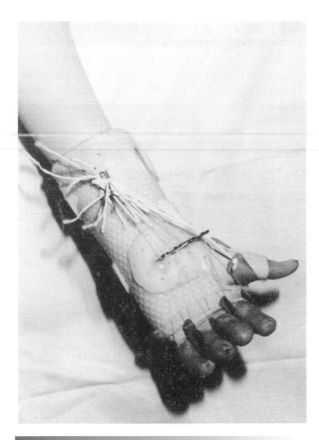

Figure 5.4 Dynamic finger MCP joint flexion and thumb abduction splint.

General points for splinting

- The position has to be effective, but not necessarily the position of function.
- Joints must not be included unnecessarily in splints.
- Tight encircling must be avoided. Splints must be bandaged on evenly.
- Grafts and flaps must not be subjected to pressure from the splint material.
- Bony prominences must be avoided where possible or require corresponding padding within the splint.
- Nerve compression must be avoided.
- Correction and prevention of deformity is essential but so too is muscular activity. Therefore, intermittent and dynamic splinting must be used where possible.

Exercises

Every joint should, where possible, be moved through full range of movement each day. An active exercise programme must be devised to achieve this. Assisted active exercises or passive movements are necessary for the damaged limbs and free active exercise for undamaged areas. If the patient is sedated and unable to perform exercises, passive movements must be carried out at regular intervals. Movement should be performed frequently to reduce oedema and resultant joint stiffness.

During bathing, the patient is immersed in water and where possible physiotherapy should be incorporated. All joints should be moved individually through full range and composite movements carried out, either actively or passively, with respect to exposed tendons and any other associated injuries, for example

the splint, thus performing passive composite flexion of the fingers (Figure 5.5).

A collar may be necessary to maintain the neck position because the skin over the anterior aspect of the neck contracts very readily, pulling the lower jaw down to the chest. A soft material may be adequate for daytime and a firmer one used at night (Figure 5.6).

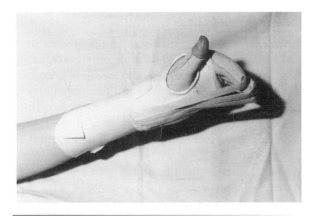

Figure 5.5 Flexor glove.

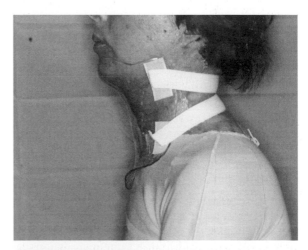

Figure 5.6 Rigid collar to maintain soft-tissue length following deep dermal burns to the neck and chest.

fractures. The exercise programme can be started on the day of the burn and must take place daily.

Exercise can be very painful; where possible treatment should be timetabled to coincide with the patient's medication or alternatively Entonox may be utilised. The physiotherapist may take the opportunity to mobilise restricted joints whilst the patient is under anaesthetic in the operating theatre. This is an ideal forum because the surgeon will be able to assess the need for release of scar tissue if this is causing the limited range. The range of movement gained during treatment will be controlled by the patient's tolerance level of pain and the limitations of movement of the burnt tissues.

The physiotherapist may perform passive movements through the dressings or the hand bags. If movement is restricted by the adherence of the dressings, then treatment can be carried out whilst the dressings are down. Therefore good communication and cooperation is essential between the therapists and the nursing staff.

Once the patient is alert enough and the intravenous drips and lines are minimal, the patient can be sat out and attempt standing. A tilt table may be used to gradually bring the patient into the vertical position. Once the patient is able to stand, walking is commenced. The use of a pulpit frame or Zimmer walking frame may be necessary.

As soon as possible the patient must be encouraged to be independent in self-care and activities of daily living.

Muscle strengthening

Where joints can be moved, the patient must work the muscles for each joint through full range at least twice a day. Muscles working over joints, which are fixed, can be worked isometrically. The use of small weights, graded rubber exercise bands and springs can increase muscle strength. An exercise programme can be devised for the patient to carry out during the day.

As soon as possible the patient should be up and about and following an exercise/activity programme. Where possible, an exercise circuit in the physiotherapy gym should be commenced.

Regaining maximum function

Function is the ability to perform activities of daily living at home, work and leisure. An individual circuit is worked out which involves free exercise and equipment work. Goals should be set, such as so many minutes on an exercise bike, so many repetitions without rest on skipping, jumping a height, or reaching a grip strength by a given time (in weeks). This programme continues

and is progressed as the patient improves, with modifications following grafting. Trips to the hospital shop and then to neighbouring shops and pubs may be included so that the patient starts to feel like a member of society again. A home visit may be carried out to assess the patient's mobility and level of independence. Discharge home is arranged as soon as the patient and relatives are ready.

Outpatient Physiotherapy

Some patients may require continuation of dressings once discharged from hospital, and will attend the burns outpatient clinic. The physiotherapist should be present to assess the range of movement, the healing process and scar formation. Contractures must be prevented by regular passive stretching, and mobility of scar tissue is maintained by techniques of scar management (see later). The patient can continue with the rehabilitation programme at the same time, which may involve continuing gym work. When all the wounds have fully healed and the grafts are stable, the patient is assessed and measured for pressure garments (see later).

As a member of an outreach team the physiotherapist may visit the patient near to or at the patient's home. This concept of the burns care team travelling to different sites to treat the burns patient is a new one and currently being piloted (British Burns Association 2001, p. 40).

Smaller burns
These may be treated by physiotherapy on an outpatient basis. Active exercise is just as important for small burns as for larger ones so that scar tissue is kept mobile and prevented from causing adhesions or contracting.

Return to Active Lifestyle

From the start the patient's independence is encouraged, and the entire multidisciplinary team dealing with the patient work together to encourage, sympathise and cajole. The physiotherapist has sometimes to push the patient hard, particularly where likelihood of contractures or loss of function is high, as with burns to the hands, axillae, chest, feet and anterior aspect of the neck.

Many patients with a burn injury find the transfer from hospitalisation to life in the community challenging and exhibit a whole range of problems at different times in the recovery process. Sometimes it helps to have patients meet people who have recovered from severe injuries, and self-help groups can provide invaluable long-term support. Return to work is obviously dependent on the nature of work and type of injury but generally the patient should return even if there are interruptions for release operations, follow-up appointments and pressure garment refits. Family, friends and employers have, therefore, to play a part in the restoration of a full active lifestyle.

Children

The treatment of children follows the same principles as for adults. The physiotherapist will need to teach the family how to perform exercises and stretches. The family must encourage the child to be as independent as possible (e.g. feeding). The patient will be reviewed on a regular basis during the years of growth until reaching adulthood.

INTRODUCTION TO PLASTIC SURGERY

The term 'plastic surgery' was introduced in the early nineteenth century. It describes the technique of moulding tissues. The work is largely reconstructive following trauma, excision of diseased tissue or correction of a congenital deformity. Burns are usually managed by the plastic surgeon in the acute phase and then in the correction of resultant deformities (Morgan and Wright 1986).

This chapter discusses the use of skin grafts and flaps and their management.

Definition
Skin grafts consist of slices of skin removed from one part of the body (the donor area) and applied to a raw surface in another part (the recipient site).

Skin Grafts

Skin grafts may be used for any part of the body in areas where there has been damage by burns, lacerated wounds, ulceration, pressure sores, skin cancers or healed contracted scars. A graft is used only when the recipient site is vascular (i.e. soft-tissue injuries). Types of skin graft are split-skin grafts and full-thickness grafts.

Split-skin grafts

Split-skin (Thiersch) grafts consist of a very thin layer of epidermis or thicker, up to the whole epidermis and part dermis. These grafts are transferred without blood supply.

This type of graft can be taken from several parts of the body, the most common being the volar aspect of the thigh, and the medial aspect of the upper arm.

The graft may be applied to the recipient site in strips or large sheets. If the recipient site is large and the split skin is smaller, the skin can be meshed to increase the area of coverage. The graft is passed through an instrument that shreds the skin at intervals to give an even meshwork (Figure 5.7).

Any skin that has been cut in excess of requirements can be stored at a temperature of 4°C and remains viable for later use, up to 21 days. The graft is wrapped in gauze moistened with saline and placed in a sterile closed container within the refrigerator (McGregor 1989).

The recipient site

Split-skin grafts are applied to raw surfaces or granulating wounds. The area must be as flat as possible and bleeding stopped. The graft is cut to size and applied raw surface down. It may be sutured, stapled or glued in place. Petroleum jelly gauze and crêpe bandages are applied.

Where it is necessary to hold the graft in contact with the recipient site, such as in a concave defect, the graft will be dressed with a pressure dressing or a 'tie-over' dressing. Sutures applied to the edges of the graft are left long enough to be tied over the top of the cotton wool pressure dressing, thus holding the graft down onto the bed.

For the first 48 hours nutrition is obtained from free tissue fluid of the recipient site. Capillaries grow into the graft and vascularisation is generally established after 48 hours. This is a critical time because movement of the graft destroys the capillary buds and the graft does not 'take'. Reasons for failure of a graft

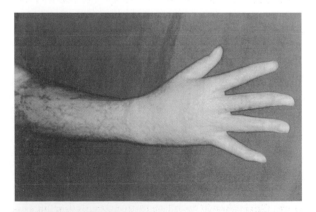

Figure 5.7   Dorsum of hand with meshed split skin 8 weeks after grafting. Note the mesh pattern in the skin surface.

may be a haematoma under the graft or 'tenting' where the graft has contracted and lifted the central area off the recipient bed.

The dressings are taken down after 24 hours to look for formation of a haematoma or seroma (space filled with serum). Grafts to the lower leg are redressed with double crêpe bandage and Tubigrip. These patients can then commence physiotherapy and mobilise.

The donor site

Donor sites are healed in 9–14 days depending on the thickness of skin removed. A donor area used for full-thickness skin has to be covered by a split-skin graft or closed primarily.

The donor area for a split-skin graft is dressed with petroleum jelly gauze and crêpe bandage and left undisturbed for 14 days. If attempts are made to remove the dressing too early the area bleeds and is very painful as the regenerating epithelium is torn away.

Once healed, the donor area is managed with moisturising cream and massage, and if necessary protected with sun block.

Full-thickness grafts

'Full thickness' (Wolfe) consists of the skin down to but excluding superficial fascia. This type of graft has little tendency to contract and it has the appearance similar to that of normal skin. Because of this these grafts are commonly used on the face or the hand (Figure 5.8).

The donor site will not heal spontaneously and will require direct closure by suture or coverage with a split-skin graft. Common donor sites are behind the ear (post-auricular) for the face, as there is a good colour match, and the upper arm, as closure is easy.

The management of full-thickness grafts is the same as for split-skin grafts. The scar management is still necessary although the graft should not contract as much.

PHYSIOTHERAPY AFTER PLASTIC SURGERY

Skin Grafts

General principles

Range of movement of the surrounding joints is maintained by exercises. If the patient is on bedrest a regime of bed maintenance exercises is implemented. Once the graft is stable the patient is instructed in active range-of-motion exercises to the joints affected by the graft. This is best carried out with the dressing removed.

The circulation to the graft should not be impaired by this activity and the therapist should observe the colour of the graft. Where the grafted area is 'squeezed' or folded, as it is in the palm of the hand on full flexion of the fingers, the circulation is intermittently occluded. The same occurs when a graft is put on excessive stretch and it will blanch. The graft should be allowed to 'pink up' in between each movement as the circulation re-establishes in the tissues. The area should not be rested with any stretching or folds to the grafted area, nor should the graft be rested upon, as this may compromise the capillary flow to the new skin.

After about 14 days, the graft begins to contract and there is danger that it will become adherent to underlying tissues. The physiotherapist must be aware of this and practice scar management techniques to maintain range of movement and soft-tissue length.

Scar management

The complications that arise from scar formation are:

- adherence of graft to underlying tissues
- contracting scar tissue
- reduced range of movement
- hard immobile tissues
- red raised areas
- discomfort of tight skin.

The objectives of physiotherapy are therefore to:

- mobilise soft tissues
- increase range of movement – passive and active
- prevent further contraction of the scar
- reduce redness and flatten raised areas
- reduce pain and discomfort
- lengthen soft tissues.

Treatment techniques
Passive stretches

Where there is restricted range of movement caused by tight scar tissue, the physiotherapist performs passive movement at the end of range to create a stretch to the scar. The amount of force applied will be controlled by the pain tolerance of the patient, the 'give' of the tissues under stretch and the circulation to the area. The physiotherapist must observe the colour changes of the scar carefully; when at full stretch it will blanch and this can be used as a guide to the effectiveness of the treatment. When the scar tissue does not respond to repeated treatments or the contraction increases, the tissues will require surgical release to regain the range of movement.

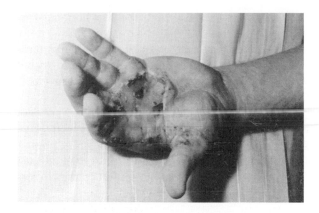

Figure 5.8   Full-thickness skin graft to the palm following fasciectomy, 2 weeks after grafting.

Massage

Once the graft is stable and the edges fully healed, massage can be commenced. A moisturising cream can be applied during this process. The massage should initially be carried out at the edges of the graft with small movements and superficial pressure. Gradually work more centrally as the graft matures. It is important to avoid pressure and sliding over the skin, as this will cause blistering of the graft. The aim is to soften and mobilise the grafted tissue to enable freedom of movement and improve nutrition and therefore restore function.

Pressure garments

These garments are made to measure and constructed from elasticated material (Figure 5.9). They are worn for nearly 24 hours a day and removed for washing and cream massage of the scars. They are used to reduce hypertrophic scarring, which is excessive formation of collagen resulting in thick, rope-like, uneven scars which both limit function and look unsightly. They

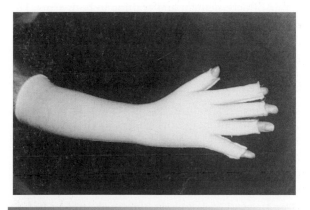

Figure 5.9   The same arm as in Figure 5.7 wearing a pressure garment.

also assist in flattening raised areas and reducing the redness of skin grafts. Pressure by an elasticated garment worn almost continuously for up to 2 years reduces this scarring.

The individual requires reassessment on a regular basis for adjustments to the garment size and shape as the person either grows or puts on weight.

The garments may be manufactured by staff on the hospital site or can be ordered from specialist suppliers. The patient is provided with sleeves, tights, vests or gloves depending on the area affected. If the garment is fitted over a concave area, for example a glove over the palm of the hand, silicon can be moulded to fit in the space in order to apply pressure.

Flaps

Definition
A flap consists of the transfer of tissue that relies on a functioning arterial and venous circulation.

Flaps may be attached to the blood supply throughout the transfer process; the part that remains attached is the pedicle or base. A flap that is detached temporarily in order to transfer the tissue is called a *free flap*. As flaps have their own blood supply they can be used to cover avascular defects, for example open joints, exposed bone, cartilage or tendon. They may consist of:

- full thickness skin – a cutaneous flap
- skin and fascia – a fasciocutaneous flap
- muscle and skin – a myocutaneous flap
- bone, muscle and skin – an osteomyocutaneous flap.

Complications of flaps include arterial insufficiency due to spasm or thrombosis, and venous thrombosis. Either will cause the flap to necrose if the anastomosis is not revised as soon as possible.

Common types of flap

- *Local flap*. This is a flap transferred from a site adjacent to the defect. It is used where the skin is pliable or loose and direct closure of the donor site is possible.
- *Transposition flap*. A square of skin is raised and moved to an adjacent defect, leaving a triangular defect which requires a split skin graft to cover.
- *Rotation flap*. A semicircle of skin is raised and rotated to cover a triangular defect. There is no secondary defect to be grafted.

- *VY advancement flap.* This is the transfer of a V shape of skin; it is moved towards the defect leaving a Y-shaped closure. It is commonly used to cover fingertip injuries.
- *Distant flap.* This is used to cover an area not adjacent to the flap. For example a defect on the hand may be covered by a flap raised from the groin. The donor area is covered with a split-skin graft or closed directly. The hand remains attached to the groin by the pedicle (through which passes the artery and vein). This remains intact for 3 weeks, after which the pedicle is divided.
- *Myocutaneous flap.* The skin and the underlying muscle is harvested to cover the recipient site. A common example of this is the latissimus dorsi muscle used in the reconstruction of the breast.
- *Osteomyocutaneous flap.* This may be taken from the forearm and used for maxillofacial reconstruction. The donor site is covered with a split-skin graft and a protective plaster of Paris applied for 4–6 weeks. The wrist and hand requires mobilising, as would a fractured radius.

Free flaps

With a free flap the skin and underlying tissues are raised, together with the artery and vein, and detached from the body. The vessels are then anastomosed to the vessels of the recipient area. These operations are performed with the use of a microscope – hence the term 'microsurgery'.

As mentioned above, these free flap transfers can involve bone and muscle as well as skin. The free flap should be elevated postoperatively, but not in high elevation, and care must be taken to eliminate any pressure applied to the vessels proximal to the flap.

Physiotherapy following flap transfer
The respiratory system

Breathing exercises with huffing or coughing to clear the lung fields may be necessary – especially after the long time under an anaesthetic when microsurgery is performed. The patient may well return to the intensive care unit following such procedures. The treatment of these patients as a whole is as for any other surgical patient on the unit.

Exercises

If the patient is sedated the physiotherapist will carry out passive movements to all joints. Care must be taken when moving the areas adjacent to, and involving the flap. The flap must not be compressed for any length of time, nor must the vessels to the flap be kinked or stretched.

Any splints that are required for positioning joints or immobilising parts must be constructed in such a way as to avoid compression of the flap or the vessels proximal to the flap.

When a pedicle flap has been used and the patient's arm or leg is attached to another part of the body, stiffness of the joints of that limb will develop. The physiotherapist must assist the patient to move the affected joints as much as possible with respect to the circulation of the flap.

Scar management

The same principles apply as for skin grafts. The flap may well be bulky and raised because of the fat layer, and this will not respond to pressure therapy. An operation may be performed some months later to de-bulk such a flap. A flap involving muscle tissue will reduce in size over time as the muscle fibres atrophy.

CASE STUDY

A 22-year-old man caught in a house fire sustained burns to his face, back, arms, legs, buttocks, hands and feet, and was admitted to the regional burns unit. The burns were partial thickness and the total percentage area of burns was 35%. Approximately 4% of these burns were full thickness. The man had no previous medical history.

First operation

On admission to the burns unit the patient underwent surgery for debridement of burns and escharotomies to both hands. See Table 5.2 for the initial assessment.

Second operation

One week later further surgery was carried out, consisting of debridement and grafting to both arms. The patient developed chest infection with oxygen saturation levels of 96% with 60% O_2 via face mask. See Table 5.3 for the new assessment.

Operation three

Two weeks later the person returned to the operating theatre for grafting to upper limbs, application of skin grafts to raw areas, and left-hand PIP joints K-wired in extension. See Table 5.4 for the new assessment.

Complications

Over a period of 4–8 weeks after the burning incident the patient developed reduced range of movement at the right elbow joint, which was painful. Heterotrophic

Table 5.2 Case study: assessment 1.

Problems	Active needs	Treatment plan
Potential for decreased ROM in affected joints due to burn	Increased ROM in all affected joints until fully healed. Maintain full active movement of unaffected joints	Passive exercises while patient sedated, progress to active Twice daily
Swelling due to burn	Prevent swelling until healed	Elevate affected areas especially hands and feet
Pain	Reduce pain to a tolerable level to allow exercises	Liaise with nursing staff on pain control
Potential deformity or contracture of joints	Prevent contractures and deformities while scar tissue forms and matures	Hand-resting splints and foot-drop splints Passive and active exercises twice daily
Potential respiratory problems due to smoke inhalation	Prevent respiratory problems and maintain clear airway	Breathing exercises and coughing two to three times daily
		Encourage fluid intake

ossification of the elbow joint was confirmed with an MRI scan. The exercise regimen for the elbow was limited to active movements within the limits of pain. A night splint was worn to hold the elbow in extension to maintain soft-tissue length on the anterior aspect of the elbow joint.

Bone exposed at the tip of the left index finger was corrected by terminalisation of the index finger at the level of the DIP joint.

The web space of the left thumb began to contract thus limiting abduction of the thumb and therefore reducing function of the left hand. Passive stretches of the thumb into palmar abduction and active abduction exercises were carried out by the physiotherapist and the family to achieve the desired range of movement. A 'C' splint was fitted to the first web space and the patient instructed to wear it between treatment and at night.

Progression

At 1 month the patient commenced standing between two physiotherapists. This was carried out twice daily and progressed to walking once the patient had acquired standing balance. The distance walked was gradually increased, as the patient was able. A stair assessment was carried out and followed with a home visit as the patient lived within the locale of the burns unit.

At 10 weeks the patient was discharged from the unit with follow-up appointments at the burns dressing clinic. These appointments were three times a week and involved 1 hour of physiotherapy in the rehabilitation room.

Once areas of grafting had healed and the condition of the skin allowed, the patient was assessed for the provision of pressure garments. These were manufactured by the senior therapy assistant who then fitted the garments and instructed the patient how to use them. The left glove was converted into a flexor glove to combine the pressure therapy with passive flexion of the fingers. This garment was worn for intervals of approximately 30 minutes followed by active flexion and extension exercises of the fingers. In between the flexor glove the patient wore a glove and a dynamic MCP joint flexion splint. Gradually the range of flexion

Table 5.3 Case study: assessment 2.

Problems	Active needs	Treatment plan
Respiratory problems due to anaesthetic and previous smoke inhalation	Improve O_2 saturation levels to 98% with oxygen @ 35% via facemask	Breathing exercises and coughing two to three times daily Encourage fluid intake
Potential for reduced ROM in joints due to the immobilisation of joints adjacent to grafts	Increase ROM in all affected joints until fully healed	Active and passive exercises once the grafts stable Twice daily

Table 5.4 Case study: assessment 3.

Problems	Active needs	Treatment plan
Potential respiratory problems due to anaesthetic	Prevent respiratory problems and maintain clear airway	Breathing exercises and coughing two to three times daily Encourage fluid intake
Pain due to surgery	Reduce pain to a tolerable level	Liaise with nursing staff on pain control
Potential for decreased ROM in joints due to the immobilisation of joints adjacent to grafts	Increase ROM in all affected joints until fully healed	Active and passive exercises once the grafts stable Twice daily
Decreased ROM of wired joints	Increase ROM of PIP joints when wires removed after 5 weeks	Passive flexion each joint and active exercises, 10 hourly Dynamic splintage if necessary

improved at the MCP and PIP joints of the left hand and function increased.

Over a period of several weeks the patient attended the rehabilitation room for intensive treatment to return to function. Activities including balance work, cycling, dressing, writing, playing cards and therapeutic putty exercises. The treatment was adapted as progress was made and the pressure garments reviewed at regular intervals as the scar tissue matured.

Discussion

The recovery period following such extensive burns is a long and arduous one; it requires a great deal of cooperation and commitment from all members of the multidisciplinary team, which includes the patient and relatives. In order for the patient to regain as much function as possible, clear objectives must be set out at the beginning and all members must be included in the decision-making process. It is essential once the patient is discharged from the hospital that the burns care continues on an intensive level by specialists.

FURTHER READING

Leveridge A (ed.) 1991 Therapy for the Burns Patient. Chapman & Hall: London

Morgan B, Wright M 1986 Essentials of Plastic and Reconstructive Surgery. Faber & Faber: London

Settle JAD (ed.) 1996 Principles and Practice of Burns Management. Churchill Livingstone: Edinburgh

REFERENCES

British Burns Association 2001 National Burn Care Review. BBA: London

CSP (Chartered Society of Physiotherapy) Therapy Standards Working Group 2000 Standards for Burns. CSP: London

McGregor IA 1989 Fundamental Techniques of Plastic Surgery. Churchill Livingstone: Edinburgh

Morgan B, Wright M 1986 Essentials of Plastic and Reconstructive Surgery. Faber & Faber: London

Muir IFK, Barclay TL 1962 Treatment of burn shock. In: Burns and Their Treatment. Lloyd Luke: London

Settle ADJ 1986 Burns – the First Five Days. Smith & Nephew Pharmaceuticals Ltd

Wachtel TL, Berry CC, Wachtel EE, Frank HA 2000 The inter-rater reliability of estimating the size of burns from various burn area chart drawings. Burns 26(2): 156–70

Biomechanics

Jim Richards

SCOPE OF THIS CHAPTER

This chapter will take you through an introduction to clinical gait analysis, definitions and detailed descriptions of the movement and force patterns found during walking, and the mathematical basis of how muscle force and power may be calculated. The book Appendix has a section devoted to background mathematics and self-assessed questions to help you practice the principles. More information about biomechanics is available in an online textbook *Functional Biomechanics in Clinic and Research*, available at the University of Salford website (www.biomechanics.org.uk).

Clinical Gait Analysis

In 1953, Saunders and co-workers referred to the major determinants in normal gait and applied these to the assessment of pathological gait. Inman (1966, 1967) and Murray (1967) both published detailed analyses on the kinematics and conservation of energy during human locomotion, and these are resources still frequently referred to. Inman et al. (1981) later published *Human Walking*, a comprehensive textbook on human locomotion.

Brand and Crowninshield (1981) highlighted the distinction between the use of biomechanical techniques to 'diagnose' or 'evaluate' clinical problems. The authors stated: 'Evaluate, in contrast to diagnose, means to place a value on something. Many medical tests are of this variety and instead of distinguishing diseases, help determine the severity of the disease or evaluate one parameter of the disease. Biomechanical tests at present are of this variety'. Brand and Crowninshield also gave a guide of six criteria for tools used in patient evaluation:

1. The measured parameter(s) must correlate well with the patient's functional capacity.
2. The measured parameter must not be directly observable and semi-quantifiable by the physician or therapist.
3. The measured parameters must clearly distinguish between normal and abnormal.
4. The measurement technique must not significantly alter the performance of the evaluated activity.
5. The measurement must be accurate and reproducible.
6. The results must be communicated in a form which is readily identifiable.

Brand and Crowninshield stated: 'It is clear to us that most methods of assessing gait do not meet all of these criteria. We believe that it is for this reason that they are not widely used.'

Advances in biomechanical assessment in the last 20 years have been considerable. The description of normal gait in terms of movement and forces about joints is now commonplace. The relationship between normal gait patterns and normal function is also well supported in both scientific papers and textbooks (Bruckner 1998; Rose and Gamble 1994; Perry 1992). This allows deviations in gait patterns to be studied in relation to changes in function in subjects with particular pathologies. It is possible for a clinician or physician to subjectively study gait, but the value and repeatability of this type of assessment is questionable owing to poor inter- and intra-tester reliability (Pomeroy et al. 2001). It is impossible for one individual to study, by observation alone, the movement pattern of all the main joints involved during an activity like walking, simultaneously. Studying movement patterns using objective motion analysis allows information to be gathered simultaneously with known accuracy and reliability. In this way changes in movement patterns due to intervention by physical therapists and surgeons may be assessed unequivocally.

Most motion analysis systems now report on the joint kinematics for the individual recorded, and also contain information for the mean for normal on the same graph allowing a direct comparison of the individual's movement pattern in relation to a pre-defined normal. Such information is also available on the Internet at sites such as 'Clinical Gait Analysis' maintained by Dr Chris Kirtley:
(http://guardian. curtin.edu.au/cga/data).

Patrick (1991) reviewed the use of movement analysis laboratory investigations in assisting decision-making for the physician and clinician. Patrick concluded that the reasons for the use of such facilities not being widespread were due to:

- the time of analysis being considerable
- bioengineers designing systems and presenting results for researchers and not clinicians
- a lack of understanding by physicians and clinicians of applied mechanics and its relevance to assessment of treatment outcome.

Since 1991 the movement analysis laboratory has become more widely accepted by physicians, and the time needed for analysis is ever decreasing, resulting in new laboratories appearing in the clinical setting. One example of this is Glasgow Caledonian University's Clinical Research Centre, at the Southern General Hospital (Bell et al. 1996). Winter (1993) reviewed techniques of gait analysis; this was a reply to the criticisms from Brand and Crowninshield. Winter gave evidence to show that clinical gait assessments can give a valuable contribution to: diagnostic information to assist surgeons in planning orthopaedic procedures; planning of rehabilitation; and the assessment of prosthetic devices. Winter also demonstrated the use of a generalised strategy and diagnostic checklist developed for all pathologies. This checklist did not focus on a particular pathology, but rather targeted gait problems, which may be common to many pathologies. Winter demonstrated the use of such a checklist using five case studies: knee arthroplasty, below-knee amputation; cerebral palsy hemiplegia; above-knee amputation; and patellectomy. The paper concluded by stating that assessment of pathological gait is not an easy task, and can require considerable expense in equipment, software and specialised personnel. Winter also stressed the need for a database of normal data for children, adult and elderly subjects.

A common argument against movement analysis laboratories has been cost. The cost of movement analysis equipment and its potential use in the clinical setting has been reported (Bell et al. 1996). A broader question indeed could be put to any clinical assessment or treatment that requires the use of technology. One example of this is the relative cost of radiography to movement analysis equipment, which in comparison is modest. Gage (1994) claimed that gait analysis costs are comparable with MRI or CAT scans. Gage also stated that the use of movement analysis, as a detailed form of assessment, may have wider cost benefits and improve clinical services more than first realised.

Bell et al. (1995) highlighted the use of an holistic approach to motion analysis including muscle performance, joint range of motion, as well as kinematic and kinetic parameters of gait. This holistic approach may be applied to many pathologies to give a detailed assessment of pathology and the subsequent effects of treatment.

Many of the techniques of collection and analysing human locomotion have been applied to clinical practice. This has led to more detailed clinical assessment of therapeutic and surgical intervention, which is becoming increasingly important in the age of evidence-based practice.

The Development of Equipment

Movement analysis

In the late nineteenth century the first motion picture cameras recorded patterns of locomotion of both humans and animals. In 1877, Muybridge demonstrated, using photographs, that when a horse runs there is a moment when all of the animal's hooves are off the ground and in 1887 published *Animal Locomotion*. Muybridge later used 24 cameras to study the movement patterns of a running man and in 1901 published *The Human Figure in Motion*. Marey, a French physiologist, used a photographic rifle to photograph movement of animals in 1873, and in 1882 and 1885 to record displacements in human gait to produce the first stick figure of a runner.

In the second half of the twentieth century many systems capable of automated and semi-automated computer-aided motion analysis were developed. One of the first systems to become commercially available was the Ariel Performance Analysis System, which required the operator to manually identify the location of each marker used for each frame. Since then the problems of automatic marker identification have been at the forefront of the development of computer-aided motion analysis. In 1974 SELSPOT, became commercially available, which allowed automatic tracking of active LED (light-emitting diode) markers. Later Watsmart and Optotrak used a similar technique. VICON, a television-camera based system, became commercially available in 1982. Since then many systems based on television-camera technology have been developed; these include the Motion Analysis Corporation system, Elite, and ProReflex by Qualisys.

Force analysis

Force platforms are devices which measure the ground reaction forces acting beneath the feet. Force platforms are considered as a basic but fundamentally important tool for gait analysis. The first force measurements date back as far as the late nineteenth century, when Marey used a wooden frame on rubber supports. Elftman (1938) used a similar method with a platform on springs. However it was not until the advancement of computers and electronic technology that the readings could be accurately measured. In 1965, Peterson and co-workers developed one of the first strain-gauge force platforms. A plethora of publications now exists on the applications of such devices in both clinical research and sports.

Since 1965 forces platforms have undergone considerable development by three internationally accepted manufacturers, Kistler Instruments, AMTI and the Bertec Corporation. Advances have been in the form of making the platforms more accurate (reducing crosstalk), increasing sensitivity (increasing the natural frequency), and making the platforms portable.

KINEMATICS

The Gait Cycle

For normal walking the obvious division is the duration when the foot is in contact with the ground and the period when it is not. These are known as 'stance phase' (approximately 60% of the gait cycle) and 'swing phase' (approximately 40% of the gait cycle) respectively.

> **Definition**
>
> The *stance phase* can be subdivided into: heel strike, foot flat, mid stance, heel off, and toe off. The *swing phase* can be subdivided into: early swing, mid swing, and late swing.

Spatial and Temporal Parameters of Gait

The simplest way to look at walking patterns is by studying distances and times while the foot is in contact with the ground.

Spatial parameters

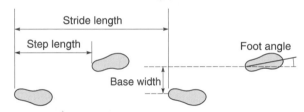

Figure 6.1   Spatial parameters.

The spatial parameters of foot contact during gait are (Figure 6.1):

- *step length* – the distance between two consecutive heel strikes
- *stride length* – the distance between two consecutive heel strikes by the same leg
- *foot angle or angle of gait* – the angle of foot orientation away from the line of progression
- *base width or base of gait* – the medial lateral distance between the centre of each heel during gait

Temporal parameters

Temporal parameters are (Figure 6.2):

- *step time* – the time between two consecutive heel strikes
- *stride time* – the time between two consecutive heel strikes by the same leg, one complete gait cycle
- *single support* – the time over which the body is supported by only one leg
- *double support* – the time over which the body is supported by both legs

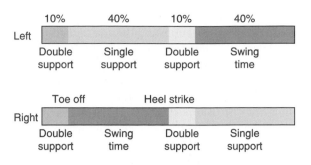

Figure 6.2   Temporal parameters.

- *swing time* – the time taken for the leg to swing through while the body is in single support on the other leg
- *total support* – the total time a foot is in contact with the ground during one complete gait cycle.

Two other parameters may easily be calculated using this information; these are *cadence* and *velocity*. The cadence is the number of steps taken in a given time, usually steps per minute. Velocity may be calculated by the formula below:

$$\text{Cadence (steps/min)} = \frac{\text{Number of Steps}}{\text{Time (min)}}$$

$$\text{Velocity (m/s)} = \frac{\text{step length (m)} \times \text{cadence (steps/min)}}{60 \text{ (number of seconds in one minute)}}$$

Symmetry can also be found by dividing the value of a parameter found for the left over that of the right:

$$\text{Symmetry of step length} = \frac{\text{step length for the left}}{\text{step length for the right}}$$

These parameters, although simple, can be a very useful means of outcome assessment. It must be noted, however, that these may not always be appropriate for some more complex pathological gait patterns (Wall et al. 1987).

Analysis of Joint Motion

Calculation of segment angles and joint angles

Normal movement patterns during gait

Human walking allows a smooth and efficient progression of the body's centre of mass (Inman 1967). To

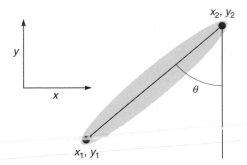

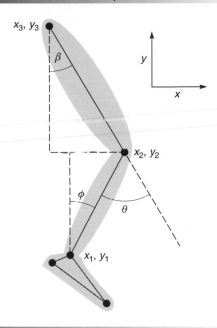

Figure 6.3   The segment angle.

Figure 6.4   Joint angle definitions.

Definition

Segment angle is defined as the angle of the body segment away from the vertical axis (Figure 6.3). The segment angles can be calculated by knowing the coordinates of the proximal and distal ends of a body segment in a particular plane. The angle can then be found by trigonometry.

$$\text{Tan } \theta = \frac{x_2 - x_1}{y_2 - y_1}$$

This is referred to as 'segment angle'.

Definition

Joint angle is defined as the angle between the line of the proximal and distal segments of a joint. The example shown in Figure 6.4 is the knee joint angle, which is usually defined such that full extension is zero degrees and an increase in flexion is positive. This may be calculated by the equation shown below.

$$\text{Tan } \phi = \frac{x_2 - x_1}{y_2 - y_1} \quad \text{Tan } \beta = \frac{x_2 - x_3}{y_3 - y_2} \quad \text{Joint Angle } \Theta = \pm\beta \perp \phi$$

However, care must be taken as the formula changes depending on which quadrant the body segments are acting in. This may result in the segment angles needing to be added or subtracted to find the true joint angle.

achieve this there are a number of different movements of the joints in the lower limb. The correct functioning of the movement patterns of these joints allows a smooth and energy efficient progression of the body. The relationship between the movements of the joints of the lower limb is critical. If there is any deviation in the coordination of these patterns the energy cost of walking may increase and also the shock absorption at impact and propulsion may not be as effective.

Joint motion patterns commonly reported include: ankle plantar-dorsiflexion, foot rotation, knee flexion/extension, knee valgus/varus, knee rotation, hip flexion/extension, hip abduction/adduction, hip rotation, pelvic tilt, pelvic obliquity, and pelvic rotation. Although all these movement patterns are of interest, only major movement patterns of the lower limb are covered here. These include:

- plantar and dorsiflexion of the ankle joint
- knee flexion/extension
- hip flexion/extension
- motion of the pelvis in the coronal plane
- motion of the pelvis in the transverse plane.

Motion of the ankle joint

The movement about the ankle joint is of great importance as it allows shock absorption at heel strike, progression of the body forwards during the stance phase, as well as being vital in the 'push off' or propulsive stage immediately before the toe leaves the ground. During the swing phase the motion of the ankle joint allows foot clearance, which can be lacking in some pathological gait patterns and is generally known as 'drop foot'.

The range of motion, which occurs in walking, varies between 20 degrees and 40 degrees, with an aver-

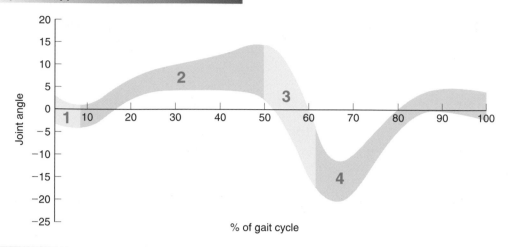

Figure 6.5   Ankle plantar/dorsiflexion.

age value of 30 degrees. However, this does not tell us how the motion of the ankle varies throughout gait. During gait the ankle has four phases of motion (Figure 6.5).

Phase 1

At initial contact, or heel strike, the ankle joint is in a neutral position; it then plantarflexes to between 3 and 5 degrees until foot flat has been achieved (Figure 6.6). This is sometimes referred to as 'first rocker' or 'first segment', which refers to the foot pivoting about the heel or calcaneus. During this period the dorsiflexor muscles in the anterior compartment of the foot and ankle are acting eccentrically, controlling the plantarflexion of the foot. This gives the effect of a shock absorber and aids smooth weight acceptance to the lower limb.

Phase 2

At the position of foot flat the ankle then begins to dorsiflex. The foot becomes stationary and the tibia becomes the moving segment, with dorsiflexion reach-

ing a maximum of 10 degrees as the tibia moves over the ankle joint (Figure 6.7). The time from foot flat to heel lift is referred to as 'second rocker' or 'second segment', which refers to the pivot of the motion now being at the ankle joint with the foot firmly planted on the ground. During this time the plantarflexor muscles are acting eccentrically to control the movement of the tibia forwards.

Phase 3

The heel then begins to lift at the beginning of double support, causing a rapid ankle plantarflexion reaching an average value of 20 degrees at the end of the stance phase at toe off (Figure 6.8). The ankle plantarflexes at a rate of 250 degrees/s. This rapid movement is associated with power production. During this propulsive phase of the gait cycle the plantarflexor muscles in the posterior compartment of the foot and ankle concentrically contract, pushing the foot into plantarflexion and propelling the body forwards. This is referred to as 'third rocker' or 'third segment' as the pivot point is now under the metatarsal heads.

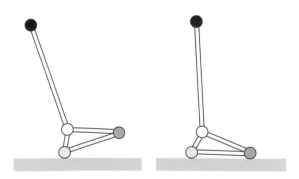

Figure 6.6   Motion of the ankle joint phase 1.

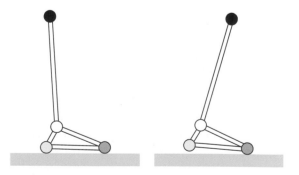

Figure 6.7   Motion of the ankle joint phase 2.

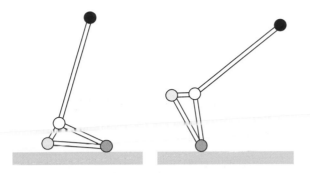

Figure 6.8   Motion of the ankle joint phase 3.

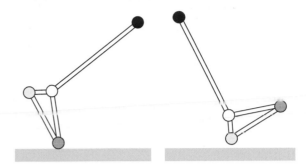

Figure 6.9   Motion of the ankle joint phase 4.

Phase 4

During the swing phase the ankle rapidly dorsiflexes (150 degrees/s) to allow the clearance of the foot from the ground (Figure 6.9). A neutral position (0 degrees) is reached by mid swing, which is maintained during the rest of the swing phase until the second heel strike. This is referred to as the 'fourth segment'. It has been recorded that there is sometimes a 3–5 degree dorsiflexion during the swing phase. During this phase the ankle dorsiflexors concentrically contract to provide foot clearance from the ground and prepare for the next foot strike.

Motion of the knee joint

During gait the knee joint moves in the sagittal, transverse and coronal planes. However, the majority of the motion of the knee joint is in the sagittal plane, which involves the flexion and extension of the knee joint. The flexion and extension of the knee joint is cyclic, and varies between 0 and 70 degrees, although there is some variation in the exact amount of peak flexion occurring. These differences may be related to differ-

ences in walking speed, subject individuality, and the landmarks selected to designate limb segment alignments. There are five phases (Figure 6.10).

Heel strike

At heel strike, or initial contact, the knee should be flexed (Figure 6.11). However, people's knee posture can vary between slight hyperextension (–2 degrees) to 10 degrees of flexion, with a mean value of 5 degrees.

Phase 1

After the initial contact there is a flexion of the knee joint to about 20 degrees when the knee is flexed under maximum weight-bearing load. The knee joint flexes to absorb the loading at a rate of 150–200 degrees/s. This occurs at the same time the ankle joint plantarflexes, with a net effect to act as a shock absorber during the loading of the lower limb. During this time the knee extensors are acting eccentrically.

Phase 2

After this first peak of knee flexion the knee joint extends at a rate of 80–100 degrees/s to almost full

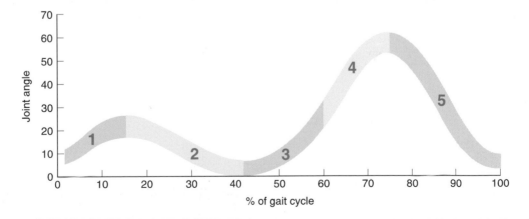

Figure 6.10   Knee flexion/extension.

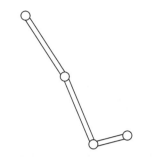

Figure 6.11   Motion of the knee joint – heel strike.

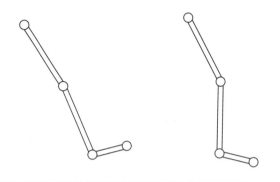

Figure 6.12   Motion of the knee joint – Phase 1.

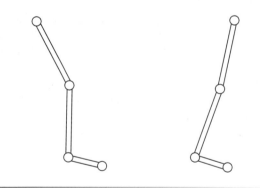

Figure 6.13   Motion of the knee joint – Phase 2.

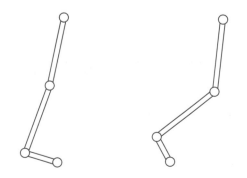

Figure 6.14   Motion of the knee joint – Phase 3.

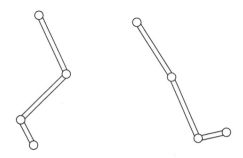

Figure 6.15   Motion of the knee joint – Phase 4 and 5.

extension. This is concerned with a smooth movement of the body over the stance limb.

Phase 3

The knee then begins its second flexion, which coincides with heel lift. During this second flexion the lower limb is in the propulsive phase of the gait cycle. The knee undergoes a rapid flexion in preparation for swing phase, sometimes referred to as pre-swing.

Phase 4

Toe off occurs when the knee flexion is approximately 40 degrees, at which time the knee is flexing at a rate of 300–350 degrees/s. This flexion, coupled with the ankle dorsiflexion, allows the toe to clear the ground. During initial to mid swing the knee continues to flex to a maximum of 65–70 degrees.

Phase 5

During late swing, the knee undergoes a rapid extension, 350–400 degrees/s to prepare for the second heel strike.

Motion of the hip joint in the sagittal plane

During walking the leg flexes forward at the hip joint to take a step and then extends until push off. This motion forms an arc starting at initial contact and finishing at toe off.

The motion of the hip joint is quite simple. The pattern may be described as follows (refer to Figure 6.16).

Maximum hip flexion occurs during terminal swing (3), this is followed by a slight extension before initial contact, (1) (Figure 6.17). After initial contact (1) the hip then extends as the body moves over the limb at a rate of 150 degrees/s. Maximum hip extension occurs just after opposite foot strike (2) (Figure 6.18), weight is then transferred to the forward limb and the

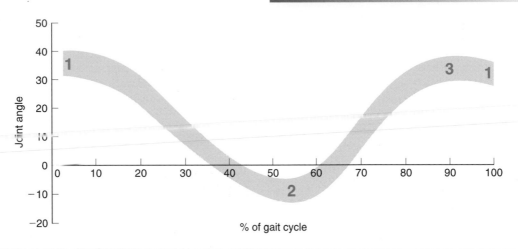

Figure 6.16   Hip flexion/extension.

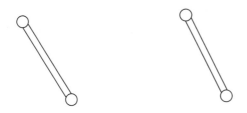

Figure 6.17   Motion of the hip joint 1.

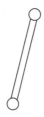

Figure 6.18   Motion of the hip joint 2.

trailing limb begins to flex at the hip. This is the pre-swing period. The toe leaves the ground at 60% of the gait cycle and the hip flexes rapidly at a rate of 200 degrees/s. This can be seen from the slope of the angle against time plot below, to progress the limb forward and prepare for the next initial contact (1).

Motion of the pelvis in the coronal plane (pelvic obliquity)

During the early stance phase the contralateral side of the pelvis drops downward in the coronal plane. In order for foot clearance to be achieved the knee undergoes rapid flexion. In normal gait the peak pelvic obliquity (drop down) occurs just after opposite toe off, which corresponds to the early stance phase on the weight-bearing limb.

Pelvic obliquity serves three purposes: to aid shock absorption, to allow limb length adjustments, and to

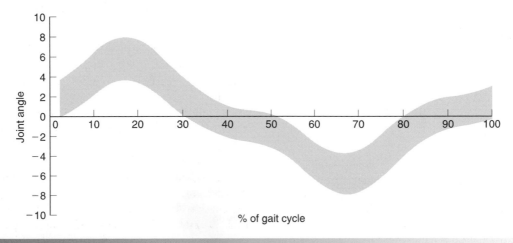

Figure 6.19   Pelvic obliquity.

reduce the vertical excursions of the body (improving efficiency).

To illustrate these points we consider an above-knee amputee gait. In above-knee amputees the pelvic obliquity does not always follow the normal pattern, as normal control of the knee joint had been lost. Hitching up the contralateral side of the pelvis often ensures foot clearance. In this way pelvic obliquity can be used to shorten the effective limb length when required. However, this may have energy costs as it increases the excursion of the vertical body.

Motion of the pelvis in the transverse plane (pelvic rotation)

During normal level walking the pelvis rotates about a vertical axis alternately to the left and to the right (Figure 6.20). This rotation is usually about 4 degrees on each side of this central axis, the peak internal rotation occurring at foot strike and the maximal external rotation at opposite foot strike. This rotation effectively lengthens the limb by increasing the step length and prevents excessive drop of the body, making the walking pattern more efficient. Pelvic rotation has the effect of smoothing the vertical excursion of the body and reducing the impact at foot strike.

Linear Motion

> ### Terminology
> s = displacement
> v = final velocity
> u = initial velocity
> a = acceleration
> t = time

Definitions

Displacement

Displacement is the average velocity multiplied by time. The average velocity may be found by adding the initial and final velocities and dividing by two:

$$\text{average velocity} = \tfrac{1}{2}(u + v).$$

Velocity

Velocity is the rate of change of displacement; that is, the distance covered in a particular time:

$$\text{velocity} = \text{change in displacement/time.}$$

Acceleration

Acceleration is the rate of change of velocity; that is, the change in velocity over a given time:

$$\text{acceleration} = \text{change in velocity/time.}$$

> ### Self-assessed task
> *Motion of the upper limb during a reaching*
> From the displacement data shown in Figure 6.21 and Table 6.1, the linear velocity and acceleration of the hand may be found. The data was collected at 10 readings per second. Calculate the velocity and acceleration of the hand and plot the displacement, velocity and acceleration on graph paper.

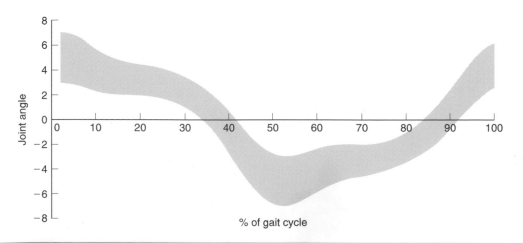

Figure 6.20   Pelvic rotation.

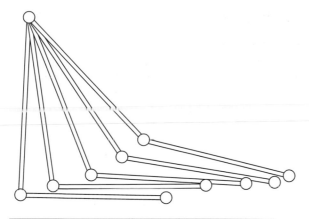

Figure 6.21   Motion of the upper limb during reaching.

Table 6.1 Data for self-assessment task.

Time	Displacement	Velocity	Acceleration
0	0.003973		
0.1	0.005293		
0.2	0.007077		
0.3	0.028080		
0.4	0.089244		
0.5	0.171660		
0.6	0.235259		
0.7	0.267247		
0.8	0.281803		
0.9	0.289150		
1.0	0.291820		

Linear displacement graph

This graph is drawn from knowing how the linear position of the hand varies over time. The graph in Figure 6.22 shows how the hand starts at a position zero and moves forward in a reaching motion. The gradient of the curve indicates the velocity at which the hand is moving throughout the task.

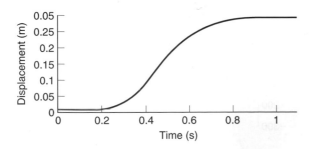

Figure 6.22   Linear displacement of the hand.

Linear velocity graph

The velocity graph is found by measuring the change in the linear displacement over each successive time interval. The linear velocity graph for the hand during reaching shows a bell-shaped curve (Figure 6.23). Initially the velocity of the hand is zero; the hand then accelerates to its maximum velocity at approximately the mid-point of the reaching movement. The hand now decelerates, as the hand gets closer to its target; this takes slightly longer than the acceleration phase to ensure accuracy of hand position.

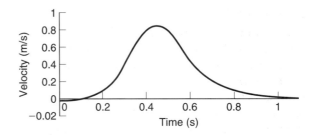

Figure 6.23   Linear velocity of the hand.

Linear acceleration graph

The acceleration graph is found by measuring the change in the linear velocity over each successive time interval. The graph in Figure 6.24 shows an initial acceleration peak early in the movement. The acceleration then decreases to zero as the hand reaches its maximum velocity. The hand then goes into a deceleration phase as the hand reaches its target. The peak deceleration is lower than the acceleration phase, but it lasts for a longer period of time as shown with the velocity curve; again this is to ensure accuracy of positioning the hand at the target.

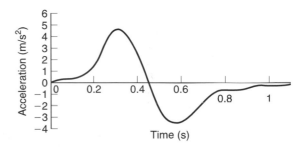

Figure 6.24   Linear acceleration of the hand.

The difference between displacement, velocity and acceleration graphs

The information presented above for displacement, velocity and acceleration comes from exactly the same original numbers. However, it is important to realise that each of these graphs tells us different information about the movement strategy. The process of finding velocity from displacement and acceleration from velocity is called *differentiation*.

Angular Motion

Definitions

Angular displacement (θ)

Angular displacement can be measured in two ways, either in degrees or in radians. There are 360 degrees in a full circle, or 2π radians. Pie (π) is the ratio of the circumference of a circle to its diameter (a ratio that is for all circles) and is very close to 3.1416. So 1 radian is approximately 57.3 degrees.

Angular velocity(ω)

Angular velocity is the change in angle over time.

$$\omega = \frac{\text{Change in } \Theta}{\text{Time}}$$

Angular velocity can be expressed in degrees/s or radians/s.

Angular acceleration (α)

Angular acceleration is the change in angular velocity over time.

$$\alpha = \frac{\text{Change in } \omega}{\text{Time}}$$

Angular acceleration can be written in degree/s² or radians/s².

> ### Self-assessed task
>
> *Motion of the knee during walking*
> From the data in Table 6.2, calculate the knee angular velocity and angular acceleration. Plot the angular displacement, velocity and acceleration on graph paper.

Knee angular displacement

The description of the angle against time graph can be found in 'Normal movement patterns during gait'. This graph is drawn from knowing how the angle between

Table 6.2 Data for self-assessment task.

Time	Displacement (degrees)	Velocity (degrees/s)	Acceleration (degrees/s²)
0	6		
0.1	18		
0.2	24		
0.3	20		
0.4	12		
0.5	25		
0.6	50		
0.7	65		
0.8	55		
0.9	27		
1.0	6		

the femoral and tibial segments varies over time (Figure 6.25).

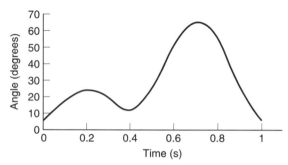

Figure 6.25 Knee angular displacement.

Knee angular velocity

The velocity graph is found by measuring the change in the angular displacement over each successive time interval. This graph (Figure 6.26) shows the speed of movement into flexion or extension during walking. This tells us more about how the movement is achieved. A flexing angular velocity is defined as being positive, and extension angular velocity negative. These graphs have been used to determine the performance of the joint and have been used to determine functional deficits in different pathologies (Richards 2002).

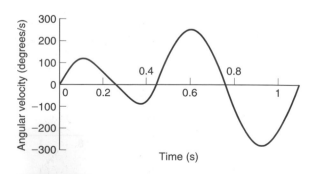

Figure 6.26 Knee angular velocity.

Knee angular acceleration

The acceleration graph is found by measuring the change in the angular velocity over each successive time interval. This graph (Figure 6.27) shows the smoothness of movement and can give information about the control of the movement.

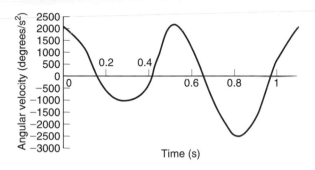

Figure 6.27   Knee angular acceleration.

Solutions to the self-assessed tasks

The solutions are shown in Tables 6.3 and 6.4.

Table 6.3 Answer to self-assessment task – motion of the upper limb during reaching.

Time	Displacement	Velocity	Acceleration
0	0.003973	0	0
0.1	0.005293	0.0132	0.132
0.2	0.007077	0.01784	0.0464
0.3	0.028080	0.21003	1.9219
0.4	0.089244	0.61164	4.0161
0.5	0.171660	0.82416	2.1252
0.6	0.235259	0.63599	−1.8817
0.7	0.267247	0.31988	−3.1611
0.8	0.281803	0.14556	−1.7432
0.9	0.289150	0.07347	−0.7209
1.0	0.291820	0.02670	−0.4677

Table 6.4 Solutions for self-assessment task – motion of the knee during walking.

Time	Displacement (degrees)	Velocity (degrees/s)	Acceleration (degrees/s^2)
0	6	0	2100
0.1	18	120	1200
0.2	24	60	−600
0.3	20	−40	−1000
0.4	12	−80	−400
0.5	25	130	2100
0.6	50	250	1200
0.7	65	150	−1000
0.8	55	−100	−2500
0.9	27	−280	−1800
1.0	6	−210	700

BASIC KINETICS: NEWTON'S LAWS

Forces

Forces make things move, stop things moving, or make things change shape. They can either push or pull. Force is a *vector*, which simply means it has both direction and magnitude. All forces thus have two characteristics, magnitude and direction, and both need to be stated in order to describe the force fully.

In *statics* we apply the fundamental concepts of mechanics, forces and moments, to the analysis of objects. A good place to start is with the laws formulated by Sir Isaac Newton. In 1687 Newton published three simple laws, which together enshrine the fundamental principles of mechanics.

Newton's first law

If an object is at rest it will stay at rest. If it is moving with a constant speed in a straight line it will continue to do so, as long as no external force acts on it. In other words, if an object is not experiencing the action of an external force it will either keep moving or not move at all (Figure 6.28).

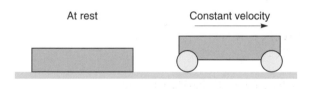

Figure 6.28   Newton's first law.

This law expresses the concept of *inertia*. The inertia of a body can be described as being its reluctance to start moving, or stop moving once it has started.

Why not perpetual motion?

Why does a car slow down when rolling on a flat road? The answer is that there are a number of external forces that need to be considered, such as wind resistance and friction in the bearings of the wheels and axle. This means we have to be careful to consider *all* the forces that are acting on an object in order to find out how it is going to move.

Newton's second law

The rate of change of velocity is directly proportional to the applied external force acting on the body and takes place in the direction of the force (Figure 6.29). Therefore forces can either cause an acceleration or deceleration of an object. *Acceleration* is usually defined as being positive and *deceleration* as being negative.

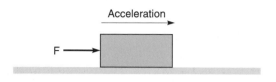

Figure 6.29   Acceleration of an object with a constant force.

If *F* is the applied force (in newtons), *m* is the mass of the body (kg) and *a* is the acceleration of the body (m/s^2), then $F = ma$. Therefore 1 N is that force which produces an acceleration of 1 m/s^2 when it acts on a mass of 1 kg.

> ### Key point
> In the SI system of units, forces are measured in Newtons (N).

Newton's third law

If the box shown in Figure 6.30 exerts a force on the table top (*action*), then the table will exert an equal and opposite force on the box (*reaction*). This does not mean the forces cancel each other out, because they act on two different objects.

The action of a force on the ground receives an equal and opposite reaction force. This is known as a *ground reaction force* (GRF).

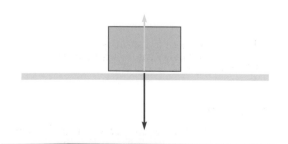

Figure 6.30   Newton's third law.

Mass and Weight

Mass

Mass is the amount of matter an object contains. This will not change unless the physical properties of the object are changed, wherever the object is moved.

Weight

Weight is a force. This depends on both the mass of the object and the acceleration acting on it. Weight is often interpreted as being the force acting beneath our feet (i.e. scales measure this force, although they never use the correct units which are Newtons).

Therefore a good way to lose weight is to stand in a lift and press the down button. You will lose weight (the ground reaction force will reduce) as the lift accelerates downwards. Unfortunately when the lift comes to a stop you will gain weight again as the lift decelerates downwards.

Another example of the difference between mass and weight is to consider astronauts. When they are in space they are weightless, but this does not mean they have gone on an amazing diet, only that there is no acceleration acting on them. Therefore weight watchers should really be called mass watchers.

Acceleration due to Gravity

Wherever you are on planet Earth there is acceleration due to gravity acting on you. This does vary a small amount but the value is generally close to 9.81 m/s^2. For the purposes of rough calculations this is often rounded up to 10 m/s^2. It is acceptable to use 10 m/s^2 for the biomechanics covered in this book. However, to get the best possible accuracy 9.81 m/s^2 should be used.

Static Equilibrium

The concept of static equilibrium is of great importance in biomechanics as it allows us to calculate forces that are unknown.

Newton's first law tells us that there is no resultant force acting if the body is at rest – i.e. the forces balance. Therefore if an object is at rest, the sum of the forces on the object, in any direction, must be zero. So when we resolve in a horizontal and vertical direction the resultant force must be zero.

Free-Body Analysis

Free-body analysis is a technique of looking at and simplifying a problem. The example below considers someone pulling a box along the ground with a piece of string at an angle to the horizontal (Figure 6.31a). We now break down what force must be acting on the box and form a simplified picture of just the box. The forces

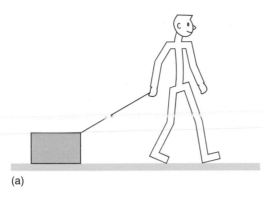

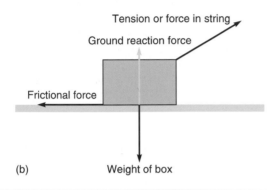

(a)

(b)

Figure 6.31 Free-body analysis.

acting are the tension in the string, the frictional force, the weight of the box, and the ground reaction force (Figure 6.31b).

Worked example

With reference to Figure 6.32, find the horizontal acceleration and the ground reaction force.

Horizontal forces
Horizontal force in string $= 10 \cos 30° = 8.66$
Therefore $8.66 - 2.66 = $ mass $\times$ acceleration
$$6 = 4 \times a$$
$$1.5 \text{ m/s} = a$$

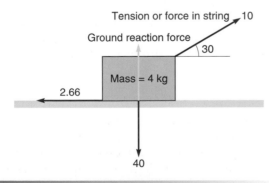

Figure 6.32 Worked example of Newton's laws.

Vertical forces
Vertical force in string $= 10 \sin 30 = 5$
Ground Reaction Force $+ 5 - 40 = 0$
Ground Reaction Force $= 40 - 5 = 35$ N.

KINETICS IN BODILY MOVEMENTS

Ground Reaction Forces

> ### Definition
> A ground reaction force is the force that acts on a body as a result of the body resting on the ground or hitting the ground.

If someone stands on a floor without moving, the person is exerting a force (the person's weight) on the floor, but the floor exerts an equal and opposite reaction force on the person. That is an example of the simplest ground reaction force, but it never happens as easily as that with human balancing, because of sway.

When standing we naturally sway backwards and forwards and from side to side. As we rock like that there are horizontal forces acting as well as the vertical force (Figure 6.33). The *centre of pressure* (CoP) is the point at which the force is acting beneath the feet. The centre of pressure moves forwards, backwards and side to side between the two feet.

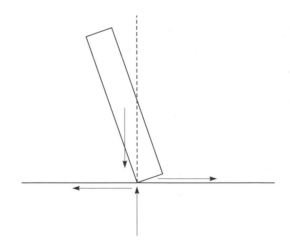

Figure 6.33 Postural sway during balance.

Force platforms

Are devices that measure and record ground reaction forces and their point of application at the centre of pressure (Figure 6.34).

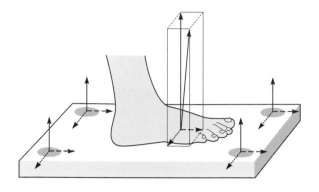

Figure 6.34   A force platform.

A ground reaction force is made up of three forces acting in three directions at the centre of pressure vertical, anterior–posterior, and mediolateral. At each corner of the force platform there is a load cell or transducer. These measure the forces in the three directions at each corner. To find the total force acting in an anterior–posterior direction, for example, all the anterior–posterior forces measured by the load cells will be added to give the total force in that direction.

Ground Reaction Forces during the Gait Cycle

Vertical force component

The vertical component of the ground reaction force can be split into four sections (refer to Figure 6.35).

Heel strike to first peak

This is where the foot strikes the ground and the body decelerates downwards, and transfers the loading from the back foot to the front foot during initial double support. The first peak should be in the order of 1.2 times the person's bodyweight.

First peak to trough

The knee extends, so raising the body. As the body approaches its highest point it is slowing down (decelerating the body) in its upward motion. This reduces the vertical ground reaction force. This has the same effect as going over a hump-backed bridge in a car: as you reach the top of the hump you feel very light, because the contact force between you and the seat is reduced. The trough should be in the order of 0.7 times the person's bodyweight.

Trough to second peak

The centre of mass now falls as the heel lifts and the foot is pushed down and back into the ground by the action of muscles in the posterior compartment of the ankle joint. Both the deceleration downward and propulsion from the foot–ankle complex cause the second peak. The second peak should be in the order of 1.2 times the person's bodyweight.

Second peak to toe off

The foot is unloaded as the load is transferred to the opposite foot.

Anterior–posterior force component

The anterior–posterior component may also be split into four sections (refer to Figure 6.36).

Clawback

Clawback is an initial anterior force, which is not always present during walking. This is caused by the swinging limb hitting the ground with a backwards velocity, thus causing an anterior reaction force as it decelerates. Clawback is often exaggerated during marching as the swing limb is driven back to meet the ground.

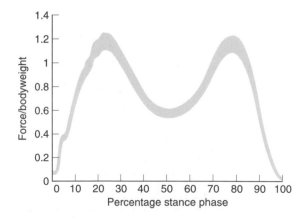

Figure 6.35   Vertical force during normal walking.

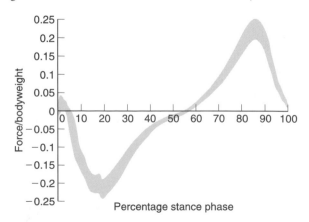

Figure 6.36   Force in the anterior/posterior direction during normal walking.

Heel strike to posterior peak

After the initial clawback (if present) the heel is in contact with the ground and the body decelerates, causing a posterior shear force. Imagine you are walking on a thick carpet, loading your front foot, and suddenly you are transported to an ice rink – your leg would slide forwards. This is because the frictional force between the ice and your foot is very low, whereas the carpet can provide a much larger posterior reaction force that stops your leg from slipping forwards. The posterior peak should be in the order of 0.2 times the person's bodyweight.

Posterior peak to crossover

The posterior component reduces as the body begins to move over the stance limb, reducing the horizontal component of the resultant ground reaction force.

Crossover to anterior peak

The heel lifts and the foot is pushed down and back into the ground by the action of muscles in the posterior compartment of the ankle joint. This has the effect of producing an anterior component of the ground reaction force, which propels the body forwards. The anterior peak should be in the order of 0.2 times the person's bodyweight.

Anterior peak to toe off

This is now the period of terminal double support where the force is being transferred to the front foot. The anterior force therefore reduces.

Mediolateral force component

The mediolateral component may be split into two main sections (refer to Figure 6.37). Initially at heel strike there is a lateral thrust during loading; during this time the foot is working as a mobile adaptor. After the initial loading, the forces push in a medial direction as the body moves over the stance limb. Small lateral forces are often seen during the final push-off stage.

The mediolateral forces are the most variable of the three components, and can easily be affected by footwear and foot orthotics. Normal maximum medial force is between 0.05 and 0.1 times the person's bodyweight. The maximum lateral force should be less than the maximum medial force.

How to study the measurements taken from these graphs

For each of these measurements the percentage difference can be studied between the left and right sides, and between the subject tested and non-pathological data. This will not only identify what differences are present in the walking patterns, but also how big the differences are.

Pedotti Diagrams

The interaction of the vertical and anterior–posterior forces described above may be shown with a Pedotti diagram. This shows the magnitude of the resultant ground reaction force.

Pedotti diagrams rely on the information provided by force platforms. To construct a Pedotti diagram we need to know the vertical and horizontal forces and the positions of the forces beneath the foot in the plane of interest for each moment in time.

As a subject walks, the forces during the stance phase move forward from under the heel to the toe, so the position of the force moves from posterior to anterior. As we have seen in the previous section, the vertical and horizontal ground reaction forces are continually changing during the stance phase, so

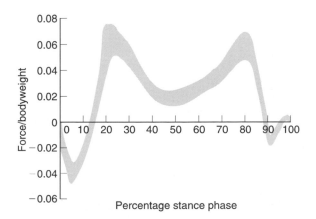

Figure 6.37   Force in the mediolateral direction during normal walking.

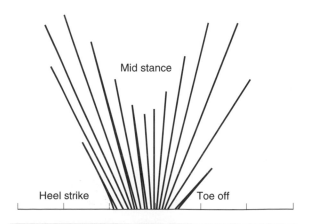

Figure 6.38   Pedotti diagram during normal walking.

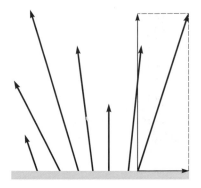

Figure 6.39   Vertical, horizontal and resultant ground reaction forces at heel off.

Table 6.5 Data for the self-assessment task.

Position (m)	Anterior–posterior force (N)	Vertical force (N)
0	−8	66
0.04	−155	678
0.08	−180	878
0.12	−54	622
0.16	−13	457
0.2	26	564
0.24	106	889
0.28	180	626
0.32	10	16

changing the direction and magnitude of the resultant ground reaction force (Figure 6.38).

Figure 6.39 shows the vertical, horizontal and resultant ground reaction force components being drawn at heel off. The centre of pressure has moved forwards from the heel to the forefoot and the new vertical, hor-

izontal and resultant ground reaction force components are drawn from the new position. This process is repeated throughout the stance phase, producing a butterfly-like diagram.

Video Vector Generators

The video vector generator is a piece of equipment that combines the information from a force platform with a video image. The resultant force can be superimposed on top of the video information, giving a picture of the action of the ground reaction forces (Figure 6.42). This uses the same information as displayed in the Pedotti diagram, but also allows the action of the forces to be seen with respect to the joints of the lower limb. This information may be used to identify biomechanical pathologies and monitor gross changes due to treatment.

Self-assessed task

Construct a Pedotti diagram

Use the data in Figure 6.40 and Table 6.5 to plot a Pedotti diagram on graph paper.

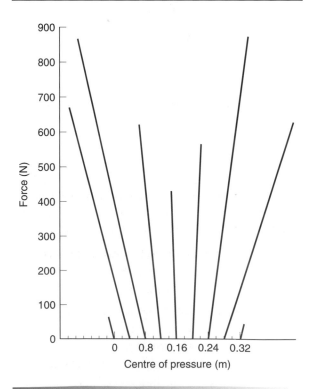

Figure 6.40   Data for the self-assessment task.

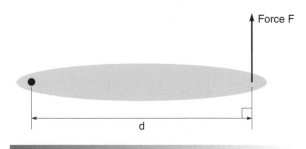

Figure 6.41   The moment of a force.

Definition

A moment (*M*) is defined as the magnitude of force *F* (how hard you push) multiplied by the perpendicular distance *d* of the force away from the pivot. So $M = Fd$ (Figure 6.42).

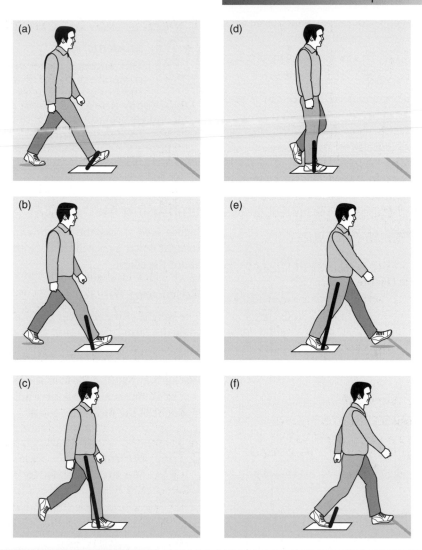

Figure 6.42 Output of a video vector generator, showing the ground reaction force (GRF) at (a) heel strike; (b) just after heel strike; (c) at foot flat; (d) at mid stance; (e) at heel off; and (f) just before toe off.

INVERSE DYNAMICS: MOMENTS

When a force acts on a body some distance away from its pivoting point, a turning effect is set up. Consider opening and closing a door, whereby you are creating sufficient force to turn the door on its hinges. The force required to do this action multiplied by the distance away from the hinges is referred to as the *moment* (also sometimes called torque).

Now consider the see-saw in Figure 6.43a. It is clear that the see-saw will not balance. However, if the 10 kg mass is moved so it is half the distance away from the pivot (point of rotation), as in Figure 6.43b, it will balance. This is explained below.

To solve problems with moments we have to consider the action of each force in turn. To do this we

consider if it will rotate the object (in this case a see-saw) in a clockwise or anticlockwise direction. If it is in a clockwise direction it is considered to be in a positive direction, and if anticlockwise it is considered to be in a negative direction (these are abitrary choices).

Force = mass × acceleration due to gravity

$$F1 = 10 \times 9/81$$
$$F1 = 98.1 \text{ N}$$

(this will try and turn the see-saw anti-clockwisse)

$$F2 = 5 \times 9.81$$
$$F2 = 49.05 \text{ N}$$

(this will try and turn the see-saw clockwise)

If the see-saw balances then the sum of the clockwise turning effects and anti-clockwise turning effects must be zero. If we say that anti-clockwise moments are negative and clockwise ones are positive, then:

Sum of the Moments = –(F1 × 0.5) + (F2 × 1)
Sum of the Moments = –(98.1 × 0.5) + (49.05 × 1) = 0

i.e. If the sum of the moments on the see-saw is zero then the see-saw will balance.

Although there seems to be little effect when we consider the see-saw vertically, we have a mass on each side giving a total force of 98.1 + 49.05 = 147.15 N downwards. From Newton's third law we know that there must be an equal and opposite reaction at the pivot of 147.15 N acting up on to the pivot of the see-saw.

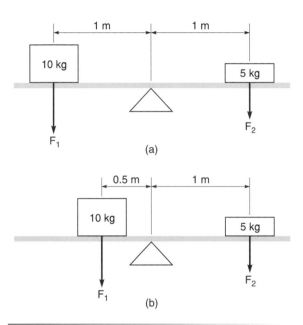

Figure 6.43 Two ways of balancing a see-saw.

CALCULATION OF MOMENTS ABOUT JOINTS

These can be found in the same was as finding moments acting on a see-saw, as in the preceding section. Therefore all we need is the forces acting about a joint and the distances at which they act from the joint.

However, forces seldom act at 90 degrees to body segments. Therefore we invariably need first to *resolve* the forces. There are two methods we can use:

- method 1 – the component of force at 90 degrees to the body segment
- method 2 – the horizontal and vertical components of the force relative to the ground.

Students' note

This author's preference is to use the component of force at 90 degrees to the body segment *for upper limb and upper body* (trunk) problems, and the horizontal and vertical components of the force relative to the ground for *lower limb* problems which involve ground reaction forces.

Calculation of moments in the upper limb using method 1

Figure 6.44 shows the weight of the forearm acting straight down. This will produce an extending moment about the elbow.

Resolving the force

The weight of the forearm is not acting perpendicular to the forearm so we cannot use it to find the moment. However, if we find the component of the weight acting perpendicular to the forearm then we can. See 'Background Maths' for help with resolving.

The component acting perpendicular to the forearm = weight of the forearm × cos Θ.

Information

See the Appendix for help with resolving forces.

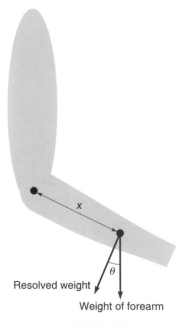

Figure 6.44 Moments in the upper limb using method 1.

Moments about the elbow

The component of the weight is acting a perpendicular distance of x away from the elbow. Therefore:

Moment about the elbow
= weight of the forearm $\times \cos \Theta \times x$.

Calculation of moments in the lower limb using method 2

Figure 6.45 shows the resultant ground reaction force seen at foot flat in a normal subject. The resultant force can be broken up into two separate components, one in the vertical direction and the other in the horizontal direction.

If we consider the moments about the knee, we need to find out the effects of both the vertical and horizontal components of the resultant ground reaction force.

Resolving the forces

Vertical component = Resultant $\times \sin \Theta$
Horizontal component = Resultant $\times \cos \Theta$.

Moments about the knee

To find the moment about the knee we are going to consider each of these forces separately.

- The horizontal force (Resultant $\times \cos \Theta$) is passing a perpendicular distance y below the knee. This force will try to turn the knee in a clockwise direction.

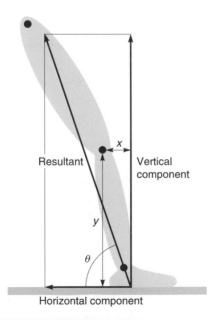

Figure 6.45   Moments in the lower limb using method 2.

- The vertical force (Resultant $x \sin \Theta$) is passing a perpendicular distance x in front of the knee. This force will try to turn the knee in an anticlockwise direction.

If we say all moments going clockwise are positive and those going anticlockwise are negative, then moments about the knee may be written:

Moment about the knee
= Resultant $\times \cos \Theta \times y$ – Resultant $\times \sin \Theta \times x$.

CALCULATION OF MUSCLE AND JOINT FORCES

Students without a maths background should not become too worried as this section uses exactly the same principles dealt with in previous sections.

Muscle forces may be considered in the same way as balancing forces on a see-saw, and joint forces may be considered in the same way as the force at the pivot in the middle of the see-saw.

Muscle Forces

One way to calculate the moment due to a force inclined at an angle is to break the force up into two perpendicular components. This is usually necessary in biomechanics calculations where the muscle acts at an angle to a body segment, as in the example in Figure 6.46. The muscle force has components along and perpendicular to the axis of the arm.

- The *rotary component* is the force that tries to turn the body segment around the proximal joint (e.g. flexing or extending the elbow joint), and balances the external moments acting on the body segment.

   Rotary component = muscle force $\times \sin$ A

- The *stabilising component* is the force that acts along the body segment (e.g. the forearm) forcing into, or pulling out of, the joint.

   Stabilizing component = muscle force $\times \cos$ A

The first of these component forces acts through the pivot and has zero moment; the second will produce a moment about the proximal joint.

Joint Forces

To find the joint force we first need to think back to the see-saw, where the force at the pivot was equal to the

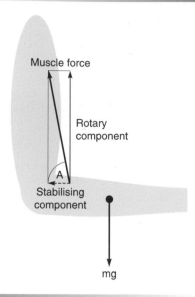

Figure 6.46   Components of muscle force.

sum of the two forces acting downwards. We shall adopt the same technique here (Figure 6.47).

First we need to find all the forces acting in a vertical direction (including the vertical component of the muscle force). The only force we will not know is the vertical force at the joint. The sum of all these forces must be zero.

Then we need to find all the forces acting in a horizontal direction (including the horizontal component of the muscle force). The only force we will not know is the horizontal force at the joint. The sum of all these forces must also be zero.

Worked Example 1: Calculation of Muscle and Joint Forces in the Upper Limb

Consider the tuning moments about the elbow joint while holding a pint of beer (Figure 6.48). Assume that the weight of a pint of beer is 7 newtons (N) and the weight of the forearm and hand is 25 N. The distance d_1 from the elbow joint to the centre of mass of the forearm and hand is 0.15 m, and the distance d_2 from the elbow joint to the beer is 0.4 m.

Finding the moment about the elbow joint

Moment = force × perpendicular distance. Therefore:

Moments about the Elbow Joint
= (weight of forearm × com)
+ (weight of beer × length of forearm)

Moments about the Elbow Joint
= $(25 \times 0.15) + (7 \times 0.4)$

Moments about the Elbow Joint
= 3.75 + 2.28 = 6.55 Nm.

Finding the force in the muscle

Assume that the muscle is inclined to the forearm at 80 degrees (angle A) and the muscle insertion point is 0.04 m away from the elbow joint (Figure 6.49).

The muscle must provide an equal and opposite moment to support the weight of the arm and the

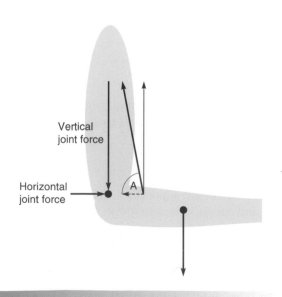

Figure 6.47   Components of joint force.

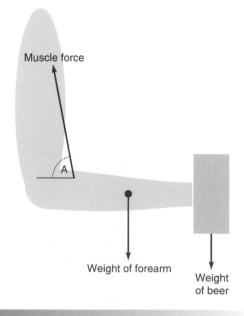

Figure 6.48   Schematic for worked example 1.

weight of the beer. However, the muscle is inclined to the forearm so the muscle force needs to be resolved so that it is perpendicular to the distance from the elbow joint.

If the muscle force is given the symbol m_f so the vertical component (or rotary component) of it will be $m_f \sin 80°$.

As the muscle produces an equal and opposite moment, the clockwise component must equal the anticlockwise component, i.e. the muscle must provide an equal and opposite moment to

Moments about the elbow joint = 6.55 Nm
Therefore:

$$m_f \sin 80° \times 0.04 = 6.55$$
$$m_f = 6.55 / (\sin 80° \times 0.04)$$
$$m_f = 166.3 \text{ N}.$$

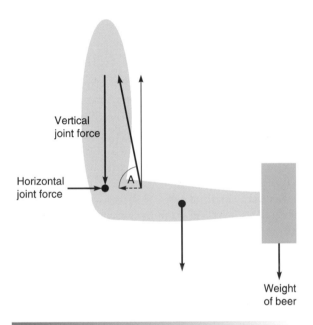

Figure 6.49 Resolving the horizontal and vertical forces.

Finding the joint force

Vertical forces

In the problem above the vertical forces include: $m_f \sin 80°$ (163.75 N), weight of beer (7 N), weight of the forearm (25 N), and the vertical joint force. If the force is acting up we will call it positive, if it is acting down we will call it negative. Therefore:

$$163.75 - 7 - 25 - \text{vertical joint force} = 0$$
$$163.75 - 7 - 25 = \text{vertical joint force}$$
$$131.75 \text{ N} = \text{vertical joint force}$$

Horizontal forces

The horizontal forces in this problem are easier; the only forces which will have a horizontal component are the muscle force and the joint force:

$m_f \cos 80°$ (28.9 N) and the horizontal joint force.

If the force is acting to the right we will call it positive, if it is acting to the left we will call it negative.

$$\text{Horizontal joint force} - 28.9 = 0$$
$$\text{Horizontal force} = 28.9 \text{ N}.$$

Resultant joint force

There is one last step. What we want to find is the total effect on the joint, or the resultant joint force. This can simply be found using Pythagoras:

$$131.75^2 + 28.9^2 = R^2$$
$$134.9 = R = \text{Resultant Joint Force}$$

Worked Example 2: Calculation of Moments in the Lower Limb

Figure 6.50 shows the ground reaction force acting at heel strike. The point of application of the ground reaction force, and the position of the ankle, knee and hip joints are known. We wish to calculate the moments produced by the ground reaction force about (i) the ankle joint, (ii) the knee joint, and (iii) the hip joint.

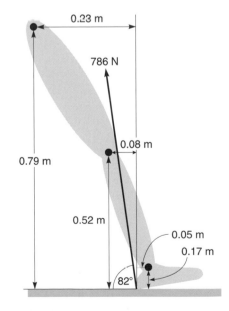

Figure 6.50 Schematic for worked example 2.

First resolve forces vertically and horizontally:

$$786 \times \cos 82 = \text{horizontal force}$$
$$786 \times \sin 82 = \text{vertical force}$$
$$\text{horizontal force} = 109 \text{ N}$$
$$\text{vertical force} = 778 \text{ N}.$$

Moments about joints

$M_{\text{ankle}} = 778 \times 0.05 + 109 \times 0.17 = 57 \text{ Nm}$
$M_{\text{knee}} = -778 \times 0.08 + 109 \times 0.52 = -6 \text{ Nm}$
$M_{\text{hip}} = -778 \times 0.23 + 109 \times 0.79 = -92 \text{ Nm}.$

Worked Example 3: Calculation of Muscle and Joint Forces on the Base of the Spine

A person lifts a weight of 600 N, as shown in Figure 6.51a.
Mass of trunk = 52.5 kg
Mass of head = 8.5 kg
Mass of upper arms = 5.8 kg
Mass of forearm = 3.4 kg.

(i)   If the centre of mass of the trunk, arms and head is a horizontal distance of 0.2 m from L5–S1 (the base of the spine) and the weights being lifted are a horizontal distance of 0.42 m from L5–S1, find the moment about L5–S1.
(ii) If this moment were supported entirely by the muscle E acting 0.07 m away from L5–S1, what would be the force in the muscle?
(iii) Find the resultant force at L5–S1 if the force E is acting at 40 degrees to the vertical.

Solution

(i) $M = 600 \times 0.42 + 702 \times 0.2 = 392.4$ Nm.
(ii) $392.4 \text{ Nm} = E \times 0.07$
      $392.4 / 0.07 = E$
      $5606 \text{ N} = E$
(iii) Force E is acting at an angle to vertical and horizontal, so we find the vertical and horizontal component by resolving:
      $E_{\text{v}} = 5606 \times \cos 40 = 4294$ N
      $E_{\text{h}} = 5606 \times \sin 40 = 3603$ N

Total force vertical = 4294 + 600 + 702 = 5596 N
Total force horizontal = 3603 N

Resultant = sq root $(5596^2 + 3603^2)$
Resultant = 6655 N.

LINEAR WORK, ENERGY AND POWER

Linear Work

> **Definition**
> Work is a product of a force applied to a body and the displacement of the body in the direction of the applied force (Figure 6.52). Work = force × displacement ($W = Fs$).

Linear work does not refer to the muscular or mental effort. Work is basically a force overcoming a resistance and moving an object through a distance. If, for example, an object is lifted from the floor to the top of a

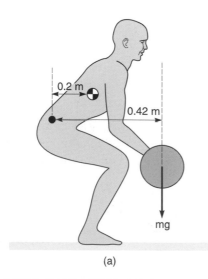

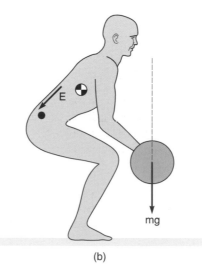

(a)   (b)

Figure 6.51   Schematic for worked example 3.

Key point

Holding a book steadily at arm's length does not involve any work, irrespective of the effort required, because there is no movement of the applied force.

table, work is done in overcoming the downward force due to gravity. On the other hand, if a constantly acting force does not produce motion, no work is performed.

The units of work are newtons × metres, or *joules* (J).

Linear Power

Power is the *rate* of performing work or transferring energy. So power measures how quickly the work is done.

Suppose a person pushes a box from one end of the room to the other in ten seconds, then pushes the box back to its original position in five seconds. In each trip across the room, the force applied and the distance the box is moved is the same, so the work done in each case is the same. But the second time the box is pushed across the room, the person has to produce more power than in the first trip because the same amount of work is done in five seconds rather than ten.

Power = Work done/Time taken

The units of power are joules per second (J/s), or *watts* (W).

Linear Energy

While work is done on a body, there is a transfer of energy to the body, and so work can be said to be 'energy in transit'.

Energy has the same units as work (*joules*), as the work done produces a change in energy.

Energy is the capacity of matter to perform work as the result of its motion or its position in relation to forces acting on it. Energy related to position is known as *potential energy*, and energy associated with motion

is known as *kinetic energy*. A swinging pendulum has maximum potential energy at the terminal points; at all intermediate positions it has both kinetic and potential energy in varying proportions.

Conservation of energy

Energy can be transformed but it cannot be created or destroyed. In the process of transformation either kinetic or potential energy may be lost or gained, but the sum total of the two remains always the same.

Potential energy

This is stored energy possessed by a system as a result of the relative positions of the components of that system. For example, if a ball is held above the ground, the system comprising the ball and the earth has a certain amount of potential energy; lifting the ball higher increases the amount of potential energy the system possesses. This is expressed mathematically as $PE = mgh$ (mass times gravity times height).

Work is needed to lift the ball up, giving the system potential energy. It takes effort to lift a ball off the ground. The amount of potential energy a system possesses is equal to the work done on the system.

Potential energy also can be transformed into other forms of energy. For example, when a ball is held above the ground and released, the potential energy is transformed into kinetic energy.

Kinetic energy

This is energy possessed by an object, resulting from the motion of that object. The magnitude of the kinetic energy depends on both the mass and the speed of the object according to the equation $KE = \frac{1}{2}mv^2$.

Angular Work and Power

Angular work

Work = force × distance moved

The distance the force is moved is not in a straight line as with linear work, but in an arc. To find the angular work the length of the arc must first be found.

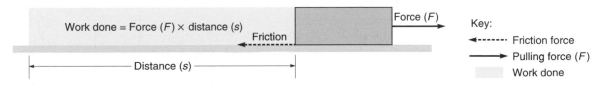

Figure 6.52 Linear work.

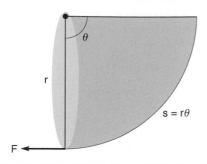

Figure 6.53   Angular work.

The length of the arc is affected by the radius of the arc, and the angle moved through.

$$\text{Length of an Arc} = \text{Radius} \times \text{Angular Displacement}$$
$$\text{Length of an Arc} = r\Theta$$

Note: The angular displacement must be measured in Radians (Rads), 1 radian = 57.3°

$$\text{work} = Fs$$
$$\text{Angular work} = Fr\Theta$$

However

$$\text{Force} \times r = \text{Moment (M)}$$

Therefore

$$\text{Work} = \text{Moment } (M) \times \Theta$$

Angular power

$$\text{Power} = \frac{\text{Work done}}{\text{Time taken}}$$

$$\text{Power} = \frac{\text{Force} \times \Theta \times r}{t}$$

or

$$\text{Power} = \frac{\text{Moment } (M) \times t}{\text{Time taken}}$$

$$\text{Power} = \frac{M \times \Theta}{t}$$

However

$$\Theta/t = \omega \text{ (angular velocity)}$$

so

$$\text{Power} = M\omega$$
$$\omega \text{ is in Radian/s (rad/s)}$$

STRENGTH TESTING AND TRAINING

When a physiotherapist evaluates muscle strength, the records taken are not direct measures of the actual strength of the muscle or muscle group. What is usually recorded is the effective *moment* being produced by the muscle, as described fully in the preceding section. What is hard to find out is the actual load taken by an individual muscle.

Most measures taken in the clinical setting do not go as far as to estimate actual muscle forces. However, there are a number of methods of *indirect evaluation*. The indirect evaluation of the power produced by a muscle is influenced by several factors, which may be grouped into: position, type of contraction, and speed of contraction.

Position
The position of the body segment

The position of the body segment changes the effective moment caused by gravity. As the body segment is moved away from the horizontal position the moment due to the weight of the body segment will decrease (Figure 6.54).

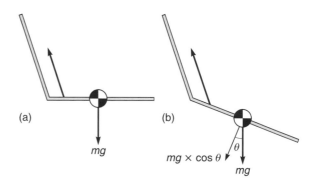

Figure 6.54   Position of the body segment.

The position of the applied load

If you position a load at the end of a subject's arm to see whether he or she can support it, the turning force will depend on the size of the load and the subject's limb length (Figure 6.55). When assessing muscle strength both these factors should be measured and taken into account with respect the function of that muscle group.

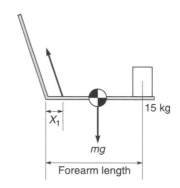

Figure 6.55   Position of the applied load.

Type of muscle contraction

The type of muscle contraction affects the resistance that can be controlled, held, or overcome.

- *Concentric contraction.* The muscle shortens during the activity. These are generally the weakest muscle contractions, requiring more recruitment than isometric and eccentric contractions for a particular load.
- *Isometric contraction.* This is a stabilising contraction where the muscle length remains virtually constant.
- *Eccentric contraction.* The muscle lengthens during the activity. These are generally the strongest muscle contractions, requiring less recruitment than isometric and concentric contractions for a particular load.

Speed of contraction

- *Isotonic.* A constant load is applied but the angular velocity of the movement may change.
- *Isokinetic.* The angular velocity of the movement is kept constant, but the load may be varied.
- *Isometric.* The muscle length remains the same, so no movement occurs.

REFERENCES

Bell F, Ghasemi M, Rafferty D, Richards J, Weir E 1995 An holistic approach to gait analysis: Glasgow Caledonian University's CRC. Gait Posture 3: 185

Bell F, Shaw L, Rafferty D, Rennie J, Richards J 1996 Movement analysis technology in clinical practice. Phys Ther Rev 1: 13–22

Brand RA, Crowninshield RD 1981 Locomotion studies: caves to computers (abstract). J Biomech 14: 497

Bruckner J 1998 The Gait Workbook: a Practical Guide to Clinical Gait Analysis. SLACK Inc.

Elftman H 1938 Forces and energy changes in the leg during walking. Am J Physiol 125: 339–56

Gage JR 1994 The role of gait analysis in the treatment of cerebral palsy. J Pediatr Orthoped 4: 701–2

Inman VT 1966 Human locomotion. Can Med Assoc J 94: 1047–54

Inman VT 1967 Conservation of energy in ambulation. Arch Phys Med Rehab 40: 404–9

Inman VT, Ralston HJ, Todd F 1981 Human Walking. Williams & Wilkins: Baltimore

Marey EJ 1873 Animal Mechanism: a Treatise on Terrestrial and Aerial Locomotion. Appleton: New York [republished as vol. XI of the International Scientific Series]

Murray MP 1967 Gait as a total pattern of movement. Am J Phys Med 40: 290–333

Muybridge E 1887 Animal locomotion. In: Brown LS (ed.) 1957 Animals in Motion. Dover: New York

Muybridge E 1901 The Human Figure in Motion. Chapman & Hall: London

Patrick J 1991 Gait laboratory investigations to assist decision making. Br J Hosp Med 45: 35–7

Perry J 1992 Gait Analysis: Normal and Pathological Function. SLACK Inc.: Thorofare, NJ

Peterson WA, Brookhart JM, Stone SA 1965 A strain-gage platform for force measurements. J Appl Physiol 20:1095–7

Pomeroy VM, Pramanik A, Sykes L, Richards JD, Hill E 2003 Agreement between physiotherapists on quality of movement during functional activity. Clin Rehabil (in press)

Richards JD, Pramanik A, Sykes L, Pomeroy VM 2003 Towards clinical measures of quality of movement: a comparison of knee kinematic characteristics of stroke patients and aged matched healthy volunteers performing three lower limb tasks. Clin Rehabil (in press)

Rose J, Gamble JG 1994 Human Walking. Williams & Wilkins: Baltimore

Saunders JBDM, Inman VT, Eberhart HS 1953 The major determinants in normal and pathological gait. J Bone Joint Surg 35A: 543–58

Wall JC, Charteris J, Turnbull G 1987 Two steps equals one stride equals what? Clin Biomech 2: 119–25

Winter DA 1993 Knowledge base for diagnostic gait assessments. Med Prog Technol 19(2): 61–81

7

Physiotherapy in Women's Health

**Gill Brook, Eileen Brayshaw, Yvonne Coldron,
Susan Davies, Georgina Evans, Ruth Hawkes,
Alison Lewis, Pauline M. Mills,
Daphne Sidney, Ros Thomas,
Jacquelyne Todd, Kathleen Vits and
Pauline Walsh**

INTRODUCTION

This chapter offers an overview of the role of the physiotherapist in women's health. Some of the expert contributors are members of the Association of Chartered Physiotherapists in Women's Health (ACPWH), a recognised clinical interest group of the Chartered Society of Physiotherapy (CSP). Originally known as the Obstetric Physiotherapists Association, it was formed in 1948, and is one of the oldest clinical interest groups.

Association of Chartered Physiotherapists in Women's Health

[www.womensphysio.com]

For general enquiries: Secretary, ACPWH, c/o CSP, 14 Bedford Row, London WC1R 4ED

For full details on ACPWH leaflets (e.g. pregnancy, birth, postnatal, continence, and relaxation): Book and Leaflet Secretary, address as above (send a stamped and addressed envelope)

The ACPWH forms a representative body that can be consulted, and will act in the professional interest of the physiotherapist working in women's health, and in the specific field of continence. By promoting relevant post-registration courses and workshops it encourages and provides means by which the physiotherapist may improve specialist therapeutic skills and understanding of the speciality. A journal is published twice a year and there is an annual conference. In order to nurture some interest in this field amongst student physiotherapists there is a student award, which provides funding to attend the annual conference. There is a lack of evidence for many of the interventions used in women's health physiotherapy and, to encourage research, support may be offered in the form of a small bursary. There is, in addition, a research officer who works closely with the CSP and other relevant funding bodies, to set the future agenda for research.

The women's health physiotherapist is a vital member of the multiprofessional team, so there is a need to foster mutual understanding between the members of the obstetric and gynaecological healthcare team and their professional bodies. An example of this is the tripartite statement, which clearly defines the role of the midwife, women's health physiotherapist and health visitor in supporting a woman and her birth partner through pregnancy, labour and the postnatal period (CSP 1995). The association continues to seek new alliances with other organisations and maintains strong ties with the Royal College of Midwives, the Association for Continence Advice and the Continence Foundation.

Health promotion is also an important aspect of this speciality and this can take the form of leading classes, advising individuals or couples, and providing a support group for an identified clientele. There is an abundance of ACPWH literature to accompany health education, and communication with other local organisations (e.g. branches of the National Childbirth Trust) can be invaluable.

The scope of practice of the physiotherapist is forever altering and the field of women's health is no exception. For example, knowledge and understanding of the assessment and treatment of incontinence has advanced considerably, and includes the male sufferer. Similarly, the needs of the partner through pregnancy, childbirth and gynaecological procedures are now recognised and must be included in any advice or treatment protocol. Cultural differences, sexuality and religious beliefs must also be considered.

ANATOMY AND PHYSIOLOGY

The physiotherapist needs a knowledge of basic anatomy and physiology of human reproduction.

Bones and joints of the pelvis

The two hip (innominate) bones meet together midline anteriorly, forming the symphysis pubis, and with the sacrum posteriorly to form the sacroiliac joints (Figure 7.1). This bony ring forms a cavity through which the fetus passes during delivery. This is made easier by a small amount of movement, which occurs at the pelvic joints during pregnancy, largely due to the hormone relaxin.

The pelvic brim or inlet divides the pelvis into the 'false' pelvis above and the 'true' pelvis below. The pelvic outlet at the base of the pelvis comprises the tip of the coccyx posteriorly, the ischial spines and tuberosities laterally, and the pubic arch anteriorly (Polden and Mantle 1990).

The shape of the female true pelvis is such that it allows the passage of the fetus during the process of birth, the head spiralling down as it moves through the pelvis, the nose turning towards the maternal sacrum as it descends and escaping under the pubic arch at vaginal delivery (Al-Azzawi 1990).

Muscles

The abdominal muscles – recti abdominis, the internal and external abdominal obliques, and transversus abdominis – form a 'four way stretch' elastic support for the abdominal contents (Figure 7.2).

The recti extend either side of the linea alba, attaching to it in midline, running from the pubis below to

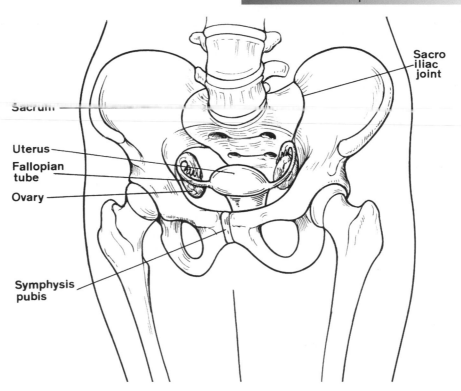

Figure 7.1   True and false pelvis: female reproductive organs.

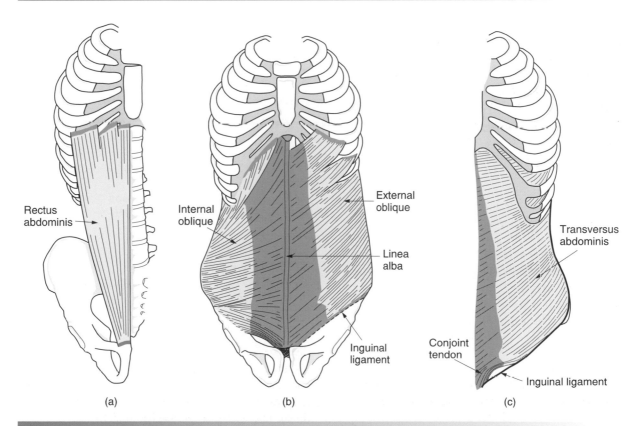

Figure 7.2   (a) Right rectus abdominis. (b) Right internal oblique and left external oblique muscles. (c) Left transversus abdominis. (Reproduced from Palastanga et al. 2002, with permission.)

the xiphoid process and lower ribs above. Towards the end of pregnancy the growing uterus stretches the abdominal muscles and can cause the recti to be separated in midline by several finger widths as the connective tissue forming the linea alba also becomes lax (Sapsford et al. 1998).

The main function of the recti is to flex the lumbar spine (Sapsford et al. 2001), whilst the obliques, interlaced diagonally in midline deep to the recti, produce side-flexion and rotation of the spine. Transversus abdominis, the deepest muscle, has horizontal fibres, which provide considerable postural support for the abdominal contents and help maintain intra-abdominal pressure, along with the pelvic floor muscles (Cresswell et al. 1992).

The pelvic floor muscles (Figure 7.3) form an elastic sling below the pelvic outlet to support the pelvic and abdominal contents. The deep pelvic floor, perforated by the openings of the genitourinary and alimentary tracts, is covered superficially by the sphincter muscles and the skin of the perineum. The deep pelvic floor muscles, the levatores ani (consisting of pubococcygeus, puborectalis, ischiococcygeus and ileococcygeus) of both sides fuse in midline and are perforated from anterior to posterior by the urethra, vagina and anus (Sapsford et al. 1998). Contraction of these muscles compresses the posterior walls of the urethra,

vagina and anus against the anterior walls, thus promoting continence. The bands of fibres interlace and sweep from the pubis to the coccyx, enclosing the whole pelvic outlet and providing a firm undercarriage of muscular support. The nerve supply to these muscles is from the sacral nerve roots and the pudendal nerve.

The superficial muscle layer forms two loops, which meet in the central perineal body. The anterior muscle loop encloses the urethra and vagina whilst the posterior loop encloses the anus. The main function of the superficial muscles is to close the sphincters. The pelvic outlet is flexible; the coccyx is able to move backwards during defaecation and parturition (childbirth). The pelvic floor muscles need to act as a whole to support the pelvic viscera but can also work separately to control the sphincters. Muscle weakness is not uncommon following pregnancy and childbirth, resulting from trauma to the pelvic floor muscles and their nerve supply. This can result in problems with continence (Schussler et al. 1994).

Organs of reproduction

The uterus and ovaries are suspended in connective tissue and peritoneum inside the true pelvis. The broad ligament of the uterus divides the pelvic cavity into two

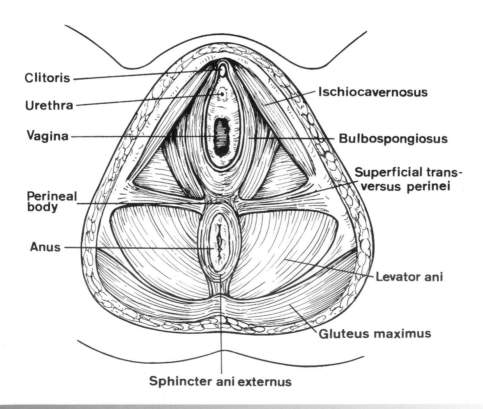

Figure 7.3   Pelvic floor muscles.

compartments – the anterior, containing the bladder, and the posterior, containing the rectum. The ovaries lie in the broad ligament on each side of the uterus. Just behind and slightly above are the trumpet-shaped open ends of the contractile fallopian tubes. Their anemone-like fringes (fimbriae) catch the ovum when it erupts from the ovary at ovulation. The free ovum is able to travel along the fallopian tube to the uterus by the beat of tiny cilia lining the tube walls. On fertilisation, the ovum is embedded in the endometrium lining the uterus. If fertilisation has not occurred, the lining is shed (menstruation).

The uterus has a remarkable capacity to grow as the fetus develops during pregnancy, able to accommodate the baby (in 1 litre of amniotic fluid within a membranous sac) and placenta, which attaches it to the uterine wall. The uterus consists of the upper part (fundus), the main part (body), and the lower part (cervix) which opens into the vagina below (Llewellyn-Jones 1999).

THE PHYSIOLOGY OF PREGNANCY

The first sign of pregnancy is amenorrhea (cessation of menstruation) following the fertilisation of the ovum. As pregnancy progresses, the uterus grows, its muscle fibres lengthening and thickening. By 12 weeks it has enlarged to become an abdominal organ. Gestational dates can be determined by the level of the uterus, which continues to rise until the latter weeks of pregnancy. Uterine activity may be felt from 20 weeks (Braxton Hicks contractions). The lower uterine segment develops, softens and stretches and collagenous supportive tissue increases, becoming more elastic.

Within the cervix, there is formation of a mucous plug, acting as a barrier to infection.

The placenta develops from 6 weeks, producing hormones to maintain pregnancy, providing nutrition for the fetus and acting as a barrier to certain noxious substances.

The fetus grows and develops within a sac, surrounded by amniotic fluid, and is nurtured by the placenta via the umbilical cord. Its heartbeat can be detected at about 14 weeks, and the mother may feel movements at 16–18 weeks.

Pregnancy is governed and controlled by hormones, which affect various systems. Some are of particular relevance to the physiotherapist:

- Progesterone decreases smooth muscle tone, initiates sensitivity to CO_2 in the respiratory centre, and causes an increase in maternal temperature, breast development, and storage of fat deposits for milk production.

- Oestrogen influences uterine and breast growth and development, prepares prime receptor sites for relaxin (e.g. pelvic joints), and causes increased water retention.
- Relaxin replaces the collagen in target areas with a modified form, which has greater pliability and extensibility. It has a softening effect on connective tissue (pelvic floor and abdominal fascia), increasing extensibility in those structures.

Pregnancy lasts on average 40 weeks and is divided into three trimesters (periods of approximately 3 months). During this time many changes occur in the body owing to the growth of the fetus, the changes effected by the above hormones, weight gain and subsequent postural alterations.

Physiotherapists treating pregnant women should be conversant with these changes and consider them during assessment, treatment or when planning or taking classes. Likewise, they should have an understanding of the complications, which might arise during pregnancy – such as placenta praevia (a low-lying placenta) or high blood pressure.

Chapter coverage
Within this text attention will be paid to the changes and complications of most relevance to the physiotherapist dealing with women during pregnancy and the postnatal period. Further reading is advised (see the end of the chapter).

MUSCULOSKELETAL CHANGES DURING PREGNANCY

Postural Changes

The overall equilibrium of the spine and pelvis alters as pregnancy progresses but there is still confusion as to the exact nature of any associated postural adaptation. With weight gain, increased blood volume and ventral growth of the fetus, the centre of gravity no longer falls over the feet and the woman may need to lean backwards to gain equilibrium (Abitol 1997). Disorganisation of spinal curves results, and adaptive postures include an increase of the lumbosacral angle, an increase (or maybe decrease) of the lumbar lordosis, or anterior displacement of the pelvis. There will be compensatory posterior displacement of the shoulders and thoracic spine and increase of the cervical lordosis. Postural changes may still be present 12 weeks postnatally (Bullock et al. 1987; Bullock-Saxton 1991).

Articular and Connective Tissue Changes

As previously mentioned, altered levels of relaxin (MacLennan 1981), oestrogen and progesterone during pregnancy result in an alteration to collagen metabolism and increased connective tissue pliability and extensibility. Therefore, ligamentous tissues are predisposed to laxity with resultant reduced joint stability. The symphysis pubis and sacroiliac joints are particularly affected to allow for birth of the baby. This ligamentous laxity may continue for 6 months postpartum.

Biomechanical changes of the joints of the spine and pelvis may involve an increase in sacral promontory, increase in the lumbosacral angle, a forward rotatory movement of the innominate bones, and downward and forward rotation of the symphysis pubis (Golightly 1982) (with resultant counternutation of the sacrum). The normal symphyseal gap of 4–5 mm shows an average increase of 3 mm during pregnancy (Abramson et al. 1934). Pelvic joint loosening begins around 10 weeks with maximum loosening near term. Joints should return to normal at 4–12 weeks postpartum (Snow and Neubert 1997). The sacrococcygeal joints also loosen.

As the uterus rises in the abdomen the rib cage is forced laterally and the diameter of the chest may increase by 10–15 cm (Polden and Mantle 1990).

Neuromuscular Changes

Abdominal and pelvic muscles contribute to spinal and pelvic stability via active tension exerted on the passive ligamentous and fascial stability structures. Passive joint instability (as seen in pregnancy) alters afferent input from joint mechanoreceptors and probably affects motor neurone recruitment. According to Bullock-Saxton (1998): 'Muscle spindle regulation may alter, resulting in decreased muscle stiffness (tension) around a joint and, therefore, a decrease in active stability.'

Rectus abdominis

As pregnancy progresses, rectus abdominis elongates by 115% and widens. Decreased stabilisation of the pelvis happens in late pregnancy and poor stability persists at 8 weeks postpartum (Gilleard and Brown 1996). The strength of gross muscle flexion has been shown to be impaired at 24 weeks postpartum.

The linea alba widens via hormonally mediated change, to allow for the growing fetus (Polden and Mantle 1990). This divarication of the linea alba during the third trimester is normally about 2–4 cm wide and 2–5 cm long, though it can split and become a diastasis.

Lateral abdominal muscles

There is very little information on the effect of pregnancy on the three lateral abdominal muscles (transversus abdominis, internal and external obliques). However, research on normal subjects has identified the importance of transversus abdominis as the prime stabiliser of the trunk (Hodges 1999).

Pelvic floor muscles

During pregnancy there is stretching to the pelvic floor, and trauma/tearing during labour and vaginal delivery. It is now thought that the function and recruitment of transversus abdominis and the pelvic floor musculature are closely associated, with voluntary activity in the deep abdominal muscles resulting in increased pelvic floor muscle activity (Sapsford and Hodges 2001).

LABOUR AND BIRTH

Definition

Labour is defined as the process by which the products of conception are expelled from the uterus after the 24th week of gestation.

Monitoring

Uterine activity, the progress of labour, and fetal condition are monitored regularly throughout labour, by abdominal palpation, vaginal assessment, and by listening to the fetal heart rate. The latter may be done by Pinard fetal stethoscope or continuous electronic monitoring (through the abdomen or via a clip electrode attached to the presenting part of the baby, with a printout on a cardiotocograph machine). Information is recorded on a partogram (progress chart), which will show any deviation from a 'normal' labour.

The mother's temperature, pulse, respiration, blood pressure, state of hydration, bladder fullness and psychological state are monitored regularly.

Onset of labour

The exact 'trigger' for labour is unknown, but there are biochemical events resulting in a fall in progesterone and a rise in oestradiol, prostaglandins and oxytocin. Signs are a 'show' of the mucous plug, rupture of membranes, and regular uterine contractions.

Stages of labour

First stage

This is from commencement of established labour to full dilation of the cervix, averaging 12 hours in a primagravid woman (one having her first baby). Contraction and retraction of the myometrial fibres of the uterus achieve effacement and dilation of the cervix. The contractions increase in intensity, duration and frequency, pulling the uterus forwards into line with the pelvic inlet and birth canal and driving the presenting part downwards.

The cervix must be fully dilated (10 cm) before pushing commences. Transition (the final part of this first stage) can be very difficult as the woman may experience mood swings, overwhelming pain, intense fatigue and a strong desire to push.

Second stage

This is the expulsive stage, from full dilation to the birth of the baby – averaging 1–2 hours in the primagravid. The fetal head must adapt to the various segments of the pelvis. The head engages in the transverse position, flexes and rotates as it strikes the pelvic floor, passes under the pubic arch, extending as it distends both the perineum and introitus maximally, and is 'crowned' and delivered with the face towards the anus. The position of the umbilical cord is checked. The head rotates back again as the anterior shoulder is born followed by the second shoulder and the body. The cord is clamped and cut.

The mother assists expulsive contractions of the uterus with short pushes, and the adoption of comfortable gravity-aided positions to widen her pelvic outlet (Russell 1982; Gardosi et al. 1989). She may be asked to pant at the crowning of the head – as the baby is being delivered.

Episiotomy

During delivery, a woman's perineum can stretch and remain intact, but it may tear. A third- or fourth-degree tear (involving the anal sphincter and mucosa respectively) may have serious implications, even faecal incontinence (Sultan et al. 1994). An episiotomy (cut) may be deemed necessary to avoid excessive trauma, to hasten the birth or to prepare for an instrumental delivery. A mediolateral incision is performed to avoid tearing into the anus.

Instrumental delivery

Delay in the second stage, or fetal or maternal distress, might be an indication for instrumental delivery, by vacumn extraction or forceps.

- With vacuum extraction (Ventouse) a suction cap is applied to the fetal scalp and traction is used with contractions.
- With forceps delivery, metal blades cradle each side of the fetal head. Traction is applied steadily during contractions. A choice of forceps allows lift out or rotation as required.

Third stage

This is the shortest stage of labour, lasting up to 30 minutes, commencing after the birth of the baby. The uterus contracts and shears the placenta off its wall, pushing it down through the vagina. The process may be aided by an injection of syntometrine at delivery and cord traction. The placenta and membranes will be examined for completeness on delivery. On occasions, part or all of the placenta and/or membranes may be retained, requiring manual removal.

CAESAREAN SECTION

This is a surgical procedure performed electively, or as an emergency, before or during labour. The baby is removed through the abdominal wall by a transverse incision through the lower uterine segment (LSCS). A vertical incision in the upper segment may be necessary, but can increase morbidity. Epidural anaesthesia or spinal block is commonly used instead of a general anaesthetic, reducing the risk of aspiration of acid stomach contents into the mother's lungs (Mendelson's syndrome).

Indications for caesarean section include fetal or maternal distress, prolonged or obstructed labour, and malpresentation of the fetus or placenta.

INDUCTION

Labour can be induced when the continuation of pregnancy is considered disadvantageous. Common indications are post-maturity (overdue), pre-eclampsia (associated with high blood pressure), diabetes, intrauterine growth retardation, and antepartum haemorrhage.

Induction may be performed by the insertion of vaginal prostaglandins (to 'ripen' the cervix), artificial rupture of membranes, oxytocin infusion, or a combination of some or all of these.

PAIN RELIEF

Henderson and Jones (1997) describe labour pain as being unique and isolating. Pain and the perception of pain will vary from individual to individual and from labour to labour.

Pain in the first stage is experienced mainly in the abdomen and lower back, becoming more intense as the contractions increase in strength and length. It is due to dilation of the cervix, contraction and distension of the uterine muscle, and pressure of the uterus on other areas.

In the second stage a sharp, burning pain is caused by distension and dilation of the birth canal (vagina) and perineum.

A woman, possibly using pain management techniques taught at antenatal classes, may be able to cope with the pain she experiences. However, many will request additional analgesia.

Drugs

Entonox is a mixture of 50% nitrous oxide and 50% oxygen, inhaled and administered by the woman via a mask or mouthpiece. There are no known adverse effects to her or the fetus. It may be particularly useful in the later part of the first stage and during the second stage. The analgesic effect is delayed, so inhalation from the start of a contraction is required.

Pethidine and diamorphine are opioid drugs readily available and easily administered by intramuscular injection. Possible disadvantages include nausea and vomiting, and neonatal respiratory depression, which may be corrected by administration of naloxone.

Epidural is a local anaesthetic introduced into the lumbar epidural space, reducing or eradicating the pain of uterine contractions (Howell and Chalmers 1992) without affecting uterine activity. It is an invasive procedure administered by an anaesthetist. Other potential disadvantages include reduced mobility for the mother, prolonged second stage with higher risk of a forceps delivery, vasodilation in the lower limbs necessitating an intravenous infusion, and urine retention. Headaches (due to dural puncture at the time of administration), backache, bladder malfunction, infection and neural damage might follow delivery. Epidural may be advised when operative delivery is suspected (e.g. with multiple births). It can also be an advantage for women with high blood pressure, as its administration reduces BP.

Transcutaneous electrical nerve stimulation

TENS (or TNS) can be used in labour. A low-frequency high-intensity current of 2–10 Hz is thought to increase the production of endorphins and encephalins. This is applied throughout labour, and a high-frequency low-intensity current at 100–200 Hz which activates the pain-gate mechanism (Melzack and Wall 1982) is used during the more intense contrac-

tions. A special two-channel battery-operated obstetric machine enables the woman to change from one frequency to the other by depression of a button. The current is introduced through coupling gel via four electrodes placed over the nerve roots to the uterus (T10 to L2) and the pelvic floor and perineum (S2 to S4). The two channels enable individual control of each pair of electrodes.

TNS is easy to apply, non-invasive with no known side-effects on mother or baby. It allows mobility, and affords the woman control of her analgesia. Bortoluzzi (1989) reported a reduction in use of narcotics. It cannot be used in water, and may on occasion interfere with the cardiograph tracings.

Alternative methods of pain control

These include the use of water (birthing pool), hypnotherapy, acupuncture, aromatherapy and reflexology.

The Puerperium

Puerperium describes the first 6 weeks after childbirth. Some body systems return to the non-pregnant state, and other changes are initiated (e.g. lactation). Within this period the uterus involutes (returns to its pre-pregnant size and position). As the site of the placenta heals, and the endometrium regenerates, the woman experiences a discharge (lochia), initially bloody, for up to 8 weeks.

Potential complications during this period, which might involve the women's health physiotherapist, include perineal or wound swelling or bruising, musculoskeletal problems, urinary incontinence, faecal incontinence, and constipation (see also the section on postnatal physiotherapy).

PHYSIOTHERAPY IN THE CHILDBEARING YEAR

The women's health physiotherapist works as part of the multidisciplinary team caring for the pregnant woman, along with obstetricians, general practitioners, midwives, health visitors, occupational therapists, social workers or other physiotherapists. Contact with the pregnant woman may be in the community, health centre, leisure centre or the physiotherapy department.

The role of the women's health physiotherapist is to:

- educate the pregnant woman for pregnancy, labour and beyond (see the section on antenatal classes)
- advise on safe and appropriate exercise (see the section on exercise and pregnancy)
- identify, assess and treat musculoskeletal problems (dealt with in this section).

Pelvic Floor Dysfunction

See the section on urogenital dysfunction. During pregnancy, physiotherapists may consider it prudent to limit their intervention to advice.

Spinal and Pelvic Pain

Spinal and posterior pelvic (sacroiliac) pain is common during pregnancy with an incidence described variously as ranging from 50% to 70% (Mantle et al. 1977; Fast et al. 1987; Berg et al. 1988; Ostgaard et al. 1991; Mantle 1994; Russell et al. 1996; Heiberg and Aarseth 1997). It is often regarded as 'a normal part of pregnancy' but, without appropriate treatment, a minor episode may develop into a chronic problem. A third of women report severe back pain that interferes with daily life and compromises their ability to work (Ostgaard et al. 1991; Mens et al. 1996). Most backache resolves in the first few weeks postpartum, but for some may continue for 18 months (Ostgaard and Andersson 1992), or may present postpartum for the first time (Russell and Reynolds 1997). Some patients may experience a relapse around menstruation and in a subsequent pregnancy (Mens et al. 1996).

The anatomical origins of peripartum spinal and pelvic pain vary and are difficult to determine and diagnose (Nilsson-Wikmar and Harms-Ringdahl 1999). Women describe pain variously as occurring in the low back, sacral, posterior thigh and leg, pubic, groin and hip areas. These may occur simultaneously or separately, antenatally, during delivery or postnatally (Heiberg and Aarseth 1997). There is often associated cervical, thoracic or coccygeal pain. Sciatic pain is common and may be of lumbar origin or from sacroiliac joint involvement as the L5 and S1 components of the lumbosacral plexus run immediately anterior to the sacroiliac joints.

Postural adaptations, fatigue, increased joint mobility, increased collagen volume causing pressure on pain sensitive structures, weight gain, and pressure from the growing fetus may all contribute to spinal and pelvic pain (Polden and Mantle 1990). Poor passive stability from lax joints plus poor active stability from altered muscle recruitment and stretched pelvic and abdominal muscles probably contribute to spinal and pelvic pain (Watkins 1998; Coldron and Vits 2001). Other musculoskeletal factors include physically strenuous work and work involving bending, twisting, lifting and sitting (Heiberg and Aarseth 1997), large abdominal sagittal and transverse diameters and a naturally large lumbar lordosis (Heckman and Sassard 1994), pre-pregnancy low back pain, and decreased fitness level before pregnancy (Ostgaard et al. 1993). Pelvic pain appears to be associated particularly with high mean relaxin values (Kristiansson 1997) or a susceptibility to relaxin and the other hormones of pregnancy (MacLennan and MacLennan 1997), parity (Heckman and Sassard 1994), weight of the newborn, and smoking (Ostgaard 1997).

Conclusive association between new-onset postpartum backache and epidural analgesia has not been demonstrated. (Breen et al. 1994; Macarthur and Weeks 1995), though the masking effect on pain may lead to women adopting unsuitable positions in labour (Macarthur et al. 1990; Russell et al. 1993).

Management of spinal and pelvic pain and dysfunction

Advice, posture, education and general exercise

Antenatal education on posture and back pain by a physiotherapist has been shown to reduce back and pelvic pain, reduce sick leave and continue to benefit women in the postnatal period (Noren et al. 1997). Advice in pregnancy includes adopting comfortable resting positions, advice on moving out of bed, chair or car, advice on postures in walking and standing, and advice on lifting and handling. In addition, postnatal advice includes positions for breast-feeding, nappy changing, bathing and handling the growing baby.

Treatment of articular/joint dysfunctions

Peripartum spinal and pelvic pain often responds to manual therapy, though correct assessment of the spine and pelvis is imperative to enable treatment to be targeted at the correct structures. Common conditions include unilateral sacroiliac dysfunction, symphysis pubis dysfunction, minor lumbar disc herniation, lumbar zygapophyseal joint problems, thoracic spine pain and coccydinia.

Manual therapy techniques used for joint hypomobility/dysfunction in the non-pregnant population can be utilised, but with appropriate precautions. Abdominal, spinal and pelvic muscle recruitment needs to be retrained to stabilise an unstable spinal segment or sacroiliac joint.

TENS may be used postnatally, but the use of TENS antenatally is controversial. Current advice recommends that TENS should not be used before 37 weeks gestation because of unknown effects on the fetus and the hypothetical risk of possible induction of premature labour.

The use of a sacroiliac/trochanteric belt for sacroiliac and symphysis pubis instability both ante- and postnatally may decrease pain (McIntosh 1995; Fry and Tudor 1997) and substitute the work of the internal oblique muscle (Snidjers et al. 1998). A large tubular bandage for the abdomen, or maternity belt, may give added support.

Costal margin pain along the anterior surface of the lower ribs (possibly related to pressure from the ascending uterus, and commonly called 'rib flare') may be accompanied by thoracic spinal and lateral chest pain. This may be relieved by side flexion manoeuvres away from the pain, and manual therapy techniques.

Muscle re-education

Non-obstetric research on patients with spinal instability problems and low back pain has shown active trunk stabilisation programmes to be of benefit (Richardson et al. 1990; Richardson et al. 1993; Jull et al. 1993; O'Sullivan et al. 1997; O'Sullivan 2000). In addition, postpartum rehabilitation of pelvic and abdominal muscles is believed to increase active stability of the pelvis (Vleeming et al. 1992).

Rehabilitation exercises antenatally and postnatally should concentrate initially on correct recruitment of both pelvic stabilising muscles (gluteus medius and maximus) and prime spinal stabilising muscles (transversus abdominis, lumbar multifidus, pelvic floor muscles). Exercise for global stabilising muscles such as the oblique abdominals, erector spinae, latissimus dorsi, and iliopsoas should follow, though probably only postnatally.

Divarication of the recti abdominis should gradually reduce after delivery, so exercises at 6 weeks postnatally should include those that shorten the muscle. Once core stability has been gained, the woman should be encouraged to increase her strength, and general aerobic and cardiovascular fitness.

Rehabilitation exercises need to be functional, as many women cannot regularly attend a physiotherapy department owing to family commitments.

Symphysis Pubis Dysfunction/Diastasis

Symphysis pubis dysfunction (SPD) is a relatively common complaint with varying incidence figures of 1 in 300 (Kubitz and Goodlin 1986) to 1 in 800 (Scriven et al. 1995). It may occur antenatally or during delivery, and cause severe social difficulties (Fry 1999).

SPD may occur because of an abnormal separation of the symphysis pubis (diastasis). However, the amount of symphyseal separation does not always correlate with symptoms (Snow and Neubert 1997) and not all symptomatic patients have an increased gap. The abnormal symphyseal gap may vary from 10 mm

to 35 mm and vertical mobility may be more than 50 mm (Gamble et al. 1986). The width is less important than reduction of the gap over time in determining likely outcome of the condition.

Common complaints are severe pain in the groin, anterior thigh and sacroiliac joint, pain on abduction of the thighs, shuffling or waddling gait, severe symphyseal tenderness, and an inability to weight-bear unilaterally (Fry 1999). Minor trauma may cause pelvic joint asymmetry. A forward rotation and oblique slip of the innominate caused by overactivity in the adductor muscles of the thigh may contribute to SPD (Röst 1999). With poor use of the glutei and lack of force closure of the pelvis, disruption of the self-locking mechanism of the pelvis ensues.

Management of SPD

SPD is often associated with sacroiliac joint dysfunction and can be treated by all of the methods described above with the aim of restoring pelvic ring stability (Fry 1999). Special attention should be paid to overactive pelvic adductors, underactive abductors, unilateral iliac displacement (Röst 1999) and poor pelvic and spinal stabilising muscles. Advice regarding unilateral weight-bearing activities and hip abduction should be given. Crutches, or in the most severe cases a wheelchair, may be required.

Liaison with midwives is essential. Women should be aware of the masking effect of epidural and spinal anaesthesia in relation to excessive abduction of hips during labour and delivery. If possible, they should adopt the most comfortable position during labour (for example left-side-lying, or kneeling upright with support). They should be discouraged from placing their feet on attendants' hips and care should be taken if lithotomy is required. Suturing should take place in the most comfortable position for the mother (ACPWH 1996).

Diastasis Rectus Abdominis (DRA)

Diastasis rectus abdominis (DRA) is an excessive gap between the bellies of rectus abdominis at the level of the umbilicus (Boissonnault and Blaschak 1988). It normally appears in pregnancy but can occur during the second stage of labour. The gap may be as wide as 20 cm and can extend the whole length of the linea alba (Polden and Mantle 1990). There has been a reported incidence of 66% of DRA during the third trimester that may persist in 30–60% of cases in the postpartum period (Boissonnault and Blaschak 1988). The period of resolution in the postnatal period is controversial (Gilleard and Brown 1996; Hsia and Jones 2000).

Risk factors include older women, multiparity, caesarean section, multiple gestations, larger babies and greater weight gain (Lo et al. 1999). It has not been established whether DRA is a factor in low back or pelvic pain but it is thought to interfere with the supportive and expulsive functions of the abdominal wall.

Management of DRA

It is advisable for physiotherapists to examine the gap manually in postnatal women and assess the degree of separation. Advice regarding exercise should then be given, including initial training of the deep abdominal muscles (transversus abdominis) (Potter 1997) and avoidance of strong trunk curling exercises.

Nerve Compression Syndromes

Fluid retention may occur during the third trimester, which can lead to a variety of nerve compression syndromes. These include carpal tunnel syndrome (CTS), brachial plexus compression, meralgia paraesthetica (compression of the lateral cutaneous nerve of the thigh as it passes under the inguinal ligament, presenting as tingling and burning in the outer thigh) and posterior tibial nerve compression. These entrapments normally resolve postpartum.

Wrist splints and ice are useful for CTS. Postural advice can be used for brachial plexus compression. Ice and elevation may help posterior tibial nerve compression (Polden and Mantle 1990).

EXERCISE AND PREGNANCY

General Issues

Physiological, emotional, social and psychological issues influence physical fitness in pregnancy. The physiotherapist must be sensitive towards these, and be aware of other issues such as language, ethnic cultures, equal opportunities and women with special needs. The therapist's approach to the pregnant woman should be holistic, flexible, individual, and – where available – evidence-based.

Many women now incorporate regular exercise into their lifestyle, and wish to continue during their pregnancy. A significant minority of women decide to take up exercise for the first time when they become pregnant.

The research available suggests that mild to moderate exercise is beneficial to the healthy pregnant woman (Clapp 2000) and is not harmful to the fetus (Riemann et al. 2000; Clapp et al. 2000; ACOG 2002). Moderate intensity is defined as being able to talk easily, whilst increasing the heart rate to a maximum 140 beats per minute. Choice of exercise must be influenced by the physiological changes, which will occur. For example, plasma volume increases before red cell volume, leading to a decreased ability to provide oxygen in response to demand. Also, increased demand causes raised respiratory rates, cardiac output values increase during pregnancy for the same activity (over the non-pregnant woman), and there is a loss of cardiac reserve. Strenuous activity might compromise the mother's health, and that of the fetus.

Benefits and Contraindications

Potential *benefits* of exercise include:

- maintenance of cardiovascular fitness
- maintenance of healthy weight range
- improvement of body awareness, posture, coordination and balance
- improvement in circulation
- increase in endurance and stamina
- provision of social interaction with exercise, enhancing feelings of social and emotional wellbeing
- possible reduction in problems during labour and delivery
- potentially shorter labour
- possible prevention of gestational diabetes
- reduction in minor complaints of pregnancy
- more rapid postnatal recovery.

Contraindications to exercise include:

- cardiovascular, respiratory, renal or thyroid disease
- diabetes (type 1, if poorly controlled)
- history of miscarriage, premature labour, fetal growth restriction, cervical incompetence
- hypertension, vaginal bleeding, reduced fetal movement, anaemia, breech presentation, placenta praevia.

(ACOG 2002)

Advice

The advice given to regular and non-regular exercisers will differ.

Regular exercisers

- Consult your doctor or midwife before beginning exercise.
- Exercise at a moderate level most days for 30 minutes or more.
- Discontinue contact sports, and activities which carry a high risk of falling or abdominal trauma. Avoid scuba diving (ACOG 2002).

- Self-regulate both the level of intensity and duration of exercise, aiming to keep core temperature below 38°C.
- Aim for low impact activity.
- Wear suitably supportive footwear to reduce musculoskeletal stresses.
- Maintain adequate fluid intake to prevent dehydration, and avoid exercise during hot and humid weather, or with pyrexia.
- Warm up and cool down for at least 5 minutes.
- Do not use developmental stretching (because of the effects of relaxin).
- Seek professional advice on specific exercises (e.g. for the pelvic floor muscles).
- Avoid ballistic exercise, low squats, crossover steps and rapid changes of direction.
- Do not exercise in the supine position after 16 weeks gestation, to avoid aortocaval compression.
- Eat to appetite without calorific restriction.
- Work towards cross training to avoid over training, and stop exercise before fatigue sets in.

Non regular exercisers

In addition to the above, women not used to regular exercise should be advised on the following.

- Do not start an exercise programme until >13 weeks gestation.
- Consider beginning with non-weight-bearing exercises such as aquanatal.
- Progress from simple and basic levels of exercise, increasing exercise tolerance gradually, under the supervision of a suitably qualified professional.

When to stop

All women should stop exercising immediately and seek advice from a doctor if they experience:

- abdominal, back or pubic pain
- PV (from the vagina) bleeding
- shortness of breath, dizziness, faintness, palpitations or tachycardia
- difficulty in walking.

Most women will naturally reduce the amount of exercise they take during pregnancy as their weight increases, and they fatigue and become breathless more rapidly.

Types of Exercise

General categories

- *Walking and swimming.* The pace adopted should be sufficient to cause aerobic changes. If pelvic pain is a problem, avoid the kicking motion of the legs during breaststroke swimming.
- *Low impact aerobics* (or equivalent classes). The emphasis is on maintaining fitness levels.
- *Pilates or yoga* (modified for pregnancy). These cater for the non-aerobic elements of fitness – flexibility, control of breathing and relaxation.
- *Back care classes.* Core stability exercises may be taught, sometimes using a Swiss ball.
- *Gym work.* The pregnant woman may have access to a static bicycle, treadmill or cross trainer, all of which encourage aerobic activity.

Technique is especially important when strength training. Women should use light weights, with submaximal lifts, aiming to use both upper and lower body muscle groups in a variety of exercises. Weights, sets and repetitions should be decreased further as pregnancy progresses.

Aquanatal classes

Aquanatal classes – water-based exercise groups designed specifically for pregnant and postnatal women – have grown in popularity in Britain in recent years. Pregnant women find exercise and relaxation in water enjoyable and beneficial, largely because of the feeling of weightlessness and reduced jarring of the joints. It has been suggested that a woman submerged up to the level of the xiphisternum will experience only 28% of her bodyweight (Harrison and Bulstrode 1987).

Women in aquanatal classes may notice that they get relief from aches and pains, feel they have more energy after the class, and sleep better. Another important benefit is the absence of post-exercise muscle soreness because, during immersion, all muscle work is concentric (Newham 1988).

Other significant advantages are less obvious to the women themselves: exercise in water helps to tone the respiratory muscles; the leg movements of swimming and exercise in water aid venous return; and the diuretic effect of immersion is helpful to a pregnant woman troubled by fluid-retention as immersion for 20–40 minutes results in a loss of 300–400 mL of fluid (Katz et al. 1991).

Women must be screened by the teacher for any relevant musculoskeletal problem or contraindication (ACPWH 1995). Exercises can be amended to accommodate back, pelvic girdle, neck or other orthopaedic problems. Pregnant women with sacroiliac or symphysis pubis discomfort should be advised to modify their breaststroke leg movements and take small, rather than wide, steps sideways. All women should take short backward steps to avoid an increase in lumbar lordosis.

Exercises that will overstretch the already compromised abdominal muscles should be excluded.

Conversely, squatting, which is difficult on land and thought by some to be damaging, is safe in water as virtually no weight goes through the knee joints.

The aim of the class is to help maintain, not improve, a woman's level of fitness. Exercises must be safe and carefully chosen, and each included for a reason. Water exercises should be considered in their own right and not taken unchanged from exercise classes on land (Evans 2002). Standard antenatal exercises, such as pelvic tilting, pelvic floor exercises, and hip and shoulder circling (with the shoulders immersed) can usefully be included. Hydrostatic pressure on the ribcage makes exercises like gently blowing a table-tennis ball across the water valuable in toning respiratory muscles. Good posture should be taught at the beginning of the class, and participants reminded to maintain it throughout. If the water is warm enough, a relaxation session is an excellent way to end the class.

Antenatal classes

Midwives, physiotherapists and health visitors typically run antenatal classes, though the latter are more usually involved in postnatal groups. Classes can take many different formats, and vary in number and timing to suit the needs of the women and their partners.

'Early bird' groups are held around 16 weeks of gestation and consist of one or two classes by a midwife and a physiotherapist, though other speakers might be invited (e.g. dietitian). As most women will be working at this stage, these classes are usually held in the evening.

The physiotherapist's role is to discuss the changes in pregnancy, how these will affect the working woman, and how to adapt to the changes. One of the most important topics is correct postural alignment and care of the back during pregnancy, to alleviate backache and prevent long-term problems. Women's work activities will be discussed and advice on seating, lifting etc. given. The structure and function of the pelvic floor muscles and the importance of pelvic floor exercises to prevent long-term continence problems will be explained. Transversus abdominis and pelvic floor exercises will be taught and the importance of bringing these muscles into everyday functional activities discussed. Relaxation techniques can be introduced, to be used during pregnancy, labour and for the rest of the couples' lives.

The majority of the classes are held later in pregnancy from about 30 weeks onwards, and may be during the day, evening, or at the weekend. Women only or couples may attend. The classes may be for first-time mothers/parents, or for women who have had previous pregnancies. Commonly they include a mixture of both. In some large hospitals there will be classes for twin pregnancies, for elective caesarean deliveries, and teenagers. These groups will benefit from meeting other women/couples in a similar situation. Where appropriate, classes may be held for women of a particular ethnic group, in their own language if necessary.

Classes are held centrally in the hospital where the baby will be born and/or in local health centres.

The physiotherapy input to the later antenatal classes will include:

- the changes in pregnancy, good posture in standing, sitting and lying
- the practice of transversus abdominis and pelvic floor exercises, relating these to functional activities
- advice on back care and prevention of long-term problems
- exercises for the circulation
- breathing awareness and adaptations, relaxation and positions of comfort
- coping strategies for labour
- advice on sport and leisure activities
- early postnatal exercises and advice.

Midwives will discuss care in pregnancy, labour, feeding and baby care.

Ideally the classes are held once a week for 5 or 6 weeks. However, the physiotherapy content may have to be prioritised to fit into one 2-hour session, according to the availability of resources.

Postnatal physiotherapy

The role of the physiotherapist in the days, weeks and sometimes even months following the birth includes advice for the new mother on how to regain and perhaps improve her former level of fitness through appropriate exercise and education. Also included is the assessment and treatment of specific physical problems, emotional support, and health education. Contact with the new mother may be in the postnatal ward, as an outpatient in the physiotherapy department, or in community-based postnatal groups.

Although it might be considered the ideal for every woman to be advised by a women's health physiotherapist postnatally, this is becoming increasingly uncommon. Many women will not be seen by a physiotherapist, but should be given appropriate literature.

Physiotherapy intervention may be limited to some or all of the following.

Caesarean section

Education during antenatal classes may help to prepare the mother for a caesarean. Postnatally, the physiotherapist should be aware of the reasons for the caesarean and offer emotional support and advice when required. Bed exercises and mobility followed by early ambulation reduce the risk of respiratory problems, back pain or deep venous thrombosis. Wound haematomatas may respond well to ultrasound or pulsed electromagnetic energy (PEME). Abdominal and pelvic floor exercises and optimal feeding postures should be taught.

Painful perineum

A prolonged or difficult delivery, episiotomy or an extended tear may result in a bruised, painful and oedematous perineum. Physiotherapeutic interventions might include ice packs, PEME, pelvic floor exercises (to increase blood supply and aid healing), advice on supported defaecation, and the use of pillows under each buttock when sitting to prevent pressure on the wound. Scar tissue may cause longer-term pain or psychosexual problems.

Incontinence

Urinary or faecal urgency and incontinence can occur after delivery, particularly after a prolonged second stage, episiotomy, instrumental delivery, or delivery of a large baby. Initial treatment can comprise advice and pelvic floor exercises (Morkved and Bø 2000). Persistent pelvic floor dysfunction should always be assessed and treated (see the section on urogenital dysfunction).

Musculoskeletal problems

See the earlier section on musculoskeletal problems in the childbearing year.

Postnatal groups

Many new mothers find difficulty adjusting to, and caring for, a baby during the first few weeks. Extreme fatigue may result. Physiotherapists are well placed to motivate women, encouraging them to attend postnatal groups, support groups, relaxation or exercise classes. Input from a team of health professionals provides education and information on a wide range of topics, relevant to the new mother. Physiotherapists may lead a low-impact aerobics or Pilates exercise class, teach baby massage, or hold discussion/support groups. They should be aware of the development of new or previously undisclosed symptoms (e.g. postnatal depression) and be instrumental in referring the sufferer to an appropriate health professional. Postnatal groups promote a positive outlook, reinforcing healthy living for life.

UROGENITAL DYSFUNCTION

Problems relating to the female urinary and genital tracts are common and often complex. Increasingly physiotherapy is the first line of treatment. The problems encountered most frequently are bladder dysfunction and genital prolapse.

Bladder Dysfunction

Most common is urinary incontinence, which may occur at any time in a woman's life, but incidence rises with age. A study of women aged 50–74 found that some leakage of urine was reported by 47%, and regularly by 31% (Holtedahl and Hunskaar 1998); other authors report similar findings. Four categories of incontinence are described: stress, urge, retention and neurogenic, and it is important to distinguish between these.

Stress urinary incontinence

Definition
Stress urinary incontinence is defined as the complaint of involuntary leakage on effort or exertion, or on sneezing or coughing (ICS 2002).

This is the most common type and may coexist with urge incontinence. It is associated with urethral hypermobility and/or an incompetent sphincter (closure) mechanism. The urethra has to remain closed and sealed, except during voluntary bladder emptying. Continence is maintained by urethral closure pressure, which must remain higher than detrusor (bladder muscle) pressure, both at rest and on physical exertion. Physical effort causes a sudden rise in intra-abdominal pressure, which is transmitted to the bladder. When pressure in the bladder rises above that of the urethra, there will be an involuntary escape of urine. The pelvic floor muscles contribute significantly to the continence mechanism, providing about one-third of urethral closure pressure (Raz and Kaufman 1977; Rud et al. 1980).

Urge incontinence

Definition
Urge incontinence is the complaint of involuntary leakage accompanied by, or immediately preceded by, urgency; that is, a sudden compelling desire to pass urine, which is difficult to defer (ICS 2002).

This form of leakage occurs when the detrusor contracts inappropriately as the bladder fills. The literature describes detrusor inhibition mediated by peripheral reflexes, which originate in the pelvic floor, perineum and urethra. Laycock (1998) suggests that activation of the dermatomes and myotomes from S2 to S4 – for example a rapid contraction of the pelvic floor, or standing on 'tip-toe' – may have an inhibitory effect on the detrusor, and so suppress inappropriate detrusor activity, leading to a decrease in urgency.

Retention

This was originally termed 'retention with overflow' and may be acute or chronic.

In hypotonic ('floppy') bladders, the normal response to the increase in pressure, which occurs during filling, may be absent, and the detrusor fails to contract. Retention is associated with outflow obstruction (e.g. in men with prostate disease), neuropathy, low spinal cord lesions, radical pelvic surgery and multiple sclerosis, or it may be secondary to drug therapy (especially with psychotropic drugs). Incontinence sometimes, but not always, occurs with retention.

Neurogenic detrusor overactivity

This term replaces 'hyperreflexia' (ICS 2002) and describes bladder dysfunction of neurological origin.

Neurogenic detrusor overactivity occurs in the presence of a suprasacral cord lesion where the bladder is isolated from cortical control (e.g. cerebrovascular incident, tumour, spinal cord injury or multiple sclerosis). One of the earliest symptoms of multiple sclerosis may be urinary urgency and it is important that physiotherapists be aware of this.

Genital Prolapse

Pelvic organ prolapse is the descent of one or more of:

- the anterior/posterior vaginal wall (known as cystocele and rectocele respectively)
- the top of the vagina (cervix, uterus)
- or the vault (cuff) after hysterectomy.

Symptoms include the feeling of a lump ('something coming down'), low backache, heaviness and dragging sensation, or the need digitally to replace the prolapse in order to defaecate or pass urine. It can occur with other lower urinary tract dysfunction and may mask incontinence.

Prolapse occurs when the fibromuscular supports of the pelvic organs fail. Fifty per cent of parous women (those who have had children) have some degree of genital prolapse but only 10–20% are symptomatic. Severity increases with age (Sultan et al. 1996). Norton (1990) reports a link between joint hypermobility, the presence of striae ('stretch marks') and prolapse, features which are present in other connective-tissue disorders. It is suggested that some women exhibit an immature collagen type and that total collagen content may be reduced significantly (Jackson et al. 1995), leading to genital prolapse.

A trained pelvic floor will contract reflexly in response to a sudden rise in intra-abdominal pressure, thereby limiting downward movement of the organs and reducing the risk of damage to their supports. A voluntary contraction performed before such episodes (e.g. coughing, lifting) will afford protection and should become a life-long habit.

Factors Contributing to Urogenital Dysfunction

It is widely accepted that urogenital problems are associated with vaginal delivery (Wilson et al. 1996; Toozs-Hobson 1998). For many women, childbirth is probably the most significant factor contributing to the development of symptoms. Allen et al. (1990) suggest that a woman's first vaginal delivery causes muscle, fascial and nerve damage, and it is likely that further damage will occur with future deliveries. Chiarelli and Campbell (1997) suggest that forceps delivery increases this risk. There are other reported risk factors: pregnancy itself, straining at stool, heavy lifting, inappropriate exercise, chronic cough, obesity, pelvic surgery, hormonal status and ageing.

PELVIC FLOOR EXERCISES

Women with stress, stress with urge, and urge incontinence and/or genital prolapse may all benefit from specialist physiotherapy.

The pelvic floor muscles have a significant role to play in the continence and organ support mechanisms; they contribute to urethral closure pressure and provide tonic inhibition to the bladder. They are capable of a brisk forceful contraction to counteract a rapid rise in

> **Key point**
>
> A Department of Health report (1997) states that 'all women presenting with incontinence should be offered, as a minimum, one-to-one training, vaginal examination to determine correct muscle action, and three months' exercise taught by a specialist physiotherapist or other professional with specialist knowledge.'

intra-abdominal pressure or to suppress a sudden compelling need to void.

Bump et al. (1991) state that all women presenting with pelvic floor dysfunction should undergo a digital vaginal examination to ensure correct muscle action. Their research demonstrated that fewer than 50% of women were able to perform an optimal or correct pelvic floor contraction when given verbal or written instruction only, and that the feedback provided by digital examination is the only way to ensure appropriate pelvic floor muscle activity

Teaching Pelvic Floor Exercises

Many widely differing exercise protocols are described in the literature and, unfortunately, no standardised outcome measures have been employed to allow evaluation. It is generally accepted, however, that certain principles are fundamental to success. One protocol is described in the boxed text.

Exercising your pelvic floor

Imagine that you are trying to stop yourself from passing wind, and at the same time trying to stop your flow of urine in mid-stream. The feeling is one of 'squeeze and lift', closing and drawing up the back and front passages. Continue the lift for as long as you can (up to 10 seconds). Release and rest for several seconds.

Repeat as many times as you can (up to a maximum of 10 repetitions at a time). This will help to increase the endurance of your pelvic floor muscles.

It is important to do this without tightening your buttocks, holding your breath or squeezing your legs together. You may feel your lower abdomen working at the same time, in the area just above your pubic bone.

It is also important that the muscles are able to react quickly to stop leakage with coughs, sneezes etc. Practise tightening hard and fast, then relaxing immediately.

Both these exercises can be practised anywhere, at any time and in any position, but not while emptying your bladder.

Specificity, overload and maintenance

Gilpin et al. (1989) demonstrated that the pelvic floor exhibits 65% type 1 fibres and 35% type 2, although these proportions vary depending on the subject's age, parity, hormonal status and the pelvic floor muscle site which is sampled. An exercise regimen should include work for both fibre types specifically.

Type 1 fibres exhibit tonic activity and are engaged at lower levels of work and during maximum sustained contraction. Type 2 fibres are recruited during maximal pelvic floor activity, producing a brisk forceful contraction but fatiguing rapidly. Overload is developed by increasing the exercise frequency and duration appropriately as muscle function improves. Maintenance of improved function requires that exercises be continued for life.

Although sometimes suggested as an exercise, midstream stop of urine is strongly discouraged since it may contribute to incomplete emptying and infection.

The pelvic floor as a synergist

Traditionally, pelvic floor exercise has been taught in isolation of other trunk muscles. Although further studies are needed, there is some evidence that the pelvic floor forms part of the functional unit of local spinal stabilisation, acting in synergy with transversus abdominis and other segmental stabilisers (Sapsford et al. 1997; Richardson et al. 1999). Appropriate training of transversus abdominis, therefore, may facilitate re-education of the pelvic floor.

Adjuncts to Exercise

The principal aim of physiotherapy is to strengthen the pelvic floor muscles, and the basis of treatment is an individualised exercise regimen that is progressed appropriately. Bø (1995) suggests that a successful outcome depends on 5–6 months of exercise, plus contact with the therapist. Other modalities may complement this programme, and might include biofeedback, neuromuscular electrical stimulation (NMES) and behavioural modification.

Biofeedback

Biofeedback may be via electromyography or a pressure sensor. The woman receives immediate visual information regarding her pelvic floor activity and is able to modify/increase her effort accordingly. This can provide high levels of motivation. Because of the many variables involved, biofeedback does not measure muscle strength but simply monitors a trend.

Electrical stimulation

NMES is not an alternative to voluntary exercise, but an additional means of strengthening and improving the function of a weakened pelvic floor. Detrusor inhibition may be achieved by targeting the sensory afferent fibres of the pudendal nerve, using a frequency of 5–10 Hz. Higher frequencies of 30–50 Hz will reinforce cortical awareness and stimulate the type 2 fibres to produce a contraction.

Behavioural modification

Many women experience urinary frequency. Pressure from a prolapse, urgency or the belief that keeping the bladder empty of urine will prevent involuntary leakage may all be contributing factors. Bladder training aims to increase gradually both the amount of urine passed and the intervals between voiding. Normal bladder capacity is 350–500 mL, and this capacity can be sustained only if the muscular bladder remains compliant. Allowing it to fill to normal volumes will maintain its elasticity.

> ### Male lower urinary tract symptoms (LUTS)
> Bladder dysfunction is not confined to women. LUTS are present in up to 30% of men aged over 50, who have not undergone surgery (Chute et al. 1993). Physiotherapy intervention for male problems does not feature significantly in the literature but help is often sought from physiotherapists who specialise in continence management. Dorey (1998, 2000) discusses the subject in some detail and provides relevant references for further reading.

ANORECTAL DYSFUNCTION

The physiotherapist seeing patients with urogenital dysfunction might also treat anorectal dysfunctions such as faecal incontinence and constipation.

Faecal Incontinence

The problem

Faecal incontinence affects about 1% of community-dwelling adults (Nelson et al. 1995) and over 10% of those in residential care for the elderly (Tobin and Brocklehurst 1986). Causes are similar to those listed under urogenital dysfunction, the most common being obstetric trauma.

> ### Definition
> Leakage is described as *passive* (patient not aware) or *urge* (patient is aware of a need to defaecate, but is unable to control it).

Arguably of greatest significance is the consistency of stool. If this is liquid or very soft, then it is far more difficult to contain. Ideally the referring doctor will have addressed this issue before the patient attends for physiotherapy.

Anal sphincters

The internal anal sphincter comprises smooth muscle, and provides 80–85% of resting pressure. The external anal sphincter (EAS) is under voluntary control, and contracts in response to rectal distension to allow the individual to defer defaecation until an appropriate time.

Puborectalis

Puborectalis, part of the levator ani, also contributes to the continence mechanism, by forming an acute angle at the top of the anal canal (anorectal angle) to prevent the escape of rectal contents.

Physiotherapy intervention

As in urogenital dysfunction, muscle re-education is indicated – exercises to improve the function of puborectalis and the EAS, with or without biofeedback. Electrical stimulation may also be used. Enck (1993), in a review, reported a cure or improvement rate of 79% with biofeedback, while Fynes et al. (1999) suggested the addition of electrical stimulation was more beneficial than exercises and biofeedback alone.

As in all aspects of physiotherapy, appropriate advice should also be given, such as about diet, and deferment (for urge incontinence).

Constipation

The problem

> ### Definition
> Constipation may be defined as infrequent bowel motions (fewer than 3 times a week) or the need to strain at defaecation. It may be subdivided into slow-transit and obstructed defaecation.

Slow transit defaecation

This may be idiopathic, but can be a result of the avoidance or postponement of defaecation by an individual. It has been claimed (Gattuso and Kamm 1993) that up to 50% of patients with severe idiopathic constipation may have a history of childhood bereavement or of emotional, sexual or physical abuse.

Obstructed defaecation

This presents as an urge to defaecate, but an inability to empty fully. It may be associated with a failure to relax puborectalis or the EAS, or a lack of pelvic floor support (and resulting descent of the perineum) during defaecation (Markwell and Sapsford 1995). Causes are many, including obstetric trauma, pelvic surgery, and prolonged straining. It may be found in combination with slow transit (Hutchinson et al. 1993).

Physiotherapy intervention

The physiotherapist is more commonly involved in the treatment of obstructed defaecation. The aim of treatment is to teach effective defaecation without straining (Markwell and Sapsford 1995) and should include correct positioning on the toilet, relaxation of puborectalis and the EAS, and optimum abdominal muscle action with an expulsive effort. Biofeedback might also be used, and different techniques have shown varying success rates (Heyman et al. 1999).

If there is evidence of perineal descent or a rectocele, women might be advised to offer manual support to the perineum or digital support to the posterior vaginal wall, respectively, to facilitate bowel emptying.

As there is an increase in colonic transit following meals, patients can be encouraged to attempt defaecation at these times.

GYNAECOLOGICAL SURGERY

Operations

Major gynaecological surgery may be necessary for many reasons, including the removal of benign or malignant tumours, urogynaecological conditions (if they fail to respond to physiotherapy) and the treatment of problems related to fertility or ectopic pregnancy. The physiotherapist should be aware of the indication for surgery and the social and emotional implications for the woman and her family.

A list of procedures undertaken is prohibitively long for this text, but those commonly encountered by the physiotherapist include:

- hysterectomy (removal of the womb) which can be undertaken vaginally or abdominally
- Burch colposuspension (for stress urinary incontinence)
- salpingectomy (removal of a fallopian tube, often for an ectopic pregnancy)
- vulvectomy (removal of the vulva, for benign or malignant disease).

Physiotherapy

The physiotherapist working on the gynaecological ward is in a unique position to be able not only to prepare women for surgery, but also to provide health education for future life. Ergonomic advice for home and work, sports and leisure, postural care, abdominal and pelvic floor exercise and relaxation should be provided, preferably preoperatively, and ideally before admission to hospital. This will give the patient an opportunity to organise changes at home. A group setting is good use of the therapist's time and gives a forum for peer support and discussion.

The physiotherapist must know each woman's history so as to be aware of any special needs (e.g. a diagnosis of malignancy). Special attention should be given to the psychosocial and psychosexual effects of gynaecological surgery on the patient and her family. Referral to other professional groups – for example a Macmillan nurse or social worker – may be appropriate.

Preoperative assessment will give the physiotherapist an opportunity to instigate treatment for problems such as urogenital or anorectal dysfunction and musculoskeletal problems.

Preoperative care

This can include:

- assessment of risk factors (e.g. respiratory conditions)
- identification of urogenital or anorectal dysfunction
- identification of musculoskeletal problems
- exercises and strategies to promote postoperative mobility and comfort
- postoperative recovery plan, both before and after discharge from hospital
- relaxation.

Postoperative care

The presence of an intravenous infusion, urinary catheter (suprapubic or urethral), patient-controlled analgesia and vaginal pack should be noted. The physiotherapist must be aware of the findings at surgery, and their potential physical and psychological impact on the patient. There may be concerns about relationships or resuming sexual activity, and referral to the relevant professional may be appropriate (Sacco Ezzell 1999).

Respiratory function

Patients may be instructed in appropriate respiratory techniques and wound support when coughing, especially women who have undergone surgery for prolapse. Patients with predisposing factors to postoperative respiratory complications, those undergoing extensive and invasive surgery, and those who are already debilitated are at increased risk of postoperative chest problems (Webber and Pryor 1998).

Circulation

Patients considered at risk of developing deep venous thrombosis (DVT) are fitted with anti-embolus stockings, and prophylactic anticoagulant therapy is administered. Ankle and quadriceps exercises will help prepare for mobilisation postoperatively and therefore reduce the risk of DVT (Webber and Pryor 1998).

Mobility, comfort and posture

The patient should be taught correct movement patterns for bed mobility, transfer from bed to chair, movement from sitting to standing, and positions of comfort on the bed and in a chair. This will reduce strain on the operation site and facilitate mobility. Reassurance that they can do no harm to the wound, and good analgesic cover, will all contribute to early mobilisation.

Urination and defaecation

The patient should sit on the toilet or commode with feet supported. When defaecating in the early postoperative period, she will feel more confident and comfortable if supporting her wound with hands placed over a folded towel (or perineal pad following vaginal surgery).

Abdominal exercises

Contractions of transversus abdominis should be taught to maintain the musculature of the abdominal wall. Pelvic tilting and knee rolling might ease low back pain and painful flatus. Abdominal massage applied in a clockwise direction can also help the latter. These exercises and self-help strategies may be commenced as soon as the woman feels ready (e.g. the first or second day after surgery). Early mobilisation will also help to relieve these postoperative discomforts.

Pelvic floor exercises and advice

The physiotherapist should confirm with the consultant any local policy for commencement of pelvic floor exercises. Women who have undergone surgery for prolapse and/or incontinence may already have poor connective tissue. If returning to a lifestyle which may have contributed to the necessity for surgery, they should be given appropriate advice – correct lifting techniques, avoidance of standing for long periods, awareness of the role of the pelvic floor and interaction with transversus abdominis. Outpatient follow-up might be beneficial.

Going home

Women are generally anxious to return to full activity. Consideration must be given to the surgery undergone when advice is sought concerning progression of physical activity (e.g. work and sports). Discharge from hospital may be as early as 3 days following some surgery, though it can be considerably longer. Convalescence is usually for 1–2 months with a gradual increase in physical activity, but heavy lifting should be avoided for at least 2 months (Chamberlain 1995).

Relaxation

If time allows, the physiotherapist may teach relaxation, to help the patient cope with the anxieties of hospitalisation and any future stresses.

PELVIC PAIN

Acute and chronic pain

Pelvic pain in women has many varied sources, diagnoses and outcomes. It can be acute or chronic. In the most part, if the former, it has an easily identifiable cause, such as dyspareunia (pain on sexual intercourse) caused by scar tissue following childbirth. Appropriate treatment will alleviate the pain.

When pain has lasted more than 6 months it is said to be chronic. Although it may still have a well-defined cause (e.g. endometriosis), it can involve a much more complex interplay between biomechanical, behavioural, emotional and sociocultural influences, all of which need to be taken into account in the treatment. This has led to clinicians involved in treating this group of women advocating a multidisciplinary integrated approach (Steege et al. 1998).

Prevalence

The annual prevalence of chronic pelvic pain has been estimated at between 24.4 cases per 1000 women (Davies et al. 1992) and 38.3 per 1000 (Zondervan et al. 1999). It has been estimated that the economic burden to the National Health Service is £158 million, with indirect costs of a further £24 million (Davies et al. 1992).

Pelvic pain has traditionally been ascribed (from a gynaecological view) to endometriosis, pelvic inflammatory disease, adhesions secondary to infection or surgery, and – more recently – pelvic venous congestion. The most important non-gynaecological cause is irritable bowel syndrome. Other causes include ilioinguinal nerve entrapment, levator ani syndrome, coccydinia, interstitial cystitis, vulval vestibulitis/vulvodynia and musculoskeletal dysfunction.

A study by Zondervan et al. (1999) showed that 28% of the patients involved never received a diagnosis, while Mathias et al. (1996) suggested an even higher rate (61%). This is highly significant for all health professionals working with this group of patients as sufferers often feel that their pain will not be taken seriously until they have a diagnosis. This may result in a fruitless round of clinicians.

Role of the physiotherapist

The role of the physiotherapist in the management of women with chronic pelvic pain is to decrease the pain, increase function, and to treat existing (and help prevent future) musculoskeletal dysfunction.

Following a detailed musculoskeletal examination including assessment of the pelvic floor muscles, the treatment modalities used to achieve this may include: muscle imbalance work, muscle energy techniques, core stability exercises, pelvic floor rehabilitation, electrical stimulation, soft-tissue mobilisations, joint manipulation, breathing and relaxation techniques, heat/cold therapy, hydrotherapy, biofeedback, and alternative therapies.

The modalities chosen will vary according to the needs of the patient and the experience of the clinician involved. Close liaison with other members of the multidisciplinary team is essential to maximise the benefit of treatment.

MENOPAUSE

Menopause is the cessation of menstruation and marks the end of a woman's reproductive years. It has signifi-

Average life expectancy has risen significantly in the last 150 years, but the age at which menopause occurs has remained remarkably constant at 50 ¾ years. A British woman can expect to enjoy about 30 years of postmenopausal life (Belsey 1999). Biochemical and metabolic changes following menopause may cause distressing symptoms, which affect adversely her quality of life.

cant implications for a woman's health and quality of life, and so is of great relevance to the physiotherapist.

Oestrogens are the group of female hormones produced by the ovary. Oestrogen receptors are present in many tissues, and normal physiological function is dependent on the presence of this steroid. The perimenopause describes the period during which ovarian function declines. The menstrual cycle becomes erratic and a woman may seek help for symptoms of oestrogen depletion.

Vasomotor effects

Examples are hot flushes and night sweats. The cause of this vasomotor instability is complex and unclear (Bachmann 2001) and severity varies widely between individuals.

Musculoskeletal and articular effects

Osteoporosis, characterised by low bone mass, is one of the most clinically significant sequelae of oestrogen deficiency.

Articular changes may occur due to a decrease in the collagen content of ligaments and articular soft tissues (Whitehead and Godfree 1992). Muscular changes are attributed to an overall reduction in muscle mass, with a decrease in both strength and endurance of muscle tissue. These changes result in an increased risk of falls and injury, which may require physiotherapy.

Cardiovascular disease

Cardiovascular disease (CVD) is the biggest killer of postmenopausal women in western society. It has generally been accepted that postmenopausal oestrogen replacement confers protection against CVD, greatly reducing the risk (Mendelsohn and Karas 1999). However, this postulation is now questioned (Burger and Teede 2001), so more data from clinical trials are needed.

Cognitive function

Oestrogen lack is thought to be involved in alteration of neurotransmitters in the brain (Genazzani et al. 1998), with a consequent decline in cognitive function and increased incidence of dementia. These changes will have implications for the woman, her family and health professionals, including the physiotherapist, who may be involved in her care.

Urogenital oestrogen deficiency syndrome

Oestrogen receptors are present in the urogenital tract and the pelvic floor (Smith et al. 1990) and the ageing woman may experience vaginal dryness, soreness, infection and dyspareunia (pain on intercourse). Genital prolapse and urinary symptoms, including incontinence, frequency, urgency and voiding difficulties, are common (Samsioe 1998). The physiotherapist has an important role to play in the conservative management of these problems (see the section above on urogenital dysfunction).

LYMPHOEDEMA

The condition

Definition
Lymphoedema is chronic and progressive swelling caused by a low output failure of the lymphatic system, resulting in the development of a high-protein oedema in the tissues (Földi et al. 1985).

In the western world, cancer or its treatment is a common cause of this condition. Surgical removal of part of the lymphatic system, or fibrotic changes subsequent to surgery or radiotherapy, result in a partial obstruction in lymphatic drainage and the development of lymphoedema in the affected limb and associated part of the trunk. The time of onset varies and in some cases can occur many years after the initial cancer treatment (Stanton et al. 1996).

Prevalence
The prevalence of this condition remains largely unknown. However, there is some evidence to indicate that approximately one quarter of women develop lymphoedema following breast cancer treatment (Pain and Purushotham 2000).

The onset of lymphoedema is often marked by intermittent swelling and paraesthesia (Piller 1999). Initially, the oedema is soft and pitting and reduces on elevation (Keeley 2000). With time and recurrent skin infections, fibrotic changes occur both in the skin and subcutis, with a progressive swelling and distortion of shape. The skin and tissues become thickened with enhanced skin folds and increased adiposity, and the swelling becomes largely non-pitting. The size of the limb increases and is sometimes accompanied by a distortion in shape. Movement becomes restricted as the limb becomes increasingly heavy and uncomfortable.

Women with lymphoedema are predisposed to recurrent attacks of acute inflammatory episode (AIE),

often referred to as cellulitis (Edwards 1963; Mortimer 1995). These apparent skin infections are recognised by signs and symptoms including acute pain, swelling, anorexia, fevers, vomiting and rigors.

The psychosocial impact of living with lymphoedema can be profound, resulting in negative feelings such as embarrassment, loss of self-esteem, and increased feelings of anxiety and depression. Patients also experience impaired physical mobility and pain (Tobin et al. 1993; Woods 1993).

Although no curative treatment is available, a combination of physical therapies is used to control and reduce the complications associated with lymphoedema. Patient education is a primary aim of any treatment programme. Assessment and treatment is provided by specialist trained physiotherapists and nurses. A treatment plan is agreed and negotiated with the patient following a comprehensive assessment of needs. Ongoing reviews are usually required to monitor progress and to provide a new supply of compression garments.

Role of the physiotherapist

Treatment is based around four key areas (Földi et al. 1985; Jenns 2000):

- skin care
- compression/support
- exercise
- lymphatic massage.

Skin care

This involves the daily application of emollient cream and the provision of information and advice on skin care to minimise the risk of AIE. Advice includes protection of the skin from cuts, insect bites and burns (e.g. when gardening, sewing or sunbathing). Whenever possible, medical interventions such as venepuncture, or taking blood pressure, should be undertaken on the unaffected side, to minimise any potential risk.

Compression garments

These are used to limit and control swelling in the limbs. In breast cancer, a glove, sleeve or combined glove and sleeve may be used depending on the extent of the swelling. Garments are usually worn during the day, especially for exercise and when working. In some cases a bandaging system described as multilayer lymphoedema bandaging (MLLB) is used in combination with lymphatic massage to reverse complications such as severe swelling or distorted limb shape, prior to the introduction of compression garments (Todd 2000).

Pneumatic compression therapy (e.g. Flotron) is a method of treatment traditionally used, but its value in the treatment of lymphoedema is limited (Casley-Smith and Casley-Smith 1997).

Dynamic exercise

This is beneficial, as lymphatic drainage is enhanced by the effect of the muscle pump, particularly when a compression garment is worn. Gentle stretching exercises also help to maintain or improve range of movement and to facilitate good posture. Excessive exercise can increase the lymphatic load and result in further swelling, so patients are warned to introduce any new activity gradually and with caution.

Lymphatic massage

Manual lymphatic drainage (MLD) is characterised by the pressure and sequence of the technique, designed to stimulate drainage through the functioning lymphatics. This is usually the only method of care available to treat midline oedema (i.e. face, trunk). A simplified method is shown to the patient for self-treatment (simple lymphatic drainage – SLD) (Gillham 1994).

PSYCHOSEXUAL ISSUES

Sexual activity and enjoyment is essentially a psychophysical act, which can be affected by obstetric and gynaecological problems, and by emotions. The use of the term 'psychosexual' is important, as any sexual relationship involves whole people with previous experiences and feelings, attached to anatomical sexual parts.

Physiotherapists usually feel they must be 'doing' something to treat their patients. However, unless they are also able to listen and acknowledge the real problem, change will not occur. They may be the first person with whom the patient feels enough trust to share this problem. The women's health physiotherapist is one of the few professionals who may include a vaginal examination as part of their assessment. This is a very intimate procedure and a time of self-awareness for the patient. In psychosexual counselling it is referred to as the 'moment of truth' and should be approached with sensitivity and care. This may be the occasion when past feelings come to light, for example previous sexual abuse.

Childbirth is said to be the greatest emotional crisis in a woman's life and she can find it very traumatic. Some women take time to come to terms with the experience and the consequent changes to their body caused by pregnancy and birth, which may affect their sexual activity in the short or long term. The perineum can feel painful for some time after an episiotomy or tear, and intercourse may be difficult and therefore avoided. This pain and a perceived change in body image may affect any close relationship. The physiotherapist and other health professionals must encourage the woman to talk about her labour and of any feelings of disappointment or loss of control, particularly how the experience made her feel.

A woman who suffers from faecal and urinary incontinence is embarrassed and often unable to speak to anyone about the problem. She is afraid that she smells, she feels dirty and is ashamed that she leaks, so she may avoid having intercourse or close contact with her partner. This can have a devastating affect on the relationship.

Concern about a change in body image can occur after breast and gynaecological surgery, particularly for malignancy. Some women grieve for the loss of their uterus. To them, it is an intrinsic part of being a woman and its removal feels like a bereavement.

During the menopause, many changes take place, both physical and emotional. Women may suffer from loss of libido (sex drive), and vaginal tissues can become dry and cause pain during intercourse. Dyspareunia can also be the result of a surgical procedure, acute or chronic pelvic pain, as well as after childbirth.

Feelings play a large part in psychosexual problems and the physiotherapist must be prepared to listen to patients who choose to share these feelings. If the patient feels she needs further help, the physiotherapist should know what options are available for referral. It is also very important that the therapist knows to whom to go to debrief, as he or she might require experienced support with these sometimes complex issues.

FURTHER READING

Physiotherapy in women's health

Polden M, Mantle J 1990 Physiotherapy in Obstetrics and Gynaecology. Butterworth–Heinemann: Oxford
Sapsford R, Bullock-Saxton J, Markwell S 1998 Women's Health: a Textbook for Physiotherapists. WB Saunders: London

Anatomy and physiology

Veralls S 1993 Anatomy and Physiology Applied to Obstetrics, 3rd edn. Churchill Livingstone: Edinburgh

Pregnancy and childbirth

Bennett, Brown 1999 Myles' Textbook for Midwives, 13th edn. Churchill Livingstone: Edinburgh
Henderson C, Jones K (eds) 1997 Essential Midwifery. Mosby: London
Symonds EM, Symonds IM 1998 Essential Obstetrics and Gynaecology, 3rd edn. Churchill Livingstone: Edinburgh

Antenatal classes, advice and exercise

Brayshaw E, Wright P 1994 Teaching Physical Skills for the Childbearing Year. Books for Midwives Press: Hale

Nolan M 2000 Antenatal Education. A Dynamic Approach. Baillière Tindall: London

Schott J, Priest J 2002 Leading Antenatal Classes: a Practical Guide. Books for Midwives Press: Oxford

Gynaecology

Chamberlain G 1995 Gynaecology by Ten Teachers. Edward Arnold: London

Lymphoedema

Twycross R, Jenns K, Todd J (eds) 2000 Lymphoedema. Radcliffe Medical Press: Oxford

Psychosexual issues

Institute of Psychosexual Medicine: www.ipm.org.uk

Skrine RL 1997 Blocks and Freedoms in Sexual Life. Radcliffe Medical Press: Oxford

REFERENCES

Abitol MM 1997 Quadrupedalism, bipedalism, and human pregnancy. In: Vleeming A, Mooney V, Dorman T (eds) Movement, Stability and Low Back Pain. Churchill Livingstone: Edinburgh

Abramson D, Roberts SM, Wilson PD 1934 Relaxation of the pelvic joints in pregnancy. Surg Gynaecol Obstet 58: 595–613

ACOG (American College of Obstetricians and Gynecologists) 2002 Exercise during pregnancy and the postpartum period. Obstet Gynecol 99: 171–3

ACPWH (Association of Chartered Physiotherapists in Women's Health) 1995 Aquanatal Guidelines (available from the Book and Leaflet Secretary, ACPWH, c/o Chartered Society of Physiotherapy, 14 Bedford Row, London WC1R 4ED)

ACPWH (Association of Chartered Physiotherapists in Women's Health) 1996 Symphysis Pubis Dysfunction – a Guideline (available from the Book and Leaflet Secretary, ACPWH, c/o Chartered Society of Physiotherapy, 14 Bedford Row, London WC1R 4ED)

Al-Azzawi F 1990 A Colour Atlas of Childbirth and Obstetrics. Wolfe Publishing: London

Allen RE, Hosker GL, Smith AR, Warrell DW 1990 Pelvic floor damage and childbirth: a neurophysiological study. Br J Obstet Gynaecol 97: 770–9

Bachmann G 2001 Physiological aspects of natural and surgical menopause. J Reprod Med 46(3 Suppl): 307–15

Belsey J 1999 Evidence-based review of tibolone and oestrogen-based hormone replacement therapy. J Br Meno Soc 5(Suppl 1): 33–5

Berg G, Hammar M, Moller-Nielsen J 1988 Low back pain during pregnancy. Obstet Gynaecol 71: 71–5

Bø K 1995 Pelvic floor muscle exercise for the treatment of stress urinary incontinence: an exercise physiology perspective. Int Urogynecol J 6: 282–91

Boissonnault JS, Blaschak MJ 1988 Incidence of diastasis recti abdominis during the childbearing year. Phys Ther 86: 1082–6

Bortoluzzi G 1989 Transcutaneous electrical nerve stimulation in labour: practicability and effectiveness in a public hospital ward. Aust J Physiother 35: 81–7

Breen TW, Ransil BJ, Groves PA, Oriol NE 1994 Factors associated with back pain after childbirth. Anesthesiology 81(1): 29–34

Bullock JE, Jull GA, Bullock MI 1987 The relationship of low back pain to postural changes during pregnancy. Aust J Physiother 33(1): 10–17

Bullock-Saxton JE 1991 Changes in posture associated with pregnancy and the early postnatal period measured in standing. Physiother Theory Pract 7:103–9

Bullock-Saxton JE 1998 Musculoskeletal changes associated with the perinatal period. In: Sapsford R, Bullock-Saxton J, Markwell S (eds) Women's Health: a Textbook for Physiotherapists, ch. 14, pp. 134–61. WB Saunders: London

Bump R, Hurt WG, Fantl A, Wyman J 1991 Assessment of Kegel pelvic muscle exercise performance after brief verbal instruction. Am J Obstet Gynecol 165: 322–9

Burger H, Teede H 2001 Cardiovascular disease. Maturitas 40: 1–3

Casley-Smith JR, Casley-Smith JR 1997 Modern Treatment for Lymphoedema, 5th edn, pp. 288–301. Terrance Printing: Adelaide

Chamberlain G 1995 Gynaecology by Ten Teachers, ch. 13, p. 282. Edward Arnold: London

Chiarelli P, Campbell E 1997 Incontinence during pregnancy: prevalence and opportunities for continence promotion. Aust NZ J Obstet Gynaecol 37(1): 66–73

Chute CG, Panser LA, Girman CJ et al. 1993 The prevalence of prostatism: a population-based survey of urinary symptoms. J Urol 150: 85–9

Clapp JF 2000 Exercise during pregnancy: a clinical update. Clin Sports Med 19(2): 273–86

Clapp JF, Kim H, Burciu B, Lopez B 2000 Beginning regular exercise in early pregnancy: effect on fetoplacental growth. Am J Obstet Gynecol 183: 1484–8

Coldron Y, Vits K 2001 Musculoskeletal considerations and the role of physiotherapy in the management of peripartum spinal and pelvic pain. In: Maclean AB, Stones RW, Thornton S (eds) Pain in Obstetrics and Gynaecology, ch. 25, pp. 295–307. RCOG Press: London

Cresswell AG, Grundstrom H, Thortensson A 1992 Observations on intra-abdominal pressure and patterns of abdominal intramuscular activity in man. Acta Physiol Scand 144: 409–18

CSP 1995 Tripartite Statement (document PA13). Chartered Society of Physiotherapy, 14 Bedford Row, London WC1R 4ED

Davies L, Gangar KF, Drummond M, Saunders D, Beard RW 1992 The economic burden of intractable gynaecological pain. J Obstet Gynaecol 12(Suppl 2): S54–6

Department of Health 1997 Working Group on Outcome Indicators for Urinary Incontinence, Unit of Health Care Epidemiology, University of Oxford, p 42

Dorey G 1998 Physiotherapy for male continence problems. Physiotherapy 85: 556–663

Dorey G 2000 Physiotherapy for the relief of male lower urinary tract symptoms. Physiotherapy 86: 413–26

Edwards EA 1963 Recurrent febrile episodes and lymphoedema. JAMA 184: 858–62

Enck P 1993 Biofeedback training in disorded defecation: a critical review. Digest Dis Sci 38:1953–60

Evans GM 2002 Aquanatal exercise. In: Campion MR, Pattmann J (eds) Hydrotherapy: Principles and Practice, 2nd edn. Butterworth–Heinemann: Oxford

Fast A, Shapiro D, Ducommun EJ 1987 Low back pain in pregnancy. Spine 12: 368–71

Földi E, Földi M, Weisleder H 1985 Conservative treatment of lymphoedema of the limbs. Angiology 36: 171–80

Fry D 1990 Perinatal symphysis pubis dysfunction: a review of the literature. J Assoc Chart Physiother Wom Health 85:11–18

Fry D, Tudor A 1997 Pelvic support belt. J Assoc Chart Physiother Wom Health 81: 40

Fynes MM, Marshall K, Cassidy M et al. 1999 A prospective, randomized study comparing the effect of augmented biofeedback with sensory biofeedback alone on fecal incontinence after obstetric trauma. Dis Colon Rectum 42: 753–61

Gamble JG, Simmons SC, Freedman M 1986 The symphysis pubis: anatomic and pathologic considerations. Clin Orthop 203: 261–72

Gardosi J, Sylvester S, B-Lynch C 1989 Alternative positions in the second stage of labour: a randomised controlled trial. Br J Obstet Gynaecol 96B: 1290

Gatusso J, Kamm M 1993 The management of constipation in adults. Aliment Pharmacol Ther 7: 487–500

Genazzani AR, Bernadi F, Stomati M et al. 1998 Sex steroids and the brain. J Br Meno Soc 5(Suppl 1): 11–12

Gilleard WL, Brown JMM 1996 Structure and function of the abdominal muscles during pregnancy and the immediate post birth period. Phys Ther 7: 750–62

Gillham L 1994 Lymphoedema and physiotherapists: control not cure. Physiotherapy 80: 835–43

Gilpin SA, Gosling JA, Smith ARB et al. 1989 The pathogenesis of genitourinary prolapse and stress incontinence of urine: a histological and histochemical study. Br J Obstet Gynaecol 96: 15–23

Golighty R 1982 Pelvic arthropathy in pregnancy and the puerperium. Physiotherapy 68 (7): 216–20

Harrison R, Bulstrode F 1987 Percentage weight bearing during partial immersion in a hydrotherapy pool. Physiother Pract 3: 60–3

Heckman JD, Sassard R 1994 Musculoskeletal considerations in pregnancy. J Bone Joint Surg 76: 1720–6

Heiberg E, Aarseth SP 1997 Epidemiology of pelvic pain and low back pain in pregnant women. In: Vleeming A et al. (eds) Movement, Stability and Low Back Pain, ch. 32, pp. 405–10. Churchill Livingstone: Edinburgh

Henderson C, Jones K (eds) 1997 Essential Midwifery. Mosby: London

Heyman S, Wexner SD, Vickers D et al. 1999 Prospective, randomized trial comparing four biofeedback techniques for patients with constipation. Dis Colon Rectum 42: 1388–93

Hodges PW 1999 Is there a role for transversus abdominis in lumbo-pelvic stability? Manual Ther 4(2): 74–86

Holtedahl K, Hunskaar S 1998 Prevalence, 1-year incidence and factors associated with urinary incontinence: a population based study of women 50–74 years of age in primary care. Maturitas 28(3): 205–11

Howell CJ, Chalmers I 1992 A review of prospectively controlled comparisons of epidural with non-epidural forms of pain relief during labour. Int J Obstet Anesth 1: 93

Hsia M, Jones S 2000 Natural resolution of rectus abdominis diastasis: two single case studies. Aust J Physiother 46: 301–7

Hutchinson R, Notghi A, Mostafa AB, Harding LK, Kumar D 1993 Audit of transit abnormality in chronic idiopathic constipation. Gut 34(Supp 4): W49

ICS (International Continence Society) 2002 Standardisation of Terminology in Lower Urinary Tract Function. ICS: London

Jackson S, Avery N, Eckford S et al. 1995 Connective tissue analysis in genitourinary prolapse. Neurourol Urodynam 14: 412–14

Jenns K 2000 Management strategies. In: Twycross R, Jenns K, Todd J (eds) Lymphoedema, pp. 98–117. Radcliffe Medical Press: Oxford

Jull G, Richardson C, Toppenberg R, Comerford M, Bui B 1993 Towards a measurement of active muscle control for lumbar stabilisation. Aust J Physiother 39: 187–93

Katz VL, McMurray RG, Cefalo RC 1991 Aquatic exercise during pregnancy. In: Mittelmark RA, Wiswell RA, Drinkwater BL (eds) Exercise in Pregnancy, 2nd edn, pp. 271–8. Williams & Wilkins: Baltimore

Keeley V 2000 Clinical features of lymphoedema. In: Twycross R, Jenns K, Todd J (eds) Lymphoedema, pp. 44–67. Radcliffe Medical Press: Oxford

Kristiansson P 1997 S–relaxin and pelvic pain in pregnant women. In: Vleeming A et al. (eds) Movement Stability and Low Back Pain, ch. 34, pp. 421–4. Churchill Livingstone: Edinburgh

Kubitz RL, Goodlin RC 1986 Symptomatic separation of the pubic symphysis. South Med Jnl 79: 578–80

Laycock J 1998 An update on the management of female urinary incontinence. J Assoc Chart Physiother Wom Health 83: 3–5

Llewellyn-Jones D 1999 Fundamentals of Obstetrics and Gynaecology, 7th edn. Mosby: London

Lo T, Candido G, Janssen P 1999 Diastasis of the recti abdominis in pregnancy: risk factors and treatment. Physiother Can 44: 32–7

MacArthur C, Weeks S 1995 Epidural anaesthesia and low back pain after delivery: prospective cohort study. BMJ 311: 1336–9

MacArthur C, Lewis M, Knox BJ, Crawford JS 1990 Epidural anaesthesia and long-term backache after childbirth. BMJ 301: 9–12

MacLennan AH 1981 Relaxin: a review. Aust NZ J Obstet Gynaecol 21: 195–201

MacLennan AH, MacLennan SC 1997 Symptom-giving pelvic girdle relaxation of pregnancy, postnatal pelvic joint syndrome and dysplasia of the hip. Acta Obstet Gynecol Scand 76:760–4

Mantle J 1994 Back pain in the childbearing year. In: Boyling JD, Palastanga N (eds) Grieve's Modern Manual Therapy, ch. 59, pp. 799–808. Churchill Livingstone: Edinburgh

Mantle MJ, Greenwood RM, Currey HLF 1977 Backache in pregnancy. Rheumatol Rehabil 16: 95–101

Markwell SJ, Sapsford RR 1995 Physiotherapy management of obstructed defaecation. Aust J Physiother 41: 279–83

Mathias SD, Kuppermann M, Liberman RF, Lipschutz RC, Steege JF 1996 Chronic pelvic pain: prevalence, health-related quality of life, and economic correlates. Obstet Gynecol 87: 321–7

McIntosh JM 1995 Treatment note: alternative pelvic support. J Assoc Chart Physiother Wom Health 76: 28

Melzack R, Wall P 1982 The Challenge of Pain. Harmondsworth: Penguin

Mendelsohn ME, Karas RH 1999 The protective effects of oestrogen on the cardiovascular system. N Engl J Med 340: 1801–11

Mens JM, Vleeming A, Stoeckart R, Stam HJ, Snijders CJ 1996 Understanding peripartum pelvic pain. Spine 21: 1363–70

Morkved S, Bø K 2000 Effect of postpartum pelvic floor muscle training in prevention and treatment of urinary incontinence: a one year follow up. Br J Obstet Gynaecol 107: 1022–8

Mortimer PS 1995 Managing lymphoedema. Clin Expl Dermatol 20: 98–106

Nelson R, Norton N, Cautley E, Furner S 1995 Community-based prevalence of anal incontinence. JAMA 274: 559–61

Newham DJ 1988 The consequences of eccentric contraction and their relationship to delayed onset of muscle pain. Eur J Appl Physiol 57: 3353–9

Nilsson-Wikmar L, Harms-Ringdahl K 1999 Back pain in women post-partum is not a unitary concept. Physiother Res Int 4(3): 201–13

Noren L, Ostgaard S, Nielson TF, Ostgaard HC 1997 Reduction of sick leave for lumbar back and posterior pain in pregnancy. Spine 22: 2157–60

Norton P 1990 Genitourinary prolapse: relationship with joint mobility. Neurourol Urodynam 9: 321–2

O'Sullivan PB 2000 Lumbar segmental 'instability': clinical presentation and specific stabilising exercises management. Manual Ther 51(1): 2–12

O'Sullivan PB, Twomey L, Allison GT 1997 Evaluation of specific stabilising exercises in the treatment of chronic low back pain with radiological diagnosis of spondylolisis or spondylolisthesis. Spine 22: 2959–67

Ostgaard HC 1997 Lumbar back and posterior pelvic pain in pregnancy. In: Vleeming A et al. (eds) Movement, Stability and Low Back Pain, ch. 33, pp. 411–20. Churchill Livingstone: Edinburgh

Ostgaard HC, Andersson GBJ 1992 Postpartum low back pain. Spine 17: 53–5

Ostgaard HC, Andersson GB, Karlsson K. 1991 Prevalence of back pain in pregnancy. Spine 16: 549–52

Ostgaard HC, Andersson GBJ, Schuttz AB, Miller JA 1993 Influence of some biomechanical factors on low back pain in pregnancy. Spine 18: 61–5

Pain SJ, Purushotham AD 2000 Lymphoedema following surgery for breast cancer. Br J Breast Surg 87: 1128–41

Palastanga N, Field, D, Soames R 2002 Anatomy and Human Movement, 4th edn. Butterworth–Heinemann: Oxford.

Piller NB 1999 Gaining an accurate assessment of the stages of lymphedema subsequent to cancer: the role of objective and subjective information when to make measurements and their optimal use. Eur J Lymphol 7(25): 1–9

Polden M, Mantle J 1990 Physiotherapy in Obstetrics and Gynaecology. Butterworth–Heinemann: Oxford

Potter H 1997 Effect of an intense training programme for the deep anterolateral muscles on rectus abdominis diastasis: a single case study. In: Biennial Conference Proceedings of the Manipulative Physiotherapists Association of Australia. MPPA Clinical Solutions Publisher: Victoria

Raz S, Kaufman JJ 1977 Carbon dioxide urethral pressure profile in female incontinence. J Urol 117: 765–9

Richardson C, Toppenburg R, Jull G 1990 An initial evaluation of eight abdominal exercises for their ability to provide stability for the lumbar spine. Aust J Physiother 36: 6–11

Richardson C, Jull G, Toppenburg R, Commerford M 1993 Techniques for active stabilisation for spinal protection: a pilot study. Aust J Physiother 38: 105–11

Richardson C, Jull G, Hodges P, Hides J 1999 Therapeutic Exercise for Spinal Segmental Stabilization in Low Back Pain, p. 95. Churchill Livingstone: Edinburgh

Riemann MK, Kanstrup Hansen IL 2000 Effects on the fetus of exercise in pregnancy (review). Scand J Med Sci Sports 10(1): 12–19

Röst C 1999 Bekkenpijn Tijden En Na De Zwangerschap Een Programma ter Voorkoming van Chronische Bekkeninstabiliteit. Elsevier/De Tijdstroom: Maarssen

Rud T, Anderson KE, Asmusson M et al. 1980 Factors maintaining the intraurethral pressure in women. Invest Urol 17: 343–7

Russell JGB 1982 The rationale of primitive delivery positions. Br J Obstet Gynaecol 89: 712

Russell R, Reynolds F 1997 Back pain, pregnancy and childbirth. BMJ 314: 1062

Russell R, Groves P Taub N, O'Dowd J, Reynolds F 1993 Assessing long term backache after childbirth. BMJ 306: 1299–303

Russell R, Dundas R, Reynolds F 1996 Long term backache after childbirth: prospective search for causative factors. BMJ 312: 1384–8

Sacco Ezzell P 1999 Managing the effects of gynaecological cancer treatment on quality of life and sexuality. Soc Gynaecol Nurs Oncol 8(3): 23–6

Samsioe G 1998 Urogenital ageing: a forgotten problem. Meno Rev 3(1): 5–6

Sapsford RR, Hodges PW 2001 Contraction of the pelvic floor muscles during abdominal manoeuvres. Arch Phys Med Rehabil 82: 1081–8

Sapsford RR, Hodges PW, Richardson CA 1997 Activation of the abdominal muscles is a normal response to contraction of the pelvic floor muscles. International Continence Society Conference, Japan (abstract)

Sapsford RR, Bullock-Saxton J, Markwell S 1998 Women's Health: a Textbook for Physiotherapists. WB Saunders: London

Sapsford RR, Hodges PW, Richardson CA et al. 2001 Co-activation of the abdominal muscles and pelvic floor muscles during voluntary exercises. Neurourol Urodynam 20: 31–42

Schussler B, Laycock J, Norton P, Stanton S 1994 Pelvic Floor Re-education: Principles and Practice. Springer-Verlag: London

Scriven MW, Jones DA, McKnight L 1995 The importance of pubic pain following childbirth: a clinical and ultrasonographic study of diastasis of the pubic symphysis. J R Soc Med 88: 26–30

Smith P, Heimer G, Norgren A et al. 1990 Steroid hormone receptors in pelvic muscles and ligaments in women. Gynecol Obstet Invest 30: 27–30

Snidjers CJ, Ribbers MTLM, de Bakker HV, Stoeckart, R, Stam HJ 1998 EMG recordings of abdominal and back muscles in various standing postures: validation of a biomechanical model on sacroiliac joint. J Electromyogr Kinesiol 8:205–14

Snow RE, Neubert AG 1997 Peripartum pubic symphysis separation: a case series and review of the literature. CME Review 7: 438–43

Stanton AWB, Levick JR, Mortimer PS 1996 Current puzzles presented by post mastectomy oedema (breast cancer related lymphoedema). Vasc Med 1: 213–25

Steege JF, Metzger DA, Levy BS (eds) 1998 Chronic Pelvic Pain: an Integrated Approach. WB Saunders: Philadelphia

Sultan AH, Kamm MA, Hudson CM, Bartram CI 1994 Third degree obstetric and sphincter tears: risk factors and outcomes of primary repair. BMJ 308: 887

Sultan AH, Monga AK, Stanton SL 1996 The pelvic floor sequelae of childbirth. Br J Hosp Med 55: 575–9

Tobin GW, Brocklehurst JC 1986 Faecal incontinence in residential homes for the elderly: prevalence, aetiology and management. Age Ageing 15(1): 41–6

Tobin MB, Lacey HJ, Meyer L, Mortimer P 1993 The psychological morbidity of breast cancer related arm swelling. Cancer 72: 3248–52

Todd J 2000 Containment in the management of lymphoedema. In: Twycross R, Jenns K, Todd J (eds) Lymphoedema, pp. 165–202. Radcliffe Medical Press: Oxford

Toozs-Hobson P 1998 Pelvic floor ultrasonography: the current state of ultrasound imaging of the pelvic floor in relation to urogynaecology and childbirth. J Assoc Chart Physiother Wom Health 84: 18–22

Vleeming A, Buyruk HM, Stoeckart R, Karamursel S, Snijders CJ 1992 Towards an integrated therapy for peripartum pelvic instability. Am J Obstet Gynaecol 166: 1243–7

Watkins Y 1998 Current concepts in dynamic stabilisation of the spine and pelvis: their relevance in obstetrics. J Assoc Chart Physiother Wom Health 83: 16–26

Webber BA, Pryor JA 1998 Physiotherapy for Respiratory and Cardiac Problems, pp. 295–305. Churchill Livingstone: Edinburgh

Whitehead M, Godfree V 1992 Consequences of oestrogen deficiency. In: Hormone Replacement Therapy: Your Questions Answered, pp. 13–36. Churchill Livingstone: Edinburgh

Wilson PD, Herbison RM, Herbison GP 1996 Obstetric practice and the prevalence of urinary incontinence three months after delivery. Br J Obstet Gynaecol 103: 154–61

Woods M 1993 Patients' perceptions of breast cancer related lymphoedema. Eur J Cancer Care 125–8

Zondervan KT, Yudkin PL, Vessey MP et al. 1999 Prevalence and incidence of chronic pelvic pain in primary care: evidence from a national general practice database. Br J Obstet Gynaecol 106: 1149–55

8

Principles of Paediatric Physiotherapy

Alison Carter

THE AREA OF PAEDIATRIC PHYSIOTHERAPY

General Issues

This chapter provides an overview of the areas in which paediatric physiotherapists are employed and the types of conditions they commonly encounter. It also provides background information on some of the physio-

---

Association of Paediatric Chartered Physiotherapists (APCP)

[www.csp.org.uk/membergroups/clinicalinterestgroups/microsites/apcp.cfm]
[www.apcp.org.uk/]

APCP is one of the largest clinical interest groups (CIGs) affiliated to the Chartered Society of Physiotherapy. There are 1800 members, most of whom are resident in the United Kingdom but a small number are based overseas. APCP has a national committee, which meets quarterly to direct the business of the CIG. The national committee consists of chairman, vice chair, secretary, treasurer, membership secretary, public relations officer, publications officer, research officer, education liaison officer, journal editor and liaison officer.

The APCP divides the UK into eleven regions. Each region has a committee that includes a chairman, secretary, treasurer and regional representative. The regional representatives meet twice yearly and attend each national committee meeting to ensure information is devolved back to local members.

The aim of APCP is to inform the membership of professional and clinical issues relating to paediatric physiotherapy, to act as an information resource for the membership, and to be in the forefront of developing publications and guidelines particular to paediatrics. APCP issues a quarterly journal, which contains clinical articles, information about paediatric courses, and opportunities for open letters and communication between members.

APCP holds an annual conference, which is a two-day event, organised by a different regional committee with topical lectures and workshops. It plans and organises a five-day course called 'Introduction to paediatrics' each year in a different area of the UK. Each regional group holds study days and seminars several times a year. All these events are open to members, non-members and others as appropriate.

Most members work with children from birth to 18 years of age. Paediatric physiotherapists also have an important role to play in reassuring and teaching anxious parents how to most help their sick or disabled child.

Acknowledgement: With thanks to Christine Shaw, APCP Secretary

---

logical differences between adults and children and cognitive and motor development.

Paediatric physiotherapy encompasses a wide spectrum of activities and skills. The type of work undertaken by the paediatric physiotherapist is often governed by the nature and structure of the institution, school, hospital or other environment in which the person works. The role of the paediatric physiotherapist also varies from trust to trust and even within different geographical regions of the United Kingdom.

Historically, physiotherapists have been involved in every area of childcare, giving valued support and advice to families and carers and undertaking at times very structured therapy programmes and exercise regimens. The last 10 years has seen a significant shift in emphasis; physiotherapists are now questioning practices much more and chartered physiotherapists now want (and need) a stronger evidence base behind their interventions. For many of our interventions there is still not the evidence base we would like to see to support what we 'feel' or 'believe' to be having a positive effect. What is clear is that physiotherapists have a very specific role in supporting and educating parents, colleagues, carers and other people in the management of sick infants and children.

The Association of Paediatric Chartered Physiotherapists is attempting to draw together current evidence on specific topics of care, thereby to create national evidence-based guidelines which will lead to fewer discrepancies in care depending on location. In addition it will be possible to say with a greater degree of confidence whether physiotherapy is or is not appropriate in particular cases, enabling a move away from prescriptive referrals. APCP members are encouraged to write up case studies for the journal and present research findings and papers at conferences. There is also a database of members who are involved in research.

There is currently no requirement for postgraduate experience to become a paediatric physiotherapist. What tends to happen is that people get jobs in the paediatric field and then gradually gain experience; indeed some units with small paediatric requirements utilise only adult physiotherapists. All this may change. Children are not simply small adults, so an adult approach to a paediatric setting may not be the most appropriate.

Where Paediatric Physiotherapists Work

Although there are other models of paediatric physiotherapy, the following list gives an indication that not all paediatric physiotherapists will possess the experience and skills to treat all children.

- *Acute NHS trusts/former district general hospitals.* Such establishments may have one paediatric ward or several depending on the size of the hospital. Paediatric therapists who cover all types of paediatrics include outpatient, musculoskeletal, neurological, and orthopaedic. Adult physiotherapists may also have input.
- *Specialist children's hospitals.* These tend to be situated in the larger cities. They have paediatric therapists who are specialists in one or several areas. There are sometimes regional specialties such as neurology, cardiology or oncology.
- *Child development centres* (CDCs). The same therapist sees all children from 0–16 years of age, encountering musculoskeletal, acute, respiratory, rehabilitation and ongoing input for children with birth trauma, syndromes, or developmental issues of unknown aetiology.
- *Community trusts/CDCs.* These have input to schools, nurseries and home visiting. Paediatric therapists are involved with rehabilitation and monitoring of children with mild to severe neurological or orthopaedic impairment, developmental delay and other problems, to support them in their home and school environments.
- *Combined acute and community trusts.*
- *GP practices.* These may have paediatric/adult therapists who treat children with musculoskeletal disorders or trauma.
- *Special schools, residential and non-residential.* A specialist paediatric therapist is attached to individual schools or several schools.
- *Private practice.*

Paediatrics is an exciting area in which to work, with great potential, and experience gained in working in one of the above areas will greatly enhance the ability to work in another.

Parent Support Groups

These are groups set up so that families of children with specific conditions can meet other parents in the same situation. They help parents share experiences and strategies for coping and managing the challenges of their child's condition. The groups have been particularly helpful at linking parents with children who have rare conditions.

Within the groups parents can feel that their situation is understood and can in return provide that understanding to others. The groups provide a safe place to talk and can alleviate the isolation often experienced by parents. Such groups should be encouraged to actually direct and support therapists.

The Multidisciplinary Team

Children must be managed with a holistic approach. The team, which should have shared goals and regular communication, may include: nurse, doctor, paediatrician/neurologist/metabolic specialists etc., physiotherapist, occupational therapist, play therapist, speech and language therapist, psychologist, pharmacist, dietitian, teachers – and students of any of the above professions.

'NORMAL' CHILD DEVELOPMENT

> ### *Key point*
> As with all aspects of physiotherapy, an understanding of the 'normal' is necessary before the abnormal can be identified. Although the end-product of normal child development is the same, the processes by which children attain that development can be very variable indeed.

We use the adjective 'normal' with development, but it is important to recognise that the rate of growth and mobility of a child is affected by the differing experiences of the child, and provided the child is continuing to develop along a line, many parental anxieties can be allayed. An example of this is the fact that prone lying is no longer recommended by the Department of Health (because of 'cot death' worries); this has led to a decreased experience of babies on their fronts. In some stages of play we have seen whole stages of development being omitted or bypassed. There is anecdotal evidence that this links with decreased central/core stability, leading some infants to tip-toe walk in order to stabilise themselves, or to have subsequent problems with balance and coordination with secondary musculoskeletal pains as the child grows.

> ### *Key point*
> Ratliff-Schaub et al. (2001) commented: 'Supine sleeping has been associated with decreased risk for sudden infant death syndrome, but compensatory strategies while awake may be needed to avoid delayed acquisition of head control.'

Normal (usual) development must be described with caution, especially in cases where the infant has been critically ill in the early months of life. Indeed, opinions and views regarding the development of motor behaviour of infants and children are significantly changing (Helders et al. 2001).

TYPICAL CHILD DEVELOPMENT

Tables 8.1 to 8.4 summarise the major features of development in the first 5 years of life. The information is adapted from Khot and Palmer (2002).

Motor Development in the First Year

Key point

The developing brain can be remarkably plastic (adaptable) and 'underlies all skill learning and is a part of CNS function in healthy and brain damaged individuals at any age' (Leonard 1998).

All physiotherapists, paediatric or otherwise, should have a working knowledge of the development of the infant and child. This is because any prenatal or subsequent trauma will potentially affect this development.

What initially may appear to be devastating changes on MRI or CT scans can have little developmental effect on the child. Conversely some infants with few visible changes can be severely developmentally challenged. This situation differs from brain injury in a mature adult.

Psychological Aspects of Treating Children

In order to approach children with the most appropriate manner, a basic knowledge of child psychology is important. Knowing what a child might understand at each stage in his or her development can make the difference between a successful and unsuccessful treatment session. An understanding of the role of play is also important.

Children with neurological impairment, various syndromes and congenital abnormalities may have varying degrees of mental impairment and lack of understanding. This is a huge challenge for the physiotherapist. Appropriate approaches must be adopted and adapted to make sure that fears, anxieties and a

Table 8.1 Typical development from birth to 16 weeks.

	0–4 weeks	**6–8 weeks**	**12–16 weeks**
Social behaviour	Watches mother, may smiles	Responsive smile by 6 weeks, vocalises	Recognises family shows pleasure
Motor ventral suspension	Head hangs down until 3 or 4 weeks, then up momentarily	Head held horizontal, briefly up by 8 weeks	Head maintained well above plane of body by 12 weeks
Prone	Head to side, pelvis high, knees drawn up under abdomen	Chin up intermittently at 6 weeks	Head and shoulders up, chest up by 16 weeks Takes weight on forearms
Supine	Head to side, limbs flexed or ATNR posture	ATNR posture common but head to midline by 8 weeks	ATNR declining Head and hand to midline Slight head lag
Pull to sit	Complete head lag	Less head lag	Back is straighter
Held sitting	Walking, placing reflexes present until 6 weeks old	Sags at hips and knees	Increasingly bears weight on legs
Hands	String grasp reflex, hands often closed	Grasp reflex present but slight by 8 weeks Fingers extend more frequently	Grasp reflex fades from 12–16 weeks Can hold a rattle briefly
Vision	Eye righting reflex random movements but is able to fixate	Smoother conjugate eye movements Fixates on face/objects	Hand regards common
Vocalisation and hearing	Cries, startles to sounds	Eyes turn to sound, starts vocalising	Coos, squeals and laughs

ATNR, asymmetric tonic neck reflex.
From Khot A, Palmer A, 1999 Practical General Practice. Butterworth–Heinemann: Oxford.

Table 8.2 Typical development from 4 months to 10 months.

	4–10 months	6–8 months	8–10 months
Social behaviour	Responds to all-comers Smiles in a mirror Excited at approach of food	Knows the difference between family and strangers Attracts attention	Wary of strangers Waves bye-bye Uses a spoon
Gross motor	No head lag Rolls from prone to supine Back straight in supported sitting	Lifts head up in supine Rolls supine to prone Bears weight on feet at 5–8 months	Sits steadily Gets from prone to sitting Pulls self to standing
Fine motor and vision	Reaches and grabs toys Plays with toes	Transfers a block hand to hand	Pincer grasp developed Releases objects
Language and hearing	Varied sounds and squeals	Turns to sounds May say da-da	Varied babble Indicates and understands 'no' Can locate sounds

From Khot A, Palmer A 1999 Practical General Practice. Butterworth–Heinemann: Oxford.

lack of understanding are catered for. In some areas of paediatric work, severe behavioural problems can mean that specialist training is required.

Levels of Cognitive Development

Piaget argued that cognitive development undergoes stage-like changes that affect all aspects of children's cognitive functioning (e.g. Lee Kang 2000). He also thought that all children go through the same four stages in an unchanging order:

- the sensorimotor stage (up to 2 years)
- the preoperational stage (2–7 years)
- the concrete operational stage (7–11 years)
- the formal operational stage (11+ years).

This is summarised in Table 8.5.

The physiotherapist should have an understanding of these stages since it is important to teach a child at their level of understanding. In many cases, the use of play can facilitate this.

Play as Therapy

Key point

Play-based therapy is beneficial in the treatment of balance disorders and may enhance skills, improve function and inspire and motivate the child (Yaggie and Armstrong 1999).

Table 8.3 Typical development from 12 to 24 months.

	12–15 months	18–24 months
Personal and social behaviour	Shows affection May be shy Indicates needs and wants May manage a cup and spoon	Becomes egocentric, clinging and resistant Enjoys domestic mimicry Helps undress
Gross motor	Walks holding on at 8–12 months Walks alone at 11–15 months	Walks well at 12–18 months Climbs stairs, kneels at 14–22 months
Fine motor and vision	Fine pincer grip Bangs bricks together Scribbles	May show hand preference after 15 months
Language and hearing	'Mama' and 'dada' with meaning at 9–15 months	Can point to three parts of the body Has 6–20 words of jargon at 15–24 months

From Khot A, Palmer A 1999 Practical General Practice. Butterworth–Heinemann: Oxford.

Table 8.4 Typical development from 2.5 years to 5 years.

	2.5 years	3–4 years	5 years
Personal and social skills	Enjoys solitary play Possessive, some tantrums Feeds neatly using spoon and fork May be continent by day	Plays with peers Enjoys make-believe Shows concern for other people Mostly dry at night Can wash hands and undress by age 4	Plays complicated co-operative games Makes friends Almost independent in self-help skills Can run simple errands
Gross motor	Very mobile Runs and kicks a ball Tries to throw Walks up and down stairs Propels a tricycle with feet	Goes upstairs one foot at a time Can walk on tip-toe Enjoys climbing	Can walk on tip-toe Enjoys running, jumping and climbing Can stand on one leg
Fine motor and vision	Neat prehension and controlled release Scribbles Builds a tower of 6–8 bricks	Tower of 9–10 bricks Awkward tripod Pencil grasp	Can write name Draws person with details. Can fold paper Performs Snellen chart type of vision test
Language and hearing	Listens to simple stories Can say 50–100 single words Asks many questions	Intelligible but immature speech with 3–5 word sentences Knows age and address	Enjoys riddles and jokes Understands negatives Gives long descriptions and explanations

From Khot A, Palmer A 1999 Practical General Practice. Butterworth–Heinemann: Oxford.

Play is the work of a child. It assists in the development and perfection of social, cognitive and emotional skills. It often helps to relax children when they are in a strange environment, and it is safe for children since they often consider themselves to be expert at it.

There are thought to be two types of play, normative and therapeutic.

- *Normative play* is spontaneous and pleasurable. It is child-led, with no intrinsic goals. It also maintains normality in an otherwise strange environment.
- *Therapeutic play* is led by a professional. There are goals to achieve. This promotes physical and emotional well-being in hospitalised children.

Three types of therapeutic play have been identified:

- *Emotional outlet play* is good in difficult situations.
- *Instructional play* is preparation for forthcoming procedures. For example, it is important to illustrate that changes are reversible, such as hair loss following chemotherapy. The interaction gives an opportunity to ask questions.
- *Physiologically enhancing play* is particularly relevant to physiotherapists who get children to do exercises or actions to improve their condition but

which they are unlikely to do when asked more formally. The exercises need to be age-appropriate; examples include blowing bubbles, in respiratory care (Vessey and Mahon 1990).

MUSCULOSKELETAL CONDITIONS IN THE OUTPATIENT SETTING

Typical musculoskeletal conditions are listed in Table 8.6.

CHILDREN AS INPATIENTS

A great diversity of conditions will be seen within a hospital ward setting, ranging from neurological to respiratory to musculoskeletal disorders. This section looks at some typical paediatric conditions that the student can expect to encounter.

Respiratory Conditions

Acute conditions

Table 8.7 lists the most common conditions encountered in paediatric acute respiratory care.

Table 8.5 Stages of cognitive development.

	Cognitive development	Child's understanding of illness or hospitalisation
Sensorimotor stage	Babies are discovering the relationship between what they do and their consequences. Learning through senses and physical activity A sense of objective permanence is evolving which is not present in younger infants In infants beyond 1 year old this has developed implications (e.g. cry for mother when she is out of sight)	
Pre-operational stage	Child is prone to invest an object with life and personal identities (talks of an 'unhappy knee' not a 'bad knee') Use of language to symbolise or represent things and events within their world Centre on own point of view or perspective – egocentrism	Children see causes of illness as external, concrete and remote from them, out of their control as a result of their wrongdoing Focus on individual aspects of experience without reference to the whole
Concrete operational stage	Can form internal pictures of a series of actions Able to see relationships with things Can see things in relative terms (e.g. hurts a little, hurts a lot) Understanding is still in relation to absolute objects, not to events or relationships which have happened	Body equated with surface (e.g. a child with juvenile chronic arthritis may equate feeling unwell with a visibly swollen red joint) A child will not be worried by thoughts of what might be going wrong internally
Formal operational	Can think beyond concrete and think abstractly Able to imagine and hypothesise abstract alternatives Reasoning can be done symbolically without the need for things or events to be present	Gaining an idea of the interaction between external cause and internal body response Understanding that the thoughts and feelings can affect the way the body feels (e.g. use of distraction to reduce pain) Children over 12 years may show growing concern about internal disease process Pain will be more difficult to cope with in some adolescents as cognitive development allows them to imagine the more sinister implications of pain

From Khot A, Palmer A 1999 Practical General Practice. Butterworth–Heinemann: Oxford.

Anatomical and physiological issues

Some anatomical and physiological differences between respiration in children and adults, and the implications for the physiotherapist, are listed in Table 8.8.

Signs of respiratory distress in infants include (Kendall 1987):

- increased respiratory rate (over 60/minute)
- nasal flaring
- intercostal and sternal recession
- grunting on expiration (to generate positive end-expiratory pressure – PEEP)
- cyanosis.

Acute Neurology

This is one of the most diverse and complex areas of paediatrics. It is possible to have two children with the same illness but presenting in a very different way depending on the part of the brain or central nervous system affected, and their age. Additionally, areas of

Table 8.6 Typical paediatric musculoskeletal conditions seen within an outpatient department.

	Condition	Approach principles
Musculoskeletal	After trauma, fracture or soft-tissue injury Postural backache Thoracic and lumbar problems Anterior knee pain Osgood Sschlatters disease Slipped upper femoral epiphysis (SUFE)	Rehabilitation following musculoskeletal assessment Postural alignment, core stability assessment of tight muscle groups, muscle imbalance Growth related issues, self help
Orthopaedic anomalies	Flat feet Intoeing Genu valgum and genu varum Persistent femoral neck anteversion Tibial torsion	Holistic assessment Postural alignment Core stability Explain and reassure parent and child with regard to normal variance in the population Pain management Limited evidence of intervention – natural course self-limiting on the whole
Congenital orthopaedic problems	Talipes equinovarus Calcaneovalgus Vertical talus Congenital dislocation of hip (CDH) Brachial plexus lesions incl. Erb's palsy (NB with Erb's palsy there is a high incidence of litigation) Torticollis/plagiocephaly Arthrogryphosis Hand contractures and other abnormalities Other conditions such as Perthes' disease and juvenile chronic arthritis	Congenital orthopaedic problems Physiotherapy management approach is centre-specific – local guidelines should be followed Identify the aims of treatment May use correction Maintenance of ROM exercises, hydrotherapy, gait re education Splinting or surgery Monitoring of the condition is important if the abnormality will affect overall development as well

Table 8.7 Acute respiratory care in paediatrics.

	Condition	Approach/role
Ward-based	Cystic fibrosis (CF) chest infection Pneumonia Bronchiolitis Asthma	Management of secretion retention Lobar collapse Anatomical differences between children and adults Treatment techniques include positioning, humidification Adjuncts to treatment including pep mask etc.
Intensive care	Multiple trauma (road traffic accidents) Near drowning Cerebral palsy Encephalitis Meningitis Post acute illness/surgery Guillaime Barre syndrome Asthma Metabolic disorders After cardiac surgery After organ transplant	Appropriate respiratory assessment Neurological assessment Splinting Positioning Passive movements Monitoring rehabilitation referral/liaison with other members of the team

Table 8.8 Anatomical and physiological differences between respiration in children and in adults.

Variance	Implication for physiotherapist
Obligatory nose breathers	If nose becomes blocked by mucous, oedema or tubes may lead to respiratory distress
Average infant trachea diameter is 5–6 mm compared with 14–15 mm in an adult	Oedema of upper airways leads to significant narrowing and increased work of breathing
Bronchial wall structure differs, more glands and cartilage and less smooth muscle	Poor response to bronchodilators in infants under 1 year of age
Ribs almost horizontal Lack bucket handle movements Ribs soft AP and transverse diameter cannot be increased	Diaphragm very important Impairment of diaphragm can cause respiratory insufficiency
Heart and other organs relatively large	Relatively less room to breathe
Pre-term infant's cilia are immature	Accumulation of secretions has a more marked effect exacerbated by relatively small airway diameter
Muscle of respiration fatigue quickly Infants have fewer type 1 fibres (fatigue resistant) within the diaphragm	Children may exhibit signs of distress in minimal illness Short treatments may be advisable with adequate oxygenation
Lung compliance does not change but is proportional to size Chest wall compliance is high due to soft rib cage	Weak force to oppose action of the diaphragm and maintain function residual capacity (FRC)
Intercostal muscle inhibition during REM (rapid eye movement) sleep	Allows paradoxical movement of soft chest wall, and a further decrease in FRC may lead to apnoea (cessation of breathing) attacks in infants, especially pre-term
Collateral circulation is not fully established	Makes atalectasis (collapse) more likely to occur in association with pneumonia etc.
Infants have higher metabolic rate for oxygen consumption	Hypoxaemia develops rapidly Infant response to this is bradycardia (slowing of heart rate) possibly due to hypoxia and acidosis

undamaged brain may take over function in some individuals who have seemingly gross impairment. Plastic changes within the nervous system are associated with this spread of activity, including activation of brain regions that are not typically involved (Moller 2001).

Common treatment approaches

Approaches vary according to the chronicity of the condition. The approach may be intensive in a period of rapid recovery, or more directed to maintenance at other times.

- Acute conditions seen include meningitis, epilepsy, encephalitis, metabolic disorders, neuromuscular disorders and cerebral palsy. Approaches need careful assessment by the team and the involvement of community teams.

- Chronic conditions include cerebral palsy, fits, reflux and aspiration conversion disorders, ME and postviral syndromes, and acquired brain injury. Such cases again need careful team coordination, including speech and language therapy, occupational therapy, plus psychological, nursing and play therapy. These children often have cognitive and perceptual deficits.

General principles of treatment

Some specific treatments

Neurodevelopmental treatment (the Bobath approach)

- Developmental sequences.
- Inhibition of abnormal patterns.

- Attention to key points of control.
- Sensory stimuli.
- Facilitation of normal postural control.
- Sensory stimulation for activation and inhibition of movement.

Conductive education

This concentrates on all aspects of life with a 'conductor' supervising the child. It is very intensive.

The Margaret Rood technique

This consists of manipulations to activate/inhibit motor activity:

- stimulation by stroking – superficial
- stretching – deep.

The Temple Fay technique

Developmental sequences or movement are used to activate normal patterns.

The Kabat–Knott–Voss technique

This consists of proprioceptive neuromuscular facilitation (PNF). It makes use of functional patterns of movement. All movements include rotatory and diagonal components.

The Doman–Delecato technique

This consists of repeated passive patterning and developmental sequences of movement. It facilitates use of dormant pathways in the central nervous system and brain

Orthopaedic Conditions

Common orthopaedic problems are listed in Table 8.9.

Children with orthopaedic abnormalities will often need a period of postoperative immobilisation. They are admitted for rehabilitation or this may be undertaken on a community basis.

Key point

Many paediatric physiotherapists working in this field also have a significant role in pre-admission and follow-up clinics, being involved in the assessment for the need of surgery and assessing functional outcomes. This has considerably enhanced the status of paediatric neuromuscular orthopaedics.

COMMUNITY PAEDIATRICS

Some children will need to be seen throughout their lives, for adaptation and progression of programmes as their needs change. Others may be seen on a review basis and receive short spurts of therapy as their need dictates, whilst others will have a finite time requirement for physiotherapy and then are discharged. In many circumstances, community physiotherapists are able to assess, treat and advise on needs for children at home, in schools, or in the community. They work as part of a closely coordinated team which includes the patient and the family, to ensure the best possible integration of the child into the community taking into

Table 8.9 Orthopaedic conditions.

	Condition	Approach
Upper and lower limb trauma	Traction, surgery: open reduction internal fixation (ORIF) Manipulation under anaesthesia (MUA) Plaster of Paris or other splinting materials	Assessment Exercises Advice re self-care, mobility Note: Children under 5 years cannot usually coordinate the use of crutches effectively Hydrotherapy, community follow up, braces and casts Congenital abnormality: correction talipes equinovarus Vertical talus
Elective (cold) orthopaedics	Congenital dislocation of hip (CDH) Other orthopaedic abnormalities with or without neuromuscular involvement Soft-tissue release Bony reconstruction Spinal surgery for scoliosis	

account the educational, social and cultural needs of the individual.

FURTHER READING

APCP publications

Baby Massage
Evidence-Based Practice in Paediatrics
Guidelines for Calculating Caseloads
Haemophilia Booklet
Hip Dislocation in Children with Cerebral Palsy: a Guide to Physiotherapy Management
Human Postural Reactions: Lessons from Purdon Martin by Dr John Foley
Obstetric Brachial Plexus Palsy: a Guide to Physiotherapy Management
Paediatric Manual Handling: Guidelines for Paediatric Physiotherapists
Paediatric Physiotherapy: Guidance for Good Practice, revised 2002 [booklet includes principles of paediatric physiotherapy, issues of consent and communication, documentation, assessment, continuing professional development, and other topics]
Statutory Assessment of Children with Special Educational Needs
Tests and Measures Resources Pack, 2nd edn
The Children Act 1989: a Synopsis for Physiotherapists

General

Hussey J, Prasad SA 1995 Paediatric Respiratory Care: a Guide for Physiotherapists and Health Professionals. Singular Publishing Group: Chapman & Hall: London

Prasad SA, Hussey J, Campling J 1994 Paediatric Respiratory Care. Nelson Thornes: London
Sheridan MD, Frost M, Sharma A 1997 From Birth to Five Years. Routledge: London
Staheli LT 1992 Fundamentals of Paediatric Orthopaedics, 2nd edn. Lippincott Williams & Wilkins: Baltimore

Play and child psychology

Edwards M, Davis H 1997 Counselling Children with Chronic Medical Conditions. Blackwell: Oxford

REFERENCES

Helders PJ, Engelbert RH et al. 2001 Paediatric rehabilitation. Disabil Rehabil 23: 497–500

Kendall L 1987 A comparison between adult and paediatric intensive care. Physiotherapy 73: 495–9.

Khot A, Palmer A 2002 Practical General Practice. Butterworth–Heinemann: Oxford

Leonard CT 1998 The Neuroscience of Human Movement. Mosby: St Louis

Moller AR 2001 Symptoms and signs caused by neural plasticity. Neurol Res 23: 565–72

Lee Kang (eds) 2000 Piaget's theory: childhood cognitive development. In: Essential Readings in Developmental Psychology, pp. 33–47. Blackwell: Malden

Ratliff-Schaub K, Hunt CE et al. 2001 Relationship between infant sleep position and motor development in preterm infants. J Dev Behav Pediatr 22: 293–9

Vessey JA, Mahon MM 1990 Therapeutic play and the hospitalized child. J Pediatr Nurs 5: 328–33

Yaggie JA, ArmstrongWJ 1999 The use of play-therapy in the treatment of children with cerebellar dysfunction. Clin Kinesiol 53(4): 91–5

Osteoarthritis

Stuart B. Porter

INTRODUCTION

Synovial joints are subjected to tremendous forces throughout our lives. In a healthy joint, the layer of hyaline articular cartilage lining the bone ends and only a few millimetres thick is able to cope perfectly well with these demands.

Osteoarthritis (OA) is the most common synovial joint disease and it has existed since prehistoric times, affecting the dinosaurs and modern humans alike. Even the great pharaoh Rameses II was not spared from this disabling condition, and in life suffered from osteoarthritis of the hips (El Mahdy 1989).

Osteoarthritis is still not fully understood and it is a disease worthy of ongoing study and research, particularly in terms of the most effective approaches to rehabilitation and the role that physiotherapy can play in its management.

The clinical features of OA make sense only when one understands how OA affects the normal functioning of a joint. This chapter begins with a profile of the structure and function of hyaline articular cartilage, and synovial fluid, since an understanding of the normal will facilitate understanding of the abnormal.

CARTILAGE AND SYNOVIAL FLUID

Articular Hyaline Cartilage

Hyaline cartilage is specialised and perfectly suited to its function. The frictional resistance of normal articular cartilage against itself may be as little as one-tenth the friction between an ice-skate and ice (Radin and Paul 1971).

In articular cartilage a precarious equilibrium exists between damage and repair. If this equilibrium is upset there are dire consequences. Adult articular hyaline cartilage has no blood, lymph or nerve supply. Articular cartilage can be compressed to one-fifth its original thickness during weight-bearing, so nerves and blood vessels cannot exist within it since they would be crushed when the cartilage is compressed. Its only source of nutrition is synovial fluid which washes across the surfaces of the joint during movement, providing nourishment. This is known as *synovial sweep*.

Another important source of nutrition occurs during joint loading, when synovial fluid is forced into the cartilage matrix. During compressive loading of the joint, the overall shape of the cartilage changes, and a joint whose articular surfaces were not fully congruent, become so.

Articular cartilage consists of 10% chondrocytes, up to 10% proteoglycans, 10–30% type 2 collagen, 50–70% water, salts, lipids and other substances. Other types of collagen contributing to the matrix include types iii, vi, ix, x xi, xii and xv (Eyre 2002). As much as 70% of the water content of articular hyaline cartilage is intercellular (between the cells), not intracellular (inside the cells), so it is free to move under conditions of joint loading. This is an important biomechanical property of hyaline cartilage, which behaves like a wet sponge, consisting of both fluid and solid phases (Nordin and Frankel 1989).

When a joint is loaded, water is squeezed out of the matrix. This pushes the proteoglycans closer together, making it more resilient to further deformation. When the load is removed, the cartilage absorbs water and returns to its resting shape.

Articular cartilage appears smooth to the naked eye, but closer examination with the scanning electron microscope reveals tiny pits on its surface, 20–40 µm in diameter. It has been theorised that these may provide a site for anchorage of filamentous glycoproteins, which assist with joint lubrication (Swann et al. 1979). The cells of articular cartilage are arranged in zones, shown in Figure 9.1.

Synovial Fluid

Synovial fluid is produced by the synovial membrane and is present in small amounts in all synovial joints. An increase in volume of synovial fluid often occurs after trauma, in the presence of infection, loose bodies, or as a response to other pathology.

> **Definition**
> Too much synovial fluid in a joint is known as an *effusion*.

Synovial fluid is a clear or straw-coloured fluid, which is thixotropic. This unusual quality means that the more quickly a joint moves, the less viscous its synovial fluid becomes. The fluid contains nutrients, and the glycoprotein hyaluronate.

While synovial fluid bathes and nourishes the joint, it also plays an important role in absorbing joint stresses. When moving from sitting to standing, stresses on the hip joint have been calculated to be in excess of 2610 pounds per square inch. Studies have shown that 90% of this load may be borne by hydrostatic pressure within the synovial fluid between the articulating surfaces. This protects the cartilage matrix from these potentially catastrophic pressures (Makirowski et al. 1994).

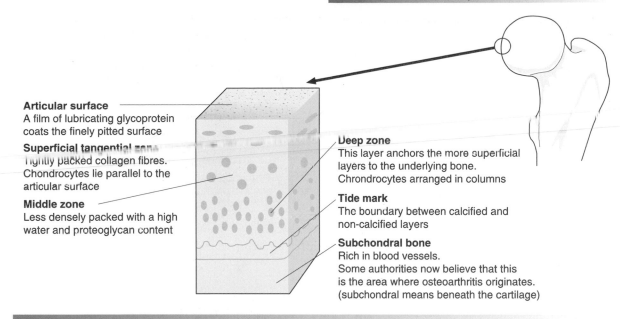

Articular surface
A film of lubricating glycoprotein
coats the finely pitted surface

Superficial tangential zone
Tightly packed collagen fibres.
Chondrocytes lie parallel to the
articular surface

Middle zone
Less densely packed with a high
water and proteoglycan content

Deep zone
This layer anchors the more superficial
layers to the underlying bone.
Chrondrocytes arranged in columns

Tide mark
The boundary between calcified and
non-calcified layers

Subchondral bone
Rich in blood vessels.
Some authorities now believe that this
is the area where osteoarthritis originates.
(subchondral means beneath the cartilage)

Figure 9.1   The structure of articular cartilage.

Intra Articular Pressures, Joint Stability and Cracking Joints

Medical illustrations usually portray synovial membrane as an expansive fluid-filled bag, but this can be misleading. The synovial cavity is a potential space containing a small amount of fluid and the sides of the synovial membrane are similar to a wet collapsed balloon whose walls are stuck together. This creates a pressure which is negative in comparison that of the atmosphere outside. This 'glues' the articular surfaces together.

The stability of synovial joints may centre on the suction effect created by these sub-atmospheric pressures within the joint. This bond is thought to keep the head of the humerus in contact with the glenoid, for example. When an effusion is present, pressure inside the joint rises to a positive level compared with atmospheric pressure and joint stability may be lost, predisposing the joint to further injury; hence the therapeutic importance of removing effusions quickly. This has clinical significance when surgical attempts are made to enter the synovial cavity by arthroscopy, which may destroy the sub-atmospheric pressure and inherent stability of the joint.

The cause of cracking joints is thought to be the rupture of the aforementioned bond and the formation of a bubble of gas within the joint. The joint cannot be cracked again for several minutes, as the gases need to dissolve back into solution (Chen and Israelachvili 1991). Experiments where distraction is applied to the metacarpophalangeal joints of the finger show that a pull of 10 kg is needed to cause the familiar knuckle crack (Simkin 1993). After the crack has occurred, true separation of the articular surfaces can occur and the collateral ligaments have to take up the strain.

Key point
This cracking is not the same as crepitus, which is a prolonged, repeatable, and often painful creaking of joints. Crepitus is a pathological state.

DEFINITION AND CLASSIFICATION OF OSTEOARTHRITIS

Definition

Osteoarthritis is one of the most common causes of pain and disability in the western world and it affects up to 80% of people over the age of 65 (Brandt 2000). Despite numerous research studies, the exact pathways and triggers involved in OA are still the cause of some debate.

Definition
Osteoarthritis is 'morphologic, biochemical, molecular and biochemical changes of both cells and matrix which lead to softening, fibrillation, ulceration and loss of articular cartilage, sclerosis, and eburnation of subchondral bone, osteophytes and subchondral cysts' (Keuttner and Goldberg 1995).

OA is sometimes known as 'degenerative joint disease'. There has been debate over the years about whether *osteoarthrosis* or *osteoarthritis* is the appropriate term. It is now known that OA also has reparative and re-modelling components. Both men and women are affected but the joint distribution pattern is different. In men, hip, wrist and spine are most commonly affected; in females, multiple joint involvement is more common.

Classification

There are two main types of OA, primary and secondary.

Primary OA or generalised OA (GOA)

There is no obvious cause. It is due to an intrinsic alteration of the articular tissues themselves. It affects joints in a classical pattern and is common in post-menopausal women who typically exhibit Heberden's and Bouchard's nodes (bony swellings of the distal and intermediate interphalangeal joints respectively; see Figure 9.2). The classical pattern of joint involvement is illustrated in Figure 9.3.

Secondary OA

This arises as a consequence of another condition. The causes of secondary OA can be divided into one of the following four categories: metabolic, anatomic, traumatic or inflammatory.

OA appears to be more common in people with a previous injury or fracture to a particular joint (Coggon et al. 2001). Repeated minor trauma may lead to micro fractures and subsequent OA. Occupational factors are thought to be important in the development of secondary OA. Miner's knees are at risk, as are tailor's first carpometacarpal and metacarpophalangeal joints, and the elbows and shoulders of pneumatic drill operators.

Joint infection puts a joint at risk of OA, as does deformity, for example following fractures which cause biomechanical anomalies or direct cartilage damage if the fracture included the articular surface.

The relationship between obesity and OA is complex and still not fully understood. Being overweight is linked to development of OA in some joints but not in others. There is a correlation between high body mass index and knee osteoarthritis, which may be due to varus deformities in obese persons (Sharma et al. 2000), but the correlation is less strong between obesity and OA of the hip, and with generalised OA (Sturmer et al. 2000). Being overweight may result in premature muscle fatigue which in turn leads to abnormal kinematics and the subsequent development of OA. The relationship seems to be much stronger in women. Increased load across the joints clearly plays a role, but hormonal abnormalities associated with obesity may

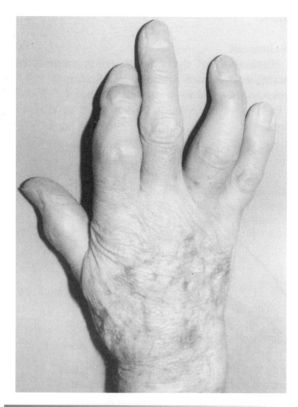

Figure 9.2   Heberden's and Bouchard's nodes (bony swellings of the distal and intermediate interphalangeal joints respectively) in primary OA. (Reproduced from Dandy and Edwards 1998, with permission.)

also be to blame, as suggested by an increase, albeit modest, in hand OA in obese women.

Haemophilia, acromegaly and hyperthyroidism all predispose joints to secondary OA, as does Charcot's joints – the phenomenon of joint destruction which follows as a result of loss of joint proprioception and sensation, leading to abnormal stresses and joint positions.

Key point
Interestingly there is overlap between primary and secondary OA. People who develop secondary OA also appear to have a predisposition to primary OA (Doherty et al. 1983).

AETIOLOGY

Definition
Osteoarthritis is a 'mechanically driven but chemically mediated disease process' (Sowers 2001).

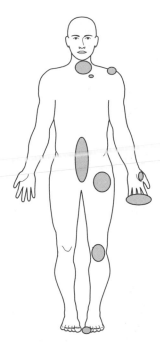

- Intervertebral joints and facet joints particularly in the lower cervical and lower lumbar areas.
- Distal interphalangeal joints of the fingers
- Metatarsophalangeal joint of the big toe
- First carpometacarpal joint of the thumb
- Temperomandibular joints
- Sternoclavicular joint, acromioclavicular joint
- Hip joint
- Knee joint including patellofemoral joint

Primary OA is not common in the wrists, shoulders, or ankles

Figure 9.3   The joints commonly affected by primary OA.

A single pathway to adequately explain all the pathological features of osteoarthritis has not yet been identified, and many authorities now consider it to be the final common pathway of a number of diverse conditions. Cartilage seems to possess a functional threshold. Within this threshold it is able to cope and function normally. OA develops when this threshold is surpassed.

Osteoarthritis was once considered to be a disease of hyaline cartilage. This is now being called into question, and evidence has emerged to suggest that the disease process does not originate in the cartilage, but that it begins with changes in the subchondral bone. These changes include redistribution of blood supply with hypertension in the subchondral bone marrow, oedema and micro-necrosis, which may result in secondary hyaline cartilage degeneration (Imhof et al. 1997). The accumulation of micro-fractures in the subchondral bone makes it more brittle, which in turn places greater stress upon the articular cartilage (Radin and Rose 1986).

Osteoarthritis does not develop exclusively as a result of the amount of weight that a joint has to bear. If it did, all people would suffer from OA of the ankles, and OA of the hands would be unheard of. Osteoarthritis is not simply a disease of the elderly either; autopsy specimens show evidence of the disease in the second decade of life, and there are many elderly persons with no evidence of it.

Joints that do not move are prone to develop OA. Lower proteoglycan content is found in the cartilage of immobile joints along with a decrease in synovial fluid volume; these are changes that are associated with cartilage degeneration. Abnormal movement of a joint predisposes joints to OA, such as in the knee joint following rupture of the anterior cruciate ligament. Joint hypermobility correlates positively with the risk of developing OA (Bird et al. 1978).

Daily exercise seems to prevent early cartilage degeneration (Otterness et al. 1998), but controversy persists about the relationship between exercise and OA and establishing causal factors remains problematic. People with early OA may cease to exercise because of their pain, so giving the false impression that OA is more common in people who do not exercise. It is also difficult to correlate causal relationships between poor posture and the development of OA.

Genetic factors are involved in primary OA, Heberden's nodes are 10 times more common in females than males, and mothers and sisters of affected females are 2–3 times more likely to be affected by primary OA. Increased frequency of human leucocyte antigen (HLA) A1 and B8 occurs in people with OA. Proinflammatory cytokines may be involved in the process, and there is increasing evidence that nitric oxide, which is an inorganic free radical, may play a role in cartilage degradation (Pelletier et al. 2001). Climate does not seem to be directly linked to the pathological changes of OA, but individuals who live in cold, damp climates often perceive their pain to be greater.

Defective lubricating mechanisms and uneven nutrition of the articular cartilage may initiate OA, for example following surgical removal of a meniscus (meniscectomy), where decreased synovial sweep may predispose the knee joint to accelerated degeneration.

EFFECTS OF OSTEOARTHRITIS

Definition
Osteoarthritis may be thought of as 'failure of the joint as an organ' (Lozada and Altman 2001).

Effect on articular cartilage

Fibrillation, or minute cracks and loss of water content occur which lead to softening, splitting and fragmentation of the cartilage. This occurs in both weight-bearing and non-weight-bearing areas of the joint surfaces. Collagen fibres split and there is a disorganisation of the normal proteoglycan–collagen relationship. As a result, water is attracted into the cartilage matrix, causing further softening and flaking. These flakes of cartilage break off, float freely within the joint, and may be impacted between the joint surfaces causing locking, inflammation, and synovial irritation. Proliferation occurs at the periphery of the cartilage and chondrocytes attempt damage repair, but the final product is not as resilient to stress as the original cartilage was.

This sets off a cascade of pathological processes in other tissues, which are discussed below.

Effect on bone

In osteoarthritis there is a degree of bony remodelling and attempts at repair. This remodelling can be seen in subchondral bone, which becomes eburnated (ivory-like and polished) and on X-ray takes on a white, dense, sclerotic appearance (Figure 9.4). The bone ends become hard and abnormally dense, as protection from the overlying cartilage is lost. Cysts may form in the subchondral bone and because eburnated bone is brittle, micro fractures occur, allowing the passage of synovial fluid into the deeper bone.

Venous congestion occurs in the subchondral bone, and osteophytes (bony spurs) form at the margins of the articular surfaces where they may project outwards or into the joint, capsule and ligaments causing sharp stabbing pains. If osteophytes are large enough they cause a mechanical obstruction to joint movement. Osteophytes are useful to a joint in the sense that they may increase the load-bearing area of a joint, dissipating pressure, but more often they cause problems since they restrict joint movement and are themselves liable to cause pain if nipped.

Bone of the weight-bearing joints alters in shape. The femoral head becomes flattened or mushroom shaped for example, and if this progresses it may cause loss of joint space and limb length changes.

Effect on synovial membrane

Synovial membrane undergoes hypertrophy and becomes oedematous. The many minute flakes of cartilage which have broken off act as an irritant to the synovial membrane, and cause repeated effusions.

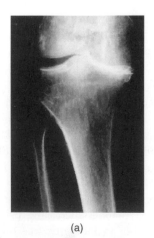

(a)

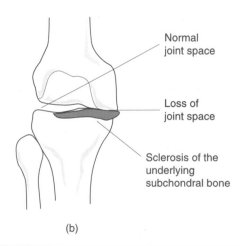

Normal joint space

Loss of joint space

Sclerosis of the underlying subchondral bone

(b)

Figure 9.4   Osteoarthritis of the medial compartment of the knee joint.

Effect on the joint capsule and ligaments

These undergo fibrous degeneration and adaptive shortening if the disease is advanced. Low-grade chronic inflammatory changes are often seen, although OA by definition is degenerative and not inflammatory. Ligaments undergo the same changes as the capsule and, according to the aspect of the joint, become either contracted or elongated. If joint space is diminished to a significant degree, ligaments that were once of adequate length may become effectively too long as joint space is diminished and they are no longer able to support the joint or provide adequate proprioceptive feedback.

There is controversy about how other soft tissues are involved in osteoarthritis, and whilst OA is not inflammatory in the strictest definition, villous hypertrophy and fibrosis of the synovium is commonly seen. Higher than normal levels of C reactive protein may also be found, suggestive of an inflammatory response.

CLINICAL FEATURES RELATED TO PATHOLOGY

Pain

Causes of pain in OA are discussed later in this chapter. The causes are multiple and the presentations multifactorial.

Heat/redness

This cannot always be detected, especially in the deeper joints such as the hip joint. Superficial joints such as the knee can become warm to palpation, signifying active inflammation.

Joint effusions/swelling

Effusion is swelling confined to a synovial cavity. 'Swelling' is a more general term.

Muscle spasm

Spasm is a protective mechanism. Movement causes pain so the body attempts to stop movement, but spasm often occurs out of all proportion to the underlying pathological cause. Prolonged spasm causes pain due to metabolite accumulation, and fatigue itself may limit joint movement. It may also interfere with sleep. Adaptive shortening of muscles may also occur (e.g. hamstrings if the knee is held in flexion for prolonged periods).

Stiffness (articular gelling)

Stiffness refers to the impairment of quality of movement, not quantity. Stiffness is present after rest and takes a little time to wear off with movement. It may be due to loss of joint lubrication, chronic oedema in the periarticular structures, swelling of the articular cartilage, or possibly the accumulation of hyaluronate in the capsule and synovium.

Loss of movement

This is due to adaptive soft-tissue shortening or lengthening, alteration of joint contour, or osteophytes

Radiographic findings

X-ray changes may not correlate with pain or disability levels. The visible changes include:

- loss of joint space
- sclerosis
- altered bone end shape
- osteophytes.

> **Key point**
> The term 'joint space' is a misnomer. Hyaline cartilage is invisible on X-ray so appears only as a space.

Figure 9.5 shows an example of a normal hip joint and one with clear signs of OA of both hips.

Muscle atrophy

Either through disuse or because of pain inhibition, muscles become weak, often on the aspect of the joint that is opposite to contractures (e.g. the hip extensors in cases of hip flexion deformity).

Joint enlargement

Chronic oedema of synovial membrane and capsule makes the joint appear large. Osteophytes and chronic effusions also contribute. Muscle atrophy may also make the joint look bigger, for example affecting the vastus medialis

Crepitus

Crepitus can range from mild creaking (which may also indicate synovitis), to loud cracking sounds in advanced disease. The flaked cartilage and eburnated bone ends grate against each other with a characteristic sound on movement.

Joint instability

Loss of proprioception, loss of ligamentous control, and loss of negative pressure within the joints as a result of effusions all contribute to joint instability in OA.

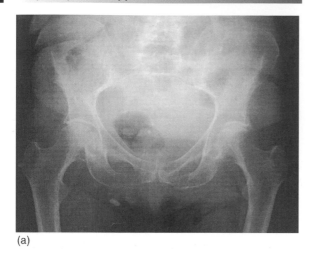

(a)

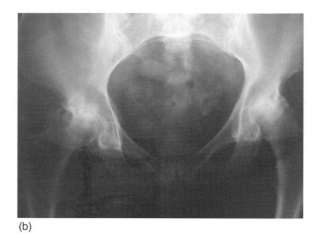

(b)

Figure 9.5 (a) X-ray of a normal pelvis and hips. Note the joint space and the spherical shape of the joints. (b) Osteoarthritis of both hips. Note the loss of joint space, flattening of the femoral head, and the sclerotic appearance.

Loss of function and deformity

The pathology is a combination of all the above clinical features. Each joint adopts a characteristic deformity or restriction of movements, known as the *capsular pattern*.

The capsule of a joint affected by osteoarthritis over a prolonged period behaves in a predictable way. Movements are lost in a classical pattern as the joint capsule contracts (Table 9.1). Knowledge of capsular patterns can provide useful diagnostic clues for the presence of some form of arthritis (capsular pathology).

PAIN IN OSTEOARTHRITIS

Causes and Sites of Pain

Articular hyaline cartilage does not contain nerve endings, so it cannot generate pain. The pain of OA occurs as an indirect consequence of the damage to the cartilage (Lozada and Altman 2001).

- Synovium possesses nerves so may be a source of pain, especially if infiltrated by inflammatory cells, and irritated by flakes of broken off cartilage.
- Subchondral bone may be a source of ischaemic pain.
- Bony remodelling, micro fractures and increased arterial pressures within the bone have also been proposed as sources of pain in OA.
- Osteophytes and effusions stretch the periosteum, capsule and ligaments, causing pain.
- Bursitis and muscle spasm are common secondary causes of pain.
- Joint instability causes pain as ligaments are over-stretched and traumatised.
- Effusions and increased subchondral vascular pressure causes throbbing pains.
- Release of inflammatory mediators results in pain.
- Sleep loss and other psychosocial variables may result in perceived increased pain.
- Other causes of pain include periosteal elevation, enzyme release, and an increase in volume of

Table 9.1 The capsular pattern of movement disorders.

Joint	Capsular pattern (largest restriction listed first)
Shoulder (glenohumeral)	Lateral rotation > abduction > medial rotation
Elbow	Flexion > extension
Wrist	Flexion and extension equally
Fingers	Flexion most of all
Trapeziometacarpal	Abduction > extension
Hip	Flexion > abduction > medial rotation
Knee	Flexion > extension
Ankle	Plantarflexion > dorsiflexion
Subtalar	Loss of varus

synovial fluid, which acts as a reservoir for inflammatory by-products.

Patterns of Pain

Early in the disease, the pain is usually intermittent and of low intensity. Individuals describe the pain of OA as an ache following weight-bearing, often worse at night after an active day. This is due to stresses on ligaments and synovial membrane and later due to the exposed bone surfaces coming into direct contact with each other.

Aching becomes more constant as the condition progresses. This is thought to be due to venous congestion in the bone ends. Referred pain is described as passing down a limb distally from the affected joint. For example OA hips often refer pain to the knee or down the anterior of the shin. Sharp stabbing pains are usually associated with loose bodies becoming impacted within the joint cavity, or osteophytic nipping. Larger loose fragments may cause locking of the joint. A detached fragment of articular cartilage will not be visible on X-ray unless it carries with it a piece of subchondral bone, which is opaque to X-rays.

Figure 9.6 shows common anatomical sites of pain.

CLINICAL FEATURES IN THE HIP, KNEE AND ANKLE JOINTS

The Hip

Pain over the abductor aspect or groin is referred down the anterior aspect of the thigh to the knee and shin.

Muscle spasm occurs in the adductor, flexor and lateral rotator muscles. A capsular pattern is commonly seen, with the resulting deformity of flexion, adduction and lateral rotation.

Muscle weakness occurs in all muscles, but the most functionally restricting is the weakness of the extensors and abductors. Loss of function includes difficulty in getting up from sitting and in walking far. The normal human hip joint possesses only 10–15 degrees of extension, so if this is lost the functional consequences are severe, leading to inability to push off during gait, stand erect, and rise from sitting.

The characteristic gait is Trendelenburg (see Figures 2.42 and 2.43) due to weakness of the hip abductor muscles. When the person stands on the affected leg the pelvis drops to the non weight-bearing side because the hip abductors are too weak to stabilise the pelvis in the horizontal plane. To balance and to maintain the line of gravity passing through the base, the trunk is side-flexed over to the side of the affected leg.

Crepitus may be heard as loud 'cracks'. In later stages, decreased joint space in extreme cases leads to leg length inequality and may result in compensatory scoliosis or flexion of the opposite knee.

Management note

It is fair to say that by far the most successful long-term management option when joint shape and function are compromised is replacement arthroplasty, which is now an extremely commonplace and successful operation.

The Knee

Osteoarthritis is most common in the medial compartment of the knee. Pain is described as round and through the joint, and may be referred down the shin to the ankle. Osteophytes may be palpable and muscle

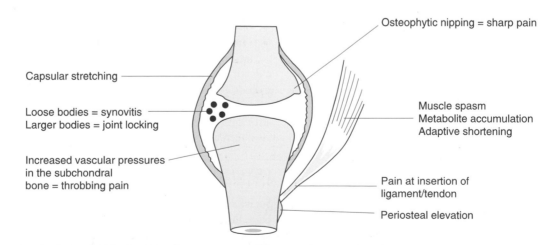

Capsular stretching

Loose bodies = synovitis
Larger bodies = joint locking

Increased vascular pressures in the subchondral bone = throbbing pain

Osteophytic nipping = sharp pain

Muscle spasm
Metabolite accumulation
Adaptive shortening

Pain at insertion of ligament/tendon

Periosteal elevation

Figure 9.6   Anatomical sites of pain in OA.

spasm may be present in the hamstring muscles. Patellofemoral crepitus is common.

The capsular pattern is loss of flexion then extension. Prolonged hamstring spasm combined with the fact that the joint is more comfortable in slight flexion (loose packed) may produce a flexion deformity and there is often valgus or varus deformity. Loss of full knee extension is functionally disabling, as the knee requires full extension – the close packed position, for prolonged standing with minimal muscle activity.

The joint is often enlarged and there is commonly quadriceps atrophy especially of the vastus medialis. There is an antalgic gait due to pain and a tendency for the joint to give way especially during stepping down. Collateral ligaments become effectively too long as a result of loss of joint space, so they are ill-equipped to control varus and valgus movements (Sharma 1999). This instability may cause permanent deformity and contracture with adaptive shortening or lengthening of various tissues.

Management note

Recent advances in arthroscopic surgery and arthroscopic washouts have proved valuable in removing debris from the synovial cavity, and it is possible to shave off rough bone arthroscopically.

The Ankle

Surprisingly, in view of the amount of load this small joint has to withstand, primary OA affecting the ankle is not common. Far more common is secondary OA following fracture or fracture dislocations of the ankle resulting in altered biomechanics – hence the need for these fractures to be correctly reduced anatomically.

Management note

Ankle joint replacement is now becoming more established as an alternative to arthrodesis (surgical fusion).

PROGNOSIS AND MANAGEMENT

Key point

People with osteoarthritis often show marked variations in their response to treatments (Creamer 2000), so a universal treatment recipe does not exist. There is no 'cure' for OA.

Since osteoarthritis might be thought of as a failed repair process (Piperno et al. 1998), and articular cartilage has limited regenerative abilities, efforts are now being made to stimulate the repair process in articular cartilage. Double-blind placebo-controlled trials (Pavelka et al. 2000; Reginster et al. 2001) suggest that glucosamine sulphate may control the symptoms of osteoarthritis of the knee, and may also be associated with a reduction in the progressive narrowing of joint space. Similar findings are reported for chondroitin sulphate (Michel et al. 2001).

Cartilage transplantation and synthetic articular cartilage is being developed (Oka et al. 2000), and synovial fluid replacement is also emerging.

With an holistic approach to management, sensible diet, joint protection advice and appropriate rest/exercise balance there can be good function preservation. Function can also be regained by joint arthroplasty in more advanced disease states. Temporary relief is often afforded through arthroscopic techniques and steroid injections.

As with all healthcare, an effective multidisciplinary team (MDT) is essential. Each team member will have his or her own distinctive role but there will always be overlap. Good communication is vital and needs to include the patient at the head of the MDT (Kelley and Ramsey 2000). The team consists of the person with the condition (often not automatically included in the team!), doctor, dietitian, pharmacist, occupational therapist, surgical appliance officer, specialist nurse practitioners or advisers, and chartered physiotherapist. The general practitioner prescribes and monitors drugs, and acts as a conduit for further referrals. The rheumatologist may be consulted as the condition advances. The orthopaedic surgeon may perform appropriate surgery.

Patients may need advice on weight reduction and healthy diet. There are many analgesics on the market and all have side-effects to varying degrees. A pharmacist can help the patient recognize side-effects and advise on the alternative drugs. The patient will need aids for daily living if there is severe disability. This may include provision of aids, for example for dressing or adaptations to the house for mobility. Surgical appliance officers may be involved. Self-help groups have also been employed with success.

PSYCHOSOCIAL ISSUES

Social support plays an important role in moderating pain, functional limitation, and depression (Blixen and Kippes 1999). Most published studies have taken the perspective of an individual or groups of experts rather than that of the patient (Bellamy et al. 2001) but there

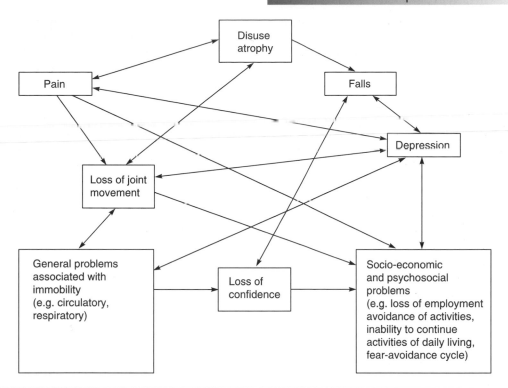

Figure 9.7   The interrelationships between various aspects of OA.

is now widening acknowledgement of the fact that progression and outcome in arthritis may depend on a complex set of psychosocial factors, as well as biological ones (Dieppe et al. 2000; see Figure 9.7). For example, Creamer et al. (2000) have claimed that function in knee OA is determined more by pain and obesity than by the structural changes observable on X-ray.

USEFUL MEASURING TOOLS

WOMAC index

Angst F, Aeschlimann A, Steiner W, Stucki G 2001 The responsiveness of the WOMAC osteoarthritis index as compared with the SF36 in patients with osteoarthritis of the legs undergoing a comprehensive rehabilitation intervention. Ann Rheum Dis 60: 834–40

Arthritis Impact Measurement Scales (AIMS)

Meenan RF, Gertman PM, Mason JH, Dunaif R 1982 The Arthritis Impact Measurement Scales: further investigations of a health status measure. Arth Rheum 25: 1048–53

AIMS2:

Meenan RF, Mason JH, Anderson JJ, Guccione AA, Kazis LE 1992 AIMS2: the content and properties of a revised and expanded Arthritis Impact Measurement Scales health status questionnaire. Arth Rheum 35: 1–10

Arthritis Self-Efficacy Scale (ASES)

Lorig K, Chastain RL, Ung E, Shoor S, Holman HR 1989 Development and evaluation of a scale to measure perceived self-efficacy in people with arthritis. Arth Rheum 32: 37–44

Functional Status Index (FSI)

Jette AM 1980 Functional Status Index: reliability of a chronic disease evaluation instrument. Arch Phys Med Rehabil 61: 395–401

Health Assessment Questionnaire (HAQ)

Fries JF, Spitz P, Kraines RG, Holman HR 1980 Measurement of patient outcome in arthritis. Arth Rheum 23: 137–45

British Modification of the HAQ

Kirwan JR, Reeback JS 1986 Stanford Health Assessment Questionnaire modified to assess disability in British patients with rheumatoid arthritis. Br J Rheumatol 25: 206–9

McGill Pain Questionnaire (MPQ)

Melzack R 1975 The McGill Pain Questionnaire: major properties and scoring methods. Pain 1: 277–99

Multidimensional Health Locus of Control Scale

Wallston KA, Wallston BS, DeVellis R 1978 Development of the Multidimensional Health Locus of Control Scales. Health Educ Monogr 6: 161–70

Nottingham Health Profile

Hunt SM, McKenna SP 1991 The Nottingham Health Profile: User's Manual, revised edn. Galen Research and Consultancy: Manchester

REFERENCES

Bellamy N, Carr A, Dougados M, Shea B, Wells G 2001 Towards a definition of 'difference' in osteoarthritis. J Rheumatol 28: 427–30

Bird HA, Tribe CR, Bacon PA 1978 Joint hypermobility leading to osteoarthrosis and chondrocalcinosis. Ann Rheum Dis 37: 203–311

Brandt KD 2000 The role of analgesics in the management of osteoarthritis pain. Am J Ther 7(2): 75–90

Blixen CE, Kippes C 1999 Depression, social support, and quality of life in older adults with osteoarthritis. Image J Nurs Sch 31(3): 221–6

Chen YL, Israelachvili J 1991 New mechanism of cavitation damage. Science 252: 1157–60

Coggon D, Reading I et al. 2001 Knee osteoarthritis and obesity. Int J Obes Relat Metab Disord 25: 622–7

Creamer P 2000 Osteoarthritis pain and its treatment. Curr Opin Rheumatol 12: 450–5

Creamer P, Lethbridge-Cejku M, Hochberg MC 2000 Factors associated with functional impairment in symptomatic knee osteoarthritis. Rheumatology (Oxf) 39: 490–6

Dandy DJ, Edwards DJ 1998 Essential Orthopaedics and Trauma, 3rd edn, p. 367. Churchill Livingstone: New York

Dieppe P, Cushnaghan J, Tucker M, Browning S, Shepstone L 2000 The Bristol 'OA500 study': progression and impact of the disease after 8 years. Osteoarth Cartil 8(2): 63–8

Doherty M, Watt I, Dieppe P 1983 Influence of primary generalised osteoarthritis on the development of secondary osteoarthritis. Lancet ii: 8–11

El Mahdy C 1989. Mummies Myth and Magic. Thames & Hudson: London

Eyre D 2002 Collagen of articular cartilage. Arth Res 4: 30–5

Imhof H, Breitenseher M, Kainberger F, Trattnig S 1997 Degenerative joint disease: cartilage or vascular disease? Skeletal Radiol 26: 398–403

Kelley MJ, Ramsey ML 2000 Osteoarthritis and traumatic arthritis of the shoulder. J Hand Ther 13(2): 148–62

Keuttner KE, Goldberg V (eds) 1995 Osteoarthritic Disorders, pp. 21–5. Academy of Orthopedic Surgeons: Rosemont, IL

Lozada CJ, Altman RD 2001 In: Koopman WJ (ed.) Arthritis and Allied Conditions: a Textbook of Rheumatology. Lippincott Williams & Wilkins: Philadelphia

Makirowski T, Tepic S et al. 1994 Cartilage stresses in the human hip joint. J Biomech Engng 116: 106–7

Michel B, Vignon E, de Vathaire F et al. 2001 Oral chondroitin sulphate in knee OA patients: radiographic outcomes of a 2-year prospective study. Osteoporos Int 9(Suppl): S68

Nordin M, Frankel VH 1989 Basic Biomechanics of the Musculoskeletal System. Lippincott Williams & Wilkins: Philadelphia

Oka M, Ushio K et al. 2000 Development of artificial articular cartilage. Proc Inst Mech Engng 214H: 59–68

Otterness IG, Eskra JD et al. 1998 Exercise protects against articular cartilage degeneration in the hamster. Arth Rheum 41: 2068–76

Pavelka K, Gatterova J, Olejarova M et al. 2000 Glucosamine sulfate decreased progression of knee osteoarthritis in a long-term randomized placebo-controlled, independent, confirmatory trial. Arth Rheum 43(S38): 1908

Pelletier JP, Pelletier JM, Howell DS 2001 Etiopathogenesis of osteoarthritis. In: Koopman WJ (ed.) Arthritis and Allied Conditions: a Textbook of Rheumatology. Lippincott Williams & Wilkins: Philadelphia

Piperno M, Reboul P et al. 1998 Osteoarthritic cartilage fibrillation is associated with a decrease in chondrocyte adhesion to fibronectin. Osteoarth Cartil 6: 393–9.

Radin EL, Paul IL 1971 Response of joints to impact loading. I: In-vitro wear. Arth Rheum 14: 356

Radin EL, Rose RM 1986 Role of subchondral bone in the initiation and progression of cartilage damage. Clin Orthop 213: 34–40

Reginster JY, Deroisy R, Rovati LC et al. 2001 Long-term effects of glucosamine sulphate on osteoarthritis progression: a randomised, placebo-controlled clinical trial. Lancet 357: 251–6

Sharma L, Hayes KW et al. 1999 Does laxity alter the relationship between strength and physical function in knee osteoarthritis? Arth Rheum 42: 25–32

Sharma L, Lou C et al. 2000 The mechanism of the effect of obesity in knee osteoarthritis: the mediating role of malalignment. Arth Rheum 43: 568–75

Simkin PA 1993 Synovial physiology. In: McCarty DJ, Koopman WJ (eds) Arthritis and Allied Conditions, 12th edn, pp. 199–212. Lea & Febiger: Philadelphia

Sowers M 2001 Epidemiology of risk factors for osteoarthritis: systemic factors. Curr Opin Rheumatol 13: 447–51

Sturmer T, Gunther KP et al. 2000 Obesity, overweight and patterns of osteoarthritis: the Ulm Osteoarthritis Study. J Clin Epidemiol 53: 307–13

Swann DA, Radin EL, Hendren RB 1979 The lubrication of articular cartilage by synovial fluid glycoproteins. Arth Rheum 22: 665

Common Chronic Inflammatory Polyarthropathies

J. A. Goodacre and I. Stewart

10

This chapter provides an introduction to some of the common types of chronic polyarthropathy. The main clinical features of these conditions are described, focusing in particular on the symptoms, signs and investigative findings that are of most value for diagnostic and monitoring purposes in clinical practice. The key principles of clinical management are also discussed, highlighting issues that have generic applicability to all forms of chronic arthritis as well as those that apply more specifically to each of the types of rheumatic disease described here.

Effective and integrated multidisciplinary approaches to clinical management are of paramount importance in these long-term conditions in order to achieve optimal health outcomes.

TYPES OF CHRONIC INFLAMMATORY POLYARTHROPATHY

There are many different types of chronic inflammatory polyarthropathy. They all cause pain, swelling and functional impairment of several joints, and are frequently associated with extra-articular and systemic symptoms and signs. Development of the process of chronic inflammation in and around the joints is often, although not invariably, accompanied by structural damage to joint cartilage and bone, as well as to other tissues associated with the joint.

The rate and extent of joint damage is highly variable and is determined by the outcome of a complex array of interacting cellular and molecular mechanisms, leading to breakdown or repair of tissue. In recent years, much research has been aimed at understanding these pathways and mechanisms, and this has led to the identification of an increasing number of promising new molecular targets for use in treating the chronic polyarthropathies. These advances, together with the increasing availability and use of genetic information to improve the definition of patient subgroups, and the opening up of the possibility that in the future it may be possible to use genetic information to predict clinical outcomes to therapies in these diseases, have led to major and exciting new approaches in the treatment of people with chronic arthritis.

Categories of Symptoms and Signs

The following categories of symptoms and signs provide a useful clinical framework for distinguishing the different types of chronic arthritis:

- the features and distribution of joint involvement

- the presence and characteristics of extra-articular and systemic features
- the presence of other previous or concomitant associated diseases
- a family history of arthritis or other associated conditions
- results from laboratory investigations and bone or joint imaging.

Diagnostic Issues

Some types of polyarthropathy display characteristic *patterns of joint involvement*, and this provides an important basis for diagnosis. The pattern of joint involvement, combined with other features of the history, examination and results of investigations, enables different diagnostic groups to be distinguished. Other types of polyarthropathy are less distinctive in terms of the types of joint involved.

Even within particular diagnostic types, however, there can be a remarkable degree of individual heterogeneity in terms of the onset, progression and outcome of these diseases. Furthermore, it is common to find that the clinical features in individual patients may not conform neatly or distinctly to the characteristics of any of the recognised diagnostic categories.

Clinical note

It is important to appreciate that the clinical features of the chronic polyarthropathies may evolve and change over periods of months or years, sometimes therefore requiring the passage of time before the correct diagnosis can be made with any degree of certainty.

Irrespective of the type of arthropathy involved, all people with chronic arthritis experience variable and usually unpredictable levels of joint pain and swelling, which inevitably not only leads to various degrees of functional impairment but also engenders significant concerns and anxieties about their state of health, their employment capability, and their capacity for independence and social functioning in both the short and long term. The overall effects of chronic polyarthropathies on health almost always, therefore, involve many aspects of physical, psychological and social well-being.

Consequently, the processes of clinical assessment and monitoring of patients by health professionals need to take account of key factors within each of these domains. For example, in addition to the need for careful observation and documentation of the physical symptoms and signs, and accurate and appropriate interpretation of the investigative findings, it is essential for health professionals to assess the patient's mood and coping capacity, together with the level and effectiveness of social support available. Factors such as personal goals and work or social needs can often have a very important bearing on disease expression and progression, as can knowledge, beliefs and expectations formed by gleaning information from traditional or Internet-based sources of written information, shared experience or anecdote.

The Multidisciplinary Team and Evidence-Based Therapies

The members of the multidisciplinary care team have the important task of drawing together the different elements of diagnosis and assessment in order to synthesise and formulate a plan for management and monitoring. The plan should be based on goals that are relevant, realistic and feasible.

Whilst it remains the case that some aspects of clinical management of the chronic polyarthropathies must continue to involve decisions based on clinical experience, common sense and general consensus rather than proven evidence, there are now an increasing number of circumstances in which clinicians working in this field should, as far as possible, utilise the rapidly developing base of published evidence in order to guide their decisions in clinical management. In the future, it is likely that clinical management teams will need to give increasing consideration to the use of new biological therapies for several of these conditions, as well as to give greater attention to ways of identifying patient subgroups to facilitate effective and selective targeting of different medical and non-medical therapies as appropriate, and to ways of synergising the increasing number of different treatment modalities in order to achieve optimal benefit. This era is therefore one of unprecedented excitement and opportunity for all working in the field.

Successful translation of new knowledge from many disciplines within the life, clinical and social sciences into clinical practice will require tomorrow's health professionals in rheumatology to utilise a generic and advancing base of knowledge across these disciplines, as well as to acquire and maintain specialist knowledge and skills in their chosen area of expertise. Although these issues present major challenges – not only for students and healthcare professionals but also for the many sectors and institutions involved in undergraduate and postgraduate education and healthcare provision – they nevertheless point the way towards how substantial improvement in the health of patients with chronic arthritis is becoming increasingly feasible and attainable.

RHEUMATOID ARTHRITIS

The *multisystem autoimmune diseases*, of which the most common is rheumatoid arthritis (RA), are associated with marked systemic upset and involvement of other organs and tissues in addition to the presence of chronic joint disease. These diseases are all characterised by high titres of autoantibodies and many other features of immune activation and regulation.

Key point
Rheumatoid arthritis affects about 1% of adults and is characterised by a peripheral, symmetrical erosive polyarthritis, frequently associated with extra-articular tissue involvement. It is the cause of substantial levels of morbidity, disability and economic burden worldwide.

Pathogenesis of RA

The causes of RA are unknown, but it is recognised as a type of autoimmune disorder. RA is a long-term condition, usually involving unpredictable cycles of exacerbation and remission.

The pathogenesis of RA involves chronic synovitis in which large numbers of a wide range of types of inflammatory and immune cells migrate into synovial tissue. This process, and its consequences, involves endothelial cells together with the several different types of cells resident not only in synovium but also in adjacent bone and cartilage, such as fibroblasts, osteoclasts and chondrocytes. Although many of the key molecular pathways, which drive and perpetuate this process, have been identified in recent years, the fundamental reasons why RA inflammation develops and persists remain unknown. Nevertheless, it is clear that complex cellular and molecular interactions between infiltrating inflammatory cells and resident cells, mediated by a variety of cell surface receptors, cytokines, chemokines, extracellular enzymes and other inflammatory mediators, results in persistent chronic synovitis and breakdown of cartilage and bone.

It is well established that the pathogenesis of RA involves an important component of *genetic susceptibility*, although non-genetic factors, as yet unidentified, play the predominant role. For example, RA disease concordance in identical twins has been reported to be as low as about 15%. Susceptibility to RA involves several genes, of which the highly polymorphic HLA

DRB1 gene is known to impart the most significant contribution. Detailed structural analyses of the DRB1 gene alleles which confer susceptibility to RA have led to the theory that the key disease mechanisms may depend upon aspects of the activation and function of T lymphocytes, since DRB1 genes are known to have an important role in these pathways. These findings have also provided further support to the concept that RA is an autoimmune disease.

This view was based originally on the fact that RA involves the production of various autoantibodies, of which rheumatoid factor is an example. Rheumatoid factors are antibodies, which recognise epitopes in the constant regions of IgG molecules; that is, they are antibodies, which recognise and bind to other antibodies. Rheumatoid factors are often found in high concentrations in RA sera (which are consequently termed 'seropositive') and are therefore used as one of the diagnostic criteria for RA.

However, some people with RA are termed 'seronegative', since they do not have raised concentrations of rheumatoid factor in their sera. Furthermore, rheumatoid factor is quite frequently found in other chronic inflammatory diseases besides RA. Other autoantibodies besides rheumatoid factors can also be found in RA, and in recent years it has been shown that such auto antibodies include antifilaggrin, antikeratin and anticitrullinated peptide antibodies.

Whilst the pathogenic significance of these findings remains unclear, there continues to be considerable interest in the possibility that measurement of these antibodies in a patient's serum may provide a useful additional diagnostic tool in RA.

Clinical Features of RA

The clinical features of RA manifest as joint pain, swelling and stiffness, accompanied by severe fatigue and systemic disturbance. The onset can be either rapid or insidious, and usually begins in the hands and/or feet. The elbows, knees and cervical spine are also commonly involved. In the early stages the disease can sometimes undergo quite prolonged periods of remission. Chronic synovitis may be accompanied by effusion and joint function may be compromised. There may also be an associated lymphadenopathy.

In addition to joint symptoms there is marked systemic upset and severe fatigue. For many patients the fatigue is often the most troublesome and frustrating aspect of the disease. Loss of muscle bulk and strength, loss of appetite, and intermittent fever may also occur.

Outside the joints themselves, rheumatoid nodules may appear, for example on the extensor surfaces of the elbows, and other symptoms may result from involvement of extra-articular tissues. A wide range of other tissues and organs may be involved in RA, among

Table 10.1 The 1987 American College of Rheumatology diagnostic criteria for rheumatoid arthritis. At least four criteria must be fulfilled for the diagnosis of RA.

	Criterion	Comment
1.	Morning stiffness	Morning stiffness in and around the joints lasting at least 1 hour
2.	Arthritis in three or more joint areas	Arthritis in three or more joint areas, involving the PIP, MCP, wrist, elbow, knee, ankle or MTP joints on the right or left Soft-tissue swelling or fluid (but not bony overgrowth) observed by a physician, present simultaneously for at least 6 weeks
3.	Arthritis of the hand joints	Swelling of wrist, MCP or hand joints for at least 6 weeks
4.	Symmetrical arthritis	Simultaneous involvement of the same joint areas (defined in 2 above) on both sides of the body (bilateral involvement of PIP, MCP or MTP joints is acceptable without absolute symmetry) for at least 6 weeks
5.	Rheumatoid nodules	Subcutaneous nodules over bony prominences, extensor surfaces or in juxta-articular regions, observed by a physician
6.	Rheumatoid factor	Detected by a method positive in fewer than 5% of normal controls
7.	Radiographic changes	Typical of RA on posteroanterior hand and wrist radiographs These must include erosions or unequivocal bony decalcification localised in or most marked adjacent to the involved joints (OA changes alone do not qualify)

From Arnet FC, Edworthy SM, Bloch DA et al. 1988 The American Rheumatism Association 1987 revised criteria for the classification of rheumatoid arthritis. Arthritis Rheum 31: 315–24.

which involvement of the lacrimal and salivary glands, leading to dry eyes and dry mouth (Sjögren's syndrome), is particularly common (Table 10.2).

Establishing the Diagnosis of RA

The first step is to establish a diagnosis, using information from the history and examination together with the results of laboratory investigations and joint imaging. Classically, the presence of a peripheral and symmetrical polyarthritis, associated with systemic fatigue, with nodules, with erosive changes on X-rays of the hands or feet, and with raised titres of serum rheumatoid factor, would leave the diagnosis in no doubt. However, the absence of one or more of these features can quite often lead to the need to make a provisional, rather than a definite, diagnosis. This may particularly apply in the diagnosis of early RA. The formal and widely used American College of Rheumatology criteria for the diagnosis of RA are shown in Table 10.1.

Clinical Assessment and Monitoring

After the diagnosis has been established, a full medical and social assessment is essential, involving discussions with all the health professionals involved as well as with the patient's family, carers or friends. This should lead to the development of an appropriate treatment plan, following which further assessments should continue to be conducted at regular intervals in order to inform discussions about the efficacy of intervention(s), and to enable the treatment plan to be reviewed and modified accordingly.

Observations and investigations

Disease activity and severity is assessed using a range of subjective and objective methods aimed at providing overall measures of the inflammatory, systemic and functional components of the disease. The assessment should include evaluation of active synovitis, as measured by tender and swollen joint counts, and by measuring the erythrocyte sedimentation rate (ESR) and concentrations of serum acute phase proteins such as C reactive protein or ferritin. The acute-phase response in RA is reflected in the raised ESR which is usually found in these patients, and which is a useful objective indicator of the severity of inflammation. Similarly, haemoglobin concentrations are typically reduced, usually reflecting an anaemia of chronic illness (although other possible causes of anaemia should always be considered and sought), and platelet counts are often increased. Although useful diagnostically,

rheumatoid factor titres are a relatively poor indicator of the severity of synovitis.

Baseline laboratory investigations should include tests of hepatic and renal function. The assessment should also include measures of severity of pain, morning stiffness and fatigue, and of joint function as reflected by range of movement, instability and deformity. The presence of extra-articular features and comorbid conditions should be sought. Joint imaging should be performed routinely at an early stage, and in current practice this usually involves radiographs of the hands and feet. In the early stages, radiographs may show soft-tissue swelling, periarticular osteoporosis or loss of joint space. These changes may be followed by the development of erosion of cartilage and bone, and, in severe cases, subsequently by complete loss of the structure of the joint. Additional imaging techniques, for example magnetic resonance imaging and high-resolution ultrasound, are now increasingly available and are being extensively evaluated for their potential role in RA assessment.

Table 10.2 Common extra-articular features of rheumatoid arthritis.

Systemic	Nodules Anaemia Lymphadenopathy Amyloidosis[a] Vasculitis[b] Felty's syndrome[c]
Ocular	Keratoconjunctivitis Scleritis and episcleritis
Bone	Osteoporosis
Neurological	Peripheral nerve entrapment Peripheral neuropathy Cervical spine instability Cervical cord compression Nerve root compression
Pulmonary	Pleurisy Pleural effusion Pulmonary alveolitis and fibrosis
Cardiovascular	Pericarditis and myocarditis Pericardial effusion Conduction defects Atherosclerosis

[a] Results when amyloid protein builds up in one or more organs to cause their malfunction. The heart, kidneys, nervous system and gastrointestinal tract are most often affected.
[b] A type of inflammation of the blood vessels.
[c] Includes an enlarged spleen, and an abnormally low white blood count.

Clinical assessment scales

A variety of clinical assessment scales to score the severity of joint inflammation have been developed, among which the Ritchie Index, or one of its modified forms, continues to be used commonly, particularly in research settings. For measuring function, several quantitative scales have been developed for use both in research and healthcare settings. These include the Health Assessment Questionnaire (HAQ) and the Arthritis Impact Measurement Scale (AIMS).

A variety of composite methods of expressing overall disease activity as a single score have been developed, of which the DAS score is in most frequent use. The DAS score measures disease activity on a scale of 1 to 10 and is based on the number of swollen joints, the number of tender joints, and the ESR.

The DAS score

Since it was first introduced, the score has been modified to the simpler DAS28, which takes account of fewer joints than the original form, which involved assessment of 44 joints.

Furthermore, a variety of methods of quantifying overall change in disease status have been developed, primarily for the purpose of comparing the efficacy of different treatment interventions. The American College of Rheumatology (ACR) definition of response requires improvement in both the tender and swollen joint counts together with improvement in three of the following five parameters:

- patient's global assessment
- physician's global assessment
- pain severity
- level of disability (as measured for example using HAQ)
- levels of the acute-phase response as measured by the ESR or serum concentrations of C-reactive protein.

Responses are defined as ACR 20, ACR 50 or ACR 70, in which the figures denote percentage improvement in clinical scores compared with baseline measurements.

Clinical Management of RA

Overall, the major goals of treatment are to minimise joint inflammation and damage, prevent loss of joint function, and reduce symptoms of pain, stiffness and fatigue.

Assessment and discussion by a multidisciplinary team, with active involvement of the patient and the

Consensus guidelines

Consensus guidelines for the management and monitoring of RA were first developed by the American College of Rheumatology in the mid-1990s and have recently been reviewed and revised. These guidelines provide a useful framework of reference from which practices tailored to local conditions and resources can be developed.

family or carer, leading to the development of a coherent and coordinated plan, provides the optimal basis for long-term clinical management. It is essential that this process be underpinned by clear and effective communication between all members of the team.

The treatment plan must reflect both the nature and severity of the disease and the views and expectations of the patient. Since predicting the course of the disease and its response to treatment is uncertain, the clinicians in the team should aim to provide support that is optimistic whilst balanced with a level of realism appropriate for each individual patient.

Optimal management of RA is achieved by combining non-pharmacological and pharmacological treatments in a manner tailored to individual patient's needs and disease status.

Non-pharmacological treatments

Maintenance of joint function and overall personal function (at home, at leisure and in the workplace) are vitally important goals, and to this end all patients should, at an early stage, undergo a detailed programme of instruction and advice in the principles of joint protection and splinting, pain management, energy conservation and management, and exercise.

The importance of dynamic and aerobic exercise programmes for maintaining muscle strength and joint mobility has been widely recognised for many years, but this particular aspect of clinical management is currently gaining even further importance in the context of preventing the long-term cardiovascular sequelae of RA. The programme should also cover relevant aspects of activity planning, diet and nutrition, choice and use of appropriate footwear, and the availability of assistive technologies.

Patients should also be given advice and guidance on sources of further information and literature, and details of local, regional and national self-help and other support groups. Opportunities should be sought to involve, as appropriate, other family members or carers so that patients can benefit from informed support in the domestic setting.

The potential educative and therapeutic value of a programme which addresses the issues described here is extremely high, and this approach can often be invaluable in providing an effective means of establishing a secure basis for effective and successful care delivery in this long-term condition.

Pharmacological treatments

Pharmacological therapies for RA can be categorised according to whether the medication is aimed primarily at relief of symptoms or at disease modification, and to whether or not the medication is based upon a defined molecular target.

Complementary therapies

Use of complementary therapies is extremely common amongst people with RA. A wide variety of preparations, approaches and dietary supplements are available for use in helping to alleviate the symptoms of pain, stiffness and systemic upset.

Analgesic and anti-inflammatory medications

These include non-steroidal anti-inflammatory drugs (NSAIDs) and selective cyclo-oxygenase 2 (COX-2) inhibitors. The primary role of these medications is to achieve symptomatic improvement, rather than to alter the course of the disease or prevent joint damage. The choice of medication usually takes into account considerations of efficacy, safety and cost, as well as the issue of whether or not the patient has had any side-effects from previous use of such treatments.

Key point

In principle, patients should take only one from this class of medication at any given time. If symptoms are not satisfactorily relieved to an acceptable level the medication should be stopped before a different drug within this class is tried.

Dyspepsia and gastroduodenal ulceration are common side-effects. If the patient is found to be at risk of an adverse gastrointestinal event, the use of gastroprotective therapies (such as H_2 blockers and proton pump inhibitors) should be considered, although routine concomitant use of gastroprotective therapies is not recommended.

Disease-modifying antirheumatic drugs (DMARDs)

This category of medication includes a diverse array of drugs, which are used because of their potential to reduce joint damage. They are used in people who have persistently active synovitis, persistently elevated ESR, and radiographic joint damage.

The trend in recent years has been to commence DMARDs at an early stage in people who fulfil these clinical features. Typically it takes several weeks or months for clinical benefit to become manifest, and it is important that patients on DMARDs be closely monitored for possible side-effects.

DMARDs commonly used in RA include methotrexate, sulphasalazine and hydroxychloroquine, whilst leflunomide, azathioprine, gold salts, D-penicillamine, minocycline and cyclosporine may also be prescribed. Choice of DMARD is influenced by many factors, including patient preference, physician experience, and convenience of administration and monitoring.

Key point

There has been an increasing trend in recent years towards use of combination DMARD therapy. The possibility that this may be beneficial continues to be investigated.

Glucocorticoids

There is evidence to suggest that low-dose glucocorticoids (that is, prednisolone in doses of less than 10 mg daily) may have disease-modifying effects in RA and that patients may feel markedly better within days following commencement of such therapy. However, these factors need to be balanced against the known adverse effects of glucocorticoids, particularly osteoporosis. Similarly, glucocorticoid injection of joints and tendons continues to be used in clinical practice and can sometimes provide dramatic local, and even systemic, benefit, albeit often only temporarily.

It is important to rule out other possible causes of active synovitis in RA, such as joint infection and crystal-mediated arthritis, before injections are given, and repeated injections into the same joint or tendon should be avoided if at all possible.

Biological therapies

The feasibility of developing and utilising biological therapies in the treatment of RA has arisen from the success of a large body of research aimed at increasing our understanding of the molecular mechanisms of the disease. This has led to the identification of several well-defined target molecules. This knowledge, allied to the availability of modern techniques in molecular biology and protein chemistry, has for the first time enabled pharmacological therapy in RA to be approached on a rational scientific basis.

The first examples of such therapies to reach the clinic are based on the knowledge that two cytokines, namely tumour necrosis factor alpha (TNFα) and interleukin one (IL-1), which regulate inflammatory and immune responses, have a key role in RA pathogenesis. This has led to the design and development of therapeutic molecules which are based closely on the known natural structure of these cytokines or their receptors and which can therefore be used to modify their biological effects. Clinical trials using infliximab (a monoclonal antibody which binds TNFα), etanercept (a soluble form of one of the types of TNFα receptor found on cell surfaces) and anakinra (a soluble form of the IL-1 receptor antagonist) in RA have produced extremely promising results, such that the benefits of these therapies appear to be markedly stronger and to become manifest much earlier than those of traditional DMARDs.

Key point

Studies to determine long-term outcome and to investigate possible long-term side-effects of these therapies are in progress. Other types of biological therapies based on these and other known key target molecules in RA are currently under development and evaluation.

Surgery

Surgical procedures may be indicated in RA when the effects of severe structural joint damage lead to loss of function and/or intractable pain. Total joint arthroplasty is potentially extremely beneficial, such that many patients experience marked improvement in their function and quality of life. The longevity of joint prostheses is being gradually increased through the use of new materials for manufacturing prostheses and for use in cements, as well as through continuing improvements in surgical and perioperative techniques and experience. Other surgical procedures used in RA include synovectomy, joint fusion, resection of the metatarsal heads, and carpal tunnel release.

PRACTICE POINTS IN THE MANAGEMENT OF RA

This section describes some of the practical issues that frequently arise in the management of RA and which are of direct relevance to allied health professionals involved in the field. Many of the points raised here are not necessarily exclusive to RA and may apply equally to other types of polyarthropathy; nor are they necessarily regarded as being the only available method of treating the problems commonly faced by people with RA.

Joint Splinting: General Principles

Custom-made and proprietary splints are used frequently in the management of RA. The fabrication of splints often falls into the remit of therapists working in rheumatology.

Splints can be classified either by their design or by their function. In relation to design, splints are either static (preventing movement and resting affected joints) or dynamic (allowing movement by incorporating hinges, elastic or springs). In relation to function, the majority of splints used in the management of RA fall into three main categories: resting, functional and corrective.

- *Resting splints* are used to relieve pain, decrease inflammation, prevent the development of contractures, maintain proper joint alignment, decrease or alleviate symptoms of nerve entrapment, support ligaments and joint capsules.
- *Functional splints* are used to relieve pain, support unstable joint structures, accommodate for muscle weakness or atrophy, protect from further damage, assist in controlling inflammation, protect against nerve entrapment or tenosynovitis.
- *Corrective splints* are used to modify soft-tissue contractures.

Other types of splint are those used postoperatively to maintain joint alignment or mobility, to assist with postoperative stretching and to minimise adhesions.

A wide range of thermoplastic materials are available to custom-made splints, the choice of which is influenced by factors such as the specific requirement of the splint, the length of time for which the splint will be used, the place where the splint is being made and the equipment available, the condition of the patient's skin, and the cost of materials.

Key point

The provision of any splint should occur in conjunction with appropriate patient education to ensure that the patient understands the purpose of the splint, the need to carry out relevant exercise programmes, and the need to check for signs of an ill-fitting splint, such as the occurrence of pressure points.

Management of Specific Joints

Hands

Resting splints are used commonly to treat hand involvement in early and active RA. Fabrication of hand splints should occur only after a detailed hand assessment has been carried out to provide baseline measurements against which changes can be assessed, and to define the aims of splinting. All resting splints should be custom-made in order to ensure correct fit and joint positioning, and to be acceptable to the patient. Short-term use may still offer some symptomatic benefit and help to prevent deformity. Splints may also help to prevent deterioration of deformities such as ulnar deviation, swan-neck or Boutonnière deformities.

Local corticosteroid injections are often used as a means of reducing active synovitis in one or more PIP or MCP joint, or to treat flexor tendon nodules or flexor tenosynovitis, in which there may be limited active flexion of the fingers but nevertheless a good range of passive movement. Treatment of local flexor tendon problems by injection requires highly skilled and accurate infiltration of corticosteroid into the flexor tendon sheath.

Key point
There is often cause for concern about the potential for tendon rupture following steroid injection. This is an important issue that should be taken into account when discussing the advantages and disadvantages of this approach with the patient, whilst bearing in mind that tendon rupture may also sometimes occur as a result of the chronic inflammatory process of RA itself.

Wrists

Proprietary splints can be invaluable in helping to maintain function, reducing pain and preventing deformity of the wrists. It is important to appreciate that poor wrist function will undoubtedly contribute significantly to poor overall hand function. More rigid polythene or prefabricated splints may sometimes be considered particularly if wrist mobility is already reduced. Long-term restriction of movement should not occur, although a stiff wrist held in an optimal position may still be relatively pain-free and functional.

Carpal tunnel syndrome, due to entrapment of the median nerve, is a common associated problem in RA and may lead to hand pain and sensory symptoms. Confirmation of the diagnosis using nerve conduction studies should be obtained if possible. If symptoms do not improve despite the regular use of splints, control of the activity of the rheumatoid disease and a local steroid injection, then surgery to decompress the carpal tunnel may need to be considered.

Elbows

A programme of active exercises and education to encourage movement and prevent flexion deformities of the elbows is of paramount importance in RA. If the elbows are particularly inflamed such that the patient's capacity for conducting the recommended exercise programme is compromised, and if other causes of inflammation have been excluded, a corticosteroid injection into the joint or bursa may be given in an attempt to reduce pain and to enable maintenance of exercises in order to preserve range of movement in the joint.

Rheumatoid nodules occur in approximately 25–30% of patients with RA. Surgical removal may be considered, particularly if infection of the nodule occurs. However, nodules frequently recur after surgical removal.

Shoulders

Shoulder involvement is common in RA, and should be anticipated and addressed in the form of a specific programme of exercise and education in order to prevent loss of movement and function. Restriction of abduction and external rotation of the shoulder should be sought from an early stage and monitored closely, and the patient's exercise programme modified accordingly if the range of movement shows signs of deterioration. A painful arc of movement of the shoulder joint suggests tendonitis, which may, if diagnosed in its early stages, respond to a local steroid injection. As always, accurate localisation of the injection and skilled technique is essential.

Precise diagnosis of the structures producing shoulder pain is often extremely difficult, and imaging with ultrasound or MRI can provide invaluable assistance in identifying the inflamed structure and informing the choice of appropriate therapy.

Key point
Tendon rupture or partial tears should always be assessed by an orthopaedic surgeon.

Cervical spine

The cervical spine is commonly affected in RA and the consequent effects of this on the spinal cord may lead to serious complications or even death. Therefore, before embarking upon any course of physiotherapy, X-rays of the cervical spine should be taken in flexion, extension and with an open-mouth view. The films should be assessed carefully in order to determine the presence of atlanto-axial or sub-axial subluxation and the involvement of the odontoid peg, and the findings should be taken into account when planning the course of treatment. This issue should also be borne in mind when preparing patients for anaesthesia, and during surgery and postoperative management.

Soft and rigid cervical collars may be of symptomatic value for some RA patients with neck problems, although many patients find them uncomfortable.

Dorsal spine and lumbar spine

The lower spine is rarely affected by RA. Any episodes of sudden acute onset of pain should be investigated for possible vertebral collapse, especially if the patient has been treated with glucocorticoids.

Hips

Acute synovitis of the hips in RA is relatively rare unless it forms part of more widespread exacerbation in inflammation involving other joints. Pain arising from the hip joint itself is usually felt in the groin, whilst pain over the lateral aspect of the hip may often arise as referred pain from the lower lumbar spine or pelvis, or may indicate a subtrochanteric bursitis. An ultrasound scan or an MRI scan can be useful in confirming the presence of synovitis in the hip, for example by demonstrating the presence of fluid in the joint.

An active exercise programme, with hydrotherapy, should be used to help reduce symptoms, maintain hip movement and improve muscle strength.

Knees

Active synovitis in the knee occurs commonly in both early and chronic RA. Pain may cause the knee to adopt a flexed position. Early treatment is essential and may involve resting splints, serial plaster or thermoplastic splinting and active quadriceps exercises in an effort to maintain range of movement. As always, a strong emphasis should be placed on the prevention of deformity as well as symptom management, and the vital importance of this should be explained carefully and repeatedly to the patient from the outset.

Ankles and feet

Ankle pain may often arise from the subtalar joint, for which, if other measures have failed, brief immobilisation in a light weight-bearing plaster of Paris is still sometimes used. Similarly, use of below-knee callipers

Key point

Early involvement of a podiatrist for biomechanical assessment and provision of orthoses is an important component of the multidisciplinary management of RA. Consultation with a podiatrist is usually also an excellent opportunity for the patient to receive general advice about the use of appropriate and supportive footwear, and about other aspects of foot care.

and orthoses to immobilise the subtalar joint whilst allowing flexion at the ankle joint is still sometimes used for intractable ankle pain prior to surgery.

The metatarsophalangeal joints are frequently the first joints affected in RA, but despite this the symptoms and signs of MTP involvement are often overlooked.

Prevention of pressure areas is essential as, apart from being focal areas of pain and functional impairment, they may also serve as a portal of entry for infection.

OTHER AUTOIMMUNE POLYARTHROPATHIES

Although rheumatoid arthritis is the most common type of autoimmune rheumatic disease, there are several other members of this family of disorders. Overall, a wide variety of often-overlapping disease features are found, reflecting the fact that many different tissues and organs can be affected in these conditions.

The diverse array of clinical features is to some extent paralleled by the different types of autoantibodies present in patients' sera. Broadly speaking, different sets of clinical features can to some extent be matched to different profiles of autoantibodies, and this provides a framework for identifying distinct *diagnostic groups*. The family of autoimmune polyarthropathies includes Sjögren's syndrome, systemic lupus erythematosus (SLE), the vasculitides, scleroderma, dermatomyositis, and polymyositis. The main features are listed in Table 10.3.

All the autoimmune polyarthropathies typically undergo a course of exacerbations and remissions, associated with varying degrees of chronic inflammation, tissue damage and repair. In some instances factors which induce disease exacerbation can be identified – for example exposure to sunlight or certain medications in SLE – but in most circumstances the course is unpredictable. Occasionally, clinical deterioration in SLE, vasculitis and other conditions can be very rapid, and although such situations thankfully

Table 10.3 Clinical features and associated autoantibodies in autoimmune rheumatic diseases.

	Clinical feature	Associated autoantibodies
Sjögren's syndrome	Dry eyes Dry mouth Fatigue Fever Lymphadenopathy Raynaud's phenomenon Organ-specific autoimmune disease Arthralgia/arthritis Pulmonary disease Liver disease Renal disease	Rheumatoid factor Ro, La
SLE	Malar rash[a] Photosensitivity Oral ulcers Alopecia Serositis Arthritis Renal disease Neuropathy	Antinuclear DNA binding Sm
Antiphospholipid syndrome	Venous or arterial occlusion Recurrent fetal loss Livedo reticularis[b] Thrombocytopenia[c]	Anticardiolipin
Systemic vasculitis	Myalgia Arthralgia Purpura[d] Skin ulcers Sinusitis Dyspnoea Chest pain Gastrointestinal upset Neuropathy	Antineutrophil cytoplasmic Cryoglobulins
Scleroderma	Raynaud's phenomenon Telangiectasia[e] Skin thickening Calcinosis Oesophageal stricture Small bowel malabsorption Pulmonary hypertension	Anticentromere
Polymyositis/dermatomyositis	Proximal muscle weakness Muscle tenderness Skin rash Arthritis Pulmonary fibrosis Cardiac conduction defects Disturbed gastrointestinal motility	Jo1

SLE, systemic lupus erythromatus.
[a] Rash over the cheeks which may be butterfly-shaped.
[b] Mottling of the skin.
[c] Low platelet count.
[d] Purplish discolorations in the skin produced by small bleeding vessels.
[e] Persistently dilated blood capillaries.

occur relatively rarely it is nevertheless important to appreciate that they can be life-threatening and that deterioration may require urgent medical attention.

Broadly, the management of these conditions is based on principles similar to those applied to the management of RA. Non-pharmacological, as well as pharmacological, therapies have an important role. Traditionally, a wide range of medications and treatment protocols have been used in an attempt to achieve immunosuppression and disease remission. As is also the case for RA, recent identification of specific molecular targets in several of these conditions is currently leading to the development of an increasing number of novel biological therapies, several of which are already at the stage of clinical trial and evaluation.

It is normally the case that the diagnosis and management of these conditions should be based on a multispecialist as well as multidisciplinary approach, and effective communication within and across healthcare sectors is essential. It is particularly important, therefore, that all healthcare professionals involved should work to ensure optimal planning, coordination and delivery of care to people with these complex diseases. This applies not only in the context of therapeutic interventions, both pharmacological and non-pharmacological, but also to the important aspects of education, advice and counselling.

THE SPONDYLOARTHROPATHIES

The group of conditions called *spondyloarthropathies* were at one time thought to be related to RA, but the recognition of characteristic features of spinal involvement and the presence and pathogenic role of enthesopathy (inflammation at the site of tendon or ligament insertion) allowed the recognition of this as a distinct group of rheumatic diseases. The different types of spondyloarthropathy share particular clinical, epidemiological and genetic features, including associations with HLA B27, which is one of the genes known to be involved in the pathogenesis of these conditions.

The typical pathological feature for this group of conditions is enthesopathy. The enthesis is the site of tendon, ligament or capsule attachment into bone. The underlying lesion is a focal non-specific chronic inflammation. The cartilaginous layer of the enthesis and adjacent bone are destroyed and replaced by granulation tissue. Enthesopathy is followed by new bone formation and may subsequently lead to ankylosis (fusion) of the joint.

In the spine, changes at the insertion of the outer fibres of annulus fibrosus to the anterior and lateral margins of the vertebral body result in squaring of vertebral bodies, vertebral endplate destruction and syn-

desmophyte formation (Figure 10.1). These changes can be demonstrated on X-ray (Figure 10.2). Syndesmophytes that completely bridge the vertebral disc eventually form the so-called bamboo spine. These changes may take many years to develop.

The *spondyloarthropathies*
The major recognised types of spondyloarthropathy are ankylosing spondylitis (AS), reactive arthritis (ReA) and psoriatic arthritis. The last two are discussed later in this chapter.

ANKYLOSING SPONDYLITIS

Symptoms of AS

The symptoms of AS usually develop in adolescence or early adult life. Although the usual age of presentation is the late teens or early twenties, juvenile onset can occur. The principal symptoms are low back pain and stiffness, and the presence of stiffness often helps to distinguish AS from other causes of low back pain, such

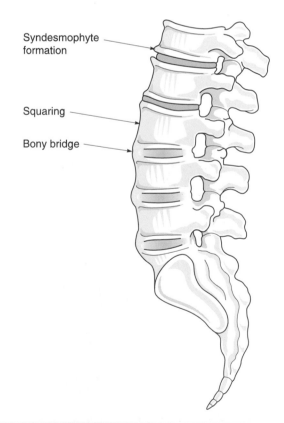

Syndesmophyte formation

Squaring

Bony bridge

Figure 10.1   Spinal involvement in ankylosing spondylitis. (Adapted from David and Lloyd 1998, with permission.)

as vertebral collapse or nerve root inflammation. One or more peripheral joints are often also involved.

Key point

Although previously thought to be more common in males, AS has undoubtedly been frequently under-diagnosed in females. Early reports of AS suggested a male/female ratio of 10:1 but more recent studies have suggested a ratio of 2.5:1. Females may have milder disease with more peripheral joint involvement.

The diagnosis of AS should always be considered in a young person presenting with low back pain, buttock pain or occasionally dorsal and chest wall pain. Stiffness is likely to be present in the morning and symptoms are made worse by inactivity and usually improved with exercises. There is often a delay in making the diagnosis, which may be due to the intermittent nature of symptoms and a lack of radiological changes.

Characteristically, involvement of the sacroiliac joints is primarily responsible for the symptoms of low back pain and stiffness. Typical sites of enthesis involvement are at the Achilles tendon, the plantar aspect of the heel, the chest wall and the pelvis. Peripheral joint involvement can be a presenting feature in about 15%, and will occur at some stage in up to 35% of people with AS. Systemic features such as pyrexia, fatigue, weight loss or anaemia should increase the suspicion for a diagnosis of AS in a young person with back pain.

Most of the extra-articular features (Table 10.4) occur in the later stages of the disease, although acute anterior uveitis presenting as a painful red eye may occur at any stage.

Genetic Susceptibility to AS

Clinical observations of familial clustering of AS and related conditions, including inflammatory bowel disease, which were subsequently confirmed in twin studies and other family studies, have shown clearly that genetic factors have an important role in AS pathogenesis.

The first, and probably the most important, gene which was found to be involved is located within the HLA class I region on the short arm of chromosome 6. As is the case for many other genes within the HLA region, the HLA B gene is remarkably polymorphic and exists in many different allelic forms within the population. The HLA B27 allele is strongly linked to ankylosing spondylitis; for example, among caucasians with AS over 95% possess this allele whereas it is found in only about 6% of the population as whole. Furthermore, the prevalence of AS in different countries broadly reflects the prevalence of HLA B27 within the population.

The fact that HLA B27 is present in such a large proportion of AS patients has led to extensive molecular and epidemiological research in an attempt to elucidate the underlying mechanisms. It is important to appreciate, however, that other genes besides B27 are likely to be involved in ankylosing spondylitis, and that most people with the B27 gene do not develop the disease. For example, HLA B27-positive relatives of HLA B27-positive AS patients are about twenty times more likely to develop AS than HLA B27-positive relatives of healthy B27-positive subjects. In other words, the B27 gene is clearly an important factor for susceptibility to AS, but other factors, both genetic and environmental, have an important role in the pathogenesis.

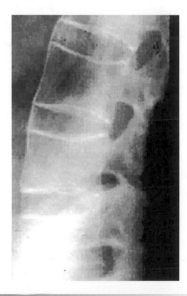

Figure 10.2   The lumbar spine in ankylosing spondylitis. Note the formation of syndesmophytes along the anterior margin of the spine.

Table 10.4 Modified New York criteria for the diagnosis of ankylosing spondylitis (1984).

1. Low back pain for at least 3 months, improved by exercise and not relieved by rest

2. Limitation of lumbar spine movement in sagittal and frontal planes

3. Chest expansion decreased relative to normal values for age and sex

4. Bilateral sacroiliitis, grade 2–4

5. Unilateral sacroiliitis, grade 3–4

The mechanisms whereby B27 determines susceptibility to AS remain unknown. There continues to be much interest in the possibility that this may be linked to the normal biological role of B27-encoded molecules, namely, in selecting and binding short peptide fragments from among the pool of intracellular self-proteins or microbial antigens, transporting them to cell surfaces and presenting them to T lymphocytes. This process is fundamentally important in the development and regulation of the immune system and in protective immune responses. Several hypotheses have been proposed to explain how this might lead to disease, including the possibility that B27 molecules might be more likely than others to present microbial peptides which are sufficiently similar to self peptides so as to evoke autoimmune responses by a mechanism termed 'molecular mimicry'. Furthermore, recent work demonstrating the propensity of B27 molecules to bind each other, and for these complexes to be expressed on cell surfaces for recognition by T lymphocytes, has raised further possibilities regarding AS disease mechanisms.

Key point

HLA B27 is also linked with the other types of spondyloarthropathy described later in this chapter, although less strongly than with AS. The associations seem generally stronger when applied to hospital-based, rather than population-based, populations, raising the possibility that the predominant effect of B27 may be on the severity of these conditions.

Establishing the Diagnosis of AS

The diagnosis is usually made primarily on clinical grounds, and clinical criteria can also be used to compare different series of patients. The only laboratory tests of use are those which measure inflammatory markers, such as the ESR or serum C-reactive protein (CRP) concentrations. Tissue typing for HLA B27 is not helpful in the routine diagnosis of AS because of the high prevalence of this gene in the population.

The earliest radiological changes may take years to develop and usually manifest as blurring of the margins of the sacroiliac joints. This may be followed by the development of sclerosis, which may be accompanied by characteristic radiological appearances of fusion of the spine due to calcification in chronically inflamed spinal joints and ligaments. Syndesmophytes (Figures 10.1 and 10.2) are the gradual ossification of the superficial layers of the annulus fibrosus following inflammation and reactive sclerosis. Destructive osteitis and repair leads to squaring of the vertebral body. Early changes may be difficult to diagnose, although further information may be obtained from isotope bone scanning or an MRI scan.

Clinical Assessment and Monitoring of AS

Assessment

Involvement of the sacroiliac joints is assessed by stressing these joints by pressure applied over the sacrum or by cross compression of the pelvis. These manoeuvres may result in pain or discomfort in the presence of active sacroiliitis. The loss of normal lumbar lordosis, with flattening of the lumbar spine in forward flexion, is the earliest clinical sign of lumbar spine involvement. Gradually, lumbar spinal movements may become restricted in all planes.

The most commonly used assessment in the clinic is the modified Schober test. A 10 cm line is drawn upwards from the L5–S1 junction (at the dimples of Venus) and the increase measured during flexion. In the normal spine an increase of 4 or 5 cm would usually be expected. Chest expansion, in the increase following full inspiration, is measured at the fourth intercostal space. Finger–floor distance is a measure of hip movement as well as spinal mobility, and hip involvement can be assessed by the standard methods of measuring ranges of movement, and monitored by measuring the intermalleolar distance. Neck movement is assessed by measuring the tragus to wall distance and rotation of the cervical spine.

Modified Schober test

See Chapter 12 on the physiotherapy management of ankylosing spondylitis for illustrations of how to perform this test.

In the later stages of the disease an abnormal posture with thoracic kyphosis and a flexion deformity of the neck may develop if early treatment has been ineffective. This is now much less common than previously due to the improvements in early diagnosis, active physiotherapy and appropriate use of medication.

Monitoring

Regular formal assessments, on at least an annual basis, are useful to monitor treatment and to determine progression or improvement of the condition. Assessments of spinal mobility, chest expansion, involvement of peripheral joints and entheses should be recorded. Several validated and convenient methods of assessment of disease activity and status in AS are now available for use in both healthcare and research settings. In addition, assessments of the severity of nocturnal pain and morning stiffness may also serve as useful measures of disease status. Overall disability can also be monitored using scoring systems such as the Bath AS Functional Index and the Health Assessment Questionnaire (HAQ).

Course of the disease

The course of AS is very variable. Some patients continue with the typical inflammatory features over decades whilst others develop a rigid spine within 10 years. The typical progression is of slowly ascending pain and stiffness with periods of remission and relapse.

The development of spinal pain with movement, eased by rest, suggests the possibility of a mechanical problem such as a spinal fracture through a syndesmophyte, or a destructive lesion of an intervertebral disc. Another possibility would be a mobile segment, which occurs where there is fusion above and below and unfused area such that movement can occur, resulting in pain This is an indication for rest and immobilisation. Spinal osteoporosis, stenosis and cauda equina syndrome are other late spinal complications of AS. The other recognised systemic complications (Table 10.5) are relatively rare but should be borne in mind if a person with AS becomes generally unwell.

Clinical Management of AS

Non-pharmacological treatments

It is now well recognised and widely accepted that the single most important aspect of clinical management

Table 10.5 Common extra-articular features of ankylosing spondylitis.

Ocular	Uveitis
	Conjunctivitis
	Synechiae[a]
	Glaucoma
Pulmonary	Upper lobe fibrosis
	Cavitation
	Aspergillosis
Cardiovascular	Aortic regurgitation
	Conduction defects
Neurological	Nerve root or cord compression
Systemic	Amyloidosis

[a] Adhesions particularly between the iris and the cornea or lens of the eye

of this condition is the practice of a clearly specified programme of regular exercises aimed at preventing the disastrous loss of spinal mobility that used to occur and which is still depicted in many medical textbooks. The potentially catastrophic and irreversible consequences of spinal immobility should be emphasised repeatedly to the patient. Some people have relatively little difficulty in undertaking a regular exercise programme and, following initial instruction and discussion, are able to incorporate such a programme satisfactorily into their domestic, work and social commitments. Others prefer to conduct an exercise programme as part of a group activity, an approach that can provide valuable additional benefits in terms of support and maintenance of morale. Self-help groups are facilitated and supported nationally by the National Ankylosing Spondylitis Society (NASS). Hydrotherapy and swimming are invaluable adjuncts to other exercise programmes.

Key point

If exercises are perceived to make a patient worse, particularly in the later stages, then investigations for a fracture or mobile segment should be undertaken and the exercise programme stopped whilst this is done.

Individual assessment and advice with regard to pain management and activities of daily living, such as driving, are also a very important part of management and health professionals often play a particularly key role in these aspects.

The use of prismatic spectacles for patients with severe upper spinal deformities can often be extremely beneficial. Spinal orthoses are not routinely used but may sometimes have a place in preventing increasing spinal deformity, and in particular to support the chin where there is a flexion deformity of the neck.

Pharmacological treatments

Many people with AS find analgesics or non-steroidal inflammatory drugs (NSAIDs) useful, particularly at times when the inflammation is active. The main aim of using these medications is to obtain relief of nocturnal pain and morning stiffness and thereby to enable the patient to undertake an exercise regimen in the morning. They are therefore usually prescribed for the evening to obtain maximum benefit in the early morning, and their use may be intermittent depending upon the pattern of symptoms.

The benefits of these medications in terms of symptom relief have to be weighed against the potential for side-effects, and their use should be monitored carefully to avoid inappropriate continual or habitual use.

Disease-modifying antirheumatic drugs (DMARDs)

These are rarely used in AS. Sulphasalazine is occasionally added to an NSAID, although most benefit is seen in the peripheral joint features rather than the spinal disease.

Biological therapy

Recent clinical trials of the biological therapy anti-TNFα in AS have reported extremely promising results, and significant benefits have also been found in the other spondyloarthropathies. It may well be that the use of anti-TNFα, and perhaps other biological therapies, in the treatment of these conditions will become increasingly established over the next few years.

Surgery

The indications for joint replacement are similar to those for patients with rheumatoid arthritis. Hip or knee joint replacement is an appropriate intervention in situations in which joint destruction is severe. Hip involvement is common in severe AS, particularly when the disease starts in early teenage life. Hip replacement, even at an early age, may dramatically reduce pain, improve mobility and improve the postural abnormalities that develop from fixed flexion deformities of the hip.

Osteotomy of the dorsal spine for severe kyphosis is sometimes considered in specialised spinal units, and although atlanto-axial instability is less common than in RA, fusion may sometimes need to be considered, as is also the case for spinal decompression in patients with cauda equina syndrome.

REACTIVE ARTHRITIS

Definition
The term 'reactive arthritis' (ReA) is used to diagnose arthritis which follows a known microbial infection and in which the microbe itself cannot be isolated in viable form from the joints.

Pathogens

Reactive arthritis has been described following a large number of bacterial and viral infections, including for example *Streptococcus pyogenes* which can lead to a variety of sequelae including ReA or rheumatic fever.

However, among the wide range of microbes recognised as having arthritogenic potential in humans, some are known to lead to rheumatic sequelae which are very similar to the features of AS and the other spondyloarthropathies. This applies in particular to different types of intracellular enteric bacteria (*Campylobacter*, *Salmonella*, *Yersinia*, *Shigella*) which are common causes of acute enteritis, and to *Chlamydia* which is a common cause of urethritis. Infection with any of these microbes can lead to ReA, and the clinical features are very similar irrespective of the causal microbe.

Symptoms of ReA

Typically, the arthritis develops between one and three weeks following the episode of infection of the urogenital tract or bowel, although infection may be asymptomatic, particularly with *Chlamydia*. The clinical features of the reactive sequelae bear close similarities to AS, although often with a greater prominence of peripheral joint involvement and enthesopathy and less severe spinal features, although low back pain and stiffness is common. The peripheral arthritis is acute, and the knees are the most commonly involved joints.

Extra-articular features of ReA are common and include sterile conjunctivitis, mouth ulcers, ulcers of the glans penis (circinate balanitis) and keratoderma blenorrhagica, a skin rash similar to pustular psoriasis. Other features of systemic involvement may be similar to those of AS, particularly in people with persistent or chronic disease.

Diagnosis and Management of ReA

The diagnosis of ReA is made predominantly on the clinical history and examination. Patients usually present several weeks after the initial infection, and it is therefore relatively uncommon for the microbe to be cultured from stool or urethral cultures. Laboratory tests may reveal raised ESR and C-reactive protein (CRP) levels as non-specific markers of inflammation. Depending on the time of presentation, demonstration of a rise in titre of antibody levels to the inciting microbe may be feasible as a means of confirming the diagnosis.

Although the majority of patients improve over a period of up to 6 months, about 15–20% may get a recurrence in symptoms and signs, and in some people the arthritis becomes more severe over a period of 10–20 years, particularly in those who have the HLA B27 gene. The extent to which this depends upon repeated infections, either overt or subclinical, following the initial episode is unknown.

Treatment of ReA is aimed at relief of symptoms, involving the standard principles of joint protection, pain management, exercise, and appropriate use of NSAIDs and analgesics as needed. Sulphasalazine, methotrexate or azathioprine is sometimes used to treat severe, persistent joint inflammation. There is evidence to suggest that antibiotic therapy may enhance recovery in post-chlamydia ReA, but there is no evidence of a similar benefit of antibiotics in the treatment of post-enteric ReA.

PSORIATIC ARTHRITIS

It is well recognised that psoriasis can occur in association with rheumatic disease, and that the onset of joint problems can occur at any stage, before or after the onset of dermatological disease.

Patterns of Disease

Among the different patterns of joint disease that have been described in psoriasis, dactylitis, enthesopathy and sacroiliitis are commonly found in these groups.

The classical patterns of psoriatic arthropathy have been described as:

- arthritis of the distal interphalangeal joints
- arthritis mutilans
- symmetrical peripheral polyarthritis, similar to RA
- asymmetrical oligoarthritis
- spondyloarthropathy.

The pattern of arthritis in an individual patient may change over time from one group to another. Psoriatic nail changes occur in 40% of people with skin psoriasis and in 90% of those with arthritis. The skin and joint involvement often have no direct relationship, and in 15–20% of cases joint involvement precedes skin psoriasis. The skin involvement may be minimal and careful examination of the scalp, flexures and umbilicus may be required in order to reveal small patches of psoriasis.

X-rays may show erosions with osteolysis and the development of a 'pencil in cup' appearance seen characteristically in arthritis mutilans. Sternoclavicular and manubriosternal joints may also be involved, this being a recognised feature of the seronegative spondyloarthropathies.

Course and Management

The course of the arthritis is typically that of periodic relapses and remissions, but fewer than 5% of cases develop very severe deforming arthritis.

The principles of clinical assessment, treatment and management of these conditions are essentially the same as those described above for other types of chronic polyarthritis. Medical treatment involves the use of NSAIDs and disease-modifying drugs as appropriate, including sulphasalazine, methotrexate and cyclosporin A. Early clinical trials data suggests that biological therapies are likely to have a useful role in the treatment of psoriatic arthritis in the future. Surgery also has a place in management in ways similar to those that apply for patients with rheumatoid arthritis.

REFERENCE

David C, Lloyd J 1998 Rheumatological Physiotherapy, p. 100. Mosby: London.

FURTHER READING

Calin A, Taurog JD (eds) 1998 The Spondyloarthritides. Oxford University Press: Oxford

Firestein GS, Panayi GS, Wollheim FA (eds) 2000 Rheumatoid Arthritis: New Frontiers in Pathogenesis and Treatment. Oxford University Press: Oxford

Klippel JH, Dieppe PA (eds) 1997 Rheumatology, 2nd edn. Mosby: St Louis

Maddison PJ, Isenberg DA, Woo P, Glass DN (eds) 1998 Oxford Textbook of Rheumatology. Oxford University Press: Oxford

11

Osteoporosis

Kirsty Carne

Physiotherapists encounter osteoporosis in a wide range of clinical situations. This chapter provides important background physiology, aetiology, diagnostic procedures and other essential information that physiotherapists need to manage and treat this increasingly common condition effectively.

INTRODUCTION

Bone is an amazing tissue. It is a tissue that is alive with the unique ability to remodel itself. It can change its density and internal architecture accordingly as we exercise more or exercise less, as it is stressed by muscles and tendons, and as our diet and health status changes.

Osteoporosis is very closely linked with the natural ageing process of human beings, but until quite recent times very little has been done to recognise it as an actual disease process, and investigate ways of treating it. Examination of medieval skeletons from a site in England found evidence of very similar age-related bone loss at the femur (Mays et al. 1998), despite the huge differences in lifestyle between then and the way we live now. Populations are on the increase and we can now expect to live well into old age, unlike our medieval ancestors. We also expect to have a much better quality of life, and greater independence during our later years. This means that osteoporosis will be an enormous problem for the modern world, and has huge implications both in terms of personal suffering and the costs to health services of treating such a condition.

Definition

At the Consensus Development Conference for the World Health Organization (CDC 1991), osteoporosis was defined as 'a progressive skeletal disorder, characterised by low bone mass and microarchitectural deterioration of bone tissue, leading to a consequent increase in bone fragility, and susceptibility to fracture.

Brittle bone disease

Note that osteoporosis is not the same as brittle bone disease (osteogenesis imperfecta), which is a genetic condition. If you require more information about brittle bone disease, write to Brittle Bone Society, 30 Guthrie Street, Dundee DD1 5BS (telephone 01382 204446), or visit www.brittle-bone.org. There is a Freephone helpline on 08000 282459 – for advice only.

Throughout childhood and our early adult years, many different aspects of skeletal growth occur. Longitudinal growth of bone ceases and each individual's peak bone size is eventually achieved. During the end of a person's third decade of life the peak bone mineral density (BMD) is also realised. These factors combine to give our skeletons the dimensions, flexibility and strength that we require to be able to function as active human beings. Skeletal growth does not then cease altogether – bone is living tissue and needs to renew itself constantly to maintain an optimal level of health. It is this process of renewal or *bone turnover* that is the important factor in osteoporosis. The action of osteogenic cells, specifically osteoclasts and osteoblasts, is key to the potential maintenance or loss of BMD.

National Osteoporosis Society

[www.nos.org.uk]
For general enquiries: National Osteoporosis Society, Camerton, Bath BA2 0PJ
Telephone: 01761 471771

The National Osteoporosis Society (NOS) is based in the United Kingdom. It campaigns to ensure that all people with, or at risk of osteoporosis receive appropriate advice and treatment to enable them to avoid fractures and enjoy a better quality of life. The NOS provides information and support for people with osteoporosis and their carers by promoting education for the public and health professionals, by lobbying government and health organisations, and by encouraging fundraising for support services and research into osteoporosis prevention and treatment.

The society offers membership packages for both lay people and health professionals. There are quarterly magazines containing the latest information and research about osteoporosis. The society also provides a medical helpline service run by nurses who are specialists in osteoporosis for health professionals and lay members alike, whether they are members or not.

The society has a large network of patient support groups around the UK. These are run by volunteers and provide an opportunity for people with osteoporosis to get together and learn about other peoples' experiences, and to hear outside speakers on a number of topics.

The society produces a wide range of publications, ranging from information booklets about all aspects of the disease, to position statements for health professionals providing guidance on certain issues. The NOS is independent of any drug company, and all information is evidence-based.

PHYSIOLOGY OF BONE TURNOVER

The skeleton comprises two types of bone: cortical bone, and trabecular or cancellous bone.

- Cortical bone is found mainly in the shafts of long bones and the surfaces of flat bones. Approximately 80–90% of the skeleton is made up of cortical bone.
- Trabecular or cancellous bone forms the internal part of flat bones, and is also found at the ends of long bones.

These two types of bone are subject to different types of forces. Trabecular bone is designed mainly to resist compression, whereas cortical bone needs to withstand twisting and bending forces as well as compression. Bone turnover or remodelling occurs throughout the skeleton at random, scattered sites. The process of remodelling takes place on the surfaces of these different bone structures, which means that the rate of remodelling in trabecular bone is significantly higher than that of cortical bone because trabecular bone has a much greater surface area.

Osteoclasts are the bone cells that are responsible for *resorption* of bone. They position themselves on the bone surface at any selected site for remodelling and absorb the old bone, creating a cavity. Following a short interval the osteoblasts then position themselves in the newly formed cavity. These are the bone-forming cells and their main function is the formation and mineral-isation of osteoid, the protein component of bone. The osteoblasts are also responsible for the regulation of some of the growth factors that are found in the protein-based bone matrix, and it is because of this fact that the osteoblasts are the cells that are generally considered to govern bone metabolism.

Key point

Although a fair amount is known about the progress of these cells, what prompts the osteoclasts to move into position at the sites that need remodelling, and causes the osteoblasts to follow behind, is still largely unclear.

Both osteoclasts and osteoblasts, like many other cells in the body, have a reasonably short life. New ones are constantly being produced and the old ones die by a process called *apoptosis*. Oestrogens and bisphosphonates (a group of non-hormonal drugs used for the prevention and treatment of osteoporosis) can promote apoptosis in the osteoclasts and inhibit this process in osteoblasts. Glucocorticoids, however, can have the opposite effect; they inhibit apoptosis in the osteoclasts, and promote the death of the osteoblast cells (Weinstein and Manolagas 2000).

The process of bone remodelling is slow, and gets even slower as we age (Figure 11.1). One complete cycle

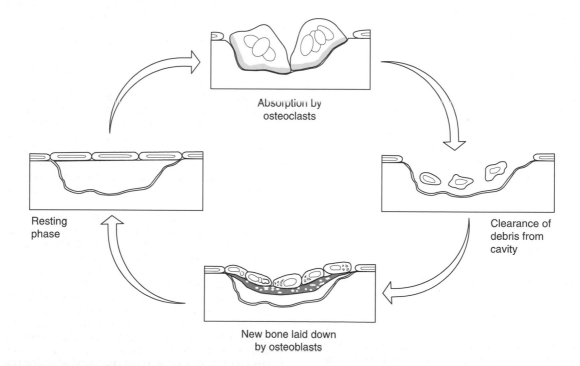

Absorption by osteoclasts

Clearance of debris from cavity

New bone laid down by osteoblasts

Resting phase

Figure 11.1   The cycle of bone turnover.

of turnover, including a resting phase, can take 3–6 months in an adult, and to replace the entire skeleton would take anything from 7 to 10 years; in children this can be completed in just 2–3 years. During this cycle any changes in bone shape and amount are barely noticeable. It is because this process is so slow that patients with osteoporosis are generally not monitored by scan more frequently than two-yearly (apart from in exceptional cases).

Ordinarily bone remodelling aims to replace exactly the same amount of bone as it takes away. When functioning correctly this is a balanced cycle (Figure 11.2a). It is when this cycle becomes unbalanced that problems occur. When the osteoclasts experience increased activity, or the osteoblasts have reduced activity, there will be a deficit in bone; more bone will be absorbed than made, leading to a loss of BMD and, potentially, osteoporosis (Figure 11.2b). As bone density decreases the structure of the bone starts to lose some of its rigidity and strength (Figure 11.3).

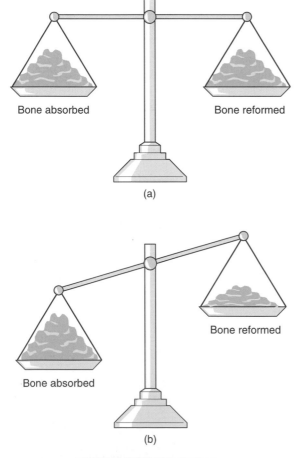

Figure 11.2   Bone remodelling: (a) normal – osteoblast activity matches osteoclast activity; (b) osteoporosis – osteoclast activity exceeds osteoblast activity.

Bone density is not the only component of bone strength. Other factors such as bone quality are equally important, but are very difficult to measure. As there is a strong inverse correlation between bone density and fracture risk, with a two- to three-fold increase in the incidence of fracture for each standard deviation reduction in BMD (see the later section on the diagnosis of osteoporosis) (Marshall et al. 1996), and BMD is measurable, it is the bone mineral density that is usually used to diagnose and monitor patients.

Loss of bone mineral density is heavily influenced by age. Studies looking at bone density levels during a lifetime period show that bone mass is steadily built up throughout childhood and the early adult years (Figure 11.4). Men achieve a higher peak bone mass than women because they generally have a larger bone structure, but both sexes achieve their peak and then maintain that level until their early to mid forties. After that point, natural age-related loss of BMD starts to occur, and this happens because the osteoclasts and osteoblasts are no longer working at quite the same rates. Several other factors such as oestrogen deficiency will also affect loss of BMD.

THE EXTENT OF THE PROBLEM

Osteoporosis is an enormous problem and has huge implications in terms of both personal suffering and the cost to the National Health Service. Osteoporosis is often referred to as a 'silent' condition. This is because having a low bone density is not a disorder that one can feel in any way. Many people do not know there is a problem until they sustain a fracture. This, combined with either a lack of awareness of the condition or a general assump-

Key point

One in three women and one in twelve men over the age of 50 will sustain a spine, hip or wrist fracture (Cooper 1999; Van Staa et al. 2001). A recent study has shown that this currently stands at around 310,000 fractures each year in the UK alone, which incurs a cost of £1.7 billion each year.

Key point

Across the world life expectancy is increasing. It is estimated that the number of people over the age of 65 will increase from the current figure of 323 million to 1555 million by the year 2050 (Cooper and Melton 1992). This will have massive implications for health services as the rates of age-related illnesses increase.

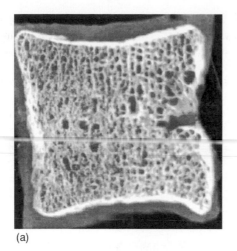

(a)

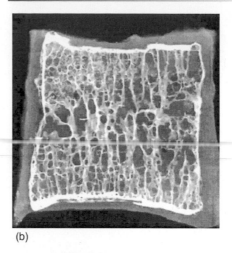

(b)

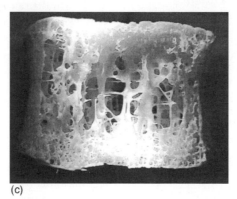

(c)

Figure 11.3   (a) Cross-section of a vertebra showing normal bone density. (b) Cross-section through an osteoporotic vertebra. (c) Lateral view of an osteoporotic vertebra.

tion that osteoporosis affects only elderly people, means that prevention is a huge challenge, and at present we may only be tackling the tip of the iceberg.

AN ANALYSIS OF RISK FACTORS

Refer to Table 11.1.

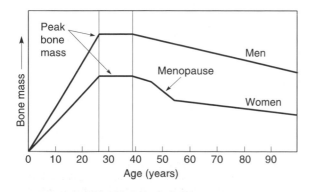

Figure 11.4   Bone mass throughout life.

Age

Many factors combine with ageing to contribute to the increasing rates of osteoporosis and associated fractures around the world. Factors directly linked to older age – such as reduced mobility and increased risk of falling – have a direct impact on the number of hip fractures. The increase in incidences of hip fracture correlates directly with increasing age, and for women from the age of 50 the risk is approximately twice that in men.

Lifestyle

New technology leading to changes in lifestyle – such as the invention of the motor car – mean that people no longer walk very far and often get very little physical exercise. Westernised diets with a heavy emphasis on convenience foods have had an enormous impact on the incidence of osteoporosis. This has led to less healthy diets, with people often not achieving recommended calcium levels for healthy bone, alongside other issues such as the consumption of fat, which

Table 11.1 Major osteoporosis risk factors in men and women.

Risk factors for women
Lack of oestrogen, caused by:

- early menopause (before the age of 45)
- early hysterectomy (before the age of 45), particularly when both ovaries are removed by oophrectomy
- missing periods for six months or more (excluding pregnancy) as a result of over-exercising or over-dieting

Risk factors for men

- Low levels of testosterone (hypogonadism)

Risk factors for men and women

- Long-term use of high-dose corticosteroid tablets (for conditions such as rheumatoid arthritis and asthma)
- Close family history of osteoporosis (maternal or paternal), particularly with history of a maternal hip fracture
- Medical conditions such as Cushing's syndrome, liver and thyroid problems
- Malabsorption problems (coeliac disease, Crohn's disease, intestinal diseases or gastric surgery
- Long-term immobility
- Heavy alcohol consumption and smoking
- Poor diet
- Low bodyweight in proportion to height

brings about more health problems. Other elements of advanced technology – such as the increasing numbers of women who have oophorectomies (removal of the ovaries), often at the time of a hysterectomy leaving them with reduced natural levels of oestrogen – increases the number of postmenopausal women who are at risk of low bone density.

Key point

There is some evidence to suggest that people are gradually growing taller when information from the last century is studied. This leads to an increase in the length of the hip axis, which may again increase a person's risk of hip fracture (Dennison and Cooper 2001).

Hormonal Changes

Loss of oestrogen

Women run a much higher risk of developing osteoporosis than do men. Not only is their peak bone density lower, but bone loss is faster owing to a decrease in the level of the hormone oestrogen. As women go through their menopause they suddenly experience a much more dramatic rate of loss of their BMD of approximately 4% in the 5–10 years after the menopause. This then slows to a more gradual rate of loss similar to that of men of approximately 1% per year (Cummings et al. 1985).

Oestrogen is known to have some 'protective' effect on bone, but exactly what that role is remains unclear. It is thought that the osteoclast and osteoblast cells may contain oestrogen receptors, although only at a very low concentration. This means that a change in oestrogen level will affect the rate of bone remodelling. A low oestrogen level results in loss of BMD or has a detrimental effect on peak bone mass obtained, through increased osteoclast activity, and simply through an increase in the rate of bone turnover.

A woman's life expectancy in the UK is 80 years, meaning many women may well spend 30 or more years of their life in a postmenopausal state with a depleted oestrogen level. In view of the fact that life expectancy is increasing, this figure is set to rise dramatically. This, combined with natural age-related loss which is also continuing for longer, could obviously have a very negative effect on bone density.

Increasing numbers of women will also find themselves experiencing premature ovarian failure for reasons other than a natural menopause. For some women, having a hysterectomy even without oophrectomy can induce spontaneous ovarian failure, and as treatments for other medical conditions such as chemotherapy and radiotherapy for cancers advance women can again experience premature ovarian failure.

Younger women, and even young girls, may also be at risk. The media bombards us with images of the stereotypical 'perfect' woman who is incredibly thin, and many women and young girls are finding themselves under pressure to conform to this ideal. Eating disorders such as anorexia nervosa and bulimia can in severe cases not only leave the sufferer malnourished in terms of minerals such as calcium, but can also lead to a decline in body function and production of hormones such as oestrogen – causing menstruation to cease. Over-exercising can also have this effect (Keay et al. 1997).

It is believed that the low energy availability caused by too little dietary energy intake in comparison to the energy used affects the hypothalamus, pituitary and thyroid glands and the amount of the hormones they produce. Amenorrhoea (absence of periods) for 6 months or more may have long-term implications for a woman's BMD, particularly if this is occurring during her younger years whilst she is still building her bone density.

Male osteoporosis

The single osteoporosis risk factor that is particular to men is hypogonadism, or low levels of the hormone testosterone. This can occur for a number of reasons, such as disorders of the testes or pituitary gland, damage to or removal of the testes, chemotherapy and radiotherapy, and alcohol abuse (Figure 11.5).

Why hypogonadism causes loss of bone mineral density is not entirely clear. It is believed that testosterone has a direct effect on BMD acting on the androgen receptors in osteoblasts, therefore influencing the remodelling of bone. It is also thought that oestrogen has an influence here. As already mentioned, osteoclasts and osteoblasts are known to be receptive to oestrogen. A small amount of testosterone in men is converted into oestrogen naturally. Therefore oestrogen deficiency may well be a contributory factor in male osteoporosis (Riggs et al. 1998; Center et al. 1999).

Although osteoporosis is far more common in women than in men, male osteoporosis should not be ignored. About 30% of all hip fractures are in men. In 1990 there were 1.66 million hip fractures worldwide, a figure expected to increase to 6.26 million by 2050 (Cooper et al. 1992; Gullberg et al. 1997), so the problem is going to increase. It has also been suggested that vertebral deformity in older men may be as common as it is in women, with a more severe degree of deformity (O'Neill et al. 1993).

> **Note**
>
> All of the remaining risk factors to be considered in this chapter apply to both men and women.

Corticosteroid Use

The influence of corticosteroid treatments on a person's bone density can be dramatic. Corticosteroids interfere with the natural lifespan of the osteogenic cells. They shorten the life of the osteoblasts and lengthen the life of the osteoblasts, which then means that the remodelling process becomes unbalanced with more bone being resorbed than built – causing a loss in BMD. Corticosteroids can also slow the rate of remodelling generally.

Moderate to high doses of oral corticosteroids taken long term will affect a person's bone density. It is also now becoming clear that other methods of administering corticosteroids, such as by means of inhalers, can still cause bone density loss (Israel et al. 2001), although this does seem to be related to dose and duration of treatment. The comparative effect of different methods of corticosteroid delivery is difficult to measure as many patients who use inhalers, for example, may have periods of more severe illness that require short durations of oral medication. Obviously most people are prescribed this sort of treatment for major illnesses or conditions that could be life-threatening, so to not take them is not for them an option. However, in view of the fact that about 40% of patients on corticosteroid treatments that are high dose or long term may experience fractures, it is important that the professionals managing such cases should be aware of the risk.

Genetics

Osteoporosis is a hereditary condition. As much as 75% of the population variance in BMD amongst age- and sex-matched individuals can be attributed to genetic or inherited factors (Gueguen et al. 1995). A woman with a family history of maternal hip fracture has nearly double the risk of developing a hip fracture herself (Cummings et al. 1995).

Many women follow the same pattern as their mother with the timing of their menopause. This means that early menopause, a risk factor for osteoporosis, can possibly run in families. Also other factors such as a small body frame can be inherited from one's parents. This is known to be a contributory risk factor for developing osteoporosis. Since these factors cannot be changed, awareness of osteoporosis is crucial to enable people to modify their lifestyle.

Other Medical Conditions

Conditions such as coeliac disease, Crohn's disease and those requiring major gastric surgery will have important implications for the person's ability to absorb essential minerals and vitamins from food. Without nutrients our bodies do not continue to function at an optimum level. Without general good health and the correct amounts of calcium and vitamin D, alongside other minerals such as magnesium and boron, our

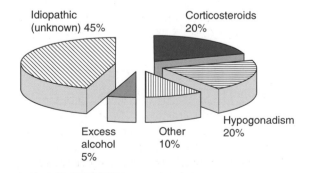

Idiopathic (unknown) 45%
Corticosteroids 20%
Excess alcohol 5%
Other 10%
Hypogonadism 20%

Figure 11.5   Causes of male osteoporosis.

bones will no longer be able to remain healthy and maintain BMD by balanced remodelling.

Disorders of the thyroid and parathyroid glands are also quite common, and can lead to a low bone density. The thyroid gland in the neck produces thyroid hormone (thyroxine) which is responsible for controlling many of the bodily functions. Hyperthyroidism occurs when the thyroid gland becomes overactive, and the excess of thyroxine that is produced causes the rate of remodelling and loss of BMD to increase. Hypothyroidism (underactive thyroid) is not a risk factor for osteoporosis unless the thyroxine medication that is given as replacement is not monitored to prevent the level becoming too high.

Hyperparathyroidism is another condition that impacts upon bone health. The parathyroid glands are situated in the neck just behind the thyroid gland. Parathyroid hormone produced by the parathyroid gland has an important role in regulating the level of calcium in the blood. If the blood calcium falls too low, then the parathyroid gland increases the level of parathyroid hormone. This then releases calcium from the bones and also allows the gut to absorb more calcium from the food, which in turn then increases the blood calcium level again. People suffering from hyperparathyroidism are producing too much parathyroid hormone and are therefore continually leaching calcium from their bones.

Diseases or disorders of the liver have an impact on bone density. The liver is responsible for filtering and processing digestive products, neutralizing toxins, secreting bile, and many other metabolic processes. If the liver becomes diseased or damaged in any way it will not be able to perform these functions properly, which in turn has a negative effect on bone density as the body is not receiving the correct amounts of nutrients or metabolism is increased greatly.

Immobility

This has particular relevance to physiotherapists. People become immobile for many reasons, some temporary and some permanent. When the body is no longer exercised in any way bone density decreases. Bone health is maintained partly by the regular stresses and load-bearing that it was designed to receive. Studies in astronauts and the effect of weightlessness of bone density have shown that approximately 1% of the skeleton is lost during each month spent in a zero-gravity environment (Holick 1998). Studies into the effect of acute immobilisation have suggested a bone loss of 1% per week, although this tended to stabilise after 6 months. Remobilisation can cause the bone density to improve again, but obviously some people are permanently unable to mobilise and are then at a very high risk of fracture, particularly if they have a fall.

Smoking and Alcohol Consumption

Smoking is believed to cause reduced bone mineral density by increasing bone resorption. This is possibly due to a reduction in the production, and acceleration of the degradation, of oestrogen. Excessive amounts of alcohol, too, cause a reduction in BMD, but this time through decreased bone formation.

Key point

Studies in this area are limited, but many have linked both smoking and heavy drinking with increased risk of fracture.

Apart from the obvious detrimental effects to health in general, smoking is also associated with premature menopause. Overton and Davies (1999) reported that women who smoke tend to have their menopause approximately two years earlier than they would have done otherwise. This means that female smokers experience two extra years of depleted oestrogen levels, which is associated with a reduction in BMD.

Smoking and excessive alcohol consumption will also affect a person's lifestyle. Smoking is known to be an appetite suppressant, and alcohol abuse often leads to a poor diet. This is associated with low nutrient intake, which contributes to poor health, and more specifically, poor bone health and loss of density.

Public awareness

Public awareness of the risk factors discussed in this section is an extremely important issue. If people are armed with the knowledge that they could be at risk of having low bone density, or of developing osteoporosis in the future, then they can seek advice, diagnosis and treatment from their doctor, and make changes towards a bone-healthy lifestyle to maximise the bone density that they have.

COMMON SITES OF FRACTURES RELATED TO OSTEOPOROSIS

The three most common sites of fracture for people with osteoporosis are:

- the wrist
- the spine
- the hip.

These parts of the skeleton are predominantly made up of cancellous bone. In Britain, fracture rates for women for hip, spine and distal forearm are 14%, 11% and 13% respectively: for men they are 3%, 2% and 2% (Dennison and Cooper 1996). This translates into over 70,000 hip fractures, 50,000 wrist fractures and 120,000 spinal fractures being seen by British doctors each year (Dolan et al. 1998, O'Neill et al. 2000, Reeve et al. 2002).

Wrist Fractures

Fractures of the distal forearm (Colles' fracture) tend to happen to women most commonly during the peri-menopausal period. In white women the incidence of Colles' fractures increases between the ages of 40 and 65, and then stabilises. In men, however, the incidence remains constant between the ages of 20 and 80. Wrist fractures are nearly always the consequence of falling onto an outstretched hand.

There is an increase of these fractures during the winter months, but this seems to be due to falls outside on icy ground rather than for any other reason. Wrist fractures do not continue to increase with age, and this is probably due to the fact that our neuromuscular coordination decreases with age, so we are less likely to put out a hand to break a fall as we get older, and land straight on to the hip instead.

Spinal Fractures

It is believed that only one-third of people with spinal fractures caused by osteoporosis come to medical attention (Cooper et al. 1993). Therefore the estimated figures of these fractures are much lower than the number of fractures in reality.

Fractures of the vertebrae can happen spontaneously and silently (no symptoms), often leaving the victim unaware of their presence until they discover that they have been gradually losing height or developing a kyphosis and wonder what has caused it. Alternatively they can occur very obviously when a person makes a specific movement, or has a fall, in which case the injury may cause intense pain.

The vertebrae that are most commonly involved tend to correspond with the weakest regions in the spine: T8, T12 and L1. With the loss of strength caused by reduced bone mineral density the vertebrae crush down into themselves. Although the bones still heal, they are unable to reform their original cubic shape and they remain in a shortened, squashed shape – causing the spine to shorten. They can also fracture irregularly to form a wedge shape, and these fractures are the cause of a kyphosis. They are often referred to as 'crush' and 'wedge' fractures (Figure 11.6).

Unlike wrist fractures, spinal fractures do seem to increase with age, particularly in women. True figures, however, are very difficult to obtain as so few of these fractures are actually reported. Firstly, as already stated, many are silent and are simply not known about. Secondly, there is nothing that can be done other than pain relief for these fractures, so many people who have experienced one do not seek medical attention for any further fractures. Studies have shown that once a person has experienced one such vertebral deformity, they are then 7–10 times more at risk of suffering further deformities.

Hip Fractures

Key point
In 1990 there were an estimated 1.66 million hip fractures worldwide. As long ago as 1993, hip fractures accounted for over 20% of orthopaedic bed occupancy in the United Kingdom (Cryer et al. 1993). Hip fractures are significantly more common in women than in men, and they are specifically associated with the very elderly.

Although hip fractures tend to happen much later in life than wrist or spinal fractures they represent the most serious consequence of osteoporosis. They are associated with considerable mortality and morbidity (subsequent illness/complications) (Cooper et al. 1993). A study by Baudoin and colleagues in 1996 showed that hip fractures are associated with a 20% mortality rate within the first year, and there is also the greater risk of functional impairment and institutionalisation. Hip fractures may require surgery or hospitalisation, and all require a long period of recovery and rehabilitation. Physiotherapists play a key role in rehabilitating people after femoral neck fractures.

Hip fractures most commonly occur following a fall from standing height. It is also not unusual for people to say that they heard the bone break before the fall, indicating that the fracture caused the fall, and not the fall the fracture. The risk of falls also increases with age. Reduced neuromuscular coordination, reduced muscle tone, strength and balance, poorer eyesight, and general increased frailty all combine to increase the likelihood of someone falling.

Other types of fracture
The three types of fracture considered in this section, although the most common, are not the only fractures that can occur in someone with osteoporosis. The disease can affect any bone anywhere in the skeleton, so fractures at other sites are possible.

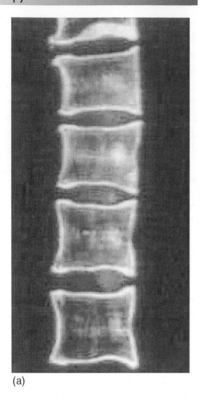
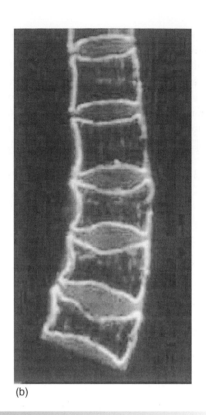

(a)   (b)

Figure 11.6   (a) Appearance of normal vertebrae on X-ray. (b) Osteoporotic vertebral column showing biconcave shape and compression fractures.

SYMPTOMS AND CLINICAL FEATURES

Silent Onset

Osteoporosis is a silent condition often giving no indication of its presence. One cannot feel changes in bone density, and without knowledge of the risk factors the first thing to alert the individual to a problem may be a fracture, by which point there has already been significant loss of bone mineral density. The fact that people do not suffer problems with pain in the early stages of the condition is a good thing, but the lack of any early warning signs often means ignorance of bone ill-health until osteoporosis is established with fractures occurring.

Having a low bone density per se does not cause pain. Although pain is very much a feature of osteoporosis, it does not generally occur until fractures happen. Obviously the pain from any recent fracture can be extremely acute for some people, often causing temporary immobility and requiring strong analgesia. For some people this pain then subsides as the fracture heals and they have no further problems. For others, permanent discomfort rising to intense, chronic pain can remain. The control of this pain then becomes the key clinical feature of that person's osteoporosis management.

Complications

Although the process of healing continues as normal in someone with osteoporosis, the fractures that people experience can then cause many associated problems as well as pain. Vertebral fractures are often the main culprit. Multiple vertebral fractures can eventually lead to kyphosis, a curvature of the top of the spine often referred to as a 'dowager's hump'. They can also cause considerable loss of height. These two factors combined can cause immense problems. A dramatic change in body image with enormous difficulty in finding clothes to fit has a huge psychological impact, causing social isolation and depression.

Spinal curvature and height loss lead in turn to reduced space for the internal organs. This tends to involve the lungs, stomach, bladder and bowel in particular. People can find themselves feeling more short of breath, as the lungs do not have the room to fill to capacity and expand properly. They will also feel easily full after small portions of food, and often lose their appetite, which can quickly lead to poor nutrition particularly in the elderly. Similarly people can find themselves needing to pass urine more frequently, and have trouble with bloating and bowel function as these organs also become squashed into a smaller space. As these organs struggle to function owing to the lack of room many people with osteoporosis develop a distended abdomen. The skeleton provides a vertical barrier confining the internal organs, so the only possible extra space to be found is by horizontal expansion at the lower abdominal area.

Investigations and Diagnosis

Osteoporosis is sometimes diagnosed purely on the strength of a persons' medical history, or even physical appearance. Plain X-rays are not particularly effective at highlighting osteoporosis, since bone loss must exceed 30–40% before it becomes visible (Johnston and Epstein 1981). Significant height loss, kyphosis, a history of low-trauma fractures and the presence of other risk factors may be enough for a doctor to diagnose osteoporosis in some patients.

Advanced technology has brought about sophisticated scanning methods that enable the measurement of bone density in people who are at high risk of the disease. Three types of scans are commonly used in the UK to examine BMD in detail:

- hip and spine dual-energy X-ray absorptiometry (DXA)
- peripheral DXA and single-energy X-ray absorptiometry (SXA)
- ultrasound.

The WHO scoring system

The World Health Organization has developed a definition of osteoporosis based on the scoring system of the DXA scan (which is discussed below). The system is now used to diagnose the condition more accurately.

These scores are expressed in 'standard deviations' (SDs) away from the normal range (Figure 11.7). The T-score, which compares the individual's BMD to that of the young adult mean, is the score that is used for diagnosis, monitoring and treatment decisions. The Z-score is where the individual's BMD is compared to the age-matched mean. This is helpful to assess the BMD of an older person.

DXA (dual-energy X-ray absorptiometry) scans

The hip and spine DXA scan

This is very much considered to be the 'gold standard' in osteoporosis scanning. For the patient it is a very simple procedure, and is low risk with the amount of radiation being approximately the same as that to which one might be exposed during a long-haul air flight. It is a quick procedure, taking only a few minutes.

The patient lies on the scanner's bed and does not even have to undress except to remove any metal items (Figure 11.8). The arm of the scanner then passes over the lower spine and non-dominant hip, producing the scan image and measurements on a screen in front of the radiographer. The scan result is sent to the radiologist for interpretation.

The peripheral scan

These are either DXA or SXA (single-energy X-ray absorptiometry). These may be performed on either the distal forearm or the calcaneus. Owing to the varying amounts of trabecular and cortical bone in these sites at different positions, these scans are not able to diagnose osteoporosis as easily as the hip and spine DXA.

Forearm scanning can use the same scoring system, if positioned correctly, and can either indicate a person's need for treatment (T-score at –2.5 SD) or indicate the need for a hip and spine DXA if the T-score is between –1 and –2.5 SD. The distal forearm is not sufficiently sensitive to be able to monitor changes in BMD with treatments and time (National Osteoporosis Society 2001). The calcaneus is a site that could potentially be used to monitor change, because unlike the distal forearm it is mainly trabecular bone. However, the threshold score of –2.5 SD is not applicable to the heel and adjustments to those scores need to be made. It is not yet clear whether those adjustments would be appropriate for different makes of scanners.

Ultrasound scans

These scans use the calcaneus. There is no ionising radiation involved in these scans, and the machines themselves are often easily portable (unlike the hip and spine DXA). They are also considerably cheaper than other scanners.

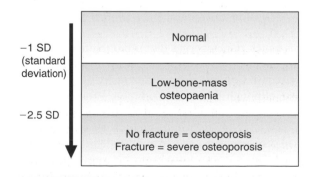

Figure 11.7   The WHO definition of T-scores (WHO 1994).

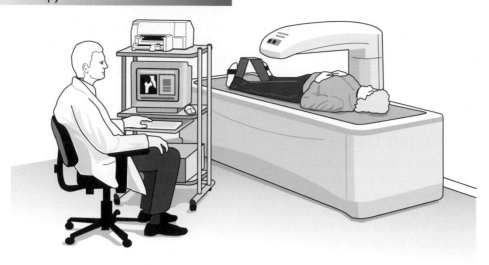

Figure 11.8   A bone density scan in progress.

Ultrasound cannot diagnose osteoporosis, as it does not measure bone mineral content or density directly. However, a low result from an ultrasound scan is recognised as an independent risk factor for future osteoporotic hip fracture. Ultrasound also cannot yet (in most cases) be used to monitor bone loss and response to treatment in an individual patient.

> **Key point**
>
> This method of scanning was designed to look at postmenopausal women, so its use in children, younger women and men is not recommended for clinical purposes.

Ultrasound scanners need to be operated by properly trained personnel in the right conditions to achieve accurate results.

Other methods of measuring bone density

It is worth remembering that other methods of scanning may be used to diagnose osteoporosis, directly or indirectly. Computerised tomography (CT) may be used, although this is not common. Plain X-rays are, however, very commonly used. Often a patient may go to have an X-ray to investigate back pain, or an unrelated problem, and a degree of bone density loss will be noted. This is not an entirely reliable way of diagnosing reduction in BMD as the development process of the X-ray film can sometimes give the appearance of low BMD, which is open to misinterpretation.

Urine testing to measure breakdown products (biochemical markers) produced during the bone remodelling process is being researched. Although this is currently available in some specialist centres, and even available in kit form (to be sent away for analysis) from supermarkets, it is not a process that has yet reached its full potential. In the future this could be a much cheaper and simpler form of monitoring a person's response to a treatment.

Methods of measuring bone density are evolving and changing with improvements in technology. It is very likely that more will be learnt about further uses of both ultrasound and DXA scanning techniques, and also the use of urine testing, making the diagnosis and monitoring of low bone density quicker, easier, cheaper and more widely available.

PREVENTATIVE MEASURES

Certain lifestyle factors, such as diet and exercise, have an influence on bone density and bone health in general. If positive population-wide lifestyle changes could be made to increase peak bone mass this would be a step in the right direction in reducing the incidence of osteoporosis.

Diet

Diet plays a major role in bone health. The protein component of bone, the osteoid, needs to be mineralised to give the bone its hardness and strength. The key mineral required in this process is calcium. Calcium is freely available in our diets with many rich food sources available.

The human body contains over a kilogram of calcium, almost all of which is in our skeleton; the remaining 1% is found in the blood stream and other body fluids. To maintain this level calcium-rich foods such as dairy products, green leafy vegetables, bony fish, cereal products and dried fruit, to name just a few, need to be included in the diet. Some people, however, are not able to achieve everything that they require from their diet alone and will use a calcium supplement to top this level up. The National Osteoporosis Society recommend that someone who has a diagnosis of osteoporosis, and is taking a treatment as well, may need to boost calcium intake to 1200 mg per day, and many people will find this amount difficult to achieve from dietary sources alone.

Calcium, however, is only one part of a bone-friendly diet. Humans need to have a healthy, balanced diet that includes all of the major food groups, to provide the essential vitamins and minerals, and the right balance of acid and alkali, required to function properly. A balanced diet should give more than adequate amounts of all the other nutrients that we require, such as boron, copper, zinc, magnesium, manganese, potassium, vitamins B6, C and K, and essential fatty acids.

Of course, there are also elements of our diet that can cause the potential deterioration of bone health. Several things can inhibit our natural ability to absorb calcium. These include caffeine, excess sodium (salt), excess protein and even phosphate, which is a preservative used in some carbonated (fizzy) drinks. There is also much scientific discussion over the possible detrimental effects of a diet that is too acidic or alkaline. The key to all of these issues is to have a balanced diet without excess.

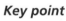

Key point

Diet is not merely an issue for adults. It is essential that children and young adults have a healthy, balanced diet too. It is during these early years that bone density is being built, and bone health is being firmly established. A good diet with all the important nutrients will ensure that person's peak bone mass is as high as possible.

Phytoestrogens are very weak plant oestrogens that are similar to one type of human oestrodiol. Isoflavones and ligans are types of phytoestrogens that are found in soya products, grains, cereals and linseed. These are becoming more interesting to scientists and researchers as it seems that populations who consume diets rich in these phytoestrogens have much lower rates of certain cancers and diseases such as osteoporosis. The use of these in the diet or in supplement form to prevent bone density loss, however, is still not proven and further research does need to be done.

Exercise

Exercise has two important roles in the prevention of fractures. Firstly it is shown to aid bone density, and secondly it tones and strengthens muscles, thereby ensuring good balance, coordination and skeletal support.

Bone is designed to bear certain stresses and loads, and appears to be at its healthiest when this functional 'use' is maintained (Lanyon 1996). A meta-analysis (overall review) of several studies looking into the effect of exercise on bone mass showed a prevention, or reversal, of bone loss of almost 1% per year (Wolff et al. 1999). However, studies looking at the effect of exercise are only relatively short term, so we do not know what the long-term effect will be. Increases in BMD may possibly plateau unless the intensity of exercise is continually increased, which is not really feasible. Maintenance of exercise will help maintenance of BMD.

Weight-bearing exercise is important when considering osteoporosis prevention. High-impact exercise such as jogging will target the hips and spine, and resistance exercises like weight lifting can target specific areas such as the wrist. Loading the skeleton with physical weights or bodyweight stimulates the osteogenic cells, giving rise to a maintenance or possible increase in BMD. A greater load provides greater stimulation. Bodyweight is multiplied during high-impact exercise (a jump where you leave the ground and then land again, compared to a step where a foot always remains on the floor for example), and this is why exercises such as jogging and aerobics have more effect than brisk walking.

Obviously exercise needs to be appropriate and safe, and high-impact exercise is not suitable for everyone. Many people are not used to doing any regular exercise and would need to start very gently and carefully. Something like walking may be appropriate despite the fact that it does not give as effective results on BMD, and something non-threatening like walking may well mean that person does some exercise instead of none at all, giving them other health benefits as well. Also many people will have other medical conditions to take into account, such as arthritis or ME, which may restrict any activity they can do.

People who have established osteoporosis with fractures and those who have very low bone density obviously need to approach exercise with care. Bone loading and impact exercises, and some stretches, such as an extreme forward flexion for example, could be dangerous for them by possibly causing further fractures. People in this situation need to do gentle muscle toning and strength building exercises instead.

Key point
There are still exercise groups that are safe for people like this to go to if they wish. Organisations such as Extend do classes involving movement to music for the over-60s, and for people with disabilities at any age.

The important features of these lifestyle factors is that they do not have to involve any major cost, and they can be done in the privacy of a person's own home. No major adjustment to a person's daily routine needs to be made, unless he or she chooses to join an exercise class or gym. They will, however, not only provide extra help for the health of a person's bones, they will also benefit overall general health and fitness too.

TREATMENT OF OSTEOPOROSIS

Drugs and Supplements

There are a wide variety of medications available for the prevention and treatment of osteoporosis, and fortunately further research and increased technology in pharmacology mean that new developments in the management of this disease are frequently occurring.

There are three commonly used types of medication for osteoporosis prevention and treatment in the UK. These are the bisphosphonates, hormone replacement therapy (HRT), and raloxifene (a selective oestrogen receptor modulator). The majority of people requiring treatment will be able to use one of these drugs, but some for various reasons will not. There are several other types of treatment available, which a specialist may consider.

The bisphosphonates

This is a family of non-hormonal drugs specifically for the prevention and treatment of osteoporosis. The three most common drugs within this family are alendronate (Fosamax), risedronate (Actonel) and etidronate (Didronel).

These drugs are antiresorptive, and work by directly inhibiting the osteoclasts, whilst allowing the osteoblasts to continue at their normal rate. They aim to slow or stop the loss of bone mineral density that is

occurring, and possibly encourage a slight increase. By doing this they reduce the person's risk of fracture.

The bisphosphonates have very strict instructions for their safe and effective administration. They must be taken on an empty stomach and must be accompanied by a glass of plain tap water. The various brands differ slightly in their instructions. Fosamax needs to be taken first thing in the morning, half an hour before the first food or drink of the day. Didronel can be taken at any time of day or night in the middle of a 4-hour fast, and Actonel can be taken by either method, but not at night. These drugs can be associated with a degree of gastric irritation so the instructions do need to be followed accurately.

The bisphosphonates are licensed for the prevention and treatment of osteoporosis in postmenopausal women. Fosamax is also licensed for use in men. They have been shown to be effective in reducing fractures of the spine, hip and other non-vertebral sites. They are also licensed for the prevention of corticosteroid-induced osteoporosis. Specialists will sometimes use these drugs outside of their licenses on younger people, or on men. For any drug to become legally licensed for use it has to undergo trials to prove its safety and efficacy. The easiest, most readily available group of people to study with osteoporosis is postmenopausal women. This does not mean, however, that these medications will not work on other groups, such as men and premenopausal women; they have not yet been studied in large trials (except for Fosamax).

Another bisphosphonate called pamidronate is sometimes used for the treatment of osteoporosis. It is not actually licensed for this use – it was developed for a different condition called Paget's disease, but again some specialists will choose to use it in their patients. This is given in the form of an intravenous drip as a day case in hospital on an intermittent basis.

Finally, there is not yet a great deal known about the long-term use of the bisphosphonates. We do not really know what the optimum duration of treatment is, or how long they may continue to offer protection to the bones even after the treatment regimen has ceased. Furthermore, newer and potentially more potent bisphosphonates are being trialled, one called ibandronate and another called zolendronate, which the manufacturers hope will be a once-a-year injection.

Hormone replacement therapy

HRT, like the bisphosphonates, is an anti-resorptive therapy and works by stimulating the oestrogen receptors on the bone cells. HRT is very commonly used in women for the prevention and treatment of osteoporosis, for two main reasons:

- Many women will start HRT whilst going through the menopause to help control the symptoms associated with the menopause, and then continue to use it for some time for bone protection.
- HRT is a more cost-effective option when targeting high-risk women at the menopause.

HRT use is, however, becoming an increasingly controversial issue. It is associated with very slight increases in the risks of developing breast cancer, venous thromboembolism (VTE), cardiovascular disease and strokes. HRT does, however, reduce the risk of spine, hip and non-vertebral fractures, although much of this evidence comes from observational data rather than large controlled clinical trials.

There is also the possibility that women who take HRT are more aware of healthy living and will improve their diet and exercise as well, which could affect their bone health.

HRT is best prescribed for the five or so years during and just after the menopause. After this time many women may wish to change to another treatment, but some may choose to stay on HRT longer.

As with any drug, the potential risks need to be weighed against the potential benefits for each individual case. Some women may feel very well whilst taking HRT, and are happy to stay on it as long as they continue to have regular health checks such as mammograms.

Selective oestrogen receptor modulators

Selective (o)estrogen receptor modulators (SERMs) are a different type of drug. Raloxifene (Evista) is the first of these drugs to be designed and licensed as a treatment for osteoporosis. Again this is licensed for post-menopausal women, and it works by acting as an oestrogen agonist in bone and an oestrogen antagonist in areas like the breast and uterus.

Evista is not a hormone replacement so will not have any of the other effects that HRT has. It does carry a similar risk of VTE to that of hormone replacement, but nothing else. Evista has been shown to reduce the risk of vertebral fractures, but no effects have been noted so far on non-vertebral sites. Evista is very convenient and easy to take at any time of the day with no food restrictions.

Calcium and vitamin D

All the clinical trials looking at osteoporosis treatments and their efficacy have ensured that the correct amount of calcium was being used as well. In some cases, however, calcium and vitamin D supplements are used as a treatment on their own.

Vitamin D is required to metabolise calcium, and we normally get most of what we need from the sunshine. Elderly people in particular are often unable to go out and about and may very well be deficient in this vitamin. Studies have shown that regular supplementation in the elderly reduces the risk of non-vertebral fractures.

Given the fact that calcium and vitamin D supplements have very few side-effects, other than some constipation with calcium, they are often a good treatment option for those people who cannot tolerate other treatments.

Other Treatments

Hip protectors are an external hip protection system comprising two hip-protecting shells, made of polypropylene, integrated into a pair of stretchy, cotton-mix pants. The shells disperse the impact of a fall into the soft tissue and muscles around the pelvis. Various research projects have been completed into the acceptability and safety of hip protectors and studies are ongoing. Hip protectors are not available on prescription and have to be purchased.

The majority of treatments available are anti-resorptive, and any gains in BMD are relatively small. A new treatment call parathyroid hormone (PTH) is currently undergoing clinical trials. If this comes through the trials and is licensed, then it will be a new approach to the treatment of this condition, as it stimulates the osteoblasts to build bone rather than preventing bone loss.

REFERENCES

Baudoin C, Fardellone P et al. 1996 Clinical outcomes and mortality after hip fracture: a 2-year follow-up study. Bone 18(3 Suppl): 149S–157S

Center JR, Nguyen TV et al. 1999 Hormonal and biochemical parameters in the determination of osteoporosis in elderly men. J Clin Endocrinol Metab 84: 3626–35

CDC (Consensus Development Conference) 1991 Prophylaxis and treatment of osteoporosis. Am J Med 90: 107–10

Cooper C 1999 Epidemiology of osteoporosis. Osteopor Int 2(Suppl): S2–S8

Cooper C, Melton LJ 1992 Epidemiology of osteoporosis. TEM 3: 224–9

Cooper C, Campion G, Melton LJ 1992 Hip fractures in the elderly: a worldwide projection. Osteopor Int 2: 285–9

Cooper C, Atkinson EJ, Jacobsen SJ, O'Fallon WM, Melton LJ 1993 Population based study of survival after osteoporotic fractures. Am J Epidemiol 137: 1001–7

Cryer et al. 1993 Injury Epidemiology in the South East: Identifying Priorities for Action. South East Institute of Public Health, South Thames Regional Health Authority.

Cummings ST, Kelsey JL, Nevitt MC et al. 1985 Epidemiology of osteoporosis and osteoporotic fractures. Epidemiol Rev 7: 178–208

Cummings SR, Nevitt MC, Browner WS et al.1995 Risk factors for hip fracture in white women. N Engl J Med 332: 767–73

Dennison E, Cooper C 1996 The epidemiology of osteoporosis. Br J Clin Pract 50: 33–6

Dennison E, Cooper C 2001 Epidemiology of Osteoporotic Fractures: Effective Management of Osteoporosis. Aesculapius Medical Press: London

Dolan P et al. 1998 The cost of treating osteoporotic fractures in the United Kingdom female population. Osteopor Int 8: 611–17

Guegan R, Jouanny P, Guellemin F et al. 1995 Segregation analysis and variance components analysis of bone mineral density in healthy families. J Bone Min Res 12: 2017–22

Gullberg B et al. 1997 Worldwide projections for hip fracture. Osteopor Int 7: 407–13

Holick MF 1998 Perspective on the impact of weightlessness on calcium and bone metabolism. Bone 22 (Suppl 5): 105s–111s

Israel E, Banerjee T, Fitzmaurice G et al. 2001 Effects of inhaled glucocorticoids on bone density in premenopausal women. N Engl J Med 345: 941–7

Johnston CC, Epstein S 1981 Clinical, biochemical, radiographic, epidemiologic, and economic features in osteoporosis. Orthoped Clin N Am 12: 559–69

Keay N, Fogelman I et al. 1997 Bone mineral density in professional female dancers. Br J Sports Med 31(2): 143–7

Lanyon LE 1996 Using functional loading to influence bone mass and architecture: objectives, mechanisms and relationship with estrogen of the mechanically adaptive process in bone. Bone 18: S37–S43

Marshall D, Johnell O, Wedel H 1996 Meta-analysis of how well measures of bone mineral density predict occurrence of osteoporotic fractures. BMJ 312: 1254–9

Mays S, Less B, Stevenson JC 1998 Age-dependent bone loss in the femur in a medieval population. Int J Osteoarchaeol 8: 97–106

National Osteoporosis Society 2001 Position Statement on the Use of Peripheral X-ray Absorptiometry in the Management of Osteoporosis. NOS: Bath

O'Neill TW, Varlow J, Cooper C et al. 1993 Differences in vertebral deformity indices between three European populations. J Bone Min Res 8 (Suppl 1): S149

O'Neill TW et al. 2000 Incidence of Colles' fracture in the UK. Abstracts of the 7th Bath Conference on Osteoporosis

Overton C, Davies M 1999 Factors which Determine the Age of the Menopause: Handbook of the British Menopause Society. BMS Publications: London

Reeve J et al. 2002 Incidence of vertebral fracture in Europe: results from the European Prospective Osteoporosis Study. J Bone Min Res 17: 716–24

Riggs BL, Khosla S et al. 1998 A unitary model for involutional osteoporosis: estrogen deficiency causes both type I and type II osteoporosis in postmenopausal women and contributes to bone loss in aging men. J Bone Miner Res 13: 763–73

Van Staa TP, Dennison EM, Leufkens HG, Cooper C 2001 Epidemiology of fractures in England and Wales. Bone 29: 517–22

Weinstein RS, Manolagas SC 2000 Apoptosis and osteoporosis. Am J Med 108: 153–4

WHO (World Health Organization) 1994 Assessment of Fracture Risk and its Application to Screening for Postmenopausal Osteoporosis. WHO technical report series 843. WHO: Geneva

Wolff I, Van Croonenborg JJ, Kemper HCG et al. 1999 The effect of exercise training programs on bone mass: a meta-analysis of published controlled trials in pre- and postmenopausal women. Osteopor Int 9: 1–12

Physiotherapy in Rheumatology

Rachel Lewis

Earlier chapters have examined the clinical aspects of osteoarthritis, rheumatoid arthritis and osteoporosis. This chapter details the valuable contribution the physiotherapist can make to the management of each of these conditions.

OSTEOARTHRITIS: BASIC ISSUES

Chartered physiotherapists play a pivotal role in the management of people with osteoarthritis (OA). The physiotherapist needs to work in harmony with other members of the multidisciplinary team to ensure optimal management. Physiotherapy needs to be geared towards enabling the individual to be independent in activities of daily living (ADL), employment and leisure activities. If patients can be functionally independent, quality of life should consequently improve.

Self-management is an important issue for individuals with OA to ensure long-term management of this chronic condition. The multidisciplinary team must educate the patient in self-management of pain, preservation of function and muscle strength, and coping strategies. Occupational therapists may be involved in helping the person to implement coping strategies and assisting patients in ADL.

During the assessment, the patient's leisure, ADL and employment needs should be discussed in order to assess the positions the patient will need to adopt at work or in the home. Individuals in some areas need to work in enclosed spaces and may need to be able to flex their trunk into a very small space and be able to rotate tools etc. with some power to fulfil their daily tasks; other people may need to care for grandchildren and so on. The physiotherapist should enquire whether any recent X-rays or further imaging have been completed to add further information to the assessment.

The patient's expectation of physiotherapy treatment is relevant. The general practitioner may have 'just sent them for physiotherapy' – this could give some indication of the person's motivation or lack of it. Frequently the patient has been given and has sought little information, and this can affect the outcome owing to a disinterest in well-being and improvement. Conversely the patient may have very specific goals – for example ascending stairs, walking the dog, going to the shops, doing up buttons and zips.

Chapter 1 introduced the concept that an important source of evidence is what patients tell us about their condition, which treatments they find effective, and the degree to which interventions improve their ability to get on with their lives. It is therefore important to ask the patient about their past experiences of physiotherapy services:

- What treatment did the person receive?
- Was it beneficial?
- Does the person still do the exercises and follow any information given by a physiotherapist?

ASSESSMENT IN OSTEOARTHRITIS

Subjective Assessment

Physiotherapists typically see patients with OA affecting the weight-bearing joints of the knee, hip and lumbar spine, or the hands. Assessment should follow the musculoskeletal guidelines set out in Chapter 2 and should include palpation, functional outcomes, pain, and joint range of movement (ROM). Muscle strength and gait should also be assessed.

A subjective assessment should be undertaken to evaluate the current difficulties experienced by the patient. It is important to enquire whether sleep is affected by pain, and if so which joint is principally causing the problem. Frequency of pain, and night postures, should be noted – especially of the lumbar spine, cervical spine and hips. Many patients sleep with a pillow under their knees to support them and alleviate pain on a temporary basis. This may lead to a fixed flexion deformity and patients should be educated on appropriate sleeping postures to minimise the risk of deformities.

A body chart should be completed (Maitland 1991). This includes information regarding the site, quality and type of pain, and aggravating and easing factors. All this will provide information on the cause of the pain – whether it is inflammatory, mechanical or neural. Severity, irritability and nature (SIN) factors can then be calculated to facilitate the objective assessment (refer to Chapter 2 on musculoskeletal assessment).

Key point
The phraseology a patient uses can also highlight psychological acceptance and understanding of the disease. The physiotherapist should be aware of these aspects and their possible impact on treatment.

Objective Assessment

The person's gait and general posture should be observed. A Trendelenburg gait may be a feature of OA of the hip. Observe any flexion of the knees, hip or spine, and look for equality and duration of stance and the swing phase. Observe how easily the patient undresses and what type of movement patterns are used. The type of footwear and the shoe wear pattern should be noted. This provides further information regarding biomechanics and gait. Other points to note are:

- Does the person have any walking aids?

- Does a walking aid improve pain control or safety, or is it used to assist balance?

Posture in standing

Refer to Figure 2.6 in Chapter 2.

- The patient may have flexion contractures. These can be very functionally disabling and are common in the hips or knees. They are often initiated by knee pain and tight hamstrings.
- Is there loss of lumbar lordosis, any kyphosis or scoliosis? If so, what is the cause? Anatomical markers such as posterior superior iliac spines, popliteal and gluteal creases should all be level.
- There may be leg length inequality.
- Valgus and varus deformities at the knees are often magnified when weight-bearing, and in some patients the limb can return to neutral in a non-weight-bearing position. X-rays may or may not have been taken with weight-bearing.
- There may be a loss of the medial arch, or toe deformities affecting weight-bearing.
- The tibia may be rotated when the patient is observed in the standing position.
- Atrophy of any muscle groups should be noted.
- Valgus/varus of the tendo-Achilles should be noted, as well as excessive pronation/supination of the feet.

Palpation in Osteoarthritis

With the back of the hand, check for temperature changes and swelling (signs of an effusion). When palpated, does the patient immediately complain of pain or withdraw the limb?

> ### Key point
> Always look at the individual's face as well to check for those key signs of pain.

Joint range of movement can be measured by manual or electrical goniometers (Williams and Callaghan 1990). Experienced physiotherapists can often quite accurately estimate joint ranges without goniometers, but early on in your career remember that it takes practice with a goniometer to obtain such accuracy.

Ligament tests should be undertaken on the joint(s) involved, along with the end feel of the joint; an osteoarthritic joint may be very swollen and physiological passive movement is often painful. The joint may not extend fully owing to soft tissue contracture, or the joint space may be narrowed resulting in bone-on-bone contact.

Joint ranges commonly lost include rotation in the hip, and extension in the knee. Proximal and distal interphalangeal joint ROM can be restricted by Heberden's nodes. The patient may resist the motion in anticipation of pain. It is sometimes easier to measure gross or composite movements such as fist, hook and opposition grips, which are good functional measures.

Functional tests can be performed such as:

- timed up and go (Podsiadlo and Richardson 1991)
- number of sits-to-stand completed in 1 minute
- standing on one lower limb (timed)
- timed heart rate during a set length of walk
- functional questionnaires such as SF36 (Ware et al. 1993)

Most relevant and sensitive to osteoarthritis is the WOMAC Osteoarthritis Index devised by Western Ontario and McMaster universities (Angst et al. 2001) which assesses only lower limb function.

Muscle strength can be graded on the Oxford scale, and isokinetic machines are now used much more following research protocols and increasing availability in departments. However, with the development of primary care groups this may be diminished by the increasing use of physiotherapists in general practitioner surgeries where there is a lack of space for bulky items of equipment.

PHYSIOTHERAPY FOR PEOPLE WITH OSTEOARTHRITIS

Types of Treatment

Students often ask 'What is the best treatment for OA?' and are dismayed to get the same answer: 'It depends on the individual.' Perhaps Figure 12.1 will explain the situation.

Most people will be somewhere between the two ends of the OA spectrum, and this illustrates the importance of an appropriate patient assessment with goals mutually agreed between therapist and patient.

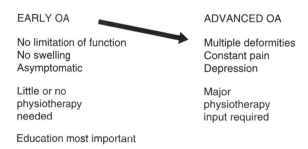

Figure 12.1   The range of clinical presentation.

Therapists should educate and prepare the individual for long-term management.

Holistic management should be upheld whenever possible, since educating the individual will enable the person to address any new joint symptoms when they arise, and consequently reduce re-referral rates to allied health professionals. However, patients could be provided with a contact or helpline number to use if they develop difficulties subsequent to their initial episode of treatment.

After the initial assessment some patients will benefit from individual treatments such as strapping for patellofemoral dysfunction, whereas other patients will benefit from group treatments. Many people with OA have reduced aerobic capacity owing to pain limiting their mobility, or comorbid factors. Once pain is more controlled, aerobic exercise capacity should be addressed.

Information should be provided regarding appropriate footwear, and walking aids provided. Since many obese patients experience OA, access to a dietitian may be helpful, either in a group setting or by means of a diet information sheet. Many patients wish to be proactive in their own self-management. The media provides a wealth of information on alleviating arthritis with various diets, herbal remedies and so on. Frequently the GP and a physiotherapist are the only healthcare professionals managing the individual with OA, so the physiotherapist is often the main source of information and advice. Therapists often spend longer with patients during treatment sessions to discuss such issues.

Issues Related to the Stage of the Condition

Consideration of the stage of the condition is important. If the patient has had an exacerbation of inflammatory OA, advice about pain relief and self-management is appropriate, with subsequent individual treatment and progression to a group situation. Possibly a review of medications and liaison with medics will be needed. Injections may be indicated if there is no or minimal improvement. One should aim to prevent deformity and maintain and improve mobility. Advice on joint protection is also important.

> ### Key point
> Patient advice should not conflict with any previous information given.

In the later stages of OA, with mechanical changes, the aims may include maintaining joint and general mobility and the prevention of further deformity in the joint affected and adjacent joints caused by altered biomechanical stresses. Orthoses may be needed, such as functional foot orthoses.

Pain can be self-limiting at this stage. Many patients have severe crepitus, yet state that they have no pain. Other patients can have severe pain caused by joint space narrowing and will proceed to total joint replacement. The physiotherapist needs to prepare the patient for surgery by maintaining and increasing muscle strength and ROM for the joint in question and adjacent joints.

Liaison with an occupational therapist is important with regard to the home situation and heights of furniture, especially for a total hip replacement. Practice with walking aids, but be aware of limitations of some walking aids in people with hand or upper limb joint involvement.

Pain relief

Keep treatments simple. This allows the patient to easily replicate and continue self-treatment at home, promoting self-maintenance. It also allows the physiotherapist to have many further treatment modalities to use if the simple ones fail! This is important because when patients have only passive treatments performed on them they tend to develop a reliance on the physiotherapist. Patients may also see the only solution to pain relief in the piece of electrotherapy equipment coming out of the cupboard! If a highly technical piece of equipment fails, a simple ice-pack has little chance of being acceptable.

Ice-pack/cryotherapy

Ice or cold therapy can be very effective as an analgesic (Yurtkuran and Kocagil 1999). It can be used to produce alternating vasodilation and constriction, thus affecting swelling. Cold also reduces the rate of neuronal firing, thus reducing the number of threshold pain responses. After the application of an ice-pack, gentle exercise can be performed with greater ease, often facilitating a greater range of movement.

Heat

Heat reduces muscle spasm, induces vasodilation and increases the circulation to the painful area. Heat can be applied with simple heat-packs such as gel or wheat and a hot water bottle. An infrared lamp can be useful, but subjectively patients appear to gain benefit from a more direct form of heat. (There appears to be no literature to support this.) Using heat-packs is also easy to replicate at home.

Key point

Patients should be told why they are using a particular modality and given some physiological basis for its effectiveness, to ensure they continue to follow their treatments. Patients are often advised to use heat for areas of muscle spasm and stiffness to reduce spasm, and consequently facilitate movement, and to use cryotherapy for more swollen areas, to reduce swelling.

These modalities should always be used in conjunction with active exercise and functional activities. The Philadelphia Panel (2001) found that there is a lack of evidence regarding efficacy for the above modalities, owing to a limited number of good relevant studies.

Wax treatment

Wax treatments are now more prevalent, and individual wax therapy units can be purchased in high street stores. Wax used for the treatment of hands with osteoarthritis remains poorly researched, but some studies have been undertaken. Subjectively patients find this modality extremely beneficial. Wax therapy is pleasant and is a useful precursor to exercise (Figure 12.2).

Electrotherapy

Many studies have attempted to evaluate the effectiveness of various electrotherapy modalities. These include pulsed electromagnetic energy (PEME). However, a study by Clark et al. (2000) showed no difference in outcome between genuine treatments with this modality and sham treatments when the machine was switched off during the 'treatment'.

TENS (transcutaneous electrical nerve stimulation) is an electrotherapy modality with a better evidence base. TENS is managed by the patient and is portable (Figure 12.3). Patients often prefer TENS as it may reduce the need for analgesia. TENS does not have the same side-effects as many of the medications given to patients. TENS plus exercise was one of the main recommendations of the Philadelphia Panel (2001). Patients should be encouraged to experiment with different frequencies to find the frequency and pattern of stimulation that is most beneficial for the individual.

Ultrasound

The Philadelphia study (2001) stated that there was too little evidence to suggest a level of efficacy for ultrasound therapy. Sub-therapeutic ultrasound has been used as a placebo for some studies on OA of the knee. In clinical practice, ultrasound has been used rarely in

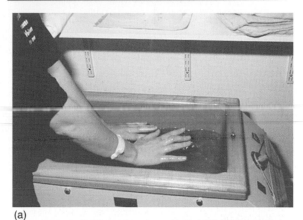
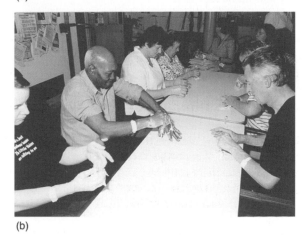

Figure 12.2 (a) Melted wax is applied to the hands from a bath. (b) The solidified wax is removed as part of the exercise programme.

recent years (Doyle et al. 2000). This has especially been the case with increased awareness of developing a dependence on the physiotherapist, and with cognitive behavioural techniques becoming more in vogue based on a good evidence base (Sinclair et al. 1998).

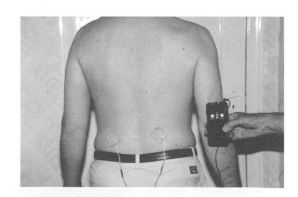

Figure 12.3 TENS is portable and can be a long-term means of pain relief in chronic arthritis.

Acupuncture

Acupuncture can be beneficial. Some studies recommend acupuncture for pain relief prior to joint surgery. Some patients even prefer to continue with episodes of acupuncture instead of joint replacement. Berman et al. (1999) reported improved WOMAC and Lequesne scores for patients with OA knee compared with those treated with 'standard treatment alone', but the standard treatments were not fully explained in the study. The benefits of acupuncture were starting to reduce 4 weeks after treatment, which questions whether treatments should be more prolonged or how frequently they should be repeated.

The Lequesne Index

Lequesne (1997) developed an index of severity for osteoarthritis of the hip. This can be used to assess the effectiveness of therapeutic interventions.

Acupuncture may reduce the initial pain and then allow patients to continue their home exercise programme more easily or allow patients to function more effectively. Acupuncture has also been shown to be effective in the treatment of low back pain (Carlsson and Sjolund 2001).

Strapping

Strapping has become popular for shoulder and knee pain in patients of all ages. Studies have shown that strapping can relieve knee pain and is a simple, safe and cheap way of providing short-term pain relief in patients with osteoarthritis of the patellofemoral joint (see Figure 12.4; Cushnaghan et al. 1994). The probable benefits of its application are the benefit of tape being both proprioceptive and facilitative to muscle fibres.

Splints can be provided for patients with difficulties within their hands. Occupational therapists and physiotherapists share splinting differently in each unit across the United Kingdom. Unlike with rheumatoid arthritis, people with OA rarely require resting splints, but dynamic splints for wrists can be very useful.

Exercise Prescription in OA

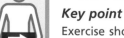

Key point

Exercise should be adapted to the individual. In the same way that a medication is always prescribed at a named and appropriate dosage, exercises should be clear and have a definite aim and repetitions. 'Go and exercise!' is not an acceptable approach.

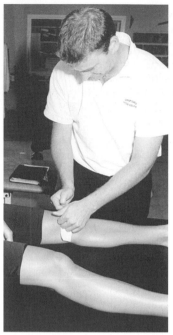

(a)

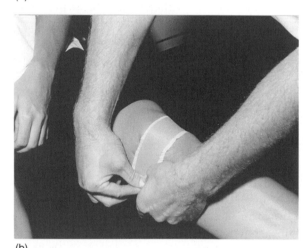

(b)

Figure 12.4   Application of strapping for patellofemoral OA.

Individuals and groups

There have been many studies comparing individual and group treatments and educational programmes for patients. These have been undertaken in both primary and secondary settings (e.g. O'Reilly et al. 1999; Maurer et al. 1999; Hart 2000; Clark 2000; Mohomed 2000; Mayer 2000; Van Baar et al. 2001; Dougados and Ravaud 2001). Some studies are unidisciplinary and some multidisciplinary.

Although patients need to be individually assessed, some imparting of information – such as methods of pain relief, coping strategies, postural advice and dietary advice – can be achieved in a group setting to utilise the physiotherapist's time most effectively. Also, patients often benefit from this group interaction, learning skills and gaining information from each other. Endorsement from other patients that treatment methods previously used were helpful can be compelling evidence for some people. Social interaction with others coping with a similar condition can be reassuring.

Compliance

Campbell et al. (2001) highlighted that loyalty to the physiotherapist is one reason for attending and increased compliance. This should probably not be underestimated and could partially account for the placebo factor. Physiotherapists are often in a unique position to capitalise on this to educate, relieve symptoms and regain function.

Compliance with exercise is, however, variable. In the literature many patients adhere to the exercise programme for the duration of the study, but as therapists what we really need to know is whether the person's beliefs and attitudes have changed enough to change the person's lifestyle to include an exercise regimen on a long-term basis. Campbell et al. (2001) found that compliance was affected by the 'willingness and ability to accommodate the exercises within everyday life, the perceived severity of symptoms, attitudes towards arthritis and comorbidity and previous experiences of osteoarthritis'. A necessary precondition for continued compliance was the perception that the physiotherapy was effective in easing the unpleasant symptoms. The study added that the reasons for non-compliance are rational but can often not be predicted by the therapist. Therefore health professionals need to understand the reasons for non-compliance if they are to provide supportive care and impact on the effectiveness of treatments.

Penninx et al. (2001) commented that a sedentary lifestyle is an important cause of disability and the prevention of disability in activities of daily living may prolong the patient's autonomy. They compared aerobic exercise programmes, resistance exercise programmes, and an attention control group for patients with OA of the knee. The aerobic and resistance exercise groups prevented ADL disability. They also noted that the lowest ADL disability risks were found for participants with the highest compliance to exercise.

Fransen et al. (2001) compared group versus individual treatments for OA of the knee in a randomised controlled trial. They concluded that both methods were effective but there were no significant differences between the two methods. Improvements were maintained for at least 2 months. Active exercise and the ability to cope was highlighted by Steultjens et al. (2001) who found that a passive coping style such as rest was found to predict a higher level of disability.

Danish patients with severe OA of the knee were included in a study assessing twice a week treatment and training for balance, fitness, coordination and muscle strength for 3 months. Pain, walking speed and muscle strength were all assessed. At 1 year follow up night pain had decreased but the number of palpable knee joint effusions had increased. They concluded that this should have further investigation. Patients did, however, have decreased pain and increased power (Rogind et al. 2001).

Hoffmann and Theiler (2001) assessed 18 studies evaluating the effectiveness of exercise therapy in OA of the hip or knee. 'All studies emphasised the general profit of exercise therapy compared to alternative programmes such as health education.' Unfortunately there were no studies comparing two or more alternative exercise programmes with regard to degree of effectiveness. Only two studies gave information about radiographic grade. Therefore effectiveness is proved only for aerobic, dynamic strengthening exercises.

Deyle et al. (2000) utilised two study arms. One group had manual therapy and exercise and the control group were given sub-therapeutic ultrasound. Unfortunately there was no exercise-only group. However, the researchers claim that treatment-group patients had statistically improved WOMAC scores and walking distance at 1-year follow-up. Whether this was due to the manual therapy, exercise, or the combination of the two is uncertain.

Points to consider when providing exercises for people with OA

Exercises for osteoarthritis may need to consider these parameters:

- maintenance of balance and coordination
- maintenance of joint range of movement
- maintenance of muscle strength
- core stability such as transversus abdominis, or erector spinae for lumbar OA
- aerobic capacity and cardiovascular fitness
- an associated weight-loss programme
- pain management
- neurodynamics
- preservation of function
- prevention of falls
- optimisation of postoperative recovery (e.g. exercises/advice prior to total knee joint replacement
- possibly delaying the need for surgery.

The exercises should be dynamic with a functional basis and include some resistance exercises such as an exercise bike. Starting positions, open and closed chain, neurodynamics and so on need to be considered when prescribing an individual exercise programme. Exercises should be kept simple and practical enough to ensure that they are maintained on a long term basis – there is little point in stipulating an exercise that is so painful or difficult for the person to undertake that it is abandoned within a week. Progressions should also be provided to allow some variety and to limit boredom.

Figures 12.5–12.8, 2.11 and 2.12 illustrate some of the principles discussed above.

Hydrotherapy

Key point

Perhaps surprisingly, there has been little research into the benefits of hydrotherapy for people with osteoarthritis. Nevertheless, the modality is often used both pre- and postoperatively in patients undergoing total joint replacement.

During hydrotherapy the weight-bearing status of the patient can be easily adapted and the resistance level can be more sensitively graded than on dry land (Harrison and Bulstrode 1987). The cardiovascular demands of exercise and hydrotherapy also make it an excellent medium to improve cardiovascular fitness, while increasing joint range of movement and muscle strength. The reduced weight bearing will help relieve pain from a condition where pain is exacerbated by weight bearing.

The physiology of immersion needs to be understood, and an extremely clear article on this is by Hall et al. (1990). The physiotherapist needs a clear under-

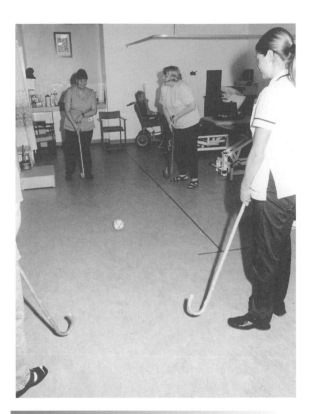

Figure 12.6   Exercise groups may also need to incorporate more general cardiovascular and coordination exercises.

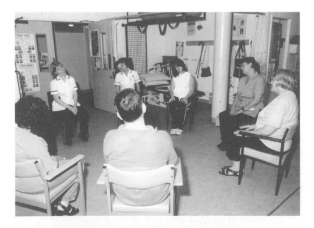

Figure 12.5   A group exercise class for OA. Such groups can be stimulating and productive if properly planned and monitored.

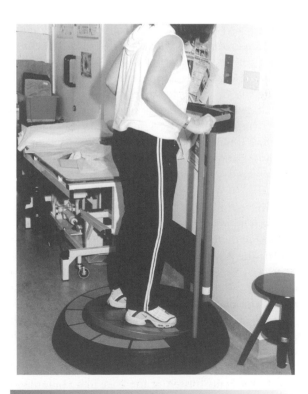

Figure 12.7   Balance work for a person with OA of the knee following an arthroscopic washout.

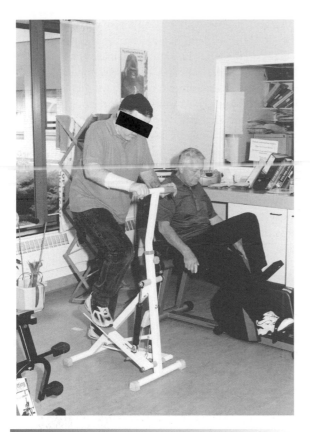

Figure 12.8   Cardiovascular and endurance exercise for OA of the knee.

standing of hydrodynamics to obtain the maximum benefit from hydrotherapy, consequently utilising the water to its maximum benefit. An example is assistance from a buoyancy aide to increase knee flexion. Many patients with multiple-joint OA who have experienced hydrotherapy are re-referred for further hydrotherapy or progression of their exercises.

Hydrotherapy groups can be very beneficial (unpublished data show improvement in WOMAC scores). After discharge, patients can then be encouraged to attend aquarobics and swimming. There are often local facilities that provide these classes and therefore provide the patient with the motivational factor, which they need. Some patients meet in a treatment group and then encourage each other to attend these sessions together, thus encouraging a more long-term exercise regimen.

Progression from buoyancy-assisted through to buoyancy-resisted exercises gives the physiotherapist access to an extensive treatment programme with sensitive grading. The Bad Ragaz patterns also reflect some of the common functional patterns utilised in ADL. The Bad Ragaz ring method can be extremely useful for strengthening muscle groups, and the physiotherapist

has an excellent opportunity to palpate the patient's strength capabilities. The physiotherapist's handling skills must be firm to ensure that the patient obtains the correct proprioceptive input and reassurance that the physiotherapist can effectively support the patient. This requires good postural stability from the physiotherapist.

Rehabilitation of the lumbar spine is often accelerated by hydrotherapy treatments, but this is only a subjective observation. When a person with multi-joint and lumbar spine OA is placed in a supine position, the back extensor musculature is often incredibly weak. This can be improved by the use of supportive positioning by the physiotherapist and the use of buoyancy devices to resist extension in supine and then progressed in other positions.

When a patient is supine, the physiotherapist can also undertake any specific joint mobilisations. For patients with hip pain, a longitudinal caudad movement through the water can decrease pain. The research evidence supporting this and the required number of repetitions remains unresearched/unpublished. In clinical practice the number of repetitions for an accessory mobilisation such as posterior–anterior movements are minimal compared to those on dry land. This could be due to the degree of muscle relaxation induced by the water temperature (Reid Campion 1990) or to buoyancy.

Isometric wrist and upper limb exercises with buoyancy-resisted apparatus can improve upper limb symptoms. Reducing the base of support while performing these (standing on one leg only for example) can improve balance. The person's balance mechanisms can also be facilitated in a relatively safe environment. The patient is constantly changing his or her metacentre and creating a degree of turbulence to contend with.

Sylvester (1989) compared hydrotherapy treatment to land exercise and short-wave diathermy in individuals with OA of the hip. This showed functional ability had improved and a higher score of life satisfaction for those treated with hydrotherapy.

OSTEOARTHRITIS: A CASE STUDY

About the patient

Mrs A was a 58-year-old retired teacher with a 4-year history of bilateral knee pain, mainly on the right side, which was limiting her function, especially walking distance. Her hobbies included gardening, walking and playing the piano. She walked with her father's wooden stick. The stick had a very narrow handle and was too high for her. Her stance phase of gait was reduced with a shortened stride length and limited use of hip extension. She wore relatively high, narrow heeled shoes, which made her slightly unsteady. All of this was observed on walking from the waiting area to the assessment area.

On questioning the patient revealed little knowledge of OA. She had received physiotherapy once before for her knee pain, about which she remembered only straight leg raises which she discontinued because they had no benefit and made her back ache. She was sent for physiotherapy by her GP and wanted to be able to garden and walk her dog on rough terrain.

Mrs A had anterior knee pain of an aching nature with occasional stabbing pains. She had a flexion deformity on the right, hamstring spasm, and knee extension limited by pain. She has started to place a pillow under her knee at night to relieve the pain. She occasionally woke with hip pain around her greater trochanter and deep within the hip joint. She had had occasional back pain for several years but felt that all her aches were deteriorating and affecting her activities of daily living. Her standing and gait duration, gardening and playing the piano, were especially limited.

Mrs A suffered from mild asthma and obesity. She took paracetamol and occasionally ibuprofen, which were helpful, but she was not keen on taking too many medications.

X-rays showed a pattern consistent with generalised OA, hands showed Heberdens and Bouchards nodes, and the CMC of the thumb was also affected, the lumbar spine showed degenerative changes and numerous osteophytes and the knees exhibited loss of joint space particularly on the medial aspect of the joint.

Objective assessment

Mrs A had a 15-degree flexion deformity on the right knee, which was making prolonged standing difficult for her, and leading to pronation of her foot with internal rotation of the hip. The deformity was not fixed and could be corrected to 5 degrees, but attempts to achieve full extension were too painful and caused her some distress. She had a mild tibial rotation on the right. The right knee had a moderate effusion and a positive patellar tap. She stood in some hip and trunk flexion with a decreased lumbar lordosis.

Her thoracic spine was mildly kyphosed but she was able to correct this. She also had multiple Heberden's nodes on her hands (see Chapter 9).

Her hip range of movement was good except for bilateral slight reduction of internal rotation that reproduced her trochanteric pain. Muscle strength and bulk was reduced in her gluteus maximus and medius.

Mrs A's pain was 7/10 using a visual analogue scale. Knee ROM was 15–80 degrees on the right side, 0–100 degrees on the left. The right knee had very tight hamstrings and gross wasting of vastus medialis. Right patellofemoral assessment reproduced her knee pain on an anteroposterior movement, and a boggy effusion was palpated. The medial patellar glide was also tight and reproduced some of her pain. Valgus stress testing at the knee showed some instability and reproduced pain over the medial collateral ligament. The wear pattern on her shoes was very lateral for heel strike.

Mrs A's muscle strength was poor, as was her posture. Quadriceps and hamstrings on both sides showed signs of atrophy and had a grade of 4 on the Oxford scale.

Mrs A's problem list

- Knee pain.
- Patellofemoral malalignment.
- Loss of knee extension (functionally disabling and a high treatment priority).
- Limited knee flexion.
- Inappropriate self-management.
- Inappropriate previous physiotherapy (straight leg raises).
- Walking aid incorrect height.
- Hand pain and stiffness.

Short-term aims of treatment

- Decrease pain to 5/10 or less on VAS within 2 weeks.
- Eliminate flexion deformity – i.e. attain full knee extension before it becomes a fixed flexion deformity.
- Improve (normalise) gait and duration/distance.
- Improve muscle strength with a simple but functional home exercise programme, particularly for the muscles having a stabilising effect upon the knee joint.
- Supply a correctly sized walking aid for use during periods of increased pain.
- Obtain a functional foot orthosis.

Long-term aims of treatment

- Refer to an osteoarthritis group.
- Advise about appropriate future self-management.

Mrs A's Treatment

The physiotherapist initially spent 10 minutes explaining the objective assessment findings to Mrs A and how they related to the pathology of her arthritis (see

Chapter 9). Mrs A was advised about the use of ice and heat at home, which she subsequently found extremely beneficial.

The right patellofemoral joint was strapped for a medial glide, taking care to ensure the tape was on the upper two-thirds of the patella and relieving pressure inferiorly. She was advised about appropriate footwear. A functional foot orthosis was discussed; a trial of new footwear relieved pain and improved lower limb biomechanics. Within ten days her pain was down to 5/10 on VAS.

Her walking stick was replaced with one of the correct height. She was given a simple but specific home exercise programme for lower limb joint mobilising and to improve strength of hip extension, abduction and vastus medialis. She was advised to place a well-wrapped hot pack on the hamstrings prior to exercise and precautions explained for knee extension since the hamstring spasm was one of the causes of her loss of knee extension. Trunk exercises were also provided such as bridging, lumbar rotation and McKenzie extension.

She was advised on transversus abdominis exercises and about the possibility of attending aquarobics, Tai Chi and Pilates groups following her discharge. She attended a hand group with other OA patients, which included wax treatment followed by gentle exercise for range of movement and strength using gel resistance exercisers etc. At one of these sessions an occupational therapist was available to discuss joint protection principles and introduce various items to aid function. Mrs A found the jar openers and kettle tippers extremely useful and she enjoyed the discussion with other patients.

Mrs A also attended the multi-joint OA group and was educated about OA, posture and pain relief. At this group she learned why it was not helpful in the long term for her to place a pillow under her knees. She purchased a TENS machine following these sessions and found it extremely useful, as was her lumbar roll for sitting at home and in the car.

She progressed her exercise in a small circuit in the gymnasium and found hip exercises with resistance bands very rewarding. She tried an exercise bike, health rider and cross-country skier which she previously thought she would never have had the ability or confidence to use.

As part of the group she also had hydrotherapy. The use of buoyancy for standing exercises and supine for the hips and trunk were very good for her hip and back pain and muscle strength. She did trunk and balance exercises with the floats for trunk rotation, isometric wrist extension, and aquarobic-type exercises while sitting on a woggle – such as alternate limb extension and cycling, and hip abduction, which also incorporate metacentric exercises.

Mrs A found the course extremely beneficial. She wore the strapping for 2 weeks by which time the facilitative benefits and home exercises had relieved much of her pain. She felt that the course had taught her much about OA and about self-maintenance, and she now had some new friends with whom to attend the local pool and possibly the gym. She was very surprised how energetically she could exercise and was beginning to loose weight. She no longer used the stick. She was glad to have the helpline number in case her condition deteriorated, but felt she could use her new knowledge of posture and pain relief to be more independently in control of her condition.

She was also aware that since the NSAID was beneficial in a flare stage, she could contact her GP for an alternative NSAID as necessary.

On discharge her strength was nearly 5 on the Oxford scale. She had regained full range of movement at her hips and knees and nearly full ROM (but full function) in her hands. Her posture was also drastically improved with some lordosis, no thoracic kyphosis, and minimal cervical protraction.

RHEUMATOID ARTHRITIS: BASIC ISSUES

The Multidisciplinary Team (MDT)

The physiotherapist is a key player in the treatment of rheumatoid arthritis (RA), but as a member of a multidisciplinary team. If the team is not cohesive, the individual's treatment will be disjointed, leading the person into a state of unease. The patient is reassured if all members of the team are aware of the current treatment regimens and aims of treatment. This is especially important when patients are started on second-line agents or disease-modifying medications. The disease-modifying drugs do not have optimal effect until approximately 12 weeks and then dosages may need to be reviewed. The physiotherapist and other team members guide the patient through this period and alert doctors to any possible deterioration and assist in the decision process to start further medications such as oral steroids or intra-articular joint injections. This liaison ensures adequate pain control for the patient during activities of daily living (ADL) and also allows the person to continue with a rehabilitation programme.

The multidisciplinary team should be freely able to refer to other members of the team, with the consultant overseeing all care. This avoids the patient repeatedly reporting the same information to different disciplines and should minimise delays in providing the most appropriate treatment.

The multidisciplinary team in rheumatology is large owing to the systemic nature of the condition. RA can affect all age groups: the young (juvenile idiopathic arthritis), young adults, mothers to be, the middle-aged and the elderly. All these client groups have different goals and aspirations in life and treatment programmes should be appropriate in this regard. For example, the team may be preparing a young adult to learn to drive, get a first job or go night-clubbing, whereas and elderly patient may want to care for grandchildren, walk the dog or simply be able to dress, and get up and down the stairs.

Key point

Other conditions seen frequently in rheumatology include psoriatic arthritis and the connective tissue diseases such as lupus, scleroderma, polymyalgia rheumatica, reactive arthritis, hypermobility and gout. Many units also manage some chronic pain conditions such as fibromyalgia, but many centres are setting up units for pain management of these patients.

The multidisciplinary team

The minimal team consists of:

- the patient's family (which should be first on the list because it has a huge effect on the patient's ability to cope with the disease)
- general practitioner
- physiotherapist
- occupational therapist
- consultant rheumatologist
- nurse.

Additional team members could include:

- orthotist
- clinical psychologist
- pain clinic staff
- community nurse/health visitor etc.
- surgeon (orthopaedic/neuro)
- consultant team: renal, cardiac, respiratory, gastroenterologist, immunologist
- radiographer/radiologist (especially for ultrasound-guided joint injections)
- social worker
- disability resettlement officer (DRO) for those with work instability or similar problems.

Increasing numbers of physiotherapists in the United Kingdom are now working as extended scope practitioners (ESPs) or lecturer practitioners in rheumatology (Carr 2001). This exciting development sees extended scope practitioners working alongside the medical teams assessing and advising on treatments for many rheumatological conditions. They also take responsibility for their own caseload. ESPs undertake management of conditions such as ankylosing spondylitis, some soft-tissue problems and OA and perform some joint injections. This is a developing role and further debate continues about the efficacy of the physiotherapist's prescribing role. At present, specialist physiotherapists or nurses advise general practitioners (GPs) on suitable medications and the GP takes the overall responsibility for the actual prescribing and assessing the possible interactions of various medications. The GP has an important role to play in monitoring of many drugs prescribed in the rheumatology department such as regular blood testing for side-effects.

General Issues

Key point

Research into physiotherapy treatment programmes in RA remains limited. Many physiotherapists attend other musculoskeletal courses and adapt skills and techniques to their own rheumatological clientele.

The trend towards specialist units for rheumatology is now increasing and this is currently reflected in the jobs section of physiotherapy professional journals. Historically, patients were seen by either outpatient teams, or by inpatient orthopaedic or medical teams. This often led to a number of therapists treating the same patient – resulting in a lack of cohesive management and direction of care for the individual patient. The introduction of specialist units has led to increased national awareness and networks for therapist to exchange ideas. This is often linked to a specialist ESP role.

Patients seen in outpatient clinics often report that they have been referred by the GP with pain in a single joint but when they attend for treatment after waiting on the waiting list they have developed more problems. Many units, however, will assess only the referred part of the person's anatomy. A focused specialist unit should assess the patient holistically. If the person is referred with knee pain, the joint above and below should be assessed, as should gait, biomechanics, footwear etc. – as in the Maitland approach or similar principles. One must also check hands, cervical spine etc. This can be achieved by a joint count. The patient should be given advice on joint protection and on maintaining strength, ROM and so on at all joints – hoping to prevent problems rather than treat them when they appear.

The art of physiotherapy in rheumatology therefore is in being one step ahead of the disease. For example, checking hand muscle imbalance prior to joint disruption can lead to proactive treatment by physiotherapy and occupational therapy, preventing or possibly delaying the onset of Swan-neck deformities in destructive disease. The use of functional foot orthoses to improve gait and address biomechanical changes can alleviate knee pain and possibly reduce lower limb deformity.

Outcome and Disease Activity Measures in RA

- **Disease Activity Score (DAS) for Rheumatoid Arthritis:** see Van der Heijde et al. (1990).
- **Modified DAS (DAS28):** see Prevoo et al. (1995).
- **Outcome Measures in Rheumatology Clinical Trials (OMERACT):** see Tugwell et al. (1992).
- **Ritchie Articular Index (RAI):** see Ritchie et al. (1968).
- **Short Form 36 (SF36) Health Survey:** see Ware et al. (1993). It is also called Medical Outcomes Study Short Form 36.
- **Health Assessment Questionnaire (HAQ)** (Fries et al. 1980).

Aims of Treatment in RA

Rheumatoid arthritis is a chronic progressive disorder with periods of exacerbation and remission. Patients need to be educated about self-maintenance so that they can cope with minor flares independently. Patients must also be advised about when it is appropriate to seek further assistance.

> **Key point**
> Many people with rheumatoid arthritis live with chronic pain and fatigue and accept quite high levels of discomfort and interference with their lifestyles before seeking help, stating 'I had a clinic appointment in two months so I didn't want to bother anyone'. Many patients are quite uncomplaining in relation to their symptoms.

Several units around the United Kingdom have helplines for patients to contact in times of increased problems or to answer any queries. Various members of the multidisciplinary team may answer the helpline: some units have nurses and others have physiotherapists who answer. However, that member of the team can seek guidance or assistance from any other member of the team to solve the patient's dilemma.

Many centres or units have formal patient education programmes, which are usually multidisciplinary. Some units have group teaching and others use a one-to-one approach. The main aims of treatment are to control pain and other symptoms to enable an independent lifestyle so that the patient can function for ADLs, employment, relationships and (importantly) leisure activities.

> **Key point**
> Loss of leisure activities is one of the main predictors for depression and subsequent loss of independence in RA (Katz and Yelin 2001).

Typical aims of treatment in RA include:

- reduction of pain – thus gaining patients' trust and confidence
- maintenance of, or increased, joint ROM
- maintenance of, or improved, muscle power
- prevention of deformity or contracture
- improvement of cardiovascular fitness
- maintenance of function
- prevention of secondary conditions such as osteoporosis
- maintenance of respiratory excursion (be alert for fibrosis and methotrexate lung)
- education with regard to self-maintenance
- maintenance of proprioception and postural stability
- prevention of falls.

ASSESSMENT IN RHEUMATOID ARTHRITIS

With the introduction of expensive anti-TNF (tumour necrosis factor) medications, a register of patients and an assessment format have been introduced to assess the efficacy of these drugs on a national basis. The register can assist in the monitoring of side-effects of long-term use of anti-TNF. This will probably lead to a national assessment process, which could also have huge implications for research and treatment outcomes. For the assessment of patients for anti-TNF therapy, various blood tests are taken to measure disease activity (mainly the erythrocyte sedimentation rate, ESR).

The 28-Joint Count and Other Measures

Visual analogue scales are used to record pain. A 28-joint count for pain and tenderness has also been developed. The 28-joint count has superseded the Ritchie or Thompson Kirwan index, and has been shown to be a reliable and valid measure for joint assessment (see Figure 12.9; Smolen et al. 1995).

> ### Key point
> A nurse or physiotherapist often undertakes the joint count prior to a clinic consultation, giving the consultant much useful information and extra time to discuss these and other important issues.

A physiotherapy assessment of an individual with RA should be similar to any other musculoskeletal assessment. The difference – which often concerns physiotherapists and students – is the multiple joint problems that occur with this type of patient. Some therapists find this intimidating. However, whereas with some pathologies in a musculoskeletal outpatient setting one small problem may prove difficult to elicit and diagnose, in RA the problems are usually more obvious to see.

The importance of having an assessment plan needs to be stressed. This plan should facilitate the minimal amount of repetitive movements to minimise pain and fatigue for the patient. A common example is that the physiotherapist will assess knee flexion, return to neutral and then assess hip flexion, return to neutral and then assess hip rotation in 90 degrees of hip flexion. All of the above could be performed as a continuous process if planned appropriately, thus leaving the patient in minimal pain if further assessment is required.

Information about difficulties in ADLs, and the patient's aims or goals of treatment, are important. The physiotherapist may wish to increase the joint ROM in a stiff joint, but the patient may be perfectly happy with this but, rather, wants to be able to drive for 50 miles.

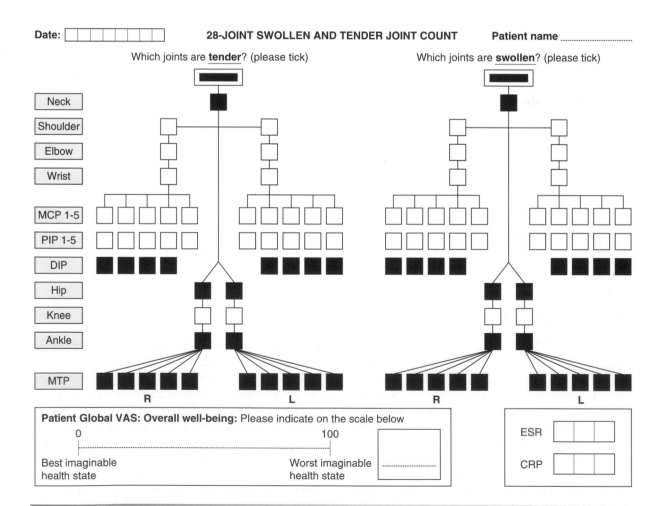

Figure 12.9   The 28-joint count form (courtesy of the British Society of Rheumatology Biologics Register).

Therefore the treatment must address the pertinent problems and educate holistically about maintaining joint ROM and power.

Functional levels of ability can be assessed subjectively with a score such as the Health Assessment Questionnaire (HAQ; Kirwan and Reeback 1986) and the Arthritis Impact Questionnaire (AIMS; Meenan et al. 1992). These can be useful in providing serial data, which can be used to monitor a patient's progress over a period of time. They are also quite quick and simple to complete.

A pain chart should be completed (see Chapter 2) and can be used to reflect back to when patients are seen in future episodes. The debate of whether patients should be assessed with accessory movements persists and evidence needs to be addressed for each joint individually. The cervical spine is the main issue. Ligamentous laxity can start very early after onset in the cervical spine. The physiotherapist will never be fully aware of the degree of laxity and red flag warning signs should warrant a flexion and extension view X-ray of the cervical spine. Some therapists mobilise when patients first appear with cervical pain and are not diagnosed with RA until the pain becomes more chronic and further investigation highlights the diagnosis. Many patients later in the disease duration state that the mobilisations performed early in disease management were extremely beneficial and request further mobilisation, but this is often when a larger extent of laxity could be present and hands-on mobilisations contraindicated. The patient then becomes more withdrawn from treatment.

Key point
Patients with RA have a reduced pain threshold to manual treatment techniques applied to the lumbar spine (Dhondt et al. 1999).

Issues Related to the Stage of the Condition

When assessing the patient with RA, the stage of pathology will become apparent and will predict the treatment required. It is also important to acknowledge and evaluate any previous treatments given to individuals. Some patients have never previously met an allied health professional and have very poor knowledge of their condition and self-management principles. At the other end of the spectrum patients may be active members of local arthritis support groups and be very well informed and just need a boost to get them back into their own supporting regimen.

The newly diagnosed

Newly diagnosed patients need to be thoroughly assessed for all problems or potential problems to ensure that they do not have any contractures or deformities. They need reassuring that they will not develop multiple deformities 'like their auntie Mary did 20 years ago'. Management of RA has improved dramatically since then, and with recent advances in medications the outlook continues to improve. Individuals need to be educated about self-management and strategies to overcome the initial flare. These can vary from very mild hand symptoms to multiple joint pain, contractures and early morning stiffness lasting all day.

Moderate joint problems affecting ADLs

Sometimes patients have one or two joints that have some biomechanical changes from erosions etc. but are not ready for joint replacement. These people may be coping with other areas. Rehabilitation, strapping, acupuncture, hydrotherapy and exercise may all have a part in the treatment programme. Liaison with other team members to facilitate such measures as provision of splints or joint injection may be appropriate.

Longstanding disease with recent flare

These patients often require a review of medications, which may not be at the correct dosage to maintain the disease; or a change of their second-line agent may be appropriate. Depomedrone injection or intravenous (IV) steroid pulse may be beneficial. A gentle exercise programme may be commenced and progressed as able. Many of these patients benefit from admission to have a rest from all the chores of family life and employment. They can then see all members of the multidisciplinary team and have intensive rehabilitation. The programme should start gently and then progress to be quite vigorous (Edmonds et al. 2001).

Longstanding disease awaiting joint replacement

These patients often need to improve their joint ROM, muscle length, strength, and position prior to surgery to ensure that preoperative function is optimal. A commonly encountered problem is fixed flexion deformity of the knees. This needs exercise and stretches to reduce the flexion contracture. Buoyancy-assisted stretches in the pool can be very beneficial. The upper limbs need to have sufficient strength and stability to facilitate use of a walking aid in the immediate postoperative period without causing further disruption to other joints. The patient can be prepared and educated about the surgery to alleviate many fears. The individual's home situation can be prepared – such as bed and bathroom access and heights of furniture. This is especially pertinent to a person about to undergo total hip replacement.

Often introducing these patients to other previously joint replacement successful candidates can be very beneficial.

Longstanding disease with multiple deformities

The mechanics of the joint often cannot be changed, and the patient may not be medically fit for surgery. Some joints can exhibit severe deformities but the person can function moderately well. Hand function is a typical example of this: sometimes the most deformed hands can function well and if operated on to improve cosmesis and deformity the functional ability might plummet. The occupational therapist can often improve ergonomics of the home situation and make ADLs as easy and least fatiguing as possible.

Early morning stiffness (EMS)

This is a common feature of rheumatoid arthritis and has been defined as 'slowness or difficulty moving the joints when getting out of bed or after staying in one position too long, which involves both sides of the body and gets better with movement' (Lineker et al. 1999). EMS is a marker of disease activity and should be checked by the therapist during assessment. This assists in the monitoring of the relatively new disease-modifying antirheumatic drugs (DMARDs).

Posture in RA

It is useful to assess the patient's posture in standing and gait prior to examining every joint. Standing usually highlights any deformities of the lower limb, which are sometimes not present in a non-weight-bearing position – such as valgus or varus knees.

- Does the patient rotate the hips in standing?
- Do the feet pronate or supinate excessively?
- Does the person wear a functional foot orthosis? If so, is it still supporting or facilitating what it should?
- Are there any rheumatoid nodules?
- Is there evidence of a Baker's cyst in the popliteal fossa?
- Are the posterior superior iliac spines, gluteal, and popliteal creases all level, or are there any signs of leg length inequality?

- Is the anterior border of the tibia rotated?
- Is the scapular position in neutral, or are they rotated or winging?
- Which muscles have allowed any imbalance to occur?
- Where else is there gross muscle atrophy?

Palpation

The affected joints should be assessed for increased temperature, synovial swelling and synovitis in the joints and tendon sheaths, to look for disease activity and guide the physiotherapist in assessment of the SIN factors (severity, irritability and nature – see Chapter 2). A hot and tender swollen joint would obviously be quite irritable and the level of severity judged. The physiotherapist should assess for ligament instability in the knee in particular. The rotator cuff is often a culprit for many problems in RA owing to inflammation within the joint leading to subsequent weakness, laxity or rupture.

When palpating the joints the active ROM should initially be assessed by goniometry (Williams and Callaghan 1990). The passive ROM should be included in the assessment as this indicates the potential for improvement. Many patients after a flare have lost huge amounts of muscle strength but have retained full passive ROM, so strengthening the muscles through ROM exercises will maintain or regain future independence. Other patients have a solid end-feel of bone grinding on bone; this should be compared with the X-rays.

If joint damage is severe, physiotherapy cannot change this and total joint arthroplasty (replacement) is required. Therefore the physiotherapist's role is to prepare this joint and any others affected by the future surgery. The patient should be given as much relevant information and literature as possible prior to surgery – many units supply their own literature. Many patients like to speak to other patients who have already successfully undergone similar joint replacement surgery.

Key point

Some assessments should include functional tests such as hand behind back and hand behind head instead of assessment in neutral. If there are problems on the functional movement the components can all be assessed individually; such as rotation. For further information see David and Lloyd (1998).

PHYSIOTHERAPY FOR PEOPLE WITH RHEUMATOID ARTHRITIS

Fixed Flexion Deformities

Fixed flexion deformities are due to shortened soft tissues. These occur when one or more joints flare and the patient rests the painful joint(s) in a shortened or flexed position to alleviate the pain. When left in one position for long periods the soft tissue contracts, and joint pain and lack of synovial lubrication on the whole joint surface exacerbate this. Joint erosions or deformities often lead to these positions as well.

Common areas to be affected by flexion contracture are knees, hips and elbows. Once the elbows start to contract and have a solid end-feel there is often limited benefit from rehabilitation, but pronation and supination must be preserved for function. One of the best ways to improve a fixed flexion deformity with minimal pain is buoyancy-assisted elbow extension in standing in the hydrotherapy pool, plus home physiological exercises. This is probably due to the muscle relaxation afforded by the water temperature, and buoyancy assisting the movement.

Treatment of other joints with flexion deformities remains very much at the discretion of each individual therapist, with minimal literature support. The use of active movements, active assisted or resisted movements can be enhanced by the use of cryotherapy or heat treatments. Hydrotherapy can be very beneficial if administered in combination with exercise. The use of splinting for a stretch of longer duration can be beneficial. Some units have splints that are dynamic and the range of movement can be altered according to need. A cheaper alternative is plaster back slabs/resting splints to maintain the stretch; a side-effect of this is that the joint can become quite stiff due to lack of movement for prolonged periods of immobilisation such as overnight. Delicate skin is a drawback, but appropriate padding can usually overcome this in most cases.

Some units also use Flowtron with variable success.

Pain Relief in RA

An important role of the physiotherapist is to help control the patient's pain. The therapist must advise about appropriate pain-relieving methods and thereby gain the patient's trust. If physiotherapeutic modalities alone cannot control the pain with the patient's current medication, the physiotherapist should liaise with the medical team to ensure adequate pain relief. Pain can cause a great deal of anxiety and affect coping strategies and consequently function. Increasing self-efficacy helps to limit anxiety (Strahl et al. 2000).

> **Definition**
> Self-efficacy is the belief of a person that he or she can successfully perform a given activity.

The patient should be educated about simple pain-relieving methods that can be easily replicated at home. These should not take up too much of the person's time and should be cost-efficient. The patient should be advised about appropriate treatment for each joint in flare at the clinic visit but the advice should also be generalised for future use independently. This empowers the patient for increased self-management, especially as many patients are not too keen to increase medication consumption. The benefit of many of the physiotherapeutic modalities is that they do not have side-effects and are easy to use at home. Often the patient will rest whilst applying the treatment, which is also important as many patients tend to care for families as a priority to their own self-management, and fatigue is a major problem for these people to overcome.

Cryotherapy

Cryotherapy (cold) is very simple and effective, but patients should be warned of the dangers of ice burns. If a joint is hot or swollen, ice will often be beneficial. The physiological and biological effects of ice are due to the reduction in temperature in the tissues, along with the relaxation of muscles. The application of cold has also been found to decrease the inflammatory reaction in experimental situations (Swenson et al. 1996). Ice uses the physiological process of the Hunting response of alternating vasodilation and constriction, which assists with swelling. The effect on neuronal tissue is to decrease the rate of neuronal firing of pain receptors; consequently the patient feels less pain. Many patients keep a bag of frozen peas in the freezer for pain relief (Fredrikus et al. 1994).

Heat

Heat treatments are very beneficial for people with RA and are very simple to use. Subjectively patients seem to gain a better response from heat placed on the body as opposed to sprays and heat lamps.

It is important to teach the patient simple methods of applying heat, otherwise the person may feel that if an infrared lamp is used by a physiotherapist that is the only method that will work. The person will then think a lamp has to be purchased for home use. Many patients are willing to spend a great deal of money on seeking the latest gadgets. Patients should be encouraged to think realistically and be selective and rational in their purchases. Advice from all the allied health professionals is important for this.

Heat can increase the circulation to the heated area and assist in the reduction of muscle spasm. This can therefore relieve some pain and perhaps inhibit overactive muscles, allowing facilitation of appropriate muscle groups in exercise rehabilitation.

Some patients have a definite preference between heat and ice. Some will state that one eases the pain and the other aggravates it. Other patients dislike ice and will always use heat; that can aggravate a swollen joint.

Wax treatment

The benefits of wax baths for hands with RA remains controversial. Patients state that they find it very beneficial, but it should be used as an adjunct or prior to exercise (see Figure 12.2).

Buljina et al. (2001) reported a reduction in joint size (which failed to reach significance, although all in the control group deteriorated compared with the wax and exercise group). A critical review of hand-treatment wax baths by Stewart (1996) showed significant improvements in ROM and grip function, while active hand exercises resulted in a reduction of stiffness and pain and increased ROM. Wax baths alone had no significant effect.

Electrotherapy

There are many electrotherapy modalities available to the physiotherapist. Each needs to be utilised with valid clinical reasoning. The evidence supporting many of these modalities in rheumatology remains limited. The use of electrotherapy also reduces the patient's own self-management, so the importance of simple treatments must also be reiterated to the patient for other joint problems.

Ultrasound

The use of ultrasound has had many phases and the dosages debated. Australian physiotherapists tend to use much higher frequencies than their British counterparts. Ultrasound can be beneficial when used in conjunction with other modalities such as exercise and strapping in some rotator cuff problems. Ultrasound tends to be more effective in the acute stages rather than prolonged chronic problems.

Pulsed electromagnetic energy

There is sparse literature in RA, but in OA the evidence in support of PEME is limited (see earlier in this chapter). Clinically PEME could be useful in the treatment of non-infected ulcers. Evidence supporting PEME, laser, ultraviolet and decompression chambers remains minimal and requires a systematic review.

Interferential therapy

Interferential therapy seems to have had its time in the limelight and been phased back into recession. The suction electrodes need to be placed carefully to avoid active synovitis, and care must be taken with the skin of patients on high-dose steroids who bruise very easily. The use of a modality such as this could lead to patient dependence on the therapist, and when a patient is experiencing multiple joint flares it would be impractical.

Transcutaneous electrical nerve stimulation (TENS)

TENS has been proven to be effective in the management of chronic pain. The patient can control it and it is portable (see Figure 12.3). The patient needs to trial different frequencies to find a suitable pattern. TENS is usually very effective or virtually useless in patients with RA; there tends to be no middle ground. Patients are often keen to utilise TENS to be in control and limit consumption of medications.

Acupuncture

There is little evidence about the benefits of acupuncture in RA. There is, however, evidence in support of its use in severe joint pain for patients with OA. Some patients even decline total joint replacement surgery and prefer to continue with acupuncture. The benefit of acupuncture may be reduced in patients who have recently taken high-dose steroids but this is not a contraindication

When there is no evidence of the degree of ligament laxity in the cervical spine and joint accessory mobilisations are contraindicated, acupuncture can be very beneficial for pain relief. This is deduced from audit data only and not from a randomised controlled trial. There remains much scope for research in acupuncture in the rheumatic diseases. Acupuncture is commonly used in clinical practice by rheumatology physiotherapists and GPs alike.

Relaxation

Patients are often taught relaxation as part of their education programme. Physiotherapists, occupational therapists, clinical psychologists or nurses can undertake this. This is variable between each unit in the United Kingdom, depending on individual knowledge and inclination. Some patients work very hard within the physiotherapy department and do not automatically associate relaxation as part of the programme, so it may be better presented by another discipline.

There are many types of relaxation. The contract–relax method can facilitate a good contraction but some patients are unable to relax fully to gain the benefits.

Many patients try various complimentary therapies. Each person has an individual response, which might be in part due to the relationship and rapport gained with the physiotherapist, which affects the outcome. Aromatherapy is subjectively beneficial when given with a gentle massage or in the patient's bath. Firm massage has been reported to aggravate symptoms.

Patients should be discouraged from trying too many different therapies in a bid to find a cure. Patient education and treatment groups can assist patient discussion on such modalities and useful local contacts. There unfortunately remains little research in this area, but this will probably change during the next decade.

ARC

The Arthritis Research Campaign (ARC) has produced a useful leaflet on complimentary therapies to advise patients. Visit the ARC website at www.arc.org.uk.

Postural training

Postural advice and education will help patients to have optimal ergonomics and facilitate everyday activities. 'Good posture' means recruitment of only the appropriate muscle fibres to limit fatigue and abnormal strains ensuing with pain.

Patients should be advised about sitting, standing and lying postures with attention to preventing contractures and further deformities. Patients can also find great benefit from advice about appropriately supporting the cervical spine at night. Some patients are also interested in postural techniques such as the Alexander method.

Postural exercises should complement the advice given. People with RA develop abnormal postures, which they think erase the pain in certain areas. These then become habit and more maladaptive practices start to occur – such as protraction and internal rotation at the shoulders.

Active and resting splints facilitate good hand posture and prevent deformity. Splinting is a key component of management of Boutonnière deformity. In the acute stage a splint maintains continuity of the central tendon to its insertion into the middle phalanx; and in the chronic stage its function is to correct the flexion contracture of the PIP joint (Massengill 1992). The importance of good hand posture cannot be exaggerated. Use of hand splinting is variable around the United Kingdom and is the role of either the occupational therapist or the physiotherapist. It is important that whoever does this splinting receives referrals swiftly for all patients requiring splints at an early stage to prevent correctable deformities from becoming fixed and non-correctable – such as ulnar deviation of the MCP with some subluxation. The passive movement should always be checked for potential for improvement.

Pacing

One of the most difficult equations for patients to balance is the need to rest with the need for activity. The recent trend has been towards pain management principles of pacing. When patients are in flare they generally need to increase their rest but put all their joints through a full range of movement every day. When coming out of flare they need to gradually progress either their exercise or level of activity. A pacing chart managed by the patient may be useful (Giorgino et al. 1994; Marks 2001; Van Lankveld et al. 2000). The person should then increase the amount of resistance or weight, and cardiovascular fitness, so as to be in optimum health before a future flare.

Education programmes

The benefit of education programmes in rheumatoid arthritis has been elicited in numerous studies (Lorig et al. 1994). The PRISM study (Program for Rheumatic Independent Self-management; Alderson et al. 1999) was an interdisciplinary programme given to patient groups to teach self-management, adult-learning case management and self-efficacy enhancement. These had beneficial effects on self-efficacy and pain. Similar results were seen by Scholten et al. (1999).

Patients do need to understand the disease process, and education is vital as it allows the person to reason both psychologically and physically with the disease, just as a health professional would clinically reason any treatment programme.

The education programme must be multidisciplinary in its presentation and have literature to support the presentations to remind patients in the future.

Joint protection suggestions

- Try to avoid becoming overweight.
- Wear splints if they have been recommended – but have periods without them to prevent ensuing weakness. Know when to utilise/stop.
- Work out how long you can sit comfortably before stiffness begins, then learn to change you position before this occurs.
- Use a firm mattress with as few pillows as possible. Do not keep a pillow under your knees for long periods.
- Spread the load over several joints. For example use both hands when lifting a kettle, and keep as much of your hands in contact with things as you can.
- Use leverage when possible, such as with long-handled equipment.
- When carrying things, use a grip which keeps fingers and wrists straight.
- Do not grip things too tightly. Tight grips produce a lot of strain on knuckles and thumb joints. You will tend to use a tight grip when you do things like writing or using a screwdriver.
- Take frequent breaks to rest your hands. Use padding to enlarge the grip on things such as your pen, knife, or toothbrush.
- Use the larger, stronger joints rather than smaller ones if possible. For example use your forearms rather than knuckles when rising from a chair.
- Avoid positions which push the joints towards deformity. See Figure 12.10 for illustration of two common deformities encountered in people with rheumatoid arthritis, i.e. swan neck and boutoniere deformities. A booklet for patients explaining the above is available from the ARC.
- Hug larger objects close to the body when carrying them.
- Use labour-saving aids and gadgets when in flare especially.
- Reduce the weight of what is lifted, and do not lift at all if the object is too heavy for you.

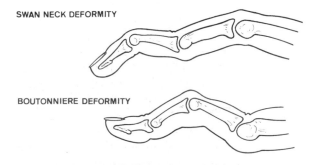

SWAN NECK DEFORMITY

BOUTONNIERE DEFORMITY

Figure 12.10   Boutonnière and swan-neck deformity.

- Slide objects along a work surface.
- Use a trolley or wheelbarrow.
- Avoid lifting heavy things with the wrists bent downwards.
- Avoid pushing down on the knuckles and avoid pushing the fingers over towards the little finger
- When working at a table or bench, sit or stand as close as you can, and reduce stretching and bending.
- If standing, keep your bodyweight so it is supported evenly through both legs.
- Pace your activities, work in short bursts.

A booklet for patients explaining the above is available from the ARC: http://www.arc.org.uk

Strapping

Strapping has become quite popular with the introduction of the McConnell concept. Strapping for entheseopthy pain and plantar fasciitis can be quite effective, or shoulder and knee taping can be an effective proprioceptive facilitator. The patient must be aware that it is a temporary device only in preparation for his or her own muscle control to utilise the information the tape provides. The taping should be used in conjunction with an exercise programme. The main contraindication to strapping is poor skin condition due to steroid therapy. The tape is only temporary and should not be used to support a rotator cuff that has totally degenerated with little hope of repair (Scholten et al. 1999).

Exercise Prescription in RA

Issues

Exercise has been one of the most researched modalities in RA. Patients should be made aware of the reasons why they must exercise, and most will feel the benefit and continue to exercise independently at some level. Exercise has obvious benefits for prevention of secondary problems such as diabetes, cardiac disease and stroke. Some patients taking steroid drugs will be slightly more prone to steroid-induced diabetes, so prevention is better than cure. The greater the strength of a muscle, the more it can protect the joint by absorbing everyday mechanical stresses. The muscle needs to be in balance with its antagonist, however, to prevent contracture; an example is balance between quadriceps and hamstrings to prevent flexion contracture of the knee. The importance of stretching muscle should be highlighted and may assist with pain relief. Consequently patients should have exercises to improve type II slow-twitch postural muscle fibres to improve postural control as a means of joint protection.

Exercise programmes should always take into consideration the systemic nature of RA. The physiotherapist should always be aware of systemic involvement and treat appropriately (Figures 12.11 and 12.12).

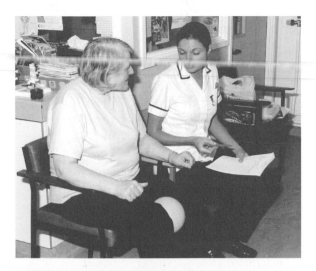

Figure 12.11   An ongoing dialogue between the physiotherapist and the individual is vital if an exercise programme is to be effective.

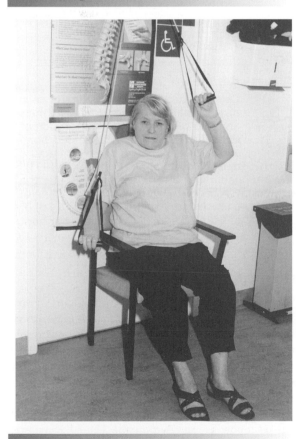

Figure 12.12   Exercise may need to be very specific, as in this case: auto assisted shoulder flexion using a reciprocal pulley system.

Aims of exercise

The physiotherapist must have clear aims for each exercise and be conscious about how much time exercises will take to complete in the patient's everyday schedule – consequently affecting the compliance.

Lineker et al. (2001) instituted a 6-week home-based exercise programme with a specialist rheumatology therapist in patients with moderate-to-severe RA and included education, exercise and pain relief modalities. At 1-year follow-up patients had improved early morning stiffness, knowledge, Stanford arthritis efficacy scale and visual analogue scale (VAS) for pain.

Some physiotherapists initially feel that RA patients are very fragile and that they need to be extremely gentle, but a study by Van den Ende et al. (2000) showed that early resistance training incorporating equipment such as an exercise bike was beneficial. The author compared an intensive exercise programme to a conservative programme with inpatients admitted for active disease. Conservative treatment included ROM and isometric exercises only; resistance included dynamic and isometric shoulder and knee strengthening exercises against resistance five times a week and conditioning exercise bike three times a week. Measures of physical functioning improved significantly for the intensive exercise group. There were no deleterious effects on disease activity. Similar results were found by Rall et al. (1996) where benefits included reduced pain and fatigue, and improved strength without any deleterious effects on joint pain or disease activity.

McMeeken et al. (1999) undertook a study to evaluate the effects of knee extensor and flexor muscle training on the timed up-and-go test (TUG). The study looked at one specific joint and exercise programme, but it is hoped that similar results will be found for other joints. The patients' HAQ and timed up-and-go improved, so specific knee muscle training can be administered safely in patients with non-acute RA and may produce functional benefits.

According to Stenstrom (1994), 'dynamic exercise requiring muscle work during joint motion appears to be superior to static or isometric exercises'.

Patient beliefs about the perceived benefits of exercise should also be addressed (Gecht et al. 1996). It is also the responsibility of the consultant to check on exercise frequency and ensure that patients continue with advice given to them (Iverson et al. 1999).

Tai Chi has had recent research and press coverage. This is a holistic exercise programme with a relaxation element. It teaches excellent posture and breathing. The Tai Chi instructor should be appropriately qualified (Chen and Snyder 1999).

To summarise, the major aims of exercise in rheumatoid arthritis are to:

- maintain joint range of movement
- reduce joint stiffness
- maintain/improve muscle power
- maintain/ improve postural control/stability
- prevent deformity
- improve cardiovascular fitness
- maintain/improve function
- improve sense of well-being
- maintain neurodynamics
- maintain bone density, especially at trabecular bone sites, wrist, hip and spine (the sites most at risk of osteoporosis)
- improve balance and coordination
- prevent falls
- maintain dexterity, especially in the upper limb
- maintain function and independence.

Hydrotherapy

When patients return for further treatment after a flare of their disease, a large percentage will state that hydrotherapy was the most useful treatment modality. Consequently many pools have local support groups that have organised evening hydrotherapy sessions for patients to continue once NHS treatment has been completed for that episode of care. This is obviously beneficial to the patient but also allows the therapist to review patients and assess any problems immediately they arise. This allows early discussion with medical teams to review problems. The physiotherapist can then utilise the properties of water to achieve desired goals with clinical reasoning (Hall et al. 1990).

Another article by Hall et al. (1996) evaluates the benefit of hydrotherapy and exercise for patients with RA. The buoyancy of the water allows the patient to have reduced weight bearing on their joints – and is depth dependent – so the person can easily over-exert. The physiotherapist should therefore deliberately under-treat the patient on the first session and evaluate the effects to gain the patient's confidence in the water and in the physiotherapist. The physiotherapist can then sensitively increase the resistance from buoyancy-assisted to buoyancy-resisted with large buoyancy devices. The only limit is the physiotherapist's imagination. The risk of joint damage from repetitive movements is minimised in the water. Large amounts of resistance can be applied to increase muscle strength. The potential to increase cardiovascular fitness is also great in the pool.

Stenstrom et al. (1991) undertook hydrotherapy research in RA patients. Patients attended weekly dynamic training in water. Those who attended required fewer admissions for RA and had higher activity levels and improved grip strength compared with controls who did not attend. Dial and Windsor (1985) reported similar findings and further studies are under way.

Key point

In today's economic climate further evidence for hydrotherapy is required, as it is an expensive treatment modality with high staff and maintenance costs.

Professional organisations in rheumatology

British Health Professionals in Rheumatology [www.rheumatology.org.uk/BHPR]

Rheumatic Care Association of chartered physiotherapists [www.csp.org.uk]

British Society for Rheumatology [www.rheumatology.org.uk]

Arthritis Research Campaign [www.arc.org.uk]

OSTEOPOROSIS: BASIC ISSUES

Definitions

Osteoporosis may be defined as a disease characterised by low bone mass and microarchitectural deterioration of bone tissue leading to increased bone fragility and a consequent increase in fracture risk (Consensus Development Conference 1991).

Osteopenia is the term used to describe the state of sufficiently reduced bone mineral density conducive to fracture following a fall or other significant trauma. It may be transient (Lundon 2000).

Introduction

Osteoporosis affects 1 in 3 women and 1 in 12 men aged over 50 years and it costs the British government approximately £1.5 billion per year. With an ageing population, the medical and social costs of skeletal fragility will cause a huge burden to our future society unless effective prophylactic and therapeutic regimens can be developed (Wolff et al. 1999).

Physiotherapy management approaches for people with osteoporosis vary within the United Kingdom. Reasons for this include different staffing levels, facilities, traditions, funding arrangements, and whether treatment is within an outpatient cubicle, in a gymnasium or in the patient's home. People may be seen individually or in groups. These differences seem to be due to differing knowledge of the pathophysiology of osteoporosis and the current evidence base, or the physiotherapist's fear of causing fractures during treatment.

Osteoporosis is encountered in many different departments within a general hospital, so who should take the main responsibility is an important question. The following specialties may all be involved:

- general medicine
- respiratory care
- care of the elderly
- gynaecology
- renal
- orthopaedics
- rheumatology
- falls services
- immunology.

Osteoporosis has been called 'the silent epidemic' in that it often does not present any signs or symptoms until a fracture occurs (Hawker 1996). Plain X-rays are not particularly effective at highlighting osteoporosis, since bone loss must exceed 30–40% before it becomes visible radiographically (Johnston and Epstein 1981).

Many physiotherapists will see patients with osteoporosis only after a fracture and aim for safe mobilising with a frame to enable discharge home. This is necessary, but such a reactive approach does little to minimise the risk of further fractures. Patients should therefore be provided with weight-bearing exercises, and measures to improve balance and coordination for the prevention of falls. People with hip fractures secondary to osteoporosis often stay in hospital for prolonged rehabilitation. This should allow physiotherapists the opportunity to assess their gait, muscle strength, balance and coordination to prevent further fractures. Preferably patients should be advised after a Colles' fracture, or even prior to any fracture aiming to prevent a hip fracture.

The familial nature of osteoporosis means that while treating the osteoporotic person there is a unique opportunity to counsel the family on fracture prevention and to optimise peak bone density in young children. Prevention of osteoporosis is especially important when one considers today's sedentary lifestyle, and the teaching of health promotion strategies for bone health is essential (Sedlak et al. 1998).

The Risks of Osteoporosis

Groups/lifestyles at risk

See Table 12.1.

Table 12.1 Groups/lifestyles at risk of osteoporosis.

- Early menopause (at age below 45 years)
- Thin body type
- Hysterectomy
- Anorexia
- Heredity component
- Rheumatoid arthritis
- High alcohol intake
- High caffeine intake
- Insufficient daily calcium and vitamin D intake (1000 mg/day with hormone replacement or 1500 mg/day without hormone replacement is recommended – NIH consensus panel 1994)
- Physical inactivity and smoking (regular exercise and not smoking are important factors in achieving maximal peak bone mass in adolescents – Valimaki et al. 1994)

Source: Taken from CSP (1999) guidelines

Anatomical sites at risk

Trabecular bone has a large surface area compared with cortical bone. Cancellous bone is more sensitive to the remodelling changes of osteoporosis. This means that the parts of the skeleton that are most at risk are the sites with a high proportion of cancellous bone. These are the neck of femur, the distal radius and the vertebral body.

ASSESSMENT IN OSTEOPOROSIS

Further to research evaluating the knowledge of Scottish and Swedish physiotherapists in interventions on osteoporosis (Ritson and Scott 1996), a set of osteoporosis physiotherapy guidelines were initiated (CSP/NOS 1999). These guidelines are a valuable source of information, but physiotherapists should also continue to continually seek further evidence and treat efficaciously. Physiotherapy training programmes for osteoporotic patients have demonstrated improved balance, better level of daily function, decreased pain and use of analgesics, and improvement in quality of life (Malmros et al. 1998)

Guidelines

The CSP/NOS (1999) guidelines give clear information on assessment. It should include:

- previous medical and social history
- metrology
- function
- pain

- general mobility
- possibly aerobic testing
- quality-of-life measures.

Assessment should take in measurement of the person's height to provide an objective measure for future comparison purposes, as patients will often lose height following each vertebral fracture. Height will vary with other factors such as diurnal rhythms. Patients will often regain some height after rehabilitation, so some of the height loss must be postural.

Tragus or occiput to wall measurement or a flexion curve should be used to assess posture and evaluate the effects of treatment interventions (Laurent et al. 1991). This can be exacerbated by weak trunk extensor muscles. Schober's trunk extension (Moll et al. 1972) and trunk lateral flexion assess spinal mobility and highlight any balance or pain limitations that are present. Some patients can appear to have quite good balance mechanisms until one is measuring lateral flexion against a wall, which inhibits many of their compensatory mechanisms.

Clinically, trunk extension does not seem to provide the physiotherapist with much useful data: the range of movement can improve but the significance of this is unclear. Most patients have only 1 cm of movement and the maximum seen in the author's unit has been 3.5 cm after rehabilitation.

Tools

There are many validated tools that can be used to assess function. The clinically important aspects of any such tools are repeatability, minimal inter-therapist variation, and speed of assessment.

One of the simplest tools is the timed up-and-go test (TUG; Podsiadlo and Richardson 1991). The TUG times a patient standing from a chair (no arms), walking 5 metres and returning to sit down; the average is 15 seconds but patients have varied from 12 seconds to over 2 minutes. This is quite easy to improve with intervention. Other tests such as functional reach, timed stairs or dressing may all be used (Lyles et al. 1993; Helmes et al. 1995).

Upper and lower limb mobility and range of movement should be assessed. Many people with osteoporosis develop a kyphosis, so glenohumeral range of movement may be inhibited with consequent limitation of function (Pearlmutter et al. 1995).

Pain levels should also be monitored, and the easiest method is a visual analogue score (Scott and Huskisson 1976; Melzack 1983). A pain or analgesia diary can also be used but is time-consuming.

Assessments

The physiotherapist should assess subjectively and objectively according to Maitland or other similar principles.

Objective assessment should not include accessory mobilisations of the spine because of the potential risk of further fracture and increase in pain. Many patients with osteoporosis experience falls; this could be due to altered proprioceptive and kinaesthetic awareness from a kyphosis or altered posture. A record should be maintained of the number of falls, reasons for falls and any injuries sustained.

PHYSIOTHERAPY FOR PEOPLE WITH OSTEOPOROSIS

General Mobility and Re-education of Balance

Balance and mobility need to be addressed to prevent falls and fractures. Often the safest place to treat these patients to prevent injury is the hydrotherapy pool. Here the risk of falling and fracture is much reduced provided the patients are safely managed in the surrounding areas. This must always be reviewed for patients with renal problems as a primary cause for their osteoporosis. Balance can be enhanced by the use of metacentric exercises using turbulence and by exercising on a woggle (Reid Campion 1990). Immersed patients often experience significant pain relief and buoyancy will assist range of movement and can then be progressed to resist movement for strengthening (Levine 1984).

All patients must be able to summon muscle control of their full range of movement. This is because when they fall they will fall into outer range of movement and if they have no muscle control they are more likely to loose control of their movement and sustain a fracture. The action of muscle and tendon 'pull' on bone will also stimulate osteoblast activity (Nordin and Frankel 1989). Whilst is it true that weight-bearing activity stimulates bone remodelling, hydrotherapy alone does not increase bone density. However, the effects of large amounts of resistance in water remains unknown. Consequently patients also need a land-based exercise programme that they can continue independently.

The high-risk areas for fracture are areas of high trabecular bone content – wrist, neck of femur and vertebral body. Treatment and exercise must be especially targeted at these at risk areas. Trunk flexion should be avoided because it poses a high risk of vertebral fracture due to the biomechanics on the trabecular tissue (Myers and Wilson 1997).

Osteoporosis patients are often not as fragile as first thought, in that they can lift surprising amounts of weight (Kerr et al. 1996).

Research

There has been a great deal of research into exercise and osteoporosis treatment and prevention in a wide age range; see for example Chow et al. (1989), Berard et al. (1997), Joakimsen et al. (1997), Wolff et al. (1999) and Kemper (2000). There has been more osteoporosis research in women than in men, but slowly more research is appearing for men; see for example Kelley et al. (2000) and Maddslozzo and Snow (2000). Frequent literature searches are important for physiotherapists working with osteoporosis to ensure that their treatments are effective.

Balance exercise are important means of fracture prevention (Gardner et al. 2000; Kannus 1999; Suomi and Koceja 2000; Steinberg et al. 2000). Tai Chi is a good postural exercise which is weight-bearing and will therefore increase bone mineral density. Tai Chi has been shown to improve balance and reduce blood pressure (Hong et al. 2000), and it is one of the few modalities that have prevented falls in the elderly population. Information about Tai Chi classes, the Alexander technique, Pilates or yoga should be investigated in the local area. Close links with these groups can be useful.

Advice on exercise to prevent osteoporosis for the rest of the family – such as racquet and team sports, skipping or weight-lifting – is very important. Families need to exercise to obtain the highest peak bone mass possible, although this is more genetically predetermined than was realised even very recently. Once obtained, bone density should be maintained with diet and lifestyle measures such as exercise to reduce the rate of loss of density.

Advice booklets such as those provided by the National Osteoporosis Society (Bassey 2000) are readily available so there is no need to reinvent the wheel. Lifestyle advice such as diet, reduction in smoking and alcohol intake is important. Many patients will not have the luxury of a dietitian to advise them, but information is available and physiotherapists should be able to facilitate referral to this or other professions to ensure holistic care. The causes of osteoporosis are multifactorial and so is the risk of fracture, so effective use of the multidisciplinary team is very important. The use of occupational therapy for difficult tasks such as dressing, ironing, vacuuming or getting in and out of

the bath is raised at every patient discussion session. Liaison with ophthalmologists and ear, nose and throat physicians may also be relevant for vestibular, vision and dizziness problems.

Physiotherapists now have a great deal of evidence in support of the use of exercise to maintain bone mineral density (BMD). Its effects are equal to that of hormone replacement therapy (HRT) and if used in conjunction with HRT the effects are enhanced (Cheng et al. 2000).

If a person's BMD is maintained and balance is improved, the risk of a fall and subsequent fracture is also reduced. General practitioners and consultants should be aware of patients at risk and refer to physiotherapy early to prevent fractures.

Many patients are referred for physiotherapy only once they are in excruciating pain from vertebral fractures or if they have harassed their doctors on multiple occasions. This is not the case with everyone but is unfortunately more frequent than prompt or preventative referrals. The physiotherapy profession is partly responsible for not undertaking large amounts of research on the holistic management of osteoporosis. This is exacerbated by clinicians working up to and beyond limitations of staffing levels in the present economic climate, and recruitment difficulties.

Specific modalities

Pain relief

People with osteoporosis need to remain active, so it is essential that their pain be adequately controlled. Following assessment of a person with osteoporosis, the physiotherapist aims to:

* control and monitor pain levels
* gain the patient's trust and confidence
* ensure compliance and willingness to persevere with treatments
* increase and maintain muscle strength, balance and cardiovascular fitness
* provide education to facilitate long-term self-management of the condition.

Patient education is important because the evidence suggests that weight-bearing exercise must be continued and progressed for at least 9 months, and once discontinued the effects are reversible (Drinkwater 1994).

Treatments should be simple enough to enable the person to continue them at home. Patients will not have a private therapist available in the middle of the night to apply interferential for example. Self-management should be a priority. The physiotherapist has a wide repertoire of pain-relieving modalities, including transcutaneous electrical nerve stimulation (TENS;

Gadsby et al. 1996), acupuncture and non-invasive acupuncture (Ernst and White 1998), heat with all adequate warnings given, hydrotherapy (Hall et al. 1996) and postural correction. Many patients try alternative treatments such as aromatherapy and reflexology, but evidence to support these is limited at present.

Postural correction

Advice should be given regarding sleeping positions with particular attention to the cervical spine and hips, which are common sites of discomfort. The use of McKenzie rolls or similar for the lumbar spine should be advised for sitting and reiterated for use when travelling to improve posture and relieve some discomfort. Ergonomic advice with regard to sitting positions should be given and the correct use of office seating, armchairs and so on should be highlighted. Information regarding local centres such as the Disabled Living Foundation should be provided for each individual. Liaison with occupational therapists or occupational health services as a means of improving ergonomics and consequently pain relief should always be considered for relevant patients, because osteoporosis does not affect only retired post-menopausal women! Further self-management advice is applicable in some instances, such as the Alexander technique.

Breathing exercises

Breathing exercises are beneficial for many patients. Some patients experience pain from vertebral fractures on deep inhalation and coughing, so they develop a reduced depth of inhalation and are at further risk of chest infection. The greater the kyphosis deformity, the greater the risk of infection. An active cycle of breathing and diaphragmatic breathing should be taught. This is especially important in patients with secondary osteoporosis from excessive steroid usage to control respiratory pathologies.

Relaxation

Relaxation can be very beneficial for patients with osteoporosis. The use of imagery and the Lara Mitchell method can be very useful (Bell and Saltikov 2000). Contract–relax methods have been subjectively reported by patients to increase pain levels, possibly because of the level of muscle tension prior to starting the relaxation technique. This is often an ideal time to introduce patients to occupational therapists who can assist them in many ways.

Pacing

The concept of pacing within pain management is important for these patients who are learning to cope with a chronic painful condition. It is important to advise patients on a gradual increase of their exercise repetitions as well as intensity, and amount of weight used. Much of this is common sense but patients may need further guidance and reassurance that they are increasing their exercise intensity correctly (Harding and Watson 2000). The pacing of activities of daily living (ADL) and planning activities can easily be undertaken by occupational therapists. Patients often feel that if they do too much exercise or mobilisation they will sustain fractures. Patients need to load the trabecular bone areas especially with gravity and weight to stimulate osteoblast activity.

OSTEOPOROSIS: A CASE STUDY

About the Patient

Ms S was a 71-year-old woman with a 3-year history of recurrent back pain. She was referred by her general practitioner with 'back pain, poor posture and kyphosis, awaiting investigations for osteoporosis'. Her referral had not been marked as urgent.

On entering the physiotherapy department Ms S had to be supported by her sister as she was standing in a stooped posture at almost a 45-degree angle. She was supporting her trunk to relieve some pain by pushing her hands on her thighs. She could sit for only 5 minutes without having to shuffle in the chair to ease her discomfort. She had never been seen previously by a physiotherapist.

Subjective examination

Ms S complained of constant lumbar and occasional buttock pain, with an intensity estimated to be 8/10. The pain would wake her every night if she lay on either side. Her pain was made worse in flexion or standing, especially if she attempted to stand upright, owing to the effort it required. Sitting with a cushion to support her lumbar spine eased the pain. Pain increased during the day and was dependent on the level of activity. She stated that she 'feels like I'm going to collapse' by the evening. This has affected her confidence and she has not been out of the house for several weeks.

Ms S had had a hysterectomy at age 46 and was not prescribed hormone replacement therapy. Didronel, a bisphosphonate drug used to rebuild bone density, was commenced 4 weeks previously.

Objective assessment

On X-ray there was partial collapse of L1 and L2. DEXA, a type of bone mineral density scan used to diagnose osteoporosis, was not undertaken.

Ms S's height was measured and her posture noted. Her gait was observed and ability to undertake functional activities such as dressing were also noted. A complete objective assessment was not possible at the first visit owing to her discomfort. Pain was recorded at 9/10 using a visual analogue scale (VAS).

Short-term aims of treatment

- Decrease pain to 5/10 on Visual analogue scale.
- Improve posture.
- Gain confidence in the therapist.
- Improve patient confidence to the point where Ms S can go out to the shops again.
- Improve trunk extensor muscle strength.

Long-term aims of treatment

- Maintain and improve bone mineral density.
- Maintain activity levels to minimise the risk of falls.
- Refer to a dietitian/advise re diet.
- Attend osteoporosis group treatment and education programme.
- Recommence leisure activities.

Ms S's Treatment

Ms S needed pain control and to quickly regain some extensor muscle strength. On her first visit she was advised about the use of heat to ease muscle spasm and given a lumbar support using a towel. In a later session she was advised about products available on the market. She was given gentle lumbar rotations to relieve pain and instructed to only undertake the movements within the pain free range of movement. She was also shown shoulder girdle retraction exercises to gain some global recruitment to attain postural stability. Use of TENS was discussed as a future option, but since frequently simple measures were effective it was not administered at this time.

Hydrotherapy

Ms S was treated individually in the hydrotherapy pool. She was initially scared of water so needed much reassurance and support. On her first hydrotherapy treatment session further rotation was undertaken and gentle physiological extension and abduction hip exercises commenced to increase her water confidence, balance and eventually muscle strength. She was encouraged to allow the physiotherapist to facilitate supine exercises for trunk extension. With reassurance this was undertaken and a large amount of pain relief was gained in a short session of approximately 10 min-

utes. The benefits of buoyancy especially supported her weak trunk and facilitated normal sensory feedback. The warmth of the water provided her with a degree of relaxation. Spinal column lengthening could be one of the reasons for her improvement.

After three sessions of hydrotherapy and the exercises noted above, peers and family reported huge improvements to Ms S's quality of life, pain control and posture. Muscle imbalance exercises were considered but, because of the patient's fear of movement, positive feedback of movement was required and patient comprehension of stability exercises can be variable so were not undertaken.

Long-term self-management

After four individual hydrotherapy sessions Ms S was prepared to join the osteoporosis group for treatment. The aim of this group is to teach patients self-management and to be in control of their own condition. It involves an education component; gym exercises and hydrotherapy. The group session lasts for one and half hours each week for 5 weeks.

The benefits of group treatments include social interaction and meeting others in a similar situation. The exchange of ideas and helpful tips are all very useful but the strength of the motivational force of exercising with others is immense. Advice aims to be holistic but with recognition of professional boundaries. Patients are encouraged to seek further advice from dietitians, general practitioners, consultants, and the nurse adviser helpline at the National Osteoporosis Society (NOS). Advice includes a description of the pathology of osteoporosis, which physiotherapists are often in a unique position to undertake as they have longer face to face interactions with patients. In a group setting this is even more cost-effective. Information on diet, smoking and alcohol consumption and exercise is given. Relatives are given the NOS at-risk questionnaire if they are concerned, and are advised to discuss the issues with their GP, thus hopefully starting the prevention cycle as soon as possible. Advice on diet and lifestyle for grandchildren can also be easily implemented to obtain the highest peak bone density.

A session is presented by an occupational therapist (OT) and patients always mention difficult tasks such as getting in and out of the bath, hoovering, and standing to prepare food or similar. The OT or other members of the group usually find practical solutions. Difficulties with driving are addressed by demonstrating various mirrors. Patients are informed of the local disabled living centre. Postural advice is always important. The biomechanical changes after a vertebral fracture are discussed and the reason for kyphosis due to anterior wedging of the vertebrae (Myers and Wilson 1997).

Ms S had never had a description like this to understand why she was so kyphosed. This helped to explain the benefits of the exercise programme. The educational aspect of the group was evaluated positively by Ms S, since it motivated her to improve her own condition. She was advised about lumbar supports and now asserts that the lumbar support used on her recent coach holiday is what made the difference between a painful journey and an enjoyable holiday.

Ms S undertook an exercise programme that followed pain management principles, a graded exercise programme and graded exposure to increased weights, resistance, and stamina (Harding and Watson 2000). Exercises in the gym start in a comfortable sitting position. Patients are then shown mat exercises such as 'angry cat' trunk extension, and thoracic mobilisation in prone kneeling and reminded that target zones are the wrist, hip and spine because of their trabecular content. Exercises in prone kneeling are encouraged as they will encourage osteoblast activity in the three vital areas all at once as Ms S exercises against gravity. Thus if patients get bored and want to do only a few exercises, all areas will be enhanced (Chow et al. 1989; Joakimsen et al. 1997; Wolff et al. 1999; Kelley 1998; Maddslozzo and Kannus 1999). No equipment is used initially in order to remind patients that they can easily continue independently at home.

Exercises with light weights starting at 0.5 kg and progressing as pain allowed were commenced, targeting wrist and hip (Kerr et al. 1996). Proprioceptive neuromuscular facilitation (PNF) patterns were utilised for their effect on many muscle groups, especially rotation at the fragile femoral neck with theraband or resistance. Finally a circuit was undertaken to increase cardiovascular fitness, muscle strength, balance, stamina and coordination. Each patient was motivated to reach their own potential and the use of similar equipment in local sports centres was reiterated. Games such as dribbling a ball around cones and basketball are used to improve balance and coordination extension of the trunk while weight-bearing on the hips and spine are encouraged (Gardner et al. 2000; Steinberg et al. 2000) The use of a ball increases automatic responses and reduces the fear of falling.

Getting up from the floor was not practised with Ms S as she started the exercises on a plinth and then in the circuit the same exercises were undertaken on a floor mat. This reduces the fear of getting on the floor and making a big issue of it. Ms S was very surprised when she was able to regain her self-esteem at being able to do this independently without thinking

As Ms S was continuing with the land programme, the hydrotherapy programme is usually one step ahead and similar muscle groups are worked in the hydrotherapy pool the week prior to the gym. There is a gradual progression from gentle movements and gait to aquarobics to increase balance and coordination and cardiovascular fitness. The pool has a dramatic effect on the cardiovascular system. The use of increasing surface area and lever length gradually increases the amount of resistance. Swimming alone will not increase bone mineral density, owing to the lack of gravity pull. Reduction of the base of support, speed and turbulence are all utilised. One of the most difficult tasks for Ms S was drawing underwater with one foot while weight-bearing on the other limb; this can be a very useful exercise for balance and coordination.

Supine exercises with increasing amounts of resistance from buoyancy devices were used for trunk extension and lateral flexion. Also very difficult for Ms S was aquastep owing to coordination difficulties, but due to the buoyancy and support offered by the water with a much-lessened risk of fracture this improved. The risk of getting her hair wet was much more daunting initially. In the pool, Ms S initially had to stand on a step of approximately 15 cm because of her height loss, but in the fifth session she was in the deep end joining in the striding exercises before she realised her great improvement in height.

Ms S was given information regarding hip protectors because of her high risk of falling, but she declined the use of these for unstated reasons. Ms S was advised of the NOS booklets, which cover all areas of self-management. She was also advised about the information sheets provided by the NOS. With several other members of the group she would sometimes attend up to one hour early to read these. Questions would then be answered and any problems with the week's home work and exercise regimen discussed. Ms S was advised of the benefits of Tai Chi and given contact details of a local centre that was undertaking research into balance in the elderly. Other members of her group have taken up yoga or Pilates.

Ms S attends the evening NOS hydrotherapy sessions on a weekly basis. This is very impressive for someone who had initially been so scared of water. She claims excellent pain relief and stiffness control and she always sleeps well the night after hydrotherapy but can be a bit 'achy' the next day. Ms S is exceptionally motivated and consistently continues her exercise programme. She undertook a demonstration of hydrotherapy one day and requested if it was all right to not do her exercises that evening as she had attended the pool; she quickly reassured the physiotherapist that she had done her home exercises twice already that day, 30 minutes each time. She continues so regularly because she states it controls her pain and maintains her posture and thus her self-esteem and respect. She has not yet purchased a TENS unit but has the purchase details.

Conclusion

One of the physiotherapist's concerns about Ms S was that, since she exercised so regularly, the programme would become too easy for her and the osteoblasts would become accustomed to the programme. Consequently variety and increased weight have been reinforced. What would have happened to this woman if she had been referred earlier is an interesting question. Would she have been so compliant with the advice given? Was the excruciating pain she had experienced preventable? Further research into the effects of hydrotherapy in osteoporosis patients is required for evidence to support very positive subjective feedback from patients, and a review of holistic care of osteoporosis would be very beneficial. Ms S's case highlights that physiotherapy has much to offer people with osteoporosis, and that this person has not fallen or sustained any further fractures is evidence in itself.

REFERENCES

Alderson M, Starr L, Gow S, Moreland J 1999 The program for rheumatic independent self-management: a pilot evaluation. Clin Rheumatol 18: 283–92

Angst F, Aeschlimann A, Steiner W, Stucki G 2001 The responsiveness of the WOMAC Osteoarthritis index as compared with the SF 36 in patients with osteoarthritis of the legs undergoing a comprehensive rehabilitation intervention. Ann Rheum Dis 60: 834–40

Bassey J 2000 Exercise and Osteoporosis, London: National Osteoporosis Society

Bell JA, Saltikov JB 2000 Mitchell's relaxation technique: is it effective? Physiotherapy 86: 473–8

Berard A, Bravo G, Gauthier P 1997 Meta-analysis of the effectiveness of physical activity for the prevention of bone loss in post menopausal women. Osteopor Int 7: 331–7

Berman BM, Singh BB, Lao L et al. 1999 A randomised trial of acupuncture as an adjunctive therapy in osteoarthritis of the knee. Rheumatology 38: 346–54

Buljina AI, Taljanovic MS, Avdic DM, Hunter TB 2001 Physical and exercise therapy for treatment of the rheumatoid hand. Arthr Rheum 45: 392–7

Campbell R, Evans M, Tucker M et al. 2001 Why don't patients do their exercises? Understanding non-compliance with physiotherapy in patients with osteoarthritis of the knee. J Epidemiol Commun Health 55(2): 132–8

Carlsson CP, Sjolund BH 2001 Acupuncture for chronic low back pain: a randomized placebo-controlled study with long-term follow-up. Clin J Pain 14: 296–305

Carr A 2001 Defining the extended clinical role for allied health professionals in rheumatology. ARC Conference Proceedings no. 12

Chartered Society of Physiotherapy/National Osteoporosis Society 1999 Physiotherapy Guidelines for the Management of Osteoporosis. Chartered Society of Physiotherapy, 14 Bedford Row, London WC1R 4ED

Chen KM, Snyder M 1999 Research based use of Tai Chi/movement therapy as a nursing intervention. J Holist Nurs 17(3): 267–79

Cheng S, Sipila S, Puolakka J, Souminen H 2000 Effects of hormone replacement therapy and high impact physical exercise on bone/muscle ratio in postmenopausal women. Osteopor Int 11: S2

Chow R, Harrison J, Dornan J 1989 Prevention and rehabilitation of osteoporosis program: exercise and osteoporosis. Int J Rehab Res 1: 49–56

Clark BM 2000 Rheumatology 9: Physical and occupational therapy in the management of arthritis. CMAJ 163: 999–1005

Consensus Development Conference 1991 Prophylaxis and treatment of osteoporosis. Am J Med 90: 107–10

Cushnaghan J, McCarthy C, Dieppe P 1994 Taping the patella medially: a new treatment for osteoarthritis of the knee joint? BMJ 308: 753–5

David C, Lloyd J 1998 Rheumatological Physiotherapy. London: Mosby

Deyle GD, Henderson NE, Matekel RL et al. 2000 Effectiveness of manual physical therapy and exercise in osteoarthritis of the knee: a randomised controlled trial. Ann Intern Med 132(3): 173–81

Dhondt W, Willaeys T, Verbruggen LA et al. 1999 Pain threshold in patients with rheumatoid arthritis and effect of manual oscillations. Scand J Rheumatol 28(2): 88–93

Dial C, Windsor RA 1985 A formative evaluation of a health education water exercise program for class II and III adult rheumatoid arthritis patients. Patient Edu Counsel 7: 33–42

Dougados M, Ravaud P 2001 Exercise therapy in patients with osteoarthritis of the hip or knee. Curr Rheumatol Rep 3(5): 353–4

Drinkwater BL 1994 The McCloy research lecture: Does physical activity play a role in preventing osteoporosis? Res Quart Ex Sport 65(3): 197–206

Edmonds S, Turnbull C, Blake D 2001 Effect of intensive exercise on patients with active RA. Ann Rheum Dis 60(4): 429

Ernst E, White A 1998 Acupuncture for back pain: a meta-analysis of randomised controlled trials. Arch Intern Med 158: 9

Fransen M, Crosbie J, Edmonds J 2001 Physical therapy is effective for patients with osteoarthritis of the knee: a randomised controlled clinical trial. J Rheumatol 28(1): 156–64

Fredrikus GJ, Oosterveld, Rasker JJ 1994 Effects of local heat and cold treatment on surface and articular temperature of arthritic knees. Arthr Rheum 11: 1578–82

Fries JF, Spitz P, Kraines G, Holman H, 1980 Measurement of patient outcome in arthritis. Arthr Rheum 23: 137–45

Gadsby JG, Bennet A, Flowerdew MW 1996 The effectiveness of transcutaneous electrical nerve stimulation and acupuncture like transcutaneous electrical nerve stimulation in the treatment of patients with chronic low back pain. In CMSG Back Module of Cochrane database of systematic reviews

Gardner MM, Robertson MG, Campbell AJ 2000 Exercise in preventing falls and fall related injuries in older people: a review of randomised controlled trials. Br J Sports Med 34(1): 7–17

Gecht MR, Connell KJJ, Sinacore JM, Prohaska TR 1996 A survey of exercise beliefs and exercise habits among people with arthritis. Arthr Care Res 9(2): 82–8

Giorgino KB, Blalock SJ, DeVellis RF et al. 1994 Appraisal of and coping with arthritis related problems in household activities, leisure activities and pain management. Arthr Care Res 7(1): 20–8

Hall J, Bisson D, O'Hare P 1990 The physiology of immersion. Physiotherapy 76: 517–20

Hall J, Skevington S, Maddison P, Chapman K 1996 A randomised controlled trial of hydrotherapy in rheumatoid arthritis. Arthr Care Res 9(3): 206–16

Harding V, Watson P 2000 Increasing activity and improving function in chronic pain management. Physiotherapy 86: 619–30

Harrision R, Bulstrode S 1987 Percentage weight-bearing during partial immersion in a hydrotherapy pool. Physiother Pract 3(2): 60–3

Hart LE 2000 Combination of manual physical therapy and exercises for osteoarthritis of the knee. Clin Sport Med 10(4): 305

Hawker GA 1996 The epidemiology of osteoporosis. J Rheumatol Suppl 45: 2–5

Helmes E, Hodsman A et al. 1995 A questionnaire to evaluate disability in osteoporotic patients with vertebral compression fractures. J Gerontol A: Biol Sci Med Sci 50(2): M91–8

Hoffmann S, Theiler R 2001 Physiotherapy in osteoarthritis: a review of literature on conservative therapy of the hip and knee osteoarthritis. Ther Umsch 58(8): 480–6

Hong Y, Li JX, Robinson PD 2000 Balance control, flexibility and cardiorespiratory fitness among older Tai Chi-practitioners. Br J Sports Med 34: 29–34

Iversen MD, Fossel AH, Daltroy LH 1999 Rheumatologist–patient communication about exercise and physical therapy management of rheumatoid arthritis. Arthr Care Res 12(30): 180–92

Joakimsen RM, Magnus JH, Fonnebo V 1997 Physical activity and predisposition for hip fractures: a review. Osteopor Int 7: 503–13

Johnston CC Epstein S 1981 Clinical, biochemical, radiographic, epidemiologic, and economic features in osteoporosis. Orthoped Clin N Am 12: 559–69

Kannus P 1999 Preventing osteoporosis, falls, and fractures among elderly people. BMJ 318: 205–6

Katz P, Yelin EH 2001 Activity loss and the onset of depressive symptoms: do some activities matter more than others? Arthr Rheum 44(5): 1194–202

Kelley G 1998 Aerobic exercise and lumbar spine bone mineral density in post menopausal women meta analysis. J Am Geriatr Soc 46(2): 143–52

Kelley GA, Kelley KS, Tran ZV 2000 Exercise and bone mineral density in men: a meta-analysis. J Appl Physiol 88(5): 1730–6

Kemper HGC, Bakker I, van Tulder MW et al. 2000 Exercise for preventing low bone mass in young males and females (protocol). The Cochrane Library, issue 4, Oxford

Kerr D, Morton A, Dick I et al. 1996 Exercise effects on bone mass in postmenopausal women are site specific and load dependent. J Bone Min Res 11: 218–25

Kirwan J, Reeback JS 1986 Stanford health assessment questionnaire modified to assess disability in British patients with rheumatoid arthritis. Br J Rheumatol 25: 206–9

Laurent MR, Buchanan WW et al. 1991 Methods of assessment used in ankylosing spondylitis clinical trials: a review. Br J Rheumatol 30(5): 326–9

Lequesne MG 1997 The algofunctional indices for hip and knee osteoarthritis. J Rheumatol 24: 779–81

Levine BA 1984 Use of hydrotherapy in reduction of anxiety. Psychol Rep 55(2): 526

Lineker S, Badley E, Charles C, Hart L, Streiner D 1999 Defining morning stiffness in rheumatoid arthritis. J Rheumatol 26(5): 1052–7

Lineker SC, Bell MJ, Wilkins AL, Bradley EM 2001 Improvements following short term home based physical therapy are maintained at one year in people with moderate to severe rheumatoid arthritis. J Rheumatol 28(1): 165–8

Lorig K et al. 1994 Arthritis and musculoskeletal patient education standards. Arthr Care Res 7: 1–4

Lundon 2000 Orthopaedic Rehabilitation Science: Principles for Clinical Management of Bone. Oxford: Butterworth–Heinemann

Lyles KW, Gold DT et al. 1993 Association of osteoporotic vertebral compression fractures with impaired functional status. Am J Med 94(6): 595–601

Maddslozzo GF, Snow CM 2000 High intensity resistance training: effects on bone in older men and women. Calcified Tiss Int 66(6): 399–404

Maitland G 1991 Peripheral Joint Assessment, 3rd edn. Oxford: Butterworth–Heinemann

Malmros BL, Mortensen L et al. 1998 Positive effects of physiotherapy on chronic pain and performance in osteoporosis. Osteopor Int 8(3): 215–21

Marks R 2001 Efficacy theory and its utility in arthritis rehabilitation: review and recommendations. Disabil Rehabil 23(7): 271–80

Massengill JB 1992 The Boutonnière deformity. Hand Clin 8: 787–801

Matthis C, Weber U, O'Neill TW et al. 1998 Health impact associated with vertebral deformities: results from the European vertebral osteoporosis study. Osteopor Int 8: 364–72

Maurer BT, Stern AG, Kinossian B et al. 1999 Osteoarthritis of the knee: isokinetic quadriceps exercise versus an educational intervention. Arch Phys Med Rehabil 80(10): 1293–9

Mayer ME 2000 Physical therapy and exercise in osteoarthritis of the knee. Ann Intern Med 132(11): 923

McMeeken J, Stillman B, Story I et al. 1999 The effects of knee extensor and flexor muscle training on the timed up and go test in individuals with rheumatoid arthritis. Physiother Res Int 4(1): 55–67

Meenan RF, Mason JH, Anderson JJ et al. 1992 AIMS2: the content and properties of a revised and expanded Arthritis Impact Measurement Scales health status questionnaire. Arthr Rheum 35(1): 1–10

Melzack R 1983 The McGill pain questionnaire. In: Melzack R (ed.) Pain Measurement and Assessment, pp. 41–46. New York: Raven Press

Mohomed NN 2000 Manual physical therapy and exercise improved function in osteoarthritis of the knee. J Bone Joint Surg Am 82(9): 1324

Moll JM, Liyanage SP et al. 1972 An objective clinical method to measure spinal extension. Rheumatol Phys Med 11(6): 293–312

Myers ER, Wilson SE 1997 Biomechanics of osteoporosis and vertebral fracture. Spine 22: 25S–31S

NIH Consensus Statement 1994 Optimal calcium intake. 12(4): 1–31

Nordin M, Frankel VH 1989 Basic Biomechanics of the Musculoskeletal System. Baltimore: Lippincott Williams & Wilkins

O'Reilly SC, Muir KR, Doherty M 1999 Effectiveness of home exercise on pain and disability from osteoarthritis of the knee: a randomised controlled trial. Ann Rheum Dis 58(1): 9–15

Pearlmutter LL, Bode BY et al. 1995 Shoulder range of motion in patients with osteoporosis. Arthr Care Res 8(3): 194–8

Penninx BW, Messier SP, Rejeski WJ et al. 2001 Physical exercise and the prevention of disability in activities of daily living in older persons with osteoarthritis. Arch Intern Med 161(19): 2309–16

Philadelphia Panel 2001 Philadelphia Panel evidence-based clinical practice guidelines on selected rehabilitation interventions for knee pain. Phys Ther 81: 1675–700

Podsiadlo D, Richardson S 1991 The timed 'up & go': a test of basic functional mobility for frail elderly persons. J Am Geriatr Soc 39(2): 142–8

Prevoo MLL et al. 1995 Modified disease activity scores that include 28 joint counts: development and validation in a prospective longitudinal study of patients with rheumatoid arthritis. Arthr Rheum 38: 44–8

Rall LC, Meydani SN, Kehayias JJ et al. 1996 The effect of progressive resistance training in rheumatoid arthritis. Arthr Rheum 39(3): 415–26

Reid Campion M 1990 Adult Hydrotherapy: a Practical Approach, pp. 3–39. Oxford: Heinemann

Ritchie DM, Boyle JA, McInnes JM et al. 1968 Clinical studies with an articular index for the assessment of joint tenderness in patients with rheumatoid arthritis. QJM 37: 393–406

Ritson F, Scott S 1996 Physiotherapy for osteoporosis. a pilot study comparing practice and knowledge in Scotland and Sweden. Physiotherapy 82(7): 390–4

Rogind H, Nielson BB, Jensen B, Moller HC 2001 A Controlled trial of training in knee arthritis. Ugeske Laeger 163(27): 3798–802

Scholten C, Brodowicz T, Graninger W et al. 1999 Persistent functional and social benefit 5 years after a multi-disciplinary arthritis training program. Arch Phys Med Rehabil 80(10): 1282–7

Scott J, Huskisson EC 1976 Graphic representation of pain. Pain 2(2): 175–84

Sedlak CA, Doheny MO, Jones SL 1998 Osteoporosis prevention in young women. Orthop Nurs 17(3): 53–60

Sinclair VG, Wallston KA, Dwyer KA et al. 1998 Effects of a cognitive–behavioral intervention for women with rheumatoid arthritis. Res Nurs Health 21(4): 315–25

Smolen JS, Breedveld, FC, Eberl G et al. 1995 Validity and reliability of the 28-joint count for the assessment of rheumatoid arthritis activity. Arthr Rheum 38(1): 38–43

Steinberg M, Cartwright C, Peel N et al. 2000 A sustainable programme to prevent falls and near falls in community dwelling older people: results of a randomised controlled trial. J Epidem Comm Health 54(3): 227–32

Stenstrom C 1994 Therapeutic exercise in rheumatoid arthritis. Arthr Care Res 7(4): 190–7

Steultjens MP, Dekker J, Bijlsma JW 2001 Coping, pain and disability in osteoarthritis: a longitudinal study. J Rheumatol 28(5): 1068–72

Strahl C, Kleinknecht RA, Dinnel DL 2000 The role of pain anxiety, coping and pain self efficacy in rheumatoid arthritis patient functioning. Behav Res Ther 38(9): 863–73

Stenstrom CH, Lindell B, Swanberg E, Swanberg P 1991 Intensive dynamic training in water for rheumatoid arthritis functional Class II: a long term study of effects. Scand J Rheumatol 20: 358–65

Stewart M 1996 Researches into the effectiveness of physiotherapy in rheumatoid arthritis of the hand. Physiotherapy 82(12): 666–72

Suomi R, Koceja DM 2000 Postural sway characteristics in women with lower extremity arthritis before and after an aquatic exercise intervention. Arch Phys Med Rehabil 81(6): 780–5

Swenson C, Sward L, Karlsson J 1996 Cryotherapy in sports medicine. Scand J Med Sports Sci 6(4): 193–200

Sylvester KL 1989 Investigation of the effect of hydrotherapy in the treatment of osteoarthritic hips. Clin Rehabil 4: 223–8

Tugwell P, Boers M 1992 OMERACT conference on outcome measures in rheumatoid arthritis clinical trials: introduction. J Rheumatol 20: 528–30

Valimaki MJ et al. 1994 Exercise, smoking and calcium intake during adolescence and early childhood as determinants of peak bone mass: Cardiovascular Risk in Young Finns Study Group. BMJ 309: 230–5

Van Baar ME, Dekker J, Oostendorp RA et al. 2001 Effectiveness of exercise in patients with osteoarthritis of hip or knee: nine months follow up. Ann Rheum Dis 60(12): 1123–30

Van der Heijde DMFM et al. 1990 Judging disease activity in clinical practice in rheumatoid arthritis: first step in the development of a disease activity score. Ann Rheum Dis 49: 916–20

Van den Ende CH, Breedveld FC, Le Cessie S et al. 2000 Effect of intensive exercise on patient with active rheumatoid arthritis. Ann Rheum Dis 59(8): 615–21

Van Lankveld W, Naring G, Van't Pad Bosch P, vande Putte L 2000 The negative effect of decreasing the level of activity in coping with pain in rheumatoid arthritis: an increase in psychological distress and disease impact. J Behav Med 23(4): 377–91

Ware JE, Snow KK, Kosinski M, Gandek B 1993 SF36 Health Survey: Manual and Interpretation Guide. Boston: The Health Institute, New England Medical Center

Williams JG, Callaghan M 1990 Comparison of visual estimation and goniometry in determination of shoulder joint angle. Physiotherapy 76: 655–7

Wolff I, van Croonenborg JJ, Kemper HC et al. 1999 The effect of exercise training programs on bone mass: a meta-analysis of published controlled trials in pre and post menopausal women. Osteopor Int 9: 1–12

Yurtkuran M, Kocagil T 1999 TENS, electroacupuncture and ice massage: comparison of treatment for osteoarthritis of the knee. Am J Acupunct 27(3/4): 133–40

Physiotherapy Management of Ankylosing Spondylitis

Juliette O'Hea

13

Physiotherapy is a key component in the management of ankylosing spondylitis (AS) and intervention should take place as early as possible following diagnosis. Owing to the chronic nature of the disease, people with AS must take control and responsibility for their own overall management. The task of the physiotherapist is to empower patients by increasing their knowledge of the disease and self-management principles. The patients need to know and believe that investment of time and energy into an exercise programme will result in a meaningful improvement in their quality of life.

AIMS OF PHYSIOTHERAPY MANAGEMENT

The overall aims are to minimise deformity and disability and to improve well-being, thereby maintaining normal function and improving the person's quality of life. Specifically these aims can be achieved by:

- advising on postural awareness and ergonomics
- reducing pain
- maintaining and improving posture and function by (a) increasing mobility of spinal, costovertebral and peripheral joints, (b) strengthening the antigravity muscles, and (c) stretching specific muscle groups
- improving and maintaining cardiovascular fitness
- monitoring posture, mobility and function through regular assessment
- devising and monitoring a home programme of specific exercises that are suitable and consistent with long-term compliance
- imparting knowledge about the disease and its management
- improving the person's psychological state, coping strategies and exercise compliance.

POSTURE

In the early stages of the disease a flattening of the lumbar curve may occur. Then, with increasing pain and a flexed posture, the thoracic curve can become more accentuated. If unchecked, this can be followed by a loss of the cervical curve and a protracted cervical spine develops as an attempt to compensate for the forward flexion. As the hips become more flexed, hip flexion contractures can occur and the knees flex to improve balance and vision. Poor posture results in muscle fatigue, weakness, disability and a poor body image. Good management of the disease should prevent poor posture from occurring, although any fusion may be delayed and not halted.

Figure 13.1 shows the typical postural deformities of advanced ankylosing spondylitis. Note especially the knee flexion and hip flexion deformities. The reason for these deformities is that, if the spine is constantly flexed as in this illustration, the patient would fall over forwards! By flexing the knees and hips, the person shifts the line of gravity back within the base to become more stable. This type of posture is biomechanically inefficient because the line of gravity falls outside the base of support, making prolonged standing a great effort.

Key point
Scoliosis does not usually exist to any significant degree in AS because pathological changes to the spinal column tend to be symmetrical.

Ergonomic considerations and postural correction

Ergonomic advice on how to maintain good posture at work, home and during leisure activities will improve the long-term outcome of the disease. The longer the patient assumes a flexed posture during the day and night, the more likely it is that the spine will assume a flexed position if the vertebrae fuse. This is particularly advisable if the patient has a job that requires a stooped

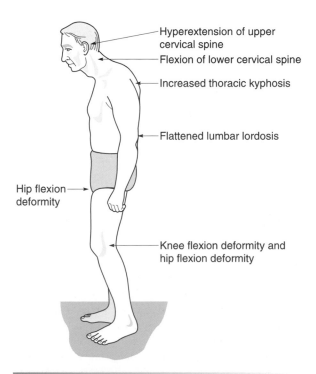

Hyperextension of upper cervical spine

Flexion of lower cervical spine

Increased thoracic kyphosis

Flattened lumbar lordosis

Hip flexion deformity

Knee flexion deformity and hip flexion deformity

Figure 13.1   The typical postural deformities of advanced ankylosing spondylitis.

posture (e.g. a dentist). The advice would be to get up and move around at regular intervals and check the posture regularly. An army officer may not need to check his posture so often! A flexed posture can relieve the pain but it ought to be discouraged.

Encourage the patient to maintain a good posture by walking tall and tucking the chin in. It may help to visualise being lifted up by a piece of string from the occiput. The posture can be checked in a mirror or by the patient standing as straight as possible against a wall, tucking the chin in. The person should try to maintain this posture when walking away from the wall.

Many of us lead sedentary lifestyles, so it is important to invest in chairs and car seats that are comfortable and supportive. Ideally any chair should provide support for the whole spine including the neck. The hips and knees should be at right-angles and the feet should be supported if they do not touch the floor. Forearms supported on arm rests can relieve tension in the neck.

Car seats that support both the neck and back are more comfortable and could reduce the risk of fracture if the person is involved in a road traffic accident. A close fit between the head and the head restraint, a head restraint that extends a minimum of 7 cm above the level of the eyes, and a restraint and seat that are designed as one system are recommended (Eriendsson 1998). Special internal and external car mirrors that can increase the field of vision can be purchased from the National Ankylosing Spondylitis Society (NASS).

For people who spend a lot of time at a computer, simple alterations such as altering the height of the computer screen and chair can make a significant difference. There are UK and EU regulations that require employers to assess the health and safety risks to employees (Health & Safety Executive 1994).

For specialist advice on seating (both at home, work and in the car), on beds and on work stations, referral to an ergonomist, to a specialist health professional or to a job centre Disability Enablement Officer (DEO) may be appropriate.

PAIN IN ANKYLOSING SPONDYLITIS

Pain may vary from low-grade discomfort to intense pain. Typically, pain is aggravated by inactivity and is often reduced by exercise. The perception of pain can be influenced by several factors, including fatigue (a common symptom of AS). Physiotherapy modalities such as ultrasound, acupuncture, transcutaneous nerve stimulation (TENS), megapulse and gentle spinal mobilisations (Bulstrode et al. 1987) can be effective, especially for localised pain. However this form of treatment should not be allowed to discourage the patient from ongoing participation in an exercise programme.

If the person has not exercised recently, exercises will need to be commenced gradually and the person warned that initially they may provoke pain. Wearing supportive shock-absorbing shoes can decrease the jarring effect of walking on hard surfaces and reduce the likelihood of aggravating the pain. Patients can be awoken at night by pain that can be alleviated with gentle exercise, heat and analgesics. The application of heat in the form of hot packs, a hot shower, bath or hydrotherapy can reduce pain by muscle relaxation and enable greater movement. Hydrotherapy is discussed later in the chapter.

EXERCISE IN ANKYLOSING SPONDYLITIS

General Issues

Regular, specific exercise is effective in the management of AS and patients should be made aware of its importance. It has a profound influence on how the disease affects the person in the long term. Non-steroidal anti-inflammatory drugs (NSAIDs) should control the pain adequately to allow exercise. Therefore, an understanding of how these medications work most effectively is important. With regular exercise, it may be possible to reduce the dose of the NSAID or stop it altogether.

Improvement in spinal mobility following exercise has been shown to be short-lived (e.g. O'Driscoll et al. 1978; Tomlinson et al. 1986; Viitanen et al. 1992) with long-term benefits remaining difficult to confirm. Exercise recommendations for people with AS differ substantially from advice given to patients with rheumatoid arthritis (Calin 1991) or osteoarthritis. Intensive physiotherapy regimens (Tomlinson et al. 1986; Viitanen et al. 1995) in a group situation (Hidding et al. 1993) and during inpatient programmes (Band et al. 1997) have been shown to be the most successful. However, it has been found that unless the exercise is supervised, intensive and sustained, progressive loss of movement can occur (Lubrano and Helliwell 1999).

Key point

A regular exercise pattern must start as early as possible following diagnosis and be performed for life. This requires a great deal of motivation on behalf of the patient. In the early more acute stages of AS, individual treatment may be preferable. The physiotherapist plays an essential role in providing the patient with ongoing education, stimulus and inspiration so that exercise becomes part of a daily routine.

Typically the symptoms of AS fluctuate. The person may experience acute exacerbations of pain and muscle spasm, chronic low-grade pain and quiescent periods. Whatever the symptoms, exercise should be continued regularly in order to prevent deterioration of posture with muscle weakness and shortening which could result in a loss of physical function. The person with AS should make the most of the relatively pain-free periods by exercising as vigorously as possible and maintaining a good general fitness level.

Joint Mobility Exercises

Flexion, extension, lateral flexion and rotation of the cervical, thoracic and lumbar spines can become limited in a person with AS owing to bony changes (formation of syndesmophytes), fibrosis and calcification of ligaments and muscle tension. Therefore, exercises should be designed to improve these movements.

Mobility exercises should put a joint through the full range of available movement. A variety of equipment can be used to make the exercises more interesting, such as a gymnastic ball. When exercising in supine, support the patient's head with the minimum number of pillows – just enough to prevent the head from tilting back. The physiotherapist should always be prepared to modify an exercise. A case study later in the chapter suggests some suitable exercises.

Breathing

As the person's rib cage mobility can be reduced owing to involvement of the costovertebral and sternocostal joints, breathing exercises should be encouraged. Singing in a choir or playing a wind instrument can be both therapeutic and enjoyable.

Strengthening Exercises

Loss of muscle strength is a feature of AS. Muscles weaken owing to postural deformity and inactivity and the associated pain (Cooper et al. 1991). Strengthening of the anti-gravity (extensor) muscle groups and abdominal muscles is important to maintain an erect posture, and it enables everyday activities to be undertaken with greater ease. Examples of extensor muscle groups are the cervical, thoracic and lumbar spine extensors and glutei. Exercises can be made harder by extending the lever arm (see Chapter 6) using gravity as a resistance or by adding weights. Strengthening of other important muscles groups such as lumbar side flexors and thoracic rotators should not be omitted. These particular muscle groups can be effectively strengthened in the hydrotherapy pool (see the case study later in this chapter). Strengthening exercises are held for several seconds and repeated at least three times.

Muscle Stretches

The muscles most commonly affected by tightness are the sternocleidomastoid and trapezius in the neck, shoulder adductors and flexors, abdominals, hip flexors and adductors, hamstrings and gastrocnemius. Much of the stiffness that patients experience is due to muscle tension. Stretching the muscles, tendons and ligaments allows more joint movement to occur and improves posture.

The contract–relax method of stretching is commonly used (Bulstrode et al. 1987). This involves a maximal isometric contraction for 3 seconds made in the position of maximum stretch of the muscle, followed by a relaxation of 2 seconds and a further passive stretch of the muscle for 6 seconds. This cycle is repeated at least three times. To improve effectiveness, it is important that the patient can feel the stretch in the correct area. The contraction can be into a firm surface or into a hydrotherapy float. If using a slow, prolonged stretch, this should be maintained for between 30 and 60 seconds (Beaulieu 1981). There are many ways to stretch each muscle group – see the case study for examples.

Cardiovascular Fitness, Stamina and Muscle Endurance

Physical fitness can be improved by cardiovascular exercise that increases the muscle strength and endurance as well as exercising the heart and lungs. This form of exercise can improve stamina, and enables people to pursue their work and hobbies with greater ease.

Circuits in the gym should include a variety of strengthening and stretching exercises interspersed with low-impact cardiovascular exercises such as the rowing machine and static bike. High-impact activities such as jogging and step-ups can aggravate the weight-bearing joints. Low-impact cardiovascular activities such as swimming, aquarobics, cycling and walking increase stamina and muscle endurance without aggravating the joints. Cardiovascular exercise can also be undertaken in the hydrotherapy pool. Contact sports such as rugby and football are best avoided as the joints can be aggravated and a fused spine can be at risk from contact with other players.

With increased respiratory excursion, cardiovascular exercise helps to mobilise the thoracic joints and maintain or improve chest expansion and vital capacity. Regular cardiovascular exercise has other benefits, including bodyweight reduction, and protection from heart disease and diabetes. It also can improve sleep, relaxation and well-being.

> ### Key point
> Effective cardiovascular exercise should be performed 3–4 times a week and built up slowly. Any prolonged joint pain is an indication that the exercise has been too vigorous.

Hydrotherapy

Hydrotherapy is an effective way of treating AS as it provides heat whilst encouraging exercise. The warmth of water can relieve pain and muscle spasm and promote relaxation. Dry-land exercises are most effective directly after hydrotherapy. The buoyancy of the water enables movements to occur which are often difficult on dry land because the pressure on weight-bearing joints is relieved (Tinsley 1997). Most patients find hydrotherapy enjoyable and it can improve morale. (See the case study for suggestions for a typical hydrotherapy session.)

> ### Key point
> Hydrotherapy is an expensive modality of treatment, so exercises should be devised to make the most of the properties of water and the time spent in the pool.

To gain further buoyancy, floatation can be used. To increase the resistance, the lever arm can be lengthened, equipment such as bats can be used, and the movement can be performed faster and in deeper water.

The type and amount of exercise should be determined by the amount of pain that the person is experiencing. A patient in flare may find gentle stretching exercises and relaxation alone to be the most beneficial. The physiotherapist should always be prepared to modify an exercise.

> ### Training
> Sufficient specific training is essential before practising hydrotherapy. A good knowledge of the properties of water and precautions is required. It is advisable to attend a foundation and a level-one course. Refer to the hydrotherapy standards in sections 17 and 18 of the Chartered Society of Physiotherapy (CSP) pack of service standards.

PHYSIOTHERAPY ASSESSMENT

Subjective assessment should be kept up to date by noting any changes to the person's circumstances. Annual objective assessment is sufficient unless the patient has needed more intervention due to active disease. Outcome measures to assess changes in mobility, disease activity, function and psychological state can also be useful.

Completion of the patient's assessment record card will show any changes in mobility and posture over time. It is important to discuss the assessment findings with each patient so that specific exercise that concentrates on the most affected areas is undertaken. Even if the patient shows minimal improvement in mobility, exercise can prevent further postural deterioration, increase muscle strength and improve well-being.

Subjective Assessment

The subjective assessment form starts by recording details of the patient's date of birth, consultant, GP and home contacts. Other essential or useful information is listed below.

Personal notes

- Occupation.
- Hobbies.
- Current exercise regimen/sports: frequency, effect on pain.
- Main problems: pain, fatigue, family, work, hobbies.
- Smoker?
- Member of local NASS group?

Medical notes

- Date of onset of symptoms/diagnosis.
- X-rays: date and result.
- HLAB27: positive, negative or unknown.
- Medical history: skin, eyes, bowels, chest, depression, other.
- Medications: present/past, frequency, side-effects.
- Effectiveness of steroid injections: joint/entheses/intramuscular/intravenous.
- Peripheral joint involvement.
- Surgery: joint(s) affected and dates.

Family history

Has there been a family history of AS, psoriasis or bowel problems?

Pain

A body chart can be used to indicate the areas, intensity, frequency and persistence of pain during a typical 24-hour period (including night pain).

Postural issues

- Seating at home, work and in the car.
- Table/desk height.
- Car head restraints.
- Type of mattress and number of pillows.

Anthropometric Assessment

Anthropometric measurements are routinely used in both research and the longitudinal assessment of patients in clinical practice (Bellamy et al. 1998, 1999).

A research group in Bath in the United Kingdom found that five objective measurements (from an original set of 20) were able to show validity, reliability and sensitivity to change. These were tragus to wall, cervical rotation, lumbar side-flexion, lumbar flexion (modified Schober's) and intermalleolar distance (see Table 13.1). Using these measurements, the Bath Ankylosing Spondylitis Metrology Index (BASMI) was designed to show clinically significant changes in spinal movement (Jenkinson et al. 1994). Chest expansion and height is often routinely measured too (Bellamy et al. 1998, 1999).

Equipment for assessment should include a neck goniometer (gravity action or spirit level), a long ruler and tape measure. In order to standardise the measurement, the assessment should ideally be made by the same physiotherapist at the same time of day and

Table 13.1   5 Anthropometric measures commonly used in AS assessment.

Measure	Starting position	Method
Tragus to wall (Figure 13.2)	This is the distance between the tragus of the ear and the wall. It is an overall measure of posture. The patient stands with bare feet together and shoulders, hips and heels as close to wall as possible. The chin is tucked in as far as possible.	The distance is measured both sides with a rigid rule. The average of the two measurements is recorded. Height can be measured at the same time.
Schober's test (modified) (Figure 13.3)	This measures the amount of lumbar spine flexion. The patient stands with bare feet.	Draw a line at the L4–L5 junction and mark 10 cm above this line and 5 cm below it. The patient bends forwards with knees slightly bent. Hold the end of the tape measure on the upper mark and measure between the two marks. Any increase beyond 15 cm is the lumbar flexion.
Cervical rotation	The patient lies supine with head at the end of the plinth and chin tucked in. Ensure shoulders do not move and the head is not tilted back.	Place the goniometer lightly on forehead. The patient rotates his/her head. Repeat on other side.
Lumbar side-flexion	The patient stands as straight as possible with bare feet and back to wall. The feet are a standardised distance apart. Keep knees straight and heels on floor.	Place a long ruler at the outer edge of left foot. The patient reaches down the ruler to left with fingers straight keeping shoulders against the wall. Measure from middle finger tip to floor. Repeat on other side.
Intermalleolar distance (hip abduction)	The patient lies supine on the floor with legs apart, knees in extension and feet turned out.	Measure between the medial malleoli.

before hydrotherapy or a gym session. To make the measurement reproducible, standardise the patient's starting position, watch for any 'trick movements', and allow time for the patient to achieve maximum stretch.

Outcome Measures

Traditionally, patient assessment was dominated by anthropometric measurements using measures that were not necessarily standardised, reliable, valid and responsive to change. Therefore, accurate assessment of improvement or deterioration was difficult to measure.

Key point

As Calin (1994) pointed out, 'without a clear understanding of outcome, we could not know whether physiotherapy or any other modality really "works" in ankylosing spondylitis'. It gives the clinician the ability to decide whether to initiate, terminate, continue or modify a treatment (Bellamy et al. 1998).

Over the years, a number of both disease-specific and generic outcome measures were developed. However, with an increasing interest in AS research, it was evident that outcome measures needed to be standardised to ensure study comparison. This was also important in clinical practice, where Bellamy et al. (1998, 1999) revealed a lack of standardisation in the selection and use of outcome measurements by rheumatologists. It was speculated that this was partly due to lack of consensus, lack of familiarity with the instruments, lack of time, lack of training, and no requirement to use the outcome measurements.

In 1995, the Assessments in Ankylosing Spondylitis (ASAS) working group was set up as a subcommittee to the larger Outcome Measures in Rheumatology Clinical Trials (OMERACT) initiative (van der Heijde et al. 1997, 1999). The group consisted of clinical experts in the field of AS, clinical epidemiologists, representatives of the pharmaceutical industry, and patients.

Based on an extensive literature review and consensus, the ASAS working group decided upon the most acceptable instruments (either generic or disease-specific) that could be used to determine changes of different domains over time. These instruments could be used in both clinical research and routine practice. The instruments had to measure what was intended, show reliability and sensitivity to change, and be simple to

complete. The domains were chosen specifically to reflect the nature of the disease and included pain, spinal mobility and functional disability. It has been argued that the domains used by ASAS were biased towards the assessment of impairment and disability and did not include important domains such as quality of life (Haywood 2000) and psychological status.

Despite the lack of consensus, examples of the instruments that are currently used in clinical practice are shown in Table 13.2. New instruments will be developed and some will need modification in due course as further research and the work of the ASAS working group continues.

EFFECTIVE PHYSIOTHERAPY FOR AS

General Issues

A person is more likely to perform an exercise effectively if it is clearly demonstrated and its rationale explained. Intentions to perform behaviours such as exercises are influenced by beliefs about their consequences (Duran and Trafimow 2000). Observing the person with constant attention to detail ensures accuracy and optimum patient effort. If targets are set, enquire about the results. Be aware of the individual's capabilities and give praise and encouragement appropriately. In a group setting, certain exercises may have to be adapted for the stiffer patients in order to ensure full participation. By using a variety of different equipment (e.g. gymnastic balls and sticks), exercise can be more interesting for the patient and there is no limit to the variety of new exercises that can be created. In the hospital setting, a mixture of both gym and hydrotherapy is used.

The physiotherapist should consider:

1 What is the exercise achieving?
2 How can I make the exercise harder?
3 How can I adapt the exercise for the stiffer patient?
4 How can I avoid trick movements?
5 Where should I fixate in order to achieve a more specific movement?
6 Is the patient confident and safe?

Partnered exercises can be fun and effective as long as both people are exercising simultaneously. This exercise could be done at home with a family member.

If you are involved in regular exercise sessions, record the muscle groups that were exercised to make sure that important mobility, strengthening or stretching exercises are not omitted. Poor performance by an individual should also be documented. Table 13.3 shows a typical record.

Table 13.2 Examples of outcome and anthropometric measurements used in AS assessment.

Domain	Instrument	Original reference
Function	Bath Ankylosing Spondylitis Functional Index (BASFI)	Calin et al. (1994)
	Revised Leeds Disability Questionnaire	Abbott et al. (1994)
	Dougados/Spondylitis Function Index	Dougados et al. (1988)
Spinal mobility	Cervical rotation	O'Driscoll et al. (1978)
	Modified Schober (15 cm)	Macrae and Wright (1969)
	Tragus to wall	Tomlinson et al. (1986)
	Lumbar side-flexion	Pile et al. (1991)
	Chest expansion	Tomlinson et al. (1986)
	Bath Ankylosing Spondylitis Metrology Index (BASMI)	Jenkinson et al. (1994)
Disease activity (includes fatigue)	Bath Ankylosing Spondylitis Disease Activity Index (BASDAI)	Garrett et al. (1994)
Depression	HAD (generic)	Zigmond and Snaith (1983)
Quality of life/well-being	Bath Ankylosing Spondylitis Global Score (BAS-G)	Jones et al. (1996b)
	AS-AIMS2	Guillemin et al. (1997)
	ASQoL	Reynolds (1999)

Self-help in AS and the Role of the Physiotherapist

Home programmes

AS is a chronic, potentially disabling condition that patients should learn to manage for themselves. National Health Service resources are not limitless and people often want to organise their own lives, rather than let their illness and disability rule it for them. Therefore, the majority of AS disease management will be controlled by the patient and undertaken at home, local sports clubs and so on.

A home programme of exercises and posture awareness that is devised should be specific to the needs and the abilities of the patient and suit the home environment. Realistic goals should be agreed between the physiotherapist and the patient to take into account fatigue and personal circumstances. A basic exercise sheet can be devised to which new exercises can be added. Memory aids such as an exercise video and a radio cassette are available from NASS. If appropriate, family members could be familiarised with the exercises by participating in the exercise classes.

To improve compliance, the exercise routine should be slotted into the most convenient time of the day depending on the patient's schedule. Exercise can also be integrated into the daily activities – for example, reaching up to cupboards or to a high clothes line, and twisting around in a static chair to a waste paper bin behind.

Patients should check their posture (see home checks), and stretch out the spine and hip flexors on a regular basis. This can be achieved by lying supine on the bed with minimal pillows under the head, the knees bent off the edge of the bed and feet on the floor or supported. The patient can also lie prone as long as the neck is comfortable, and if possible can prop himself or herself up on elbows to read or watch TV.

Education

The physiotherapist should provide advice on the disease, fatigue, pain relief, footwear, recommended sports, chairs, beds, sleeping, driving, ergonomics, etc. Literature and aids to memory should be provided wherever possible to patients. Apply to NASS for a quantity of their guidebooks that are free of charge. When a person becomes a member of NASS, further support and advice can be offered through direct communication with the charity and from their twice-yearly newsletter. Encourage the patient to attend

Key point

People who take an active interest in their condition can positively influence its outcome.

Table 13.3   A typical AS exercise record.

Date					
	Gym	Pool		Gym	Pool
WARM-UP					
Stretching:			Lumbar spine extensors		
Rectus femoris			Lumbar side flexors		
Psoas			Abdominals		
Hip adductors			Hip extensors		
Hip rotators			Hip abductors		
Hamstrings			Hip rotators		
Calf			Quadriceps		
Pectorals			Ankle and foot		
Thoracic rotators			**Mobilising:**		
Abdominals			Neck		
Neck			Temporomandibular		
Shoulder extensors			Shoulder		
Shoulder adductors			Thoracic rotation		
Shoulder rotators			Lumbar side-flexion		
Strengthening:			Lumbar flexion/extension		
Neck retractor			**Breathing exercises**		
Other neck muscles			**Posture awareness**		
Shoulder elevators			**Cardiovascular**		
Thoracic spine extensors			**Relaxation**		
Thoracic rotators			**COOL DOWN**		

By kind permission of Jane Barefoot.

regular exercise sessions either by becoming a member of the local NASS group or by attending regular daytime hospital sessions or intensive residential educational programmes, which are held at certain specialist centres.

Barriers to exercise

AS is often diagnosed at a time when work and family commitments are considerable and free time is limited. If the pain is acute and aggravated by excessive movement in the early stages, there may be little incentive to exercise. Conversely, some people experience mild pain and are not motivated to exercise. Also, people with physical jobs may suffer from fatigue by the end of the day and consider their daily activity is adequate exercise.

Santos et al. (1998) noted that, with regard to AS, adherence to a regular exercise regimen is associated with rheumatologist follow-up, belief in the benefits of exercise, and a higher education level. Consistency of exercise, rather than quantity, is of most importance. On the whole, compliance with exercise is improved when people with AS find that their pain is eased by active exercises.

Disease duration need not be a demotivating factor to people with AS, since Viitanen et al. (1995) concluded that it was possible by means of an intensive rehabilitation course to prevent, for over one year, the deterioration of spinal function and fitness in AS patients irrespective of their disease duration. Other barriers to exercise include boredom, lack of short-term gains, poor body image, lack of knowledge, aversion to exercise, and denial.

Fatigue

Persistent fatigue is now accepted as a common symptom of AS, and it is in many ways more debilitating than the pain itself. Fatigue can be the consequence of pain, anaemia, disturbed sleep, poor posture and stress. Management of this fatigue is still something of an enigma (Jones et al. 1996a). It can affect concentration and increase irritability and frustration, which can impact on relationships and cause anxiety and depression (Barlow 1994).

The National Ankylosing Spondylitis Society (NASS)

NASS was founded in 1975 by a group of patients who were keen to attend regular exercise sessions. The membership includes patients, their families and health professionals. NASS provides support, education and information in the management of social and medical aspects of the disease. It also funds research into AS.

Currently, NASS has 110 local branches around Britain. Most of the branches meet on a weekly basis at a local hospital where hydrotherapy and gym work are normally on offer. Physiotherapists with a special interest in AS supervise the sessions. The day-to-day running of the branch is organised by a committee consisting of members.

Apart from ongoing education and exercise, there are other advantages such as improving morale and encouraging the individuals to take control of their disease by providing support, understanding, encouragement, motivation and fun. The groups are cost-effective both in time and money for the hospital, patient and physiotherapists. NASS self-help group members appear to comply more with exercise treatment and also receive a valuable source of social support from fellow members.

See also the section of useful addresses towards the end of the chapter.

ANKYLOSING SPONDYLITIS: A CASE STUDY

About the Patient

Mr L had experienced intermittent low-grade back/buttock ache since he was 11. He was occasionally off games at school and it was put down to sciatica or 'growing pains'. He was sent to a physiotherapist by his GP at the age of 19. Pain in his mid thoracic spine and around his costosternal joints had become more severe. It limited his breathing and made it painful to turn in bed at night. His back was stiff in the morning for about an hour but eased off as the day progressed. He experienced a great deal of fatigue that was affecting his social life. He also had recurrent tender spots under his heels, the Achilles tendons and at

the medial collateral ligaments of the knees. He had experienced one bout of sore inflamed eyes for which he had not been treated.

The physiotherapist became suspicious at the collection of symptoms (i.e. iritis, enthesopathy pain and low back stiffness which was eased by activity) and referred Mr L to a consultant rheumatologist. Following a detailed history and X-rays of his sacroiliac joints, a diagnosis of AS was made. He was sent for blood tests that revealed that he was HLAB27 positive.

He was started immediately on a slow-release NSAID to take at night and a quicker acting NSAID in the daytime. This combination decreased his early morning stiffness and pain enough to enable him to partake in a 2-week intensive AS course at the hospital. Fortunately he enjoyed exercise and was very motivated. Although he had to give up playing amateur football, he increased his exercise tolerance until he was swimming three times a week, cycling to work and attending the local NASS group that exercised once a week in the evening. After a few months he no longer required the daytime NSAID dose. A list of exercises were recommended, as shown below in Tables 13.4–13.5.

Mr L's Hydrotherapy Session

A typical forty-minute group hydrotherapy session may include:

- a warming up with some cardiovascular (CV) content
- mobilising exercises against the side of the pool
- fun and games
- strengthening exercises in supine and prone
- trunk and leg stretches
- a cooling down with neck exercises, breathing exercises and relaxation.

Recommendations

The use of goggles can prevent aggravating the neck whilst swimming (especially in breaststroke and crawl). Goggles also protect the eyes from chlorine, which can exacerbate uveitis. A snorkel can be used if the neck is very stiff. The use of a variety of swimming strokes prevents stress and fatigue in any one area.

Warming up

Keep the neck and shoulders under water as much as possible by standing in the correct depth of water. If necessary, bend knees and hips. The faster the movement is performed, the more the turbulence and therefore the greater the resistance. Count out loud and perform the activity at least 10 times to increase the CV content and respiratory excursion still further.

1 Walk with big strides forwards, backwards or sideways around the edge of the pool. Exaggerate the arm swing and trunk movements. Change direction quickly into the turbulence created.
2 Clasp the hands together under the water straight out in front and swish the arms as far round as possible to right and left.
3 Bend the right knee and reach down to the outside of the right heel with the right hand. Repeat to other side.
4 Hop, touching the right elbow to a bent left knee. Repeat to the other side.
5 Jump, punching the right arm forwards and the left leg backwards. Repeat to the other side.

Mobilising

Lumbar and thoracic spine flexion and extension

Hold the rail with both hands straight out in front and the elbows extended. Stand two paces back facing the pool rail and with the buttocks back as far as possible. The feet should be slightly apart.

1 Push the hips forwards towards the wall (into extension) and then back out to the starting position. Keep elbows and knees straight.
2 With the same starting position as above, bring one foot up towards the wall with an extended knee. Leading with the heel and keeping the knee straight, take the heel backwards as high as possible. Repeat on the other side.

Thoracic and cervical spine rotation

1 Use the same starting position as above but with legs astride. Bend the left elbow and twist to the left to look under the elbow. Repeat to the other side.
2 Face the wall and rest the arms on the bar. Bend the knees to 90 degrees and keep the trunk, pelvis and thighs flat against the wall. Keep the knees together. Fix shoulders by holding on to the pool rail with hands and forearms. Swing both knees up to the right as far as possible until the outside of the left thigh is flat on the wall. Repeat to the other side.

Fun and games

Take care to match patients equally and ensure safety in the pool at all times.

1 Race each other across pool forwards, backwards and sideways.

2 Two opponents face each other prone with a ring or a woggle held at arms length between them. Using any swimming kick, the winner is the person who pushes the ring over to the partner's side.
3 As a race, pass a large ring over the body starting at either the head or feet.
4 Sit with a woggle between the legs. Use legs in a cycling action to race across pool.

Strengthening exercises: supine with hands holding the rail

Make sure that the neck is supported in a neck float and push the occiput into the water during the exercise. Squeeze a medium-sized ring tightly around the hips or have a woggle or polystyrene floats under the buttocks to keep them elevated. Hold the rail to fix the trunk but not so tight that it aggravates the shoulders and neck.

Lumbar/hip extensors

1 With straight knees, take both heels down towards the bottom of the pool (hip and lumbar spine extension).
2 Put a float behind the heel of one foot and take that foot down in the water until the foot is just under water. Take the other leg down in the water as far as possible and back up. Keep both knees straight.

Lumbar side-flexors

Swing the legs as far as possible to each side, side-bending at the waist and keeping knees straight and the pelvis in neutral.

Hip abductors and adductors

Take the legs apart into abduction and back together again. Keep knees straight.

Thoracic rotators

Bend the knees to 90 degrees, put a float under the soles of the feet and keep hips in neutral. Keep the knees just under the surface of the water, while swinging the feet up towards the surface of the water to each side.

Strengthening exercises: supine with feet tucked under the rail

Float supine with the neck and pelvis supported in floats. Keep the backs of hands in the water.

Shoulder abductors, adductors and flexors

Take straight arms out from the sides of the body to above the head, keeping backs of hands in the water.

Table 13.4   Mr L's mobility exercises.

Movement	Starting position	Action
Lumbar extension and flexion	Lie prone with hands under shoulders.	Push up on hands. Keep pelvis flat on floor.
	Four-point kneeling with hands under shoulders, hip and knees at 90 degrees.	(a) Hump back, clasp knee to chest and look down. (b) Hollow back, take leg straight out behind and look straight ahead
	Sit on gym ball with feet flat on floor.	Slump forwards and backwards (pelvic tilt).
Lumbar side-flexion	Stand sideways to wall bars a metre away. Hold wall bar at hip height with inside arm.	Take outside arm up over head to hold bar at head level. Push hips out to side and then in towards the wall bars.
	Lie on side over gym ball at waist level. Rest forearm and lateral side of leg on floor.	Push up on legs straightening bottom leg. Stretch top arm over head. Touch floor with hand if possible.

Table 13.4 Continued.

Movement	Starting position	Action
Thoracic rotation	Lie supine with knees bent.	Roll knees together to each side. Take arms to opposite side. Look down arms.
	Stand with back towards wall and a short distance from it. Have feet slightly apart and knees facing forwards and slightly bent.	Twist to one side, attempting to touch wall with flat hands. Can twist using ball or partner. Turn head around to look at wall
Thoracic extension	(a) Stand with back to wall with arms by side.	(b) Lift arms up, keeping back of hands in contact with wall. Try to touch hands overhead.
	Sit supported with back to wall and ball behind back. Knees bent and feet on floor.	Stretch arms obliquely to touch wall with back of hands. Push thoracic spine into ball.

Table 13.5   Mr L's strengthening exercises: thoracic spine extensors.

Starting position	Movement
Crook lie. Elbows bent by side. Shoulders and buttocks on floor.	Push down on elbows. Arch thoracic spine. Keep pelvis on floor.
Lie prone, arms by side. Grasp stick in hands behind back.	Raise stick behind back. Lift head and shoulders off floor a short distance, looking at floor.
Lie prone. Hold gym ball out in front, elbows as straight as possible.	Raise ball off ground.

Thoracic and shoulder extensors

Take the arms out to 90 degrees from the body. Hold bats in both hands and take backs of hands straight down towards the bottom of the pool.

Strengthening exercise: prone

Abdominals

Put floats around the feet and hold the rail with both hands and straight. Stretch legs straight out behind, allowing the floats to bring the feet up to the surface of the water. Push feet down in the floats to contract the abdominal muscles and then relax. Repeat at least three times.

Stretching Exercises

Key points

Trunk and leg stretches are particularly effective in the hydrotherapy pool owing to the warmth of the water and the effect of floats that, along with the buoyancy, ensure a firm passive stretch. The amount of floatation should be adjusted for each patient by either adding or removing air from the float. Again the contract–relax method can be used.

Hamstrings

Stand straight with back to the wall and arms resting on the rail. Keeping the knees straight, dorsiflex the right foot and put a float behind the heel. Allow the right foot to float up towards the surface of the water to maximum stretch.

Press the heel down into the float a short distance, relax and allow the float to take the heel back up to the surface of the water. Reach down the leg with hands for greater stretch. Repeat to the other side.

Hip adductors

Start as for the hamstring exercise above. Take the right leg out to the side with toes pointing forwards. Put a float around the right ankle and allow a full passive stretch. Stay in an upright position.

Push down the right leg into the float a short distance, relax and allow the float to take the leg up further abduction.

Quadriceps

Stand facing the wall and hold on to the rail. Keep the left leg straight and touching the wall. Bend the right knee, put a float around the right ankle and allow the foot to rise in the water. Keep the right thigh against the wall.

Table 13.6 Mr L's strengthening exercises: lumbar spine extensors/glutei.

Starting position	Movement
Supine lie. Knees bent, feet flat on floor.	Lift buttocks high off floor (bridging). Move feet further from body and/or lift leg to make more difficult. Can bridge with feet on ball or chair with straight or bent knees.
Four-point kneeling.	Lift opposite arm and leg at the same time. Keep arm and leg straight. Repeat other side.
Lie prone.	'Skydive position'. Lift head, and straight arms and legs, looking at floor.

Push the foot down into the float, relax and allow the foot to rise in the water still further. The right knee may come away from the wall a short distance.

Pectorals and abdominals

Lean back against the wall with hips flexed and feet a metre away from the wall. Take arms overhead to hold the rail.

Arch back and lift the sternum to take the back away from the wall. A float can be placed behind the back at scapula level.

Trunk rotators

Face the wall with hips bent at 90 degrees and right arm out straight, holding the rail. Hold a float with the left hand.

Twist the trunk and head by taking the float under the right elbow. Following maximum stretch, press the float down into the water a short distance, relax and allow the float to take the hand further up to the surface of the water.

Cooling down

Finish the session with a cool down. Stand with back to the wall, knees bent and neck under water. Allow the arms to float up to the surface of the water to encourage relaxation of the shoulders. Do some gentle neck and breathing exercises. Relaxation whilst totally supported with floats is very enjoyable.

HOME CHECKS

With regard to exercises, patients can record their own measurements at home. This section contains some examples of how this might be achieved.

Fingertips-to-floor

This gives a composite measurement of lumbar and hip flexion and hamstring length. The person grips a long ruler vertically between the feet and bends forwards, running the fingers down the ruler, keeping knees straight. The distance from the fingertips to the floor is recorded.

Posture check

The person stands straight with feet back against a wall and with chin tucked in to keep a book (minimum thickness) in place between occiput and wall. Ensure that the same thickness of book can be held in place on

Table 13.7 Mr L's stretching exercises.

Starting position	Movement
Neck rotators. Sit straight in a chair with shoulders back.	Turn head to right as far as possible. Place chin in palm of right hand with fingers spread along right cheek. Place left hand around back of head. Attempt to turn the head around to the left but resist the movement with the right hand. Relax and turn the head further to the right with both hands. Repeat three times.
Neck side-flexors. Same starting position as above.	Take neck sideways to right as far as possible. Take right hand across top of head to rest above left ear. Push head up into the hand but do not allow any movement. Relax and stretch the neck side-flexors with the right hand further to the right. Repeat three times.
Hamstrings. Place heel on chair seat with knees straight and foot dorsiflexed.	Stretch hamstring to maximum by reaching down leg. Push heel into seat, relax, then stretch hands down leg still further. Repeat three times.
Hip adductors. Sit on floor with soles of feet touching and knees out to side. The back may need to be supported. Rest forearms on inside of knees.	Pull knees towards each other but do not allow them to move by resisting the movement with the forearms. Relax the knees out to the side, then push knees further apart as far as possible. Repeat three times.

Table 13.7   Continued.

Starting position	Movement
Hip flexors/Quadriceps Stand straight holding right ankle with right hand. Place other hand on wall for balance.	Take right knee back to maximum stretch. Without moving the hip or knee, attempt to pull the knee forward to wall. Then relax and stretch knee back further
Calf muscles. Stand facing wall with left foot a pace back from wall and right foot directly behind in stride stand. Keep right knee straight. Place hands flat on wall.	Slowly bend left knee with heels firmly on ground. When maximum stretch of calf muscles of right leg has been achieved, attempt to lift right heel off the ground but resist the movement. Relax and bend left knee further.

each occasion. Someone else measures the person's height in this position.

Thoracic and neck rotation

The person sits firmly on a toilet seat, with elbows raised to 90 degrees to the body, hands clasped.

1 Turn trunk and head as far around as possible. Close the eye nearest to the wall and at the point where the tip of the nose appears to meet the wall, mark a point on the wall.
2 Try to improve the measurement on each occasion.

Lumbar side-flexion

The person sits on a chair with buttocks pushed well back into the back of the chair.

1 Run the fingertips of one hand down the back leg of the chair and mark the position on the chair leg.
2 Aim to reach lower on each occasion.

USEFUL ADDRESSES

Arthritis Care, 18–20 Stephenson Way, London NW1 2HD. Tel: 080 8800 4050; Web: www.arthritiscare.org.uk

Arthritis Research Campaign (ARC), Copeman House, St Mary's Court, St Mary's Gate, Chesterfield, Derbyshire S41 7TD. Tel: 0870 850 5000; Web: www.arc.org.uk

Hydrotherapy Association of Chartered Physiotherapists (HACP). Web:
www.csp.org.uk/membergroups/clinicalinterestgroups

National Ankylosing Spondylitis Society (NASS), PO Box 179, Mayfield, East Sussex TN20 6ZL. Tel: 01435 873527; E-mail: nass@nass.co.uk; Web: www.nass.co.uk

National Association for Colitis and Crohn's Disease (NACC), 4 Beaumont House, Sutton Road, St Albans, Herts AL1 5HH. Tel: 0845 1302233; Web: www.nacc. org.uk

Psoriasis Association, 7 Milton Street, Northampton, Northants NN2 7JG. Tel: 01604 711129; Web: www.timewarp.demon.co.uk/psoriasis.htm

FURTHER READING

David C, Lloyd J 1999 Rheumatological Physiotherapy. London: Mosby

NASS (online) A Positive Response to Ankylosing Spondylitis: the Guidebook for Patients. Download from www.nass.co.uk/

Russell A 1998 Ankylosing spondylitis: history. In Klippel J, Dieppe P (eds) Rheumatology, Vol. 1, 2nd edn, pp. 1–2. London: Mosby

REFERENCES

Abbott CA, Helliwell PS, Chamberlain MA 1994 Functional assessment in ankylosing spondylitis: evaluation of a new self-administered questionnaire and correlation with anthropometric variables. Br J Rheumatol 33(11): 1060–6

Band D, Jones S, Kennedy G et al. 1997 Which patients with ankylosing spondylitis derive most benefit from an inpatient management programme? J Rheumatol 24: 2381–4

Barlow J 1994 Fatigue in ankylosing spondylitis: a personal perspective. NASS Newsletter autumn/winter: 5–8

Beaulieu JG 1981 Developing a stretching program. Phys Sports Med 9(11): 59–69

Bellamy N, Kaloni S, Pope J et al. 1998 Quantitive rheumatology: a survey of outcome measurement procedures in routine rheumatology outpatient practice in Canada. J Rheumatol 25(5): 852–8

Bellamy N, Muirden K, Brooks P et al. 1999 A survey of outcome measurement procedures in routine rheumatology outpatient practice in Australia. J Rheumatol 26(7): 1593–9

Bulstrode SJ, Barefoot J, Harrison R, Clarke A 1987 The role of passive stretching in the treatment of ankylosing spondylitis. Br J Rheumatol 26: 40–2

Calin A 1991 Ankylosing spondylitis and other inflammatory disorders of the spine. In Schlapbach P, Gerber N (eds) Physiotherapy: Controlled Trials and Facts. Bern: Karger

Calin A 1994 Can we define the outcome of ankylosing spondylitis and the effect of physiotherapy management? J Rheumatol 21(2): 184–5

Calin A, Garrett S, Whitelock H et al. 1994 A new approach to defining functional ability in ankylosing spondylitis: the development of the Bath Ankylosing Spondylitis Functional Index. J Rheumatol 21(12): 2281–5

Cooper R, Freemont A, Fitzmaurice R, Alani S, Jayson M 1991 Paraspinal muscle fibrosis: a specific pathological component in ankylosing spondylitis. Ann Rheum Dis 50(11): 755–9

Dougados M, Gueguen A, Nakache J et al. 1988 Evaluation of functional index and an articular index in ankylosing spondylitis. Br J Rheumatol 15(2): 302–7

Duran A, Trafimow D 2000 Cognitive organization of favorable and unfavorable beliefs about performing a behavior. J Soc Psychol 140(2): 179–87

Eriendsson J 1998 Car Driving with Ankylosing Spondylitis. Publication available from National Ankylosing Spondylitis Society

Garrett S, Jenkinson T, Kennedy LG et al. 1994 A new approach to defining disease status in ankylosing spondylitis: the Bath Ankylosing Spondylitis Disease Activity Index. J Rheumatol 21(12): 2286–91

Guillemin F et al. 1997 The AIMS2-SF: a short form of the Arthritis Impact Measurement Scales 2. French Quality of Life in Rheumatology Group. Arthr Rheum 40:1267–74

Haywood K 2000 Health Outcomes in Ankylosing Spondylitis: an Evaluation of Patient-Based and Anthropometric Measures. DPhil thesis, University of York

Health & Safety Executive 1994 A pain in your work place? Ergonomic problems and solutions. London: HSE

Hidding A, van der Linden S, Boers M et al. 1993 Is group physical therapy superior to individualised therapy in ankylosing spondylitis? A randomised controlled trial. Arthr Care Res 6(3): 117–25

Jenkinson T, Mallorie H et al. 1994 Defining spinal mobility in ankylosing spondylitis: the Bath Metrology Index. J Rheumatol 21(9): 1694–8

Jones SD, Koh WH, Steiner A et al. 1996a Fatigue in ankylosing spondylitis: its prevalence and relationship to disease activity, sleep, and other factors. J Rheumatol 23(3): 487–90

Jones SD, Steiner A, Garrett SL, Calin A 1996b The Bath Ankylosing Spondylitis Patient Global Score (BAS-G). Br J Rheumatol 35(1): 66–71

Lubrano E, Helliwell P 1999 Deterioration in anthropometric measures over six years in patients with ankylosing spondylitis. Physiotherapy 85(3):138–43

Macrae I, Wright V 1969 Measurement of back movement. Ann Rheum Dis 28: 584–9

Pile K, Laurent M, Salmond C et al. 1991 Clinical assessment of ankylosing spondylitis: a study of observer variation in spinal measurements. Br J Rheumatol 30(1): 29–34

O'Driscoll S, Jayson M, Baddeley H 1978 Neck movement in ankylosing spondylitis and their response to physiotherapy. Ann Rheum Dis 37: 64–6

Reynolds S, Doward L, Spoorenberg A et al. 1999 The development of the Ankylosing Spondylitis Quality of Life questionnaire. Qual Life Res 8(7): 651

Santos H, Brophy S, Calin A 1998 Exercise in ankylosing spondylitis: how much is optimum? J Rheumatol 25(11): 2156–60

Tinsley M 1997 Rheumatic diseases. In Hydrotherapy Companion, pp. 255–68. Oxford: Butterworth–Heinemann

Tomlinson M, Barefoot J, Dixon A 1986 Intensive inpatient physiotherapy courses improve movement and posture in ankylosing spondylitis. Physiothcrapy 72(5): 238–40

Van der Heijde D, Bellamy N, Calin A et al. 1997 Preliminary core sets for endpoints in ankylosing spondylitis. J Rheumatol 24: 2225–9

Van der Heijde D, van der Linden S, Bellamy N et al. 1999 Which domains should be included in a core set for endpoints in ankylosing spondylitis? Introduction to the ankylosing spondylitis module of OMERACT IV. J Rheumatol 26(4): 945–7

Viitanen J, Suni J, Kautiainen H et al. 1992 Effect of physiotherapy on spinal mobility in ankylosing spondylitis. Scand J Rheumatol 21: 38–41

Viitanen JV, Lehtinen K, Suni J, Kautiainen H 1995 Fifteen months' follow-up of intensive inpatient physiotherapy and exercise in ankylosing spondylitis. Clin Rheumatol 14(4): 413–19

Zigmond A, Snaith R 1983 The hospital anxiety and depression scale. Acta Psych Scand 67: 361–70

Management of Respiratory Diseases

14

Stephanie Enright

NOTE

The reader is reminded that:

- surface marking of the lungs
- mechanics of respiration
- lung volumes
- chest radiographs
- breath sounds
- stethoscope positions

are covered in this book in the appendix, and that other relevant information such as the active cycle of breathing technique (ACBT) and basic respiratory anatomy and physiology of the lungs can be found in Chapter 16, Physiotherapy in Thoracic Surgery.

INTRODUCTION

Diseases of the respiratory system are a major cause of illness world-wide and are increasingly important as a cause of mortality and morbidity (Rimington et al. 2001). In the United Kingdom they are the most common reason for consulting a general practitioner, and result in more days lost from work than any other type of illness.

Respiratory diseases can be broadly divided into obstructive and restrictive types.

1 *Obstructive diseases* include conditions in which there is a resistance to airflow either through reversible factors such as bronchospasm or inflammation, or through irreversible factors such as airway fibrosis or loss of elastic recoil owing to damage to the airways and the alveoli.
2 *Restrictive disorders* are characterised by reduced lung compliance leading to the loss of lung volume which may be caused by disease affecting the lungs, pleura, chest wall or neuromuscular mechanisms. These diseases are therefore different from the obstructive diseases in their pure form, although mixed restrictive and obstructive conditions can occur.

Obstructive diseases are by far the most common and are secondary only to heart disease as a major cause of disability. Therefore their pathophysiology and treatment will be discussed initially in some detail. They are:

• chronic bronchitis
• emphysema
• chronic bronchitis and emphysema together
• asthma
• bronchiectasis
• cystic fibrosis.

Secondly, as the changing pattern of respiratory disease has resulted in opportunistic pneumonias which are a common presentation in patients with acquired immune deficiency syndrome (AIDS), the restrictive disorders and their management will then be considered. They are:

• pneumonia
• pleurisy
• pleural effusion
• pneumothorax
• acute respiratory distress syndrome (ARDS)
• fibrosing alveolitis.

Finally, there are other lung disorders that fit into neither of the first two categories but need to be included owing to their prevalence within the community or hospital environment. They are:

• lung abscess
• pulmonary tuberculosis
• bronchial and lung tumours
• respiratory failure.

COPD: BASIC ISSUES

Chronic obstructive pulmonary disease (COPD) is an ill-defined term that is often applied to patients who have a combination of chronic bronchitis and emphysema which frequently occur together (and may also include asthma). In the majority of cases, chronic bronchitis is the major cause of obstruction, but in some cases emphysema is predominant. There are many patients who report shortness of breath increasing in severity over several years and, on examination, are found to have a chronic cough, an overinflated chest and poor exercise tolerance. It is often difficult to assess clinically to what extent these patients have chronic bronchitis or emphysema or a mixture of both.

Patients may also present with a more episodic form of disease, which is a characteristic of an asthmatic component. Therefore, 'chronic obstructive pulmonary disease' is a convenient term which encompasses one or all of these pathological components.

Key point

Chronic bronchitis and emphysema often coexist in COPD, the disease is progressive and is characterised by acute exacerbations. It is not usually diagnosed until irreversible damage has occurred.

It is difficult to determine the exact prevalence of COPD. However, figures from general practice suggest that 5% of men and 2% of women will be diagnosed as suffering from COPD, although in the population as a whole it is estimated that 11% of men and 8% of women have evidence of obstructed airways when specifically tested by spirometry (Joint Health Surveys Unit 1996). COPD is projected to be the fifth major cause of death worldwide by 2010 (Office for National Statistics 1997).

The survival rate for COPD varies between 5 and 30 years, but eventually cardiac and ventilatory failure will occur. Avoidance of the precipitating factors listed below will tend to improve the prognosis:

• stopping smoking
• control of atmospheric pollution
• prompt treatment of all acute infections
• maintenance of good general health.

Since COPD is characterized by obstruction, the greater the obstruction the lower the chance of survival (Pearson and Calverley 1995). As obstruction to flow is measured by FEV$_1$, which stands for *forced expiratory volume in one second*. Together with age, FEV$_1$ is the most important determinant of survival (Table 14.1).

CHRONIC BRONCHITIS

Definition

Chronic bronchitis is a chronic or recurrent increase in the volume of mucus secretion sufficient to cause expectoration when this is not due to localized bronchopulmonary disease. In the definition of this disease, chronic/recurrent is further defined as a daily cough with sputum for at least 3 months of the year for at least two consecutive years and airways obstruction which does not change markedly over periods of several months (West 1995). Chronic bronchitis is a clinical diagnosis (unlike the definition of emphysema).

Aetiology of Chronic Bronchitis

This is more common in middle to late adult life and in men more than women (Clarke 1991). Cigarette smoking is the chief culprit, and although in the UK over 20% of the adult population continue to smoke (Department of Health 1997) only 15–20% of smokers develop COPD. The reason for this is probably genetic although the number of cigarettes smoked does have an effect on the progression of the disease.

Exposure to risk: pack-years

Rather than simply recording a patient's current smoking habits, a much better indicator of any potential deterioration in lung function is an assessment of pack-years, which is the number of packs (20 per pack) smoked daily multiplied by the number of years of smoking. For example, someone aged 60 years who has smoked five cigarettes per day (0.25 of a pack) since the age of 15 has a lifetime exposure equal to $0.25 \times 45 = 11$ pack-years. Another person of the same age who smoked 30 cigarettes per day (1.5 packs) between the ages of 15 and 25 (gave up till age 40, since then has smoked one pack per day) has a lifetime exposure of $(1.5 \times 10) + (1 \times 20) = 35$ pack-years.

Atmospheric pollution (e.g. industrial smoke, smog and coal dust) will also predispose to the development

Table 14.1 The relationship between age, FEV$_1$ and survival.

Age	FEV$_1$	3-year survival probability
<60	>50% of expected	90%
>60	>50% of expected	80%
>60	40–50% of expected	75%
>60	30–40% of expected	60%

of the disease, which is therefore more common in urban than in rural areas. It is more prevalent in socio-economic groups 4 and 5 and is costly in terms of working days lost annually in Britain.

Pathology of Chronic Bronchitis

The hallmark is hypertrophy of, and an increase in number of, mucous glands in the large bronchi and evidence of inflammatory changes in the small airways (Thurlbeck 1976). Some irritative substance stimulates overactivity of the mucus-secreting glands and the goblet cells in the bronchi and in the bronchioles which causes secretion of excess mucus. This mucus coats the walls of the airways and tends to clog the bronchioles, which is functionally more important. The cells increase in size and their ducts become dilated and may occupy as much as two-thirds of the wall thickness (West 1995). The airways become narrowed and show inflammatory changes, which results in mucosal oedema thus further decreasing the diameter of the airways. The ciliary action is also inhibited.

This narrowing of the lumen of the airways is further emphasised during expiration by the normal shortening and narrowing of the airways. Consequently the airways obstruction is enhanced during expiration, with resulting trapping of air in the alveoli. The lungs gradually lose their elasticity as the disease progresses. They will gradually become distended permanently, which eventually may cause extensive rupture of the alveolar walls. After repeated exacerbations due to infection there is widespread damage to the bronchioles and the alveoli with fibrosis and kinking occurring as well as compensatory overdistension of the surviving alveoli. This is closely allied to and contributory to the development of emphysema.

Clinical Features of Chronic Bronchitis

The most important clinical features are cough, sputum, wheeze and dyspnoea.

Cough

The patient will complain of a cough for many years, initially intermittent and gradually becoming continuous. Fog, damp or infection increases it. The patient may also complain of bouts of coughing occasionally on lying down or in the morning. The cough and sputum production are not associated with either mortality or disability, and are reversible in most smokers once they stop smoking. The cough is caused by either irritation of airway nerve receptors due to the release of compounds from inflammatory cells or from the presence of increased mucous production.

Sputum

This is mucoid and tenacious, usually becoming mucopurulent during an infective exacerbation.

Wheeze

Wheezing is a symptom described by as many as 80% of patients with COPD. Wheezing is a characteristic feature of COPD, although it is also reported in many other acute and chronic respiratory diseases. Wheezing is caused by the sound generated by turbulent airflow through the narrowed conducting airways and may be worse in the mornings or may be related to weather changes.

Dyspnoea or shortness of breath

This occurs in patients with COPD and, together with the energy-requiring consequences of chronic infection and inflammation, leads to increased work of breathing (Donahoe et al. 1989). The patient becomes progressively more short of breath as the disease progresses.

Other signs and symptoms
Exercise intolerance

Owing to abnormalities of respiratory function, patients with COPD ventilate excessively and ineffectively at all work levels compared with subjects with normal lung function. This limits exercise performance. Limitation of exercise tolerance is, however, determined not only by pulmonary function but also by many other factors – including motivation, muscle mass and nutritional status. Of equal importance is the impact these symptoms have on the patient's quality of life, activities of daily living and recreational activities. Patients should also be assessed for the impact that these symptoms have on:

• ability to work
• psychological well-being
• sexual function.

Deformity

These patients often develop a barrel chest due to hyperinflation and use of accessory muscles of respiration. The thoracic movements are gradually diminished and paradoxical indrawing in the intercostal spaces may develop.

Cyanosis

This is a blue coloration of the skin caused by the presence of desaturated haemoglobin due to reduced gaseous exchange. Cyanosis is also related to the development of complications, such as poor cardiac output due to ventricular failure leading to increased peripheral oxygen extraction. Cyanosis may also be due to an increase in red blood cells (polycythaemia) in response to chronic hypoxaemia.

Cor pulmonale

This may occur in the later stages of COPD. The impaired gas exchange in COPD caused by the disruption of ventilation and perfusion and the resulting hypoxia leads to widespread hypoxic pulmonary vasoconstriction. This leads to an increase in pulmonary vascular resistance resulting in pulmonary hypertension (Vender 1994). The increase in the pressure within the pulmonary artery will create a resistance, which the right ventricle must overcome. This eventually leads to hypertrophy and dilatation, a condition known as 'cor pulmonale'.

Right heart failure leads to an increased pressure in the peripheral tissues resulting in the development of peripheral oedema. The combination of renal hypoxia and the increase in blood viscosity from polycythaemia increases the systemic blood pressure (BP) and eventually leads to left heart failure. The development of pulmonary oedema, which exacerbates the hypoxia and low cardiac output in patients with COPD, leads to a terminal stage of the disease. The mechanism of this cycle is illustrated in Figure 14.1.

Lung function

There is reduction of FEV_1 and the *forced vital capacity* (FVC) is grossly reduced. The residual volume (RV) will be increased at the expense of the vital capacity (VC) because of air trapping and the inability of the expiratory muscles to decrease the volume of the thoracic cavity. The expiratory flow–volume curve is grossly abnormal in severe disease; after a brief interval of moderately high flow, flow is strikingly reduced as the airways collapse, and flow limitation by dynamic compression occurs. A scooped-out appearance is often seen.

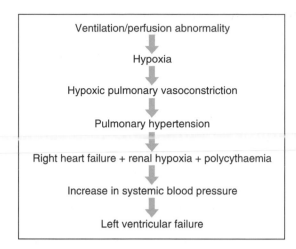

Figure 14.1   Mechanism of development of cor pulmonale and congestive heart failure in COPD.

Blood gases

Ventilation/perfusion mismatch is inevitable in COPD and leads to a low arterial oxygen pressure (PaO_2) with or without retention of carbon dioxide (CO_2). As the disease becomes severe, the arterial carbon dioxide pressure ($PaCO_2$) may rise, and there is some evidence that the sensitivity of the respiratory centre to CO_2 is reduced (Fleetham et al. 1980), which may leave the respiratory stimulus dependent upon the hypoxic drive. However, more recent evidence suggests that the administration of high levels of oxygen (>70%) in patients with COPD may increase hypercapnia owing to the reversal of pre-existing regional pulmonary hypoxic vasoconstriction, resulting in greater dead space (Crossley et al. 1997).

Auscultation signs

There will be inspiratory and expiratory wheeze with added coarse crepitations. The breath sounds are vesicular with prolonged expiration.

X-ray signs

No characteristic abnormality is seen in the early stages of the disease. If there is significant airways obstruction there may be signs of chest over-expansion (flattening of the diaphragm) and an enlarged reterosternal airspace.

EMPHYSEMA

The condition is probably highest in England when compared to the rest of Europe, especially in the major centres of industry – although often there is a family history of the disease.

Definition
Emphysema is a condition of the lung characterised by permanent dilatation of the air spaces distal to the terminal bronchioles with destruction of the walls of these airways. It is nearly always associated with chronic bronchitis from which it is difficult to distinguish during life

Causes and Types of Emphysema

Causes and predisposing factors

Congenital or primary emphysema may be caused by alpha$_1$-antitrypsin deficiency. This is a rare inherited condition, which affects one person in 4000 and results in the complete absence of one of the key antiprotease systems in the lung. The consequence is the early development of COPD, especially if the patient is already a smoker. Although alpha$_1$-antitrypsin deficiency is responsible for fewer than 1% of cases of COPD, its hereditary nature means that it is worth diagnosing. It should, therefore, be considered in any young COPD patient.

Emphysema may be secondary to other factors, such as:

- obstructive airways disease – e.g. asthma, cystic fibrosis, chronic bronchitis
- occupational lung diseases – e.g. pneumoconiosis
- compensatory to contraction of one section of the lung – e.g. fibrous collapse or removal, when the remaining lung expands to fill the space.

Types of emphysema

Definition
Centrilobular (centri-acinar) emphysema tends to affect the respiratory bronchioles with most of the alveoli remaining normal. *Panlobular* (panacinar) emphysema results in widespread destruction of most alveoli as well as respiratory bronchioles.

Primary emphysema is usually of the panacinar (panlobular) type. In centrilobular emphysema the upper zones of the lung are usually affected. This causes gross disturbance of the ventilation/perfusion relationship since there is a relatively well preserved blood supply to the alveoli but the amount of oxygen reaching the capillary is decreased owing to the damage to airways proximal to the alveoli. Panacinar emphysema predominantly affects the lower lobes. This has a less drastic effect on the ventilation/perfusion relationship since the blood supply in the damaged areas is decreased in proportion to the decreased ventilation in those areas.

Pathology of Emphysema

Smoking causes the clustering of pulmonary alveolar macrophages (which are the major defence cells of the respiratory tract) around the terminal bronchioles. These macrophages are abnormal in smokers and they release proteolytic enzymes, which destroy lung tissue locally. Polymorphonuclear leucocytes, necessary to combat infection in the lung, release an enzyme which also destroys lung tissue. The defence mechanism against the unwanted action of these enzymes lies in the serum alpha$_1$-antitrypsin, which is normally present in the airway lining fluids. Oxidants released by both cigarette smoke and the leucocytes tend to inactivate the antiproteolytic action of the alpha$_1$-antitrypsin, which causes destruction of lung tissue as seen in centrilobular emphysema.

Subsequently the walls of the airways become weak and inelastic owing to the damage from repeated infections. They tend to act as a one-way valve with the walls collapsing on expiration. This causes air trapping and consequent increase in the intra-alveolar pressure during expiration. The alveolar septa break down and form bullae (Figure 14.2).

During expiration, the pressure from the trapped air in the bullae may compress adjacent healthy tissue, thus causing occlusion and trapping of air in that tissue. The capillaries around the alveolar walls become stretched, causing the lumen to decrease and atrophy to occur. This causes an alteration in the ventilation/perfusion relationship, owing to the loss of surface area for gaseous exchange and the decrease in blood supply resulting from damage to the pulmonary capillary network.

Clinical Features of Emphysema

Progressive dyspnoea

Shortness of breath occurs initially on exertion, but as the disease progresses it will gradually occur after less and less activity and finally at rest. This disabling breathlessness is what prevents the patient from working and gradually transforms the patient into a state of severe exercise intolerance and disability.

Respiratory pattern

The patient has a 'fishlike' inspiratory gasp, which is followed by prolonged, forced expiration usually against 'pursed lips'. This creates back-pressure to try to prevent airways shutdown during expiration. Owing to increased intrathoracic pressure the jugular veins fill on expiration. A 'flick' or 'bounce' of the abdominal muscles may be seen on expiration as the outward flow of air is suddenly checked by the obstruction of the airways (Figure 14.3).

Cough with sputum

This will be present if the disease is associated with chronic bronchitis or if there is infection.

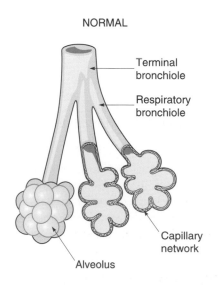
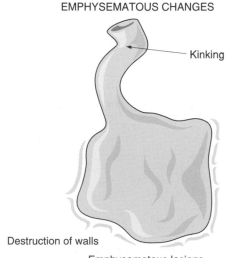

Figure 14.2   Emphysematous changes in the lung.

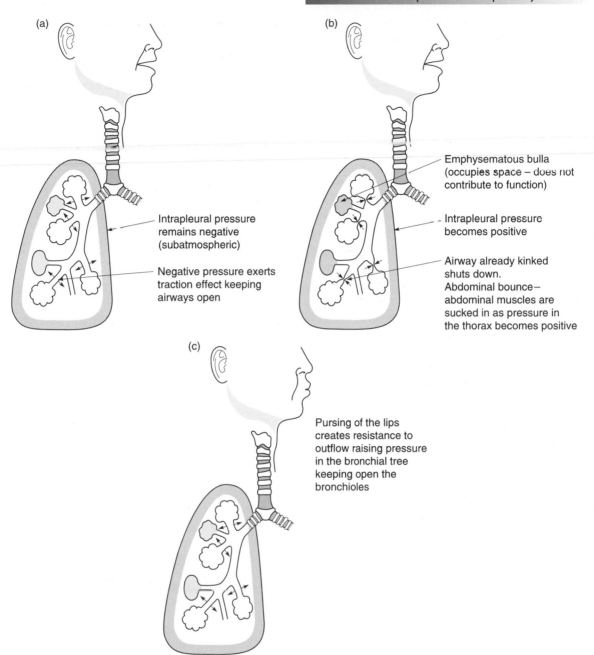

(a)

Intrapleural pressure remains negative (subatmospheric)

Negative pressure exerts traction effect keeping airways open

(b)

Emphysematous bulla (occupies space – does not contribute to function)

Intrapleural pressure becomes positive

Airway already kinked shuts down. Abdominal bounce – abdominal muscles are sucked in as pressure in the thorax becomes positive

(c)

Pursing of the lips creates resistance to outflow raising pressure in the bronchial tree keeping open the bronchioles

Figure 14.3   End of expiration: (a) normal; (b) in emphysema; (c) pursed-lip breathing.

Chest shape

The chest becomes barrel-shaped, fixed in inspiration with widening of the intercostal spaces. There may also be indrawing of the lower intercostal spaces and supra-clavicular fossa on inspiration. This is associated with the difficulty of ventilating stiff lungs through narrowed airways. The ribs are elevated by the accessory muscles of respiration and there is loss of thoracic mobility.

Poor posture

There may be a thoracic kyphosis plus elevated and protracted shoulder girdles.

Polycythaemia

This may develop if there is a prolonged decrease in PaO_2 owing to the ventilation/perfusion imbalance.

Cor pulmonale

This occurs in the advanced stages of the disease.

Lung function

The FEV_1/FVC ratio is usually below 70%. Residual volume (RV) is increased and lung volume may exceed the predicted total lung capacity (TLC) (Decramer 1989).

Examination

The percussion note will be normal or hyper-resonant due to air trapping. Auscultation will reveal decreased breath sounds and prolonged expiration. The chest radiograph shows low flat diaphragms and hyperinflation.

Prognosis of Emphysema

The patients become progressively more disabled, with death ultimately occurring from respiratory failure. Complications of the disease are pneumothorax due to rupture of an emphysematous bullae, and congestive cardiac failure.

COMBINED CHRONIC BRONCHITIS AND EMPHYSEMA

Within the spectrum of COPD, two extremes of clinical presentation are recognised: type A and type B. At one time these were classified either as 'pink puffers' (type A) or 'blue bloaters' (type B) to correlate with the relative amounts of emphysema and chronic bronchitis respectively (Figure 14.4). Whilst these definitions are over-simplistic, it is worth remembering that patients can present in dramatically different ways (Kesten and Chapman 1993).

Blue bloaters

Patients with this syndrome often show the following symptoms:

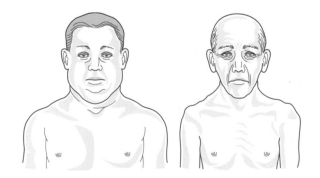

Figure 14.4   Blue bloater and pink puffer.

- obesity
- comparatively mild dyspnoea
- copious sputum which may become infected
- low PaO_2 and high $PaCO_2$ ($PaO_2 > 8$kPa; $PaCO_2 > 6.5$kPa) because they tend to hypoventilate
- central cyanosis with cor pulmonale.
- peripheral oedema
- an increased residual volume but normal total lung capacity.

Pink puffers

Patients with this syndrome often show the following symptoms:

- an anxious expression
- general thinness
- severe breathlessness
- little or no sputum production
- relatively normal PaO_2 and $PaCO_2$ ($PaO_2 < 8$ kPa; $PaCO_2$ normal/low) due to hyperventilation early on in the disease
- central cyanosis and the development of cor pulmonale in the later stages of the disease
- generally no peripheral oedema until the late stages of the disease
- an increased total lung capacity due to hyperventilation.

MEDICAL TREATMENT OF COPD

Principles of Treatment

1   *Decrease the bronchial irritation to a minimum.* The patient should be advised to stop smoking and avoid dusty, smoky, damp or foggy atmospheres. Occupation or housing conditions may need to be changed.

2   *Control infections.* All infections should be treated promptly as each exacerbation will cause further damage to the airways. The patient should have a supply of antibiotics at home and receive a vaccination against influenza each winter. The main affecting organisms are *Streptococcus pneumoniae* and *Haemophilus influenzae,* which are usually sensitive to amoxycillin or trimethoprim.

3   *Control bronchospasm.* Although bronchospasm is not a prominent feature of this disease, drugs (e.g. salbutamol) may be given to relieve the airways obstruction as much as is possible.

4   *Control/decrease the amount of sputum.* Patients with chronic bronchitis may present with excessive bronchial secretions and are usually able to eliminate this by themselves. However, during an episode

when secretions may become difficult to eliminate, physiotherapy techniques including humidification, positioning and manual techniques may aid expectoration and reduce airflow obstruction in the short term (Cochrane et al. 1977).

5 *Oxygen therapy.* Oxygen must be prescribed and should be given with great care, especially if a normal pH indicates a chronic compensated respiratory acidosis (renal conservation of bicarbonate ions (HCO$_3$) to maintain pH within 7.35 to 7.45). In this instance HCO$_3$ is raised above 24 mmol/L whilst PaO_2 is low and the $PaCO_2$ is raised. Controlled oxygen may be given via a Ventimask (or equivalent) with careful monitoring of blood gas levels.

6 *Long-term oxygen therapy* (LTOT). As respiratory function deteriorates, the level of oxygen in the blood falls leading to an increase in pulmonary hypoxic vasoconstriction and a deterioration in cardiac function. In 1981, the Medical Research Working Party examined the effects of supplementary low-concentrations of oxygen (24%) for 15 hours a day in COPD and found that it reduced 3-year mortality from 66% to 45%. The British Thoracic Society guidelines (1997) suggest that patients who have a PaO_2 of less than 7.3 kPa, with or without hypercapnia, and a FEV$_1$ of less than 1.5 litres, should receive LTOT. This therapy should be considered also for patients with a PaO_2 between 7.3 and 8.0 kPa and evidence of pulmonary hypertension, peripheral oedema or nocturnal hypoxia.

Medications

Drugs used in the treatment of respiratory disease broadly fall into two categories: relievers and preventers.

- The *relievers* are used to reduce bronchospasm and include the beta$_2$ agonists (which may be short- or long-acting), the anticholinergics and the xanthene derivatives.
- The *preventers* may be used to prevent bronchial hyper-reactivity and reduce bronchial mucosal inflammatory reactions – they include the corticosteroids.

Beta$_2$ (ß$_2$) agonists

Beta-agonists such as salbutamol (Ventolin) and terbutaline (Bricanyl) work by stimulating beta$_2$-receptors, which are widespread throughout the respiratory system. These stimulate adenylate cyclase, which leads to bronchodilation. Beta-receptors are also found in other tissues, including the heart, although these are of the beta$_1$ subtype.

Even though modern bronchodilators are designed to be beta$_2$-selective, they may still cause an increase in heart rate and other side-effects, which include fine tremor, tachycardia, hypokalaemia (low potassium) after high doses. Inhaled therapy is therefore preferred to oral, as the former limits the amount of drug that finds its way into the general circulation. The long-acting beta-agonist agents salmeterol and eformoterol offer a more favourable dose regimen, and respiratory physicians are adding a long-acting beta-agonist for patients who have not responded fully to short-acting beta-agonists and an anticholinergic used together.

Anticholinergics

Anticholinergic bronchodilators work by preventing bronchoconstriction, mediated by the parasympathetic nervous system. Two agents are currently available, ipratropium bromide and oxitropium bromide. Most studies suggest that these agents are at least as potent as beta-agonists when used alone in COPD (Tashkin et al. 1986). A short-acting bronchodilator (beta$_2$-agonist or anticholinergic) used 'as required' is recommended as initial therapy in the British Thoracic Society guidelines (BTS 1997).

Xanthene derivatives

The precise mode of action of the xanthene derivatives such as theophylline and aminophylline remains somewhat uncertain although they are moderately powerful bronchodilators. They have, however, been shown to improve symptoms in COPD by increasing the contractual ability of the diaphragm (Murciano et al. 1989).

Corticosteroids

The role of inhaled steroids (beclomethasone, budesonide) in COPD will vary from patient to patient. Steroids work by reducing inflammation and reducing bronchial hyperactivity. Trials have shown that about 10–20% of COPD patients will improve significantly following a short course of high-dose oral steroids (Gross 1995).

The most serious limitation to oral steroid therapy is the risk of long-term side-effects, which include osteoporosis, adrenal suppression, muscle wasting, poor immune response and impaired healing. However, a positive response to corticosteroids justifies the administration of regular inhaled steroids.

Drug Delivery Systems

The objective of inhaled therapy in COPD is to maximise the quantity of drug that reaches its site of action while minimising side-effects from unintended systemic absorption. Most metered-dose inhalers (which are later described in detail for asthmatic patients) are designed to deliver particles of between 0.5 and 10 microns (micrometres). Unfortunately, poor inhaler technique tends to mean that only a relatively small proportion of the drug actually reaches its site of action. It is therefore imperative that a good inhaler technique be adopted (as described for patients with asthma).

In acute exacerbations, when conventional inhalers have proved inadequate, nebulisers may be used to deliver a therapeutic dose of a drug as an aerosol within a fairly short period of time, usually 5–10 minutes (British Thoracic Society 1997). The type of nebuliser for home use consists of a compressor or pump, a chamber and a mask or mouthpiece. The compressor blows air into the chamber, where it is forced through a drug solution and past a series of baffles. The solution is converted into a fine mist, which is then inhaled by the patient through the mask or the mouthpiece.

PHYSIOTHERAPY TECHNIQUES IN COPD

General Aims of Treatment

The general aims are:

- to relieve any bronchospasm and facilitate the removal of secretions
- to improve the pattern of breathing, breathing control and the control of dyspnoea
- to teach local relaxation, improve posture and help allay fear and anxiety
- to increase knowledge of the patient's lung condition and control of the symptoms
- to improve exercise tolerance and ensure a long-term commitment to exercise
- to give advice about self-management in activities of daily living.

The treatment given must be appropriate to the stage of the disease and the patient's general health.

Treatment in the Early Stages

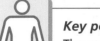

Key point
The most important themes are clearing the airways of secretions, establishing a correct breathing pattern, improving or maintaining exercise capacity, and patient education into self-management.

Removal of secretions

The active cycle of breathing technique (ACBT) (illustrated on page 374)

This is a cycle of breathing control, thoracic expansion exercises and the forced expiratory technique (FET) and has been shown to be effective in the clearance of bronchial secretions (Prior et al. 1979; Wilson et al. 1995) and to improve lung function (Webber et al. 1986).

Thoracic expansion exercises are deep breathing exercises (three or four) which may be combined with a 3-second hold on inspiration (unless the patient is very breathless when this may not be tolerated). This increase in lung volume allows air to flow via collateral channels (e.g. the pores of Kohn) and may assist in mobilising the secretions as air is able to get behind the secretions. The increase in lung volume during the inspiratory phase of the cycle may also be achieved by the patient performing a 'sniff' manoeuvre at the end of a deep inspiration. Manual techniques, for example shaking, vibrations or chest clapping, may further aid in removal of secretions.

The FET manoeuvre is a combination of one or two forced expirations (huffs) against an open glottis (as opposed to a cough, which is a forced expiration against a closed glottis). An essential part of the FET manoeuvre is a pause for some breathing control, which prevents an increase in airflow obstruction.

Postural drainage

This may also aid sputum removal and may be combined with the ACBT technique. The optimum position for effectiveness must be established with each individual, although postural drainage for the lower lobe segments may be difficult as some patients may not tolerate the head-down position or even lying flat.

Humidification

If the secretions are very thick and tenacious the patient may be given humidification via a nebuliser. Inhalations with pine oil added to near-boiling water may also be given prior to treatments to remove excessive bronchial secretions.

Improving the breathing pattern

The patient is taught how to relax the shoulder girdle in a supported posturally correct position such as crook half-lying. Breathing control is taught following clearance of secretions. If the patient is breathless, respiratory control is regained starting with short respiratory phases and allowing the rate to slow as the patient's breathing pattern improves.

Increasing/maintaining exercise tolerance

The patient may be treated as an inpatient or as an out-patient, in a health centre or at home by a community physiotherapist. It is important to see the patient regularly. Advice should be given on taking regular exercises, as for example a short walk every day. If possible, the patient should be offered participation in a multi-disciplinary comprehensive programme of pulmonary rehabilitation.

Definition

The National Institutes of Health in the USA defines pulmonary rehabilitation as 'a multidimensional continuum of services directed to persons with pulmonary disease and their families, usually an interdisciplinary team of specialists, with the goal of achieving and maintaining the individual's maximum level of independence and functioning in the community' (American Thoracic Society 1995).

There is unequivocal evidence to suggest that pulmonary rehabilitation improves both exercise capacity and health-related quality of life (Lacasse et al. 1996). In essence, the components of a pulmonary rehabilitation programme include aerobic exercise training, education about the background of the disease, smoking cessation, compliance with medication, nutritional support and energy-conserving strategies for activities of daily living (ADLs). Pulmonary rehabilitation programmes may also include psychosocial support with regard to advice on benefits, sexual function and anxiety management.

Inspiratory muscle training

The potential for fatigue of the ventilatory muscles is now recognized as an important component of ventilatory limitation in patients with COPD (Moxham 1990; Green and Moxham 1993). Fatigue may be due to a combination of:

- increased mechanical load on the respiratory muscles
- reduced muscle strength
- reduced energy supply to the respiratory muscles (Roussos and Zakynthinos 1996).

It has also been established that respiratory muscle weakness, which may be a predisposition to muscle fatigue, is present in patients with chronic obstructive

pulmonary disease (Clanton and Diaz 1995; Polkey et al. 1995). It therefore follows that training techniques, which might specifically target the respiratory muscles, may prove beneficial in patients with COPD who may develop respiratory muscle weakness due to a loss of muscle mass.

Many studies have been performed examining the benefits of inspiratory muscle training (IMT), particularly in patients with chronic obstructive pulmonary disease (Smith et al. 1992). Despite this intensive investigation, IMT has failed to become part of routine clinical practice. In part this has been due to the paucity of controlled clinical trials, but more importantly due to the nature of the training adopted. In general the trials were confounded by the nature of their training methodology in which the frequency, duration and intensity of training were less than that required to achieve a true training response (Smith et al. 1992). Therefore the training methodology employed during IMT should follow the same principles that are applied to other skeletal muscles in terms of the frequency, duration and intensity of the training.

Training methodologies should also control for the lung volume at which the training takes place, otherwise the patient may alter the lung volume at which the training is performed in order to cope with the resistive load more easily (Goldstein et al. 1993). However, recent studies which have incorporated these principles during training at 80% of maximum inspiratory pressure (MIP) have shown evidence of muscle fatigue (Chatwin et al. 2000) which indicates an appropriate training response has been applied. Furthermore, by using an appropriate training methodology, increases in exercise capacity in both moderately trained and highly trained subjects and in adult patients with cystic fibrosis have been achieved (Chatham et al. 1999, Enright et al. 2000).

Treatment in the Later Stages

It is imperative that patients with COPD be able to maintain as much independence and maximum function as is possible through the support from the hospital or community healthcare team. During acute exacerbations, the active cycle of breathing technique (ACBT) may be continued to assist clearance of secretions. Breathing control should be emphasised so that the patient can walk or climb stairs with confidence. Relaxation positions should be taught for regaining breathing control after activity has made the patient breathless. If the patient becomes very disabled, a walking frame may help to retain some degree of independence as the arms are fixed and accessory muscles of inspiration may be used.

Non-invasive positive-pressure ventilation (NIPPV)

Tracheal intubation and mechanical ventilation providing intermittent positive-pressure ventilation (IPPV) is used in intensive care units or high-dependency units to manage patients with deteriorating respiratory failure. However, tracheal intubation may result in complications, which include tracheal injury and infection. Furthermore, some patients find it difficult to stop using IPPV, resulting in a prolonged stay in intensive care.

Non-invasive positive pressure ventilation (NIPPV) is therefore indicated for the delivery of intermittent positive pressure and may be applied via the nose or mouth using a silicone mask attached to a bedside ventilator. Unlike IPPV, NIPPV can be administered on a general ward for patients in respiratory failure (Sinuff et al. 2000). The ventilator is programmed to supplement the patient's own respiratory effort and if required oxygen therapy may be given in conjunction with NIPPV. NIPPV can be used during an acute exacerbation and has been shown to improve quality of life and arterial blood gas pressures (Meecham-Jones et al. 1995) and to reduce mortality in patients with COPD (Brochard et al. 1995).

Physiotherapy will be required for short spells but frequently throughout the day and sometimes at night. Intermittent positive pressure breathing (IPPB) may also be given using a mask if the patient is too drowsy to use a mouthpiece. Postural drainage may be necessary, if tolerated, together with rigorous shaking applied during the expiratory phase of the ventilator. Patients should be positioned appropriately in order to facilitate gaseous exchange.

Suction via an airway or nasal suction may have to be used as a last resort to remove secretions if the patient is unable to cough spontaneously. If $PaCO_2$ is high and PaO_2 is low the patient should not be given a high concentration of oxygen. Two litres of oxygen through a nebuliser with the IPPB respirator driven off air gives a 25% oxygen-to-air mix which is generally suitable. Drugs such as mucolytic agents or bronchodilators may be provided through the nebuliser attached to the ventilator. The patient should be encouraged to sip drinks because dehydration makes the secretions viscid.

As the patient recovers, treatment should be directed towards that given in the 'early' stages, with special emphasis on a daily maintenance programme of regular exercise, sputum clearance and breathing exercises.

Terminal care

The main theme is to keep the patient as comfortable as possible. Treatment needs to be short and frequent.

Non-invasive nasal ventilation may be provided for home use. Inhalations may be used to loosen and liquefy secretions. Suction may be necessary and the general practitioner may provide medication for the patient if the person is being managed at home.

ASTHMA

Definition
Asthma is a clinical syndrome characterised by attacks of wheezing and breathlessness due to narrowing of the intrapulmonary airways. The severity of the narrowing varies over short periods and is reversible either spontaneously or as a result of treatment (Hargreave et al. 1990).

Types of Asthma

It has been common practice to divide asthma into *extrinsic* and *intrinsic* forms. There is a degree of overlap, and many asthmatics, particularly adults, do not fall clearly into either group.

Extrinsic asthma

Extrinsic (atopic) asthma occurs in the younger age groups and is caused by identifiable trigger factors, such as specific allergens. Patients are usually sensitive to different factors (e.g. pollen, house dust mites, feathers, fur, dust, pollution and, occasionally, food, drugs and exercise) and have a family history of similar sensitivities. Atopic subjects show an immediate skin reaction, elicited by pricking the skin through a drop of antigenic extract. Exposure to the precipitating factor causes a mucosal inflammatory allergic reaction. This type of asthma tends to be episodic. House dust mites provide the most common positive skin test in Britain, being positive in 80% of children with severe asthma. Extrinsic asthma is common in young people and is associated with a family history of asthma, hay fever and eczema.

Intrinsic asthma

Intrinsic (non-atopic) asthma tends to occur in the older patient as a chronic condition. It has no apparent allergic cause or family history. This type of asthma is precipitated by, or associated with, chronic bronchitis, strenuous exercise, stress or anxiety. Respiratory infections are also a common factor in precipitating acute attacks although the majority of these are viral in origin (Nicholson et al. 1993) – so antibiotics are inappropriate in their treatment.

Aetiology and Prevalence of Asthma

The condition can occur at any age but is most common in children, especially boys (ratio of about three to two). Approximately 10% of children under 10 years of age in the United Kingdom have bouts of coughing and wheezing related to narrowing of the airways. Asthma accounts for more absences from school than any other chronic disease, although days lost from school may be under-estimated owing to the under-diagnosis and under-treatment of childhood asthma (Speight 1983).

Childhood asthma generally remits after puberty but it may return in later life. Asthma that starts in middle age is more common in women than men and remission in this age group is rare.

The majority of cases of asthma are mild, although the course of the disease is unpredictable. The mortality rate is unacceptably high and has shown a slow rise since the 1960s to around 2000 deaths per year in England and Wales. Under-treatment and inadequate appreciation of the severity of asthma by patients and doctors are important factors, with up to 86% of asthma deaths being preventable (British Thoracic Association 1982). Those most at risk are the patients who under-estimate their symptoms. About 15–20% of asthmatics do not notice moderate changes in their airflow obstruction (Rubinfeld and Pain 1976) and may quickly deteriorate until they suddenly present with severe asthma (Kikuchi et al. 1994).

Pathology of Asthma

In all types of asthma an underlying problem seems to lie in abnormal reactivity of the airways; that is, they narrow excessively in response to stimuli which would not affect normal subjects (Bone 1996). The main pathological changes occurring during an asthmatic attack are:

- spasm of the smooth muscle in the walls of the bronchi and bronchioles (bronchoconstriction)
- oedema of the mucous membrane of the bronchi and bronchioles
- excessive mucus production and mucus plugging.

These changes result in airways obstruction. The bronchial walls become infiltrated with eosinophils and there is thickening of the epithelial basement membrane.

At the end of an attack these changes are almost totally reversible, but if attacks occur frequently then long-standing changes will occur. Such changes are hypertrophy of the smooth bronchial muscle, which increases the effect of bronchial spasm during an attack; permanent thickening of the mucous membrane with an increase in the number of goblet cells and mucous glands; over-distension of the alveoli due to trapping of air; and atelectasis of alveoli when a bronchiole, already narrowed, becomes blocked by mucus plugs.

Where the predominant factor precipitating asthma is an allergic reaction there is antigen-mediated bronchoconstriction. This means that the antigen (allergen or precipitating factor) binds to two IgE molecules (immunoglobulin antibodies) on the membranes of mast cells present in the bronchial lining. This binding releases mediators which act on receptor sites on smooth muscle cells, causing changes in intracellular cyclic AMP levels which result in muscular contraction. The mediators histamine, neutrophil chemotactic factor (NCF-A), platelet activating factor (PAF) and eosinophil chemotactic factor (ECF-A) are stored in granules within the mast cells as preformed mediators. This antigen-antibody reaction is part of the body's immune response, and previous exposure to the antigen results in greater bronchoconstriction.

Clinical Features of Asthma

Extrinsic asthma

In extrinsic asthma the onset is often sudden and paroxysmal, often at night. An attack starts with chest tightness, dryness or irritation in the upper respiratory tract. Attacks tend to be episodic, often occurring several times a year. Their duration varies from a few seconds to many months and the severity may be anything from mild wheezing to great distress. The most predominant features are summarised below.

Wheeze and dyspnoea

Dyspnoea may be intense and chiefly occurs on expiration, which becomes a conscious exhausting effort with a short gasping inspiration. Wheezing is always present on expiration but may also occur on inspiration in severe asthma.

Cough

At the initial stage of an attack the cough may be unproductive and 'barking' in nature. It causes an increase in bronchospasm and dyspnoea. As the attack subsides, the cough becomes productive of casts or plugs of sputum. Such plugs – made up of yellow viscid mucus and desquamated epithelial cells and eosinophils – are often coughed up during acute attacks, which may produce a marked relief of symptoms. Particularly in children, a cough may be the only presenting symptom of asthma (Corraco et al. 1979).

Posture

The patient will prefer to sit upright with the shoulder girdle fixed (by grasping a table or bed) to assist the accessory muscles of respiration. The chest is hyperinflated.

Pulse

This is rapid and there may be an increased drop in blood pressure during inspiration (>10 mmHg) owing to an exaggeration in intrathoracic pressure swings due to severe airways obstruction (pulsus paradoxus). However, pulsus paradoxus may be absent even in very severe attacks of asthma. When it is present, the measurement is easily performed with a sphygmomanometer and provides a guide to progress and response to treatment (Pearson et al. 1993).

Electrocardiogram (ECG)

This will show a tachycardia and may show signs of right ventricular strain or the development of a large P wave (P pulmonale). These abnormalities will return to normal as the attack subsides.

Cyanosis

This may occur at a very late stage in the progression of the disease due to worsening hypoxaemia (low PaO_2) if this is not corrected with adequate oxygen therapy.

Blood gases

Analysis of blood gases provides important information to help the management of severe asthma. The usual finding is of a low arterial PaO_2 (hypoxaemia) due to ventilation/perfusion mismatch, and a low $PaCO_2$ (hypocapnia) due to the effects of hyperventilation. Later in the disease process, the $PaCO_2$ may be found to be high because the hyperventilation fails to compensate for the fact that there are many underventilated alveoli which are distal to the blocked bronchioles. When the $PaCO_2$ is found to be increasing and the pH is low this should be a danger sign that the patient may be becoming tired and be likely to need assisted ventilation if immediate improvement cannot be achieved (British Thoracic Society 1997).

Breath sounds

These are vesicular with evidence of a prolonged expiration and high-pitched wheeze. Crackles may also be heard if sputum is present. During severe attacks with worsening obstruction, the breath sounds may be diminished and occasionally become inaudible (silent chest) due to diminished airflow.

Percussion note

The note may be hyper-resonant if the patient is hyperinflated.

Chest X-ray

Radiography is not usually helpful in the management of asthma. It usually shows only overinflation although may also show a pneumothorax if this is suspected.

Lung function

FEV_1 and FVC drop during a severe attack with little sign of reversibility (Figure 14.5). However, if FEV_1 is measured before and after giving bronchodilators and there is a 15% increase in FEV_1 – this amounts to significant reversibility. The FEV_1 may be less than 30% of FVC. Total lung capacity, FRC and RV may be increased due to overinflation of the lungs. Recovery is associated with a reduction in these lung volumes. Recordings of the peak expiratory flow rate (PEFR) for a week at home will often make the diagnosis of asthma obvious (Prior and Cochrane 1980). PEFR dips in the morning especially during the recovery phase (Figure 14.6). If the dip is severe (less than 33% of predicted) then respiratory arrest may occur (British Thoracic Society 1997). In a severe attack, the PEFR may drop below 100 litres/minute.

Between attacks

No abnormality should be detectable between attacks, although children with severe asthma may develop a pigeon chest or have a persistent, low-pitched wheeze with a productive cough.

Intrinsic (chronic) asthma

This is less paroxysmal in character than extrinsic asthma and is often associated with chronic bronchitis.

Clinical features are similar to those described above for extrinsic asthma, but wheeze and dyspnoea tend to be continuous and worse in the morning, cough produces mucoid sputum, respiratory infections occur with increasing frequency, and radiographs may show emphysematous changes.

Acute severe asthma

As asthma is by nature a paroxysmal condition, acute attacks that are resistant to bronchodilators may occur. Such attacks are potentially life-threatening, so

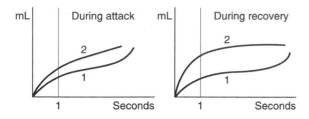

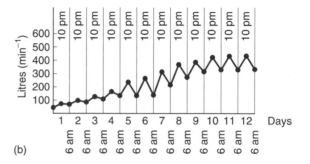

Figure 14.5   Asthma: FEV₁ and FVC reversibility during an attack and recovery. 1 = before bronchodilator; 2 = after bronchodilator.

prompt and effective treatment is imperative. In general, clinical criteria are most helpful and the recognition by the person that his or her asthma symptoms are worsening. Table 14.2 lists warning signs of an acute severe attack.

MEDICAL TREATMENT OF ASTHMA

Oxygen Therapy

Unlike patients with long-standing COPD, patients with asthma may tolerate higher levels of oxygen to correct hypoxaemia. During an acute episode it is essential that oxygen therapy be titrated according to the level of PaO_2. It may be evident on clinical examination, however, that the asthmatic patient also has evidence of COPD. In this situation examination of the blood gases will reveal whether the patient has a chronic compensated respiratory acidosis where the use of controlled oxygen will be required.

Medications

Suitable drugs are discussed in the earlier section on the management of patients with COPD. Their use is discussed here particularly with regard to the treatment of asthma.

Beta₂ (β₂) agonists

The side-effects of salbutamol (Ventolin) and terbutaline (Bricanyl) include fine tremor, tachycardia, hypokalaemia (low potassium) after high doses.

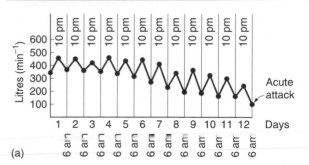

Figure 14.6   Dipping charts in asthma. (a) Recording of peak flow at home showing deterioration before onset of acute attack. Intervention when there is a chart like this can prevent the attack. (b) During recovery there is still diurnal variation. These patients are at risk and should have long-term monitoring.

Corticosteroids

In a small proportion of asthmatic people, long-term oral corticosteroids (e.g. beclomethasone and budesonide) will be necessary. In circumstances when an attack supervenes very rapidly, a short course of oral steroids (prednisolone) is required. It cannot be emphasised enough that this approach is safe and certainly much safer than a poorly controlled attack of asthma. There have been suggestions that the adverse effects associated with long-term steroids, such as osteoporosis, might be less common in asthma but this has been shown to be untrue (Adinoff and Hollester 1983). The introduction of inhaled corticosteroids in 1972 radically changed the management of asthma as side-effects from oral steroids were prevented.

Table 14.2 Warning signs of an attack of acute severe asthma.

Early warning signs	Signs of increasing severity
Increase in symptoms	Dyspnoea at rest
Sleep disturbance	Peak flow below 100 L/min
Increase in bronchodilator use	Deteriorating blood gases
Fall in peak flow	Pulsus paradoxus
Decrease in exercise tolerance	Tachycardia

Leukotriene antagonists

Oral inhibitors of leukotriene action may help to reduce the inflammatory component of asthma (Israel et al. 1993).

> **Mucolytic agents and asthma**
> There is no evidence that mucolytic agents are effective in the treatment of acute or chronic asthma (Rudolf et al. 1978).

Other agents

Other types of medication that may be useful include:

- anticholinergic agents
- long-acting beta$_2$ agonists
- theophylline
- salmeterol.

Delivery of Medication

Metered-dose inhalers

It is good practice to use inhaled therapy for asthma. This keeps the dose down and reduces side-effects.

Beta$_2$ agonists, anticholinergic agents and corticosteroids are frequently prescribed in metered-dose inhalers (MDIs). The particles leaving an MDI do so with considerable velocity and even with a perfect technique of inhalation only about 10% of the dose reaches the respiratory tract; the remainder is deposited in the mouth or swallowed (Davies 1973). The MDI does have the advantage of being small and portable and familiar to many asthmatics. The MDI can also be used with a spacer which virtually removes oropharangeal deposition, thereby increasing lung deposition to 20–30% (O'Callahan et al. 1997)

Breath-activated devices (Figure 14.7) are primed before actuation and the MDI is triggered by inspiratory airflow. The airflow required is low and the triggering of the device quiet enough not to disturb the inspiration. Beta$_2$ agonists, anticholinergic agents and corticosteroids can be prescribed in this form of inhaler.

There are various *dry powder systems* (Figure 14.8):

- The Diskhaler contains four or eight doses in one disc. Each dose is sealed to prevent problems with humidity.
- The Turbohaler is a multidose dry powder system which requires an inspiratory airflow of only 60 litres/minute. Patients therefore tend to find this system easy to use.

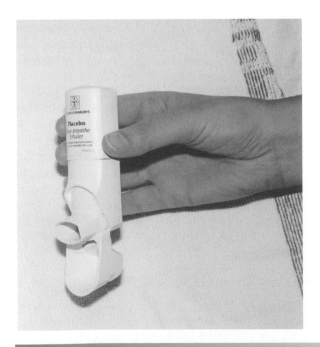

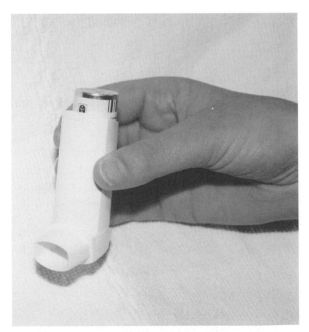

Figure 14.7   Breath-activated metered-dose inhalers. Photos courtesy Melanie Reardon and Joanne Kenyon.

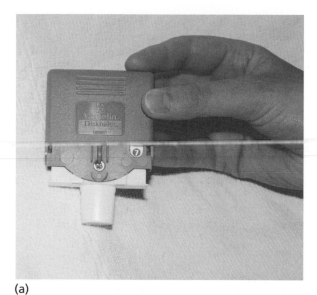

(a)

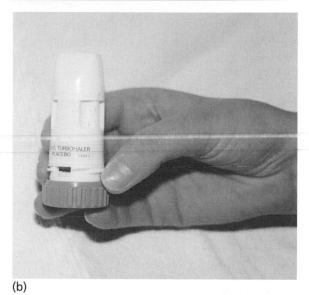

(b)

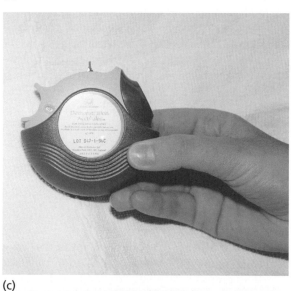

(c)

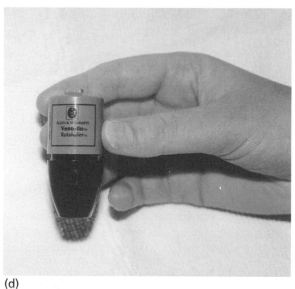

(d)

Figure 14.8 Dry powder systems: (a) Diskhaler; (b) Turbohaler; (c) Disk/Accuhaler; (d) Rotocaps. Photos courtesy Melanie Reardon and Joanne Kenyon.

- The Disk/Accuhaler is a dry powder multidose system used for the delivery of salmeterol and fluticasone propionate.
- With Rotocaps each dose of medication is loaded into the inhaler prior to use and so the inhaler needs to be stored in a dry place. Rotocaps absorb moisture and the particles can become too large to inhale.

Nebulisers

If asthma symptoms become severe, inspiratory airflow may become limited to such an extent that the contents of an MDI cannot be inhaled adequately. With a nebuliser a high-velocity jet of air or oxygen sucks liquid up

a tube and the liquid is broken into tiny particles which are inhaled and deposited in the lungs (Rees et al. 1982). Ultrasonic nebulisers may also be used to deliver medication, although currently there is insufficient data to verify their advantage over other nebulisers in the management of patients with asthma and COPD (Brocklebank et al. 2001).

Guidelines for Drug Therapy

The British Thoracic Society (1997) has recently introduced guidelines on the drug management of asthma. Steps 1 to 3 below apply to the treatment of less severe asthma, in an attempt to control symptoms. Steps 4 and 5 apply to the treatment of more severe asthma,

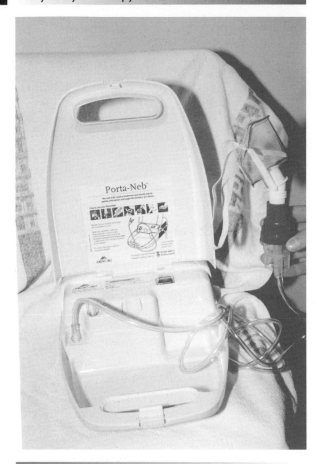

Figure 14.9   Portable nebuliser.

when it may not be possible to abolish symptoms. Stepping down and up this treatment ladder is recommended to match therapy to the person's current need.

- *Step 1*: Inhaled short-acting beta$_2$ agonists p.r.n. (when required), but not more than once daily. If needed more than once daily, move on to step 2. No prophylaxis (preventers such as inhaled corticosteroids).
- *Step 2*: Inhaled short-acting beta$_2$ agonists p.r.n. Regular low-dose inhaled steroids, such as 100–400 micrograms of beclomethasone twice daily, or budesonide daily via a large volume spacer.
- *Step 3*: Inhaled short-acting beta$_2$ agonists p.r.n. Regular high-dose inhaled steroids, such as 800–2000 micrograms of beclomethasone, or budesonide daily via a large volume spacer. In a very small number of patients who experience side-effects with high-dose inhaled steroids, either the long-acting inhaled beta$_2$ agonists option is used *or* a sustained-release theophylline may be added to step 2 medication.
- *Step 4*: Inhaled short-acting beta$_2$ agonists p.r.n. Regular high-dose inhaled steroids, such as

800–2000 micrograms of beclomethasone, or budesonide daily via a large volume spacer. Add in long-acting inhaled beta$_2$ agonists *or* sustained-release theophylline or high-dose inhaled bronchodilators.
- *Step 5*: Inhaled short-acting beta$_2$ agonists p.r.n. Regular high-dose inhaled steroids, such as 800–2000 micrograms of beclomethasone, or budesonide daily via a large volume spacer. Add in one or more long-acting bronchodilator as in step 4 *plus* regular oral prednisolone as a single daily dose.

Management between Attacks

The environment

This comprises identifying and removing the cause, if known. For example, a patient may have to avoid certain foods and damp. The home environment should be cleaned regularly, bedding vacuumed frequently, and synthetic fibres used in place of feathers for pillows and quilts. Gor-tex mattress covers are not inexpensive but are impervious to mites and their fecal particles. It may also be of benefit to avoid certain domestic animals, although getting rid of a loved family pet may provoke emotional problems in children, which can make their asthma worse. Desensitisation may be possible by injection of mild doses of the allergen, which will have been identified by a skin test although avoidance of these allergens altogether may be difficult.

Measurement of peak flow

Measurement of peak flow can be useful so that variability of lung function is clearly seen and treatment is titrated accordingly. The patient may then alter medication in order to control his or her symptoms. This is based upon the extent to which the peak flow deteriorates (60%, 40% or 30% of the patient's expected value). An example of a peak flow action plan, which will be kept by the patient for reference and which is based on the British Thoracic Society (1997) guidelines, is shown in Table 14.3.

Inhaler technique

When drugs are administered by aerosol/inhaler it is important that the patient be taught how to use the device correctly. The use of various inhaler devices requires some skill on the part of the patient and teaching the correct method of use is an essential part of the prescription of such treatment. Failure to master a metered-dose inhaler occurs in many patients of all ages. The technique for a metered-dose inhaler in which the drug is suspended in a propellant is as follows.

Table 14.3 Peak Flow Action Plan.

Daily medication	Seretide (purple inhaler) **1 suck every morning and evening**
As-needed medication	Salbutamol (blue inhaler) **2 puffs as needed**
Best peak flow reading when well	300 L/min
If unwell with cough, wheeze, breathlessness or tight chest or peak flow 310 L/min or below	Continue daily medication(s) as above Commence salbutamol (blue) **4 puffs every 4 hours** Record peak flow readings every 4 hours before taking blue inhaler
If peak flow falls to 230 L/min	Commence oral steroids **8 tablets once a day** for 3 days See your doctor within 24 hours of commencing oral steroids
If the action plan does not help relieve your child's symptoms for 4 hours or peak flow reading falls to 150 L/min, then you must seek urgent medical attention.	

1 *Shake the inhaler.* This disperses the drug uniformly throughout the propellant.
2 *Hold the inhaler upright and direct into the mouth.* If it is not held upright the metering chamber will not fill correctly.
3 *Start inspiration and press the activating mechanism.* The drug will be effective only if it is breathed in during inspiration. Although there is some controversy regarding the lung volume at which the actuation should occur (Newman et al. 1981) it is simpler to teach the person to discharge the inhaler at the beginning of inspiration.
4 *Breathe in slowly through the mouth.* The flow rate of inspiration should be slow (Newman et al. 1982). This helps to reduce impaction on the pharynx and allow for further penetration of the drug into the bronchial tree, since flow is laminar rather than turbulent.
5 *Hold the breath at maximum inspiration for 5–10 seconds.* This allows particles of the drug to settle on the airway walls. Ideally, the breath should be held for 10 seconds.
6 *Relax and allow easy expiration.* Patients need to be aware of when their inhaler is getting close to empty and patients should be instructed to shake their inhaler in order to gauge this. Another method is to place the inhaler in water. If it floats symmetrically upright then it is close to empty. It is always good advice to instruct the patient to have two inhalers at home, to avoid being caught out in an exacerbation without adequate relief.

PHYSIOTHERAPY TECHNIQUES IN ASTHMA

General Aims of Treatment

The principal aims are:

- to relieve any bronchospasm and to facilitate the removal of secretions
- to improve breathing control and the control of dyspnoea during attacks
- to teach local relaxation, improve posture and help allay fear and anxiety
- to increase knowledge of the lung condition and control of symptoms
- to improve exercise tolerance and ensure a long-term commitment to exercise
- to give advice about self-management.

The management of asthmatic patients should include maintenance of a good general fitness, and a vital part of asthma management is to educate the patient.

Patient education

All asthmatic patients and their close relatives should be aware of how to manage their asthma, and the physiotherapist is integral is the education process. Prevention of infection is important. The patient should have plenty of fresh air, avoid smoky atmospheres and keep away from people with infections such as bronchitis and influenza. Stress or anxiety must be minimised as these can precipitate an attack.

Patients must know what therapy to take and how to take it and where they should go to seek further help. All this should be carefully planned beforehand and incorporated into a written action plan and self-management strategy (refer to Table 14.3).

Acute attacks

Treatment during acute exacerbations will involve the physiotherapist in aiding removal of excessive bronchial secretions using the ACBT technique (see above), with the addition of postural drainage, if tolerated. Percussion and shakings should be applied sensitively as they may increase bronchospasm. Breathing control and the adoption of relaxed positions may be necessary.

Pulmonary rehabilitation

Pulmonary rehabilitation has largely been confined to patients with COPD, but there is now a recognition that other patient groups may benefit. The principles are the same as those previously described for patients with COPD but with some additional considerations.

Patients with asthma are younger but very commonly have a fear and inhibition of exercise (Cochrane et al. 1990) and therefore can benefit from improved cardiorespiratory fitness (Patessio et al. 1993). Also, unlike patients with COPD, individuals with asthma usually show a greater variability in airflow obstruction, and are more susceptible to exercise-induced exacerbations (EIEs). Consideration needs to be given to the prevention of exacerbations (such as by the self-administration of beta$_2$ agonists prior to exercise), although certain exercises – for example swimming – are the least likely to cause an EIE. In addition to whole-body programmes, inspiratory muscle training may also be incorporated into the exercise programme (as described previously for COPD patients).

Removal of secretions

Some patients, especially children, have constant excessive secretions and may require postural drainage with the ACBT on a daily basis. It may be essential to teach forced expiration technique for clearing secretions without increasing bronchospasm.

Relaxation

If the patient is able to practice relaxation it may be possible to ward off an attack when there has been exposure to an allergen. The onset of an attack is often preceded by a 'tickle' in the throat or a sensation of tightness in the chest. Relaxation and breathing control in an appropriate position may prevent an attack developing. 'Appropriate position' depends on where the patient is and may have to be against a wall or the back of a chair.

Breathing control

Encouraging a longer expiratory phase is helpful, but neither inspiration nor expiration should be forced. This may be helped by counting (e.g. 'in 1-2, out 1-2-3') and by manual pressure just under the xiphisternum to encourage diaphragmatic excretion. The patient must breathe at a rate and rhythm that suits him or her. Children may be taught to breathe to a nursery rhyme.

BRONCHIECTASIS

Definition
Bronchiectasis is an abnormal dilatation of the bronchi associated with obstruction and infection (Cole 1995).

The most common cause of bronchiectasis is damage to the bronchial tree after infection. Bronchiectasis may also complicate bronchial obstruction or a more widespread disorder (e.g. cystic fibrosis).

Types and Prevalence of Bronchiectasis

The condition most commonly affects the lower lobes, the lingula and then the middle lobe. It tends to affect the left lung more than the right, although 50% of cases are bilateral. The upper lobes are least affected since they drain most efficiently with the assistance of gravity. There are broadly two types of disease.

Congenital bronchiectasis

This is very rare and occurs in Kartagener's syndrome ('immotile cilia' syndrome) where there is a congenital microtubular abnormality of the cilia that prevents normal cilial beating. It is characterised by bronchiectasis, sinusitis, dextrocardia and complete visceral transposition. There may also be associated male infertility.

Acquired bronchiectasis

Bronchial obstruction and bacterial infection are the principal factors responsible for this disease. Obstruction of a bronchus, which may be due to a tumour or foreign body, will cause collapse of the lung tissue supplied by that bronchus. Bronchiectasis may also occur following an infection, which causes the production of sticky sputum leading to obstruction of multiple small bronchi. Classically this is associated with whooping cough, tuberculosis, measles and pneumonia in childhood, when the airways are smaller and therefore more easily 'plug' with sputum. Very occasionally, bronchiectasis may occur as a late complication of tuberculosis, which has affected the right middle lobe causing that segment to collapse. It may also occur following lung abscess and pneumonia and be associated with immune defects in patients with hypogammaglobulinaemia. Allergic bronchopulmonary aspergillosis, which is associated with an autoimmune response, can cause formation of mucus plugs resulting in bronchiectasis of the medium-sized bronchi.

Prevalence

The prevalence of bronchiectasis following a childhood infection is decreasing dramatically since these infections are now treated with antibiotics, but bronchiectasis is a common feature of cystic fibrosis.

Pathology of Bronchiectasis

Bronchial obstruction may be localised (due perhaps to an inhaled foreign body such as a peanut or broken tooth or obstruction due to a tumour or enlarged gland) or generalised (e.g. pneumonia that is slow to resolve owing to whooping cough or measles).

The bronchial obstruction will cause absorption of the air from the lung tissue distal to the obstruction and this area will therefore shrink and collapse. This causes a traction force to be exerted upon the more proximal airways, which will distort and dilate them. If the obstruction can be cleared and the lung re-expanded quickly then the dilatation is reversible. Secretions may collect distal to the obstruction if it is not relieved quickly and these easily become infected. This causes inflammation of the bronchial wall with destruction of the elastic and muscular tissue. These infections occur repeatedly with the walls becoming weaker and weaker. They will eventually dilate owing to the negative intrapleural pressure. As the disease advances, the bronchi become grossly dilated and pockets containing pus are formed. The elastic and muscle tissue is destroyed and the mucous lining is replaced by granulation tissue with loss of cilia. Therefore, the mucociliary transport mechanism is disrupted and passage of mucus out of the lungs is therefore hindered.

Several types are recognised pathologically: tubular, fusiform or sacular. The arterial vessels within the bronchial walls anastomose with the pulmonary capillaries and this results in the common feature of haemoptysis.

Clinical Features of Bronchiectasis

Key point
Although symptoms often begin in childhood, diagnosis is not usually made until adult life.

Cough and sputum

Patients complain of persistent cough with purulent sputum since childhood. Initially it would be present only following colds or influenza, but if the disease is allowed to progress in its severity the affected segments continually accumulate purulent secretions resulting in cough and sputum production. The sputum is usually green, often foul smelling and present in fairly large volume. The breath is fetid. The cough is particularly troublesome on a change of position and on rising first thing in the morning.

Initially the sputum culture will isolate *Haemophilus influenzae* and/or *Staphylococcus*. In the later stages of the disease *Pseudomonas aeruginosa* and *Klebsiella* may be isolated.

Dyspnoea

Shortness of breath is noticeable only if the disease is particularly severe and widespread. If the bronchiectasis is localised, other well-ventilated and perfused alveoli should maintain blood gases at a reasonable level, although bronchospasm may be a feature particularly during an exacerbation.

Haemoptysis

This occurs quite commonly, usually associated with an acute infection. It can be life-threatening if severe and may require surgical resection of the affected lung tissue.

Recurrent pneumonia

Characteristically this will affect the same sites and is a common feature.

Chronic sinusitis

This occurs in approximately 70% of the patients.

General ill-health

Patients may suffer pyrexia, night sweats, anorexia, malaise, weight loss, lassitude and joint pains.

Clubbing

In about 50% of the patients fingers and toes become clubbed. The first sign of clubbing is loss of the angle between the nail and the nail bed. This is followed by curvature of the nail, and an increase in the soft tissue of the ends of the fingers to form so-called 'drumstick' fingers.

Thoracic mobility

This gradually decreases, as do shoulder girdle movements.

Radiography

Initially the X-ray this will be normal but the patient gradually develops increase in the bronchovascular markings and sometimes shows multiple cysts with fluid levels (Armstrong et al. 1995). Bronchography is used for accurate localisation of the area affected and will reveal dilated bronchi. A CT scan will show bronchial wall thickening and dilation of the bronchi and cysts.

Prognosis of Bronchiectasis

The vast majority of these patients can lead normal lives with a nearly normal life expectancy provided the medical care is adequate. Possible complications, however, are:

- recurrent haemoptysis (common)
- pneumonia (common)
- pleurisy and empyema
- abscess formation (in lung/cerebrum) (rare)
- emphysema (rare)
- respiratory failure
- right ventricular failure (commonly develops after years of pulmonary sepsis and arterial hypoxaemia if there is widespread bronchiectasis)
- systemic amyloidosis (rare).

MANAGEMENT OF BRONCHIECTASIS

Principles of Treatment

The anatomical picture makes very little difference to the treatment of the disease.

- Relieve the obstruction before permanent damage occurs (recognition of either localised obstruction or appropriate treatment for whooping cough or measles).
- Control infection. Antibiotics are given prophylactically in all but very mild cases. The dosage of the antibiotics should be altered if an acute infection occurs. Intravenous treatment is indicated for severe infections (Currie 1997). Inhaled (delivered by a nebuliser) or continuous oral therapy may be used for chronic sepsis and more resistant pathogens (e.g. *Staph. aureus* and *P. aeruginosa*).
- Promote good health with a good diet and fresh air.
- Maintain and improve exercise tolerance as some patients with bronchiectasis become deconditioned owing to fatigue and shortness of breath.
- Inhaled steroids may be used in order to reduce inflammation and reduce the volume of sputum produced (Elborn et al. 1992).
- Surgery to remove the area of affected lung may be indicated in young patients with localised disease, although there is conflicting evidence regarding the efficacy of surgery when compared to conservative treatment (Corless and Warburton 2000).

Physiotherapy

Aims of treatment

The principal aims of physiotherapy in bronchiectasis are:

- to remove secretions and clear lung fields
- to teach an appropriate sputum clearance regimen
- to educate the patient in the pathology and management of the condition
- to promote good general health and maintain or improve exercise tolerance
- to teach the patient how to fit in home treatment within his or her lifestyle.

Clearing secretions

Postural drainage may be indicated, if tolerated for patients with excessive bronchial secretions. The position must be accurate for the areas of lung affected. Accuracy is judged by production of sputum and by identification of the affected areas on a chest radiograph. This minimises the danger of secretion overspill into the least affected side, which could cause spread of the disease or pneumonia. Percussion, shaking and vibrations with the active cycle of breathing technique (ACBT) are also necessary and must be accurately applied over the affected area of the lungs.

The patient may be taught the forced expiration technique (FET). A flutter or positive expiratory pressure (PEP) valve may be used to facilitate the move-

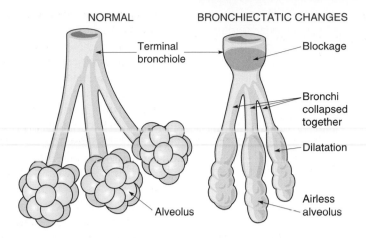

NORMAL   BRONCHIECTATIC CHANGES

Terminal bronchiole

Blockage

Bronchi collapsed together

Dilatation

Alveolus

Airless alveolus

Figure 14.10   Changes of bronchiectasis.

ment of peripheral mucus plugs and pus into the trachea from where they are cleared by coughing. The patient must perform a combination of these treatments 2–3 times daily. It is important to ensure that the patient has disposable sputum pots and polythene or paper bags to dispose of the infected sputum without the risk of reinfection or endangering other members of the family. Should the patient develop a cold or influenza, antibiotics must be readily available together with physiotherapy so that infection and secretions can be cleared promptly.

Maintaining exercise tolerance

Mobility of the thorax, good posture and good general health are achieved by the patient performing a daily exercise programme. This comprises general deep breathing, attention to maintaining a good posture and some aerobic exercise such as brisk walking. The patient may also attend a pulmonary rehabilitation programme if exercise intolerance is impairing mobility and quality of life. The patient should also be encouraged to partake in sports, such as jogging, walking, cycling, tennis or swimming.

CYSTIC FIBROSIS

Definition

Cystic fibrosis (CF) is a hereditary disorder of exocrine glands, with a high sodium chloride content in sweat and pancreatic insufficiency resulting in malabsorption. There is hypertrophy and hyperplasia of mucus-secreting glands resulting in excessive mucus production in the lining of bronchi, which predisposes the patient to chronic bronchopulmonary infection.

Cystic fibrosis is the most common hereditary disorder, being transmitted by a recessive gene, which is estimated to be present in 1 in 20 in the United Kingdom. Cystic fibrosis is the most common life-shortening autosomal recessive disorder in the Caucasian population. It is caused by mutations in a single gene on the long arm of chromosome 7 that encodes the cystic fibrosis transmembrane conductance regulator (CFTR) (Collins 1992).

Pathology of Cystic Fibrosis

Mutations in the CFTR gene result in defective chloride transport, which is accompanied by decreased transport of sodium and water in the epithelial cells in the respiratory, hepatobiliary, gastrointestinal and reproductive tracts and in the pancreas (Quinton 1990). This results in dehydration and hence an increase in the viscosity of secretions that are associated with luminal obstruction and scarring of various exocrine ducts (Oppenheimer and Esterly 1975). Other than in the respiratory system, the resultant clinical manifestations include pancreatic insufficiency, diabetes mellitus, azoospermia in affected men and evidence of biochemical liver abnormality in up to 80% of children (Ling et al. 1999).

The primary causes of morbidity and mortality in patients with CF, however, are bronchiectasis and obstructive pulmonary disease; the latter accounts for over 90% of deaths. Infants with CF have persistent endobronchial bacterial infections (Abman et al. 1991) which are associated with an intense inflammatory response that damages the airway and impairs local host defence mechanisms (Konstan and Berger 1993). Continuous inflammation coupled with thickened pulmonary secretions leads to airways obstruction and hyperinflation (Davis et al. 1996). Hyperinflation becomes a marked feature of the disorder leading to altered pulmonary mechanics, which causes the inspiratory muscles, particularly the diaphragm, to be foreshortened prior to contraction. In such cases, even a small change in breathing pattern (Bellemare and Grassino 1982) or an increase in ventilatory requirement induced by exercise could be enough to induce inspiratory muscle fatigue (Levine and Guillen 1987).

Pulmonary changes

- *Excessive mucus.* There is excess mucus production especially in the small bronchi and bronchioles. These respiratory passages are structurally normal at birth but become blocked by mucus plugs. Lung disease in CF is also characterised by impaired mucocilary clearance of secretions.
- *Viscid mucus.* The abnormality in the mucous glands results in production of mucus with a reduced water content so that the secretions produced are very viscid and stick to the bronchial walls.
- *Infection.* The accumulated mucus provides a medium for growth of bacteria and so the secretions become infected and purulent. This leads to irritation of the bronchial wall tissue, which then becomes inflamed.
- *Bronchiectasis.* Inflammation leads to weakening of the bronchial walls and dilatation occurs as in bronchiectasis.
- *Lack of development of lung tissue.* Mucus and inflammation resulting in airway obliteration inhibits the development of normal lung tissue.

Other pathological changes

Fibrosis of the pancreas causes digestive malfunction and may lead to development of diabetes. Intestinal obstruction may occur owing to gallstones or faecal impaction. In newborn babies, there is intestinal obstruction – known as 'meconium ileus' because there is excess meconium (a greenish black viscid discharge from the bowel of newborn babies) which plugs the small intestine necessitating an emergency operation. Right ventricular hypertrophy occurs owing to pulmonary congestion, which develops as fibrosis, and thickening of the pulmonary arterial walls takes place.

Prognosis of Cystic Fibrosis

With early diagnosis and good management, the life expectancy of patients with CF is increasing and sur-
vival may be to the fourth or fifth decade (Elborn et al. 1991). The majority, however, die before 40 years of age from respiratory failure related to pulmonary infection. In addition to the relentless progression of lung disease, acute exacerbations of chronic infection adversely affect the nutritional status of these patients. During the terminal phase of their life many patients with CF enter into a vicious cycle of repeated respiratory exacerbations with evidence of a deterioration in lung function measurements and declining bodyweight (Elborn et al. 1993). This evidence strongly suggests that the systemic consequences of infection and inflammation are in part responsible for weight loss in patients with CF. Chronic infection may also cause anorexia due to physical factors such as increased mucus production and the anorectic effects of cytokines.

Thus, in patients with CF there may be reduced energy intake, reduced nutrient absorption due to maldigestion, and an increase in energy expenditure resulting from abnormal pulmonary function and sepsis (Bell et al. 1996).

Clinical Features of Cystic Fibrosis

Children

At birth the infant is normal, but symptoms of organ dysfunction can appear soon after birth. The presenting features vary widely.

- *Meconium ileus.* This may present in approximately 10% of infants and is caused by the abnormally viscid nature of the meconium causing obstruction of the terminal ileum.
- *Failure to thrive and gain weight.* This results from chronic malnutrition.
- *Cough producing copious, often purulent, sputum.* Recurrent *Staph. aureus* infections are common and *Pseudomonas* and *Burkholderia capacia* colonise the respiratory tract.
- *Dyspnoea.* This is particularly evident during an exacerbation.
- *Wheezing.* This is due to airway obstruction caused by inflammation and bronchospasm.
- *High level of sodium in sweat.* Sweat sodium and chloride concentrations are elevated (sweat sodium >70 mmol/L) in children under 10 years of age. The test is reliable in older children and adults and is a reliable diagnostic sign.
- *Frequent, foul-smelling stools.* This is because of malabsorption and steatorrhoea (fat in the stools) due to secondary dysfunction of the exocrine pancreas.

Adolescents and adults

- *Progressive breathlessness.* This may be associated with infective exacerbations and increasing disease severity
- *Reduced FEV₁ and deteriorating blood gases.* Pulmonary function tests deteriorate as chronic airways obstruction develops. As the disease progresses ventilation/perfusion imbalance occurs leading to hypoxaemia and pulmonary hypertension.
- *Continued wheezing and productive cough.* This is associated with purulent sputum from which may be cultured strains of *Pseudomonas, Staphylococcus* or *Burkholderia capacia*.
- *Haemoptysis.* This occurs secondary to bronchiectasis.
- *Chest radiograph.* This will show hyperinflation and bronchial wall thickening, particularly in the upper zones and bronchiectasis.
- *Finger clubbing.* This is associated with bronchiectasis.
- *Puberty delayed.* This may be delayed for both male and female patients. Most women have normal or near-normal fertility, although pregnancy may be inadvisable if pulmonary function is less than 60% of expected.
- *Infertility in males.* This occurs owing to blockage of the vas deferens, which is either absent or blocked although they can produce sperm.
- *Lung function tests* (LFTs). There is reduction of the FEV₁/FVC ratio and the FVC is grossly reduced. The residual volume (RV) will be increased at the expense of the VC because of air trapping and the inability of the expiratory muscles to decrease the volume of the thoracic cavity.
- *Blood gases.* Ventilation/perfusion mismatch is inevitable in CF and leads to a low PaO_2 with or without CO_2 retention. As the disease becomes severe, the arterial $PaCO_2$ may rise and a diffusion abnormality will also be apparent.
- *Auscultation.* There will be inspiratory and expiratory wheeze with added coarse crepitations.
- *X-ray.* No characteristic abnormality is seen in the early stages of the disease. If there is significant airways obstruction there may be signs of chest over-expansion (flattening of the diaphragm) and an enlarged reterosternal airspace.

Complications

- *Haemoptysis.* This is usually mild but occasionally frank haemoptysis may occur.
- *Spontaneous pneumothorax.* This may occur due to rupture of emphysematous bullae.

- *Osteoporosis.* There has been a recent recognition of the high prevalence of low bone mineral density leading to osteoporosis and an increased susceptibility to fractures (Haworth et al. 1999).
- *Liver disease.* This usually presents as biliary cirrhosis and may be associated with portal hypertension and oesophageal varices.
- *Diabetes mellitus.* This results from progressive fibrosis damaging the exocrine glands that produce insulin.
- *Deformity.* These patients often develop a barrel chest due to hyperinflation with use of accessory muscles of respiration. There may be evidence of a poor posture including kyphosis and lordosis and associated musculoskeletal pain.
- *Cor pulmonale.* This may occur in the later stages of the disease.

Social–psychological problems

The disease carries with it some unfortunate social and psychological problems. Coughing and spitting are antisocial, so people, in avoiding the patient, are unwittingly unkind. The parents may feel guilty as they are carrying the gene. They have to spend a lot of time with the patient, which creates resentment in siblings. The patient on reaching adolescence may become resentful of treatment and the increasing inability to participate in a full social life. Clearly, this is only a brief mention of the total picture of which the physiotherapist must be aware.

Terminal features

The terminal features include respiratory failure, cyanosis, cor pulmonale, and severe nutritional depletion (accelerated loss of lean body mass and fat mass).

MANAGEMENT OF CYSTIC FIBROSIS

General Principles

Paediatric and adult patients with CF should receive care from a specialist CF centre. A low-fat high-calorie diet is recommended, supplemented with vitamins. In addition to maintaining or improving dietary status, treatment of CF is directed towards the correction of organ dysfunction (Davis 1996), including pancreatic-enzyme replacement and reversal of secondary nutritional and vitamin deficiencies (Ramsey et al. 1992), although the majority of treatment is directed towards the management of abnormalities of pulmonary function. This includes clearance of lower-airway secretions

(Zach and Oberwaldner 1989), treatment of persistent pulmonary infections (Turpin and Knowles 1993) and the alleviation of the symptoms of pulmonary dysfunction, especially breathlessness.

Owing to abnormalities of pulmonary function, patients with CF ventilate excessively and ineffectively at all work levels compared with subjects with normal lung function (Cerny et al. 1982). This results in loss of functional status because aerobic exercise in CF is limited by both cardiovascular and pulmonary mechanisms. Thus, maintenance of exercise capacity in patients with CF is imperative.

Medications

Antibiotics

Antibiotics are essential and the patient will be prescribed one form or another for life. There is much evidence that aggressive intravenous antibiotic therapy in children with CF has resulted in a significantly improved survival rate (Turpin and Knowles 1993). More recent investigations suggest that the use of prophylactic antibiotics is associated with a reduced requirement for additional courses of oral antibiotics and fewer hospital admissions in the first two years of life, although no effect on infant lung function has been identified (Smyth and Walters 2000). In older patients with CF, who are chronically infected with *Pseudomonas* species, no differences in lung function or mortality rate were identified between two groups of 30 patients who were given either elective or symptomatic antibiotic therapy over a 3-year period (Elborn et al. 2000).

Bronchodilators

These may be useful when there is airways obstruction which is reversible. During an acute exacerbation, a nebuliser may be used at home.

Oxygen therapy

Oxygen therapy may be appropriate in the terminal stages when there is persistent hypoxaemia.

Mucolytic agents

Because lung disease in CF is characterised by impaired mucociliary clearance, recurrent bronchial infections and inflammation, methods which may enhance the removal of retained bronchial secretions may act to lessen the destructive inflammatory process in the airways (Solomon et al. 1996).

Nebulised hypertonic saline has been shown to increase mucociliary clearance immediately after administration. This may have long-term beneficial effect, although the effect on pulmonary function tests, quality of life and frequency of exacerbations remains unclear (Wark and McDonald 2000).

Recombinant human deoxyribonuclease (rhDNase) is currently used to treat pulmonary disease in patients with CF by facilitating protein breakdown in pulmonary secretions, thereby aiding expectoration (Christopher et al. 1999). When compared to nebulised saline, evidence suggests that rhDNase may improve FEV_1 by >200 mL in 37% of patients when compared to only 3% of patients after saline when tested over a maximum of three 4-week assessment periods (Bollert et al. 1999). Also when compared to other mucolytic agents, in the short term (6 months) rhDNase has been shown to reduce the risk of respiratory exacerbations (Christopher et al. 1999), although randomised controlled trials to date have been of insufficient duration to answer important questions about long-term outcomes (Kearney and Wallace 2000). In addition to this, a large interindividual variability in response to rhDNase treatment has been documented and the benefits have been found to be unpredictable in around 50% of patients (Cobos et al. 2000).

Physiotherapy

Key point

Daily physiotherapy for life is an essential part of the treatment of the pulmonary features of cystic fibrosis, and must begin as soon as the diagnosis is made. The treatment approach should be adapted to changes in the patient's lifestyle as he or she matures and as the disease progresses.

The aims of physiotherapy are:

- to reduce bronchospasm and to clear the lung fields
- to encourage activities for maintaining physical fitness/increase exercise tolerance
- to train postural awareness and relaxation
- to educate the patient in self-management.

Clearing lung fields

This is the cornerstone of management of patients with CF, because the primary causes of morbidity and mortality are bronchiectais and obstructive pulmonary disease – the latter accounts for over 90% of deaths. It is important that the parents and the rest of the family be involved in the treatment of the child at a young age so that physiotherapy can become an accepted routine.

Chest clearance techniques in the infant include the use of postural drainage, percussion and shaking. Prior to these techniques it is useful to have an active game with a child so that he or she laughs, producing deeper respiration and then becoming breathless. This is required twice a day, every day, even when the patient is apparently well, as there is some evidence that inflammation and infection exist during infancy (Konstan et al. 1994).

Key point

During exacerbations, or when the child has an upper respiratory tract infection, these treatment sessions may have to be increased up to as much as six times a day.

A baby may be positioned on a pillow on the knee of either the physiotherapist or parent. The physiotherapist has to identify the most effective position for each individual patient and relate the treatment to the home situation. As the child grows, there comes a stage where it is necessary to position for drainage using cushions, or a newspaper parcel. A tipping frame which supports the patient totally is more comfortable for draining the anterior and lateral segments of the lower lobes, and middle lobe or lingula. Adolescents and adult patients may have blocks made so that their own bed may be tipped.

Postural drainage should be programmed to avoid mealtimes. Early morning and late evening are suitable times for most adults, but children may be treated early in the evening.

In addition to postural drainage and manual techniques, the use of a positive expiratory pressure (PEP) mask and the Flutter device can be used to facilitate the clearance of secretions by enhancing expiratory airflow (Freitag et al. 1989). Infants tend to swallow their secretions and for children under 3 years and babies the sputum needs to be cleared by a tissue. Disposal of infected sputum should be discussed with parents, relatives or patient as it is essential to avoid reinfection.

Some form of humidification is useful to reduce the viscosity of the mucus, and may be applied using a mouthpiece and nebuliser. Ultrasonic nebulisers have been shown to be preferred by cystic fibrosis patients (Thomas et al. 1991). For babies and children, a mask may be necessary. Saline solution may be used as a mucolytic agent. For home use, patients may have an electric compressor with a nebuliser.

As soon as the patient is old enough he or she should be encouraged to become involved in the treatment. The person should also be encouraged to expectorate the secretions and not to swallow the sputum as this may cause an exacerbation of the abdominal symptoms. During exacerbations of infection, patients may be admitted to hospital where intensive physiotherapy is essential.

A community physiotherapist should visit the patient's home at regular intervals and will become very well known to the involved family. The patient has to attend regular follow-up clinics to be seen by a chest specialist as well as being taken care of by the general practitioner. It is also essential that the patient be seen regularly by the physiotherapist so that treatment can be updated and problems discussed.

Maintenance of physical fitness/increasing exercise tolerance

Aerobic fitness in both children and young adults with CF can be improved by aerobic exercise training (Kaplan et al. 1991). Higher levels of aerobic fitness in patients with CF have been shown to be associated with a significantly improved length of survival (Nixon et al. 1992). Exercise has also been shown to decrease breathlessness (O'Neill et al. 1987) and to improve quality of life (de Jong et al. 1997).

Parents of an infant with CF should be encouraged to treat the child as normally as possible so that the child joins in physical activities at school and with friends at weekends. It is helpful for the parents to meet the child's teachers so that they know to encourage the child to participate fully in school life.

Adult patients may benefit from regular swimming or short sessions of jogging and if possible should be encouraged to attend the hospital or clinic when clinically stable to have their baseline exercise capacity measured. This will allow the physiotherapist to recommend a level of exercise to provide an appropriate training effect. It is also important to establish goals of an exercise programme and to tailor the programme to the patient's level of fitness and disease severity.

Postural awareness and relaxation

Children should be encouraged to join in physical education activities at school. At home, parents should be taught to recognise the typical poor posture of head forward, rounded shoulders and kyphosis of the thoracic spine and encourage the patient to stretch 'tall as a house' or 'straight as a guardsman'. Localised shoulder girdle relaxation may be taught as 'push your shoulders down and back then leave them there'. Diaphragmatic control is taught for the patient to regain quiet respiration after becoming breathless.

Terminal stages

The advanced stages of CF are characterised by repeated exacerbations and eventually respiratory failure. As the blood gases deteriorate and the $PaCO_2$ begins to rise as a result of ventilatory failure, non-invasive positive pressure ventilation (NIPPV) will be indicated. This is a distressing time for the patient, the family and the multidisciplinary team, as the patient becomes very ill and recognises that death is imminent. The family will require a great deal of emotional support from the multidisciplinary team.

The principal theme is to keep the patient as comfortable as possible, which usually means sedation using morphine or one of its derivatives to relieve the sensation of breathlessness and reduce anxiety. It is inappropriate to discontinue contact with the physiotherapist even though active treatment is no longer effective. The aim in the terminal stages of the disease is positioning of the patient in high side lying or forward lean sitting to make the person as comfortable as possible and to assist with the clearance of secretions from the upper airways if these become uncomfortable and distressing for the patient. Nasopharangeal suction is not indicated in the terminal stages of the disease.

RESTRICTIVE PULMONARY DISEASES

Pneumonia

> **Definition**
> Pneumonia is an acute inflammation of the lung tissue – the alveoli and adjacent airways.

Classification

Pneumonia may be classified in many ways, for example:

- according to its anatomical distribution (e.g. lobar, which is confined to one lobe, or bronchopneumonia, which is a more widespread, patchy infection); or
- according to its microbiological cause.

In clinical terms it may also be defined as:

- according to where the infection is acquired (i.e. in the community or in hospital)
- according to whether the patient is immunocompromised (e.g. by AIDS).

All of these factors may determine the outcome of the disease, the likely causative factors and the clinical features of the disease.

Community-acquired pneumonia

Infection is acquired through the inhalation of droplets containing the specific micro-organism, and the individual is unable to overcome the infection through the natural pulmonary defence mechanism.

Community-acquired pneumonia is a common pulmonary disease and may be responsible for over one million hospital admissions a year in the UK. The microbiological cause does, however, tend to affect different age groups:

- *Streptococcus pneumoniae* pneumonia is the most prevalent community-acquired pneumonia and affects all age groups.
- *Mycoplasm pneumoniae* pneumonia usually occurs in adolescents and young adults.
- Influenza, parainfluenza, measles and adenovirus pneumonias are more common in children and the elderly.
- Chickenpox pneumonia occurs in adults.
- Respiratory syncytial virus (RSV) is an important cause of morbidity and mortality in children under 2 years of age.
- *Legionella pneumophilia* infection (Legionnaire's disease) may occur in all age groups but is more common in men than women. It thrives in warm water and frequently contaminates badly maintained air-conditioning systems.
- *Haemophilus influenzae* may produce bronchopneumonia in those with pre-existing pulmonary disease (e.g. chronic bronchitis). It is therefore more common in the elderly.
- *Staphylococcus pyogenes, Klebsiella pneumoniae* and *Mycoplasma pneumoniae* infections are rare in healthy individuals but may commonly complicate viral pneumonia.

Predisposing factors

These are: winter or springtime, overcrowding where bacteria and viruses are easily transmitted, alcoholism, smoking (cigarette smoke and alcohol depress ciliary function and phagocytosis), atmospheric pollution, lower socio-economic groups and pre-existing respiratory disease. The disease may also occur secondary to impaired consciousness and malnutrition.

Pathological changes

The invading organism causes inflammation in the bronchioles and alveoli. The exudate spreads into neighbouring alveoli to provide a medium for rapid spread of bacteria. The alveoli become filled with red blood cells, leucocytes, macrophages and fibrin (red hepatisation) and there is congestion throughout the lobe. The overlying pleural surface is inflamed and a pleural effusion may develop. Resolution occurs when the leucocytes engulf the bacteria and macrophages clear the debris by phagocytosis (grey hepatisation).

In lobular or bronchopneumonia the inflammation is scattered irregularly in the lungs whereas in lobar pneumonia the inflammation is spread throughout but contained within one entire lobe.

Without treatment, resolution occurs by liquefaction of the consolidation, which is then expelled by coughing.

Clinical features

The onset may be sudden (lobar pneumonia) or gradual (bronchopneumonia or lobular pneumonia) and is associated with malaise, pyrexia (temperature often >40°C), rigors, vomiting, confusion due to hypoxaemia (especially in the elderly), and tachycardia.

- *Cough*. This is dry at first, but after a few days purulent sputum is produced.
- *Breathlessness*. Blood passing through the affected alveolar membranes is inadequately oxygenated so that the PaO_2 falls. Hyperventilation cannot compensate for this hypoxaemia because blood passing through the normal lung tissue is almost saturated. The inflammation that occurs makes the lung stiff and compliance is reduced, with the result that the effort of breathing is increased. Respiration therefore becomes rapid and shallow.
- *Pain*. If inflammation spreads to the pleura there is a sharp pain aggravated by taking a deep breath or coughing.
- *Radiograph*. Consolidation can be seen as an opacity especially in lobar pneumonia. There may also be evidence of a pleural effusion.
- *Auscultation*. Bronchial breathing can be heard (especially in lobar pneumonia) because the consolidated lung tissue conducts the sounds of air movement in the trachea. Whispering pectoriloquy and increased vocal resonance can be heard. Wheeze may be evident if bronchospasm is present.

Investigations

- *Haematology*. This may reveal a raised white blood cell count.
- *Biochemistry*. Arterial blood gases should be measured to reveal the extent of arterial hypoxaemia.
- *Microbiology*. Sputum should be sent for Gram staining to identify the causative organism (e.g. *Strep. pneumoniae*) and to identify which antimicrobial agents are sensitive to the organism.
- *Pleural aspiration for culture*. This should be considered if the pneumonia is complicated by a pleural effusion.

Prognosis

The outcome depends on predisposing factors, the virulence of the bacteria, and the age and general fitness of the patient. Improvement starts within 3–4 days of the patient having antibiotics, and within 10 days the sputum should be less in quantity and mucoid in nature – by which time the patient begins to feel better. In an otherwise fit person, the radiograph should be clear in 6 weeks.

Generally lobar pneumonia resolves and the patient recovers, particularly in people who are generally fit and are between the ages of 20 and 50 years. Bronchopneumonia is more serious, is often secondary to other problems, and may be the terminal illness in patients who are elderly. The disease may be fatal in the very young because the secretions readily block the narrow, underdeveloped airways.

Management

- Antibiotics are given to control infection. Specimens of sputum should be sent for culture and sensitivity as soon as possible to confirm or alter antibiotic therapy.
- Adequate fluids must be taken to ensure fluid balance.
- Analgesics are given to relieve pleuritic pain.
- Oxygen therapy may be necessary and blood gases should be monitored regularly.
- Bedrest at home may be sufficient, but an acutely ill patient should be admitted to hospital.

Complications

Possible complications of pneumonia are:

- spread to other lung areas
- delayed resolution – due to the wrong antibiotic being given, poor compliance with medication, or bronchial obstruction (e.g. due to carcinoma)
- pleural disease resulting in pleural effusion or empyema – this will require an intercostal tube and drainage (possibly surgical drainage) and antibiotics if an empyema is evident
- lung abscess – this will cause a swinging pyrexia and will require antibiotics
- cardiac failure
- septicaemia
- pneumococcal meningitis
- pneumothorax – this is particularly associated with *Staph. aureus* pneumonia and will require intercostal tube drainage.
- deconditioning due to malaise.

Physiotherapy in pneumonia

Physiotherapy is indicated when the inflammation has begun to resolve. The aims of treatment are:

- to reduce bronchospasm (if present) and to clear lung fields of secretions
- to gain full re-expansion of the lungs
- to regain exercise tolerance and fitness.

Clearing lung fields

Humidification may be necessary to moisten secretions. The method will vary according to the severity of the illness and may be by steam inhalation, nebuliser or IPPB. Clapping, shaking and breathing exercises may all be necessary in a postural drainage position appropriate to the area of the lung affected. Sometimes suction is required for the very ill patient who cannot cough or expectorate. If there is an underlying bronchospasm then a bronchodilator may be given.

Re-expansion of the lungs

Positioning should be used to increase ventilation to the affected area.

Exercise tolerance and fitness

As soon as possible, the patient should be mobilised and start walking short distances which are progressively increased in length.

Pleurisy

Definition
Pleurisy is a process whereby inflammation occurs on the visceral and parietal pleura which come into direct contact with each other to cause pain.

Aetiology and pathological changes

This condition is common in town dwellers where there is dust and grit in the atmosphere. It may also be secondary to tuberculosis or lobar pneumonia. Infection or irritation of the pleura causes inflammation and vascular congestion. A fibrinous exudate is formed within the pleural cavity and the pleural surfaces are roughened. The inflammation may resolve or develop into a pleural effusion (see below), depending upon any underlying conditions. When resolution occurs, fibrin laid down within the exudate tends to form adhesions between the two layers of the pleura.

The causes of pleurisy are:

- viral infection, which is the most common cause
- pulmonary infarction
- bronchial carcinoma
- pneumonia
- autoimmune rheumatic diseases (e.g. systemic lupus erythematosus, rheumatoid arthritis).

Clinical features

- *Pleuritic pain.* This is due to stretching of the inflamed pleura. The pain is sharp (knife-like), severe and related to movement of the chest (e.g. deep inspiration or coughing). It is usually well localised to the area of the chest under which the pleural irritation lies. Irritation of the diaphragmatic pleura, however, causes pain sensation via the phrenic nerve and this is often referred to the tip of the shoulder.
- *Pleural rub.* There is a creaking or grating sound heard through a stethoscope on both inspiration and expiration. It is localised to the affected area. This disappears if an effusion develops.
- *Cough.* Coughing may be present if respiratory infection is the cause.
- *Radiograph.* The diaphragm may be raised on the affected side.
- *Other clinical signs.* Tachycardia and pyrexia may be present depending on associated conditions.

Investigation and treatment

Haematology shows a high white cell count if infection is present. Identification and treatment of any underlying conditions is essential. Analgesics are given to relieve pain, and possibly sedative linctus reduce coughing. Rest is important to allow the inflammation to subside and to minimise the pain.

Physiotherapy in pleurisy

Physiotherapy is usually inappropriate in the early stages. During the recovery stage, however, the aims are:

- to regain full thoracic expansion
- to minimise adhesion formation between the pleural layers
- to mobilise the thorax.

Thoracic expansion is regained by teaching the patient localised expansion exercises with manual resistance over the affected area both to guide rib movement and relieve pain. General deep breathing exercises and mobility exercises, such as sitting with trunk bending side to side, are important to regain mobility of the thorax and thoracic spine.

Pleural Effusion

Definition
Pleural effusion is an excessive accumulation of fluid in the pleural cavity.

Aetiology

Pleural effusion is often secondary to conditions such as:

- malignancy of the lungs or bronchi
- pneumonia
- tuberculosis
- pulmonary infarction
- bronchiectasis
- lung abscess
- blockage of lymph vessels
- rupture of blood vessels
- left ventricular failure.

Pathological changes

Fluid accumulates in the pleural cavity, the composition of which varies according to the underlying cause. The fluid may be reabsorbed naturally or removed by surgical intervention. As the pleural layers come together they may become adherent owing to organisation of fibrin if the fluid contains plasma proteins.

Fluid may accumulate in the pleural cavity as transudate or exudate. *Transudate* occurs when there is an increased pulmonary capillary pressure (as in congestive cardiac failure) or a decreased osmotic pressure (as in hypoproteinaemia associated with malnutrition) across the pleural membrane. *Exudate* occurs when there is inflammation resulting in increased permeability of capillaries and visceral pleura together with impaired lymphatic reabsorption (as in pneumonia or malignancy).

Exudate is cloudy with a high protein content, in contrast to transudate which is clear with a low protein content. Consequently exudate tends to become consolidated whereas transudate can be reabsorbed if the underlying condition is treated.

Clinical features

- *Breathlessness*. The pressure of fluid reduces lung expansion.
- *Cyanosis*. This may be present in a large effusion.
- *Pyrexia*. This is usually associated with infection.
- *Lethargy*. The person complains of a lack of energy.
- *Pain*. The person complains of pain.
- *Thorax*. Thoracic expansion is restricted on the affected side.

Investigations and treatment

A fluid level can be identified on X-ray. There is a stony dullness on percussion over the fluid. Breath sounds are absent over the effusion (>500 mL of fluid), although bronchial breathing may be heard just above the effusion. Small effusions (220–500 mL) are revealed by chest radiography.

If the fluid does not become reabsorbed naturally, then it should be aspirated (drained surgically). Oxygen therapy may be necessary.

Physiotherapy in pleural effusion

The aims of physiotherapy are:

- to prevent the formation of disabling adhesions between the two layers of pleura
- to obtain full expansion of the affected lung
- to increase ventilation of the lungs
- to increase exercise tolerance following immobility.

The treatment must be modified to take into account any underlying condition. Following aspiration, breathing exercises should be given to encourage localised expansion of the affected side. The patient is encouraged to practice these exercises possibly with the aid of a belt.

If the patient has difficulty in localising the expansion, it may be helpful to lie on the unaffected side over a firm pillow to help stretch the affected side. Breathing exercises may also be practiced in this position several times a day. When the patient has regained lung expansion, the treatment programme should be expanded to include mobilisation of the patient and to increase exercise tolerance.

Some malignant pleural effusions may require a pleurodesis – the insertion of a powder such as tetracycline into the pleural cavity

Empyema

Definition
Empyema is a collection of pus in the pleural cavity.

Aetiology

The condition of empyema usually arises secondary to pre-existing lung disease, such as bacterial pneumonia, tuberculosis, lung abscess, or bronchiectasis. The most common cause is direct spread of infection into the pleural space in a patient with pneumonia due to *Strep. pneumoniae*. It may also arise as a result of a stab wound or as a complication of thoracic surgery.

Pathological changes

Infected material enters the pleural cavity. Both layers of pleura become covered in thick inflammatory exudate within which fibrous tissue is laid down. As this fibrous tissue contracts it acts as a physical barrier to lung expansion. The pressure of the fibrous tissue on the pus may cause rupture of the pleura and lung tissue and the pus may then be coughed up. Alternatively, an abscess may form. Healing occurs when the pus has been surgically removed or the infection has been overcome by the patient's natural antibodies, assisted by antibiotics. The layers of the pleura come together and adhesion formation may take place, restricting lung movement.

Clinical features

These include:

- pyrexia
- lassitude and loss of weight
- tachycardia
- dyspnoea
- pleuritic pain severe at first then decreasing in severity
- diminished thoracic movements.

There may be a history of pneumonia or other associated condition.

Investigations and treatment

On X-ray the empyema can be seen as a D-shaped shadow, the straight line of the D being on the lung surface. Pleural aspiration or tap will confirm the diagnosis as the sample is often thick and purulent, and may be foul-smelling. Pleural fluid cytology will reveal an exudate with pus cells and organisms.

Antibiotics are given to combat infection. Aspiration through a needle inserted into the cavity may remove sufficient pus to relieve the condition, but continuous underwater drainage may be necessary. Rib resection may be indicated if the effusion is very thick or loculated.

If the condition results in fibrosis of the pleura which severely limits lung expansion, then a rib resection may be performed and the pleura stripped off the lung (decortication).

The prognosis depends on the cause, but untreated infection can make the patient very ill from toxins absorbed into the bloodstream (toxaemia).

Physiotherapy in empyema

The aims are:

- to minimise adhesion formation within the pleura
- to regain full lung expansion
- to clear the lung fields
- to maintain good posture and thoracic mobility
- to improve exercise tolerance.

If the patient has a chest drainage tube inserted, the physiotherapy is similar to that following a thoracotomy. Good posture should be encouraged whenever physiotherapy is being given. The tendency is for the patient to protect the affected side, by side-flexing to that side. Therefore, the patient should be taught to take weight evenly on both buttocks, to keep the shoulders level and to practice stretching to the opposite side from the lesion as well as stretching backwards.

Breathing exercises to expand the lung on the affected side need to be carried out three or four times daily. Postural drainage may be indicated to clear the lungs if secretions are accumulating.

As the patient recovers, general leg, arm and trunk exercises should be taught. Walking should begin as soon as possible with breathing control practised over progressively longer distances, and going down (then up) stairs incorporated. As the patient regains lung expansion, the treatment programme should be expanded to increase exercise tolerance.

Pneumothorax

Definition
Air collects between the visceral and parietal pleura. Air in the pleural space will allow the lung to move away from the chest wall and the lung will partially deflate.

There are two types of pneumothorax, spontaneous (which may be secondary to an underlying disease) and traumatic.

Spontaneous pneumothorax

This can occur at any age but is most common in young men (a ratio of six to one) who are otherwise apparently healthy. It may also be associated with emphysema and chronic bronchitis in men over 50 years of age, or result from other underlying disease or be associated with mechanical ventilation. These spontaneous causes may be summarised as:

- airflow limitation due to asthma or bullous emphysema

- positive pressure ventilation, particularly with the use of positive end-expiratory pressure (PEEP)
- infections (e.g. *Staphylococcal pneumonia*, tuberculosis)
- cystic fibrosis
- Marfan's syndrome.

Traumatic pneumothorax

A traumatic pneumothorax may be caused by:

- penetrating injury to the chest (e.g. by stab wound or a bullet)
- non-penetrating injury to the chest wall (e.g. impact of an RTA involving the chest)
- during the insertion of an intravenous (e.g. subclavian) line
- during surgery to the chest wall
- during pleural aspiration or biopsy.

When the chest wall remains intact, the condition is termed a *closed pneumothorax*, but if the chest wall is opened following the trauma the term used is *open pneumothorax*. In the presence of an open wound, the emergency treatment is the application of a large dressing pad over the chest wall.

Pathological changes

As air escapes into the pleural cavity and reduces the subatmospheric pressure (i.e. less negative) the lung collapses. The hole in the pleura closes, the air becomes absorbed and the lung gradually re-expands. Sometimes this does not happen and the hole in the pleura becomes like a valve. Air then enters the pleural cavity on inspiration but cannot escape during expiration. The lung remains collapsed and, as air accumulates in the pleural cavity and the pressure increases, there is displacement of the heart together with compression of the other lung and great vessels. This is termed a *tension pneumothorax* and has to be treated as an emergency by needle aspiration and thereafter by insertion of a drain connected to an underwater seal.

Clinical features

The onset is often sudden with severe chest pain and progressive breathlessness. There is diminished chest movement unilaterally, and an absence of breath sounds often over the apex of the affected side.

Other clinical features may be related to the underlying pathology (e.g. emphysema). In a patient with known lung disease a pneumothorax should always be considered if the patient becomes more breathless for no apparent reason.

Subcutaneous emphysema may develop at the time of the pleural air leak or following the insertion of an intercostal drain when air may track into the subcutaneous tissues. Subcutaneous air results in a crackling sensation on palpation.

Investigations and treatment

The chest X-ray shows absence of lung markings and the edge of the collapsed lung can be seen. This will confirm the diagnosis. Inspiratory and expiratory radiographs will help define the visceral pleura where there is a small pneumothorax.

A small pneumothorax requires no treatment apart from a few days bedrest until it resolves. A large pneumothorax (i.e. more than 25% of the pleural space is filled with air) is treated by needle aspiration or by an intercostal drain which connects the pleural cavity to a drainage bottle creating an underwater seal. The drain is removed when there are no more bubbles in the drainage bottle – indicating that the pleural cavity is free of air.

Surgery is indicated for a recurrent pneumothorax. Pleurodesis comprises the insertion of a powder into the pleural cavity. This acts as an irritant to the pleural surfaces causing them to adhere to each other. Pleurectomy is the removal of the parietal pleura from the chest wall leaving a raw surface to which the visceral layer sticks. A hole in the visceral pleura may have to be stitched.

Physiotherapy in pneumothorax

A patient who has an underwater drainage system requires expansion breathing exercises to re-expand the lung. Also, full-range shoulder movements are necessary to maintain shoulder, shoulder girdle and thoracic mobility. This treatment is generally given 3–4 times daily until the drain is removed.

Following pleurodesis, expansion breathing exercises are essential to ensure that when the adhesions form between the layers of the pleura the lung is fully expanded. The patient must be taught to practice expansion breathing exercises so that thoracic mobility is maintained, otherwise there may be sharp pleuritic pain if the intrapleural adhesions become too contracted. If the lung does not re-expand within 36 hours then a second operation is required. Physiotherapy after a pleurectomy follows the same principles as for any thoracotomy.

Acute Respiratory Distress Syndrome (ARDS)

A catastrophic event can, either directly or indirectly, cause damage to the pulmonary epithelium or the alveolar capillary membrane. ARDS is, therefore, the respi-

Definition

The acute respiratory distress syndrome (ARDS) is a severe and acute form of respiratory failure precipitated by a wide range of catastrophic events – including shock, septicaemia, major trauma, or aspiration or inhalation of noxious substances (Bernard et al. 1994).

ratory manifestation of a systemic condition, which appears within 12–48 hours after the initial triggering event.

Examples of triggering events are: pulmonary aspiration, severe burns with or without inhalation injury, disseminated intravascular coagulation (a coagulation defect due to clotting abnormalities), cardiopulmonary bypass, severe trauma, massive blood transfusion, near-drowning, pre-eclampsia, septicaemia, amniotic fluid embolism (substances entering the maternal circulation usually following a vigorous labour), pancreatitis, nad fat embolism resulting from fracture of (long) bones.

Pathological changes

Activated neutrophils are thought to release a number of vasoactive mediators that damage the integrity of the alveolar membrane. As a result of increased endothelial permeability within the alveolar–capillary membrane, fluid moves from the pulmonary capillaries into the gas exchange areas of the lung. This results in alveolar oedema and extravasation of inflammatory cells. The pulmonary oedema is therefore said to be non-cardiogenic because there is normal hydrostatic pressure in the pulmonary vasculature (unlike left ventricular failure when this is raised). As this acute phase progresses, there is increasing congestion in the capillaries. The loss of functioning alveoli results in severe hypoxaemia and respiratory failure.

Clinical features

The defining features of ARDS are:

- severe refractory (resistant to treatment) hypoxaemia
- the presence of pulmonary oedema with normal hydrostatic pressure in the pulmonary vasculature
- the appearance of diffuse bilateral pulmonary infiltrates on chest X-ray
- a falling pulmonary compliance ($<50\,\mathrm{mL/cmH_2O}$).

Increasing breathlessness is evident which left untreated may lead to acute tachypnoea (>20 breaths per minute). There is evidence of the appearance of dif-

fuse bilateral pulmonary infiltrates on chest X-ray, and widespread wheezes and crackles on auscultation. Despite oxygen, the disease usually progresses to a state of severe respiratory failure, which requires the support of mechanical ventilation. The lungs become progressively stiffer and adequate oxygenation and ventilation becomes more difficult.

Investigations and treatment

On blood gas analysis the PaO_2 is reduced to critical levels. If this is not corrected the $PaCO_2$ may begin to rise.

Any underlying pathological cause is treated. Adequate ventilatory support will be necessary which may include high inspired oxygen, intermittent positive pressure ventilation, and the application of positive end-expiratory pressure (PEEP) to restore adequate function by allowing for the recruitment of hypoventilated alveoli. This will result in an improved PaO_2. High levels of oxygen may be used initially to reduce a dangerous hypoxaemia, but since oxygen is toxic at high concentrations (causing further damage to the alveolar membrane) this should be reduced to a level that will give an adequate PaO_2. Although the application of PEEP in this condition has been standard practice for over two decades, over-distension of lung tissue may result in baro- and volu-trauma with the development of pneumothorax and subcutaneous emphysema (Montgomery et al. 1985).

Complications

Nosocominal pneumonitis is a common complication in patients with ARDS on prolonged mechanical ventilation and is directly related to oropharageal colonisation of Gram-negative bacilli – the stomach being one of the possible reservoirs of these micro-organisms (Driks et al. 1987). The loss of mucosal integrity and clearance mechanisms are predisposing factors which lead to secondary infection and may contribute to worsening gas exchange.

Hence, adequate removal of retained bronchial secretions by chest physiotherapy techniques is an integral part of the management of these patients.

Prognosis

A substantial number of studies have now confirmed that the primary cause of death in patients with ARDS is not the inability to oxygenate arterial blood adequately but rather the result of the development of multiple organ dysfunction and failure (MOF) due to poor tissue oxygen extraction and altered tissue blood-flow (Montgomery et al. 1985; Fowler et al. 1985). These manifestations are associated with a high mortality rate. Approximately 30–60% of patients with

ARDS die, despite increasing awareness of the mechanisms of acute injury and the introduction of novel forms of therapy and support (Bernard et al. 1994).

Physiotherapy in ARDS

The aims of physiotherapy are:

- removal of retained secretions
- passive/active movements.

Chest physiotherapy involves four principal manoeuvers: positioning to enhance removal of secretions and to improve gas exchange; manual hyperinflation: endotracheal suctioning: and manual techniques (which include shakings and vibrations).

Passive and active exercises need to be performed regularly whilst the patient's mobility remains restricted during the critical stages of their disease, in order to maintain the mobility of joints and the extensibility of the soft tissues (e.g. the muscles, tendons and ligaments).

Fibrosing Alveolitis

Definition

In fibrosing alveolitis the alveolar walls become thickened, with an increase in type II pneumocytes and macrophages. As the disease progresses the alveolar walls fibrose and fibrosis spreads to the lung parenchyma.

The aetiology of fibrosing alveolitis is unknown (in most cases), although in some cases there is evidence of a pre-existing specific disease. These may be autoimmune (e.g. RA, systemic sclerosis), or gastrointestinal (e.g. chronic active hepatitis, ulcerative colitis).

Clinical features

- *Dyspnoea.* There is an insidious onset of breathlessness often accompanied either by a dry unproductive cough or with little clear sputum.
- *Auscultation.* A typical feature is mid-to-late inspiratory crackles, which are said to be 'metallic' in nature.
- *Finger clubbing.* As the disease progresses most patients develop gross finger clubbing.
- *Cyanosis.* This is due to impaired gas exchange.

Investigations and treatment

Blood gases reveal a progressive hypoxaemia with hypercapnia evident late in the disease. The chest radiograph will first show a ground-glass appearance mainly in the lower zones; as the disease progresses, this becomes discrete and nodular. Transbronchial or open lung biopsy shows interstitial and alveolar fibrosis. Lung function tests reveal a restrictive deficit with reduced gas transfer factor.

Chronic forms of fibrosing alveolitis are treated with high doses of oral corticosteroids. Other immunosuppressive drugs (e.g. cyclophosphamide) are sometimes used if the alveolitis is associated with an autoimmune disease. Long-term oxygen therapy (LTOT) should be considered to correct hypoxaemia which leads to pulmonary hypertension and the development of cor pulmonale. Heart–lung transplantation may be considered in younger patients.

The median survival time of patients with fibrosing alveolitis is less than 5 years, although some patients may live for much longer. In general, the earlier the onset of the disease, the worse the prognosis.

Physiotherapy in fibrosing alveolitis

Physiotherapy should be directed at teaching breathing control and maintaining exercise tolerance as the patient becomes deconditioned due to fatigue and shortness of breath.

OTHER PULMONARY DISEASES

Lung Abscess

Definition

A lung abscess is the localised formation of pus, usually surrounded by a fibrous capsule, within lung tissue.

Antibiotics and improved anesthesia have reduced the incidence of lung abscess and the condition tends now to occur secondary to bronchial carcinoma particularly in patients who are over 40 years.

Aetiology

A variety of bacteria may enter the lungs by one of the following routes:

- through the air passages due to bronchopneumonia or following inhalation of a foreign body
- through the open chest wall following a wound from a knife stab or bullet
- from the bloodstream
- to bronchial carcinoma – an abscess forms where secretions accumulate distal to the tumour.

Pathological changes

The invading organisms cause inflammation of the lung tissue. At the centre of the area there is necrosis of lung tissue with liquefaction and suppuration. The area becomes distended and fibroblasts lay down fibrous tissue around the area until there is complete encapsulation. The capsule contracts and the abscess bursts, resulting in the production of foul-smelling sputum. Sometimes the pus drains into the pleura, causing empyema, and if drainage spills into adjacent lung tissue there is a danger of bronchiectasis. Toxins from the pus can be absorbed into the bloodstream and there is then a danger of septicaemia. Healing occurs with the formation of a fibrous scar.

Clinical features

There is malaise, fever, cough and dyspnoea. The cough is at first irritable and unproductive but later is productive of foul-smelling sputum accompanied by a bad taste in the mouth. The cough may be painful if the pleura are inflamed. Haemoptysis and halitosis are further features.

Finger clubbing may become evident if the abscess becomes chronic.

Investigations and treatment

Blood analysis may reveal an increased white cell count. Cultures of sputum or lung aspirate will reveal the organism. A chest X-ray will show an area of cavitation within the lung tissue, which may contain an air-fluid level.

Most lung abscesses will respond to large intravenous doses of antibiotics to which the organism is sensitive. Drainage of the abscess may be necessary via needle aspiration or a thoracotomy. If there is an endo-bronchial obstruction caused by a foreign body, removal is essential.

Physiotherapy for a lung abscess

The site of the abscess is ascertained on the radiograph and the patient is positioned accurately for 10–15 minutes every 4 hours. Shaking is applied to the chest wall and breathing exercises are taught to regain breath control after coughing. Deep inspiration should not be encouraged because the increase in negative pressure may move the pus through healthy lung tissue.

It is important to adjust the patient's position to obtain maximum effective drainage and to ensure that precautions are taken to avoid any danger of cross-infection.

Pulmonary Tuberculosis (TB)

Definition
In pulmonary tuberculosis the bacillus *Mycobacterium tuberculosis* causes irritation of the mucous lining in the bronchioles or alveoli and inflammatory changes take place.

In 1882, Robert Koch isolated the tubercle bacillus of which there are two types, one human and the other bovine. Since then the disease has been controlled by inoculation, mass radiography, drugs and pasteurised milk.

Key point
The lungs are not the only tissues to be affected by tuberculosis. Types of tuberculosis other than pulmonary are: acute miliary (the blood is affected, with spread of the disease to spleen, liver, kidneys, meninges and lymph nodes); surgical TB; bone or joint TB; lupus vulgaris (the skin is affected); and TB adenoma (the lymph nodes are affected).

Aetiology and prevalence

Mycobacterium tuberculosis is spread by droplets during coughing and sneezing, so that a person can be infected from a patient's sputum.

Tuberculosis is common worldwide and its incidence has increased in Britain in recent years. The disease is still very common in Africa and Asia. In Europe the age group most commonly affected is middle age, but it also often occurs in elderly men. In Britain, the disease occurs mainly in the immigrant population from Ireland, Asia and the West Indies.

Predisposing factors are the environment, poor hygiene, overcrowding, lower socio-economic groups, malnutrition, smoking and alcoholism. Other factors are diseases such as diabetes mellitus, congenital heart disorder, leukaemia, Hodgkin's disease, long-term corticosteroids or immunosuppressive drugs.

Pathology

The bacilli are ingested by leucocytes and then absorbed by macrophages. More leucocytes form a barrier around this collection of cells and the complete mass is known as a 'tuberculous follicle'. The centre of the area undergoes necrosis and becomes soft and cheesy in consistency, the process being known as 'caseation'. This material may be moved into a bronchus and coughed up leaving a cavity behind. Fibroblasts lay down a capsule around the tubercle in which calcium salts become deposited and healing takes place.

Cavity formation and calcification are the features of TB with the calcified lesion remaining a potential source of infection. The bacillus may be reactivated and cause *postprimary pulmonary tuberculosis*. The danger then is that the disease may spread to other areas of the lungs including the pleura, and through the bloodstream to other parts of the body.

Clinical features

These are:

- malaise, lassitude and irritability
- loss of appetite and loss of weight
- pyrexia and tachycardia
- night sweats
- productive cough – the bacillus can be cultured from the sputum
- haemoptysis
- diminished respiratory movements with possibly some dyspnoea
- pain if there is pleural involvement.

Investigations

The chest X-ray shows cavity formation and calcification. In children these clinical features may be present to a mild degree and the disease can pass undetected. Other investigations are as follows.

- *Haematology.* The full blood count may show anaemia.
- *Immunology.* The Mantoux test is usually strongly positive in postprimary pulmonary TB, but is frequently negative in miliary TB.
- *Microbiology.* Sputum culture will show tubercle bacilli after 4–5 weeks of the primary infection. Bacilli may be cultured from the bone marrow in patients with miliary TB.
- *Diagnostic imaging.* In postprimary TB the chest X-ray may demonstrate a pleural effusion or pneumonia. A soft spreading apical shadowing is strongly suggestive of TB. In miliary TB there is widespread shadowing (i.e. small nodules 2–3 cm diameter).

Prevention

Vaccination with BCG (bacille Calmette–Guerin) greatly reduces the incidence of the disease and is currently offered to schoolchildren at 12–13 years of age. The vaccination may also be offered to people who might have contact with a patient who has active TB,

such as relatives, friends, teachers, doctors, nurses and physiotherapists. Pasteurisation of milk prevents transmission of the tubercle to humans from cows.

Treatment

Drug therapy, together with rest, is the treatment for curing tuberculosis. Anti-TB drugs used are rifampicin, isoniazid, ethambutol and para-aminosalicylic acid (PAS); these must be taken every day for up to 18 months. The antibiotic streptomycin may also be prescribed. Multiple drug regimens are used in the treatment of resistant strains. Uncomplicated pulmonary TB is treated with a relatively short course (i.e. 6–9 months). If other organs are involved a longer course of treatment may be necessary (e.g. 18 months for bone disease).

Surgery is appropriate only in a very small proportion of patients. If a patient has a resistant tubercle a lobectomy may be performed, but the patient must still be on a drugs regimen.

The prognosis is good if the patient is not immunosuppressed.

Physiotherapy in pulmonary tuberculosis

Physiotherapy is not usually indicated during the rest stage. Once the patient is ambulant, a graded programme of exercises may be required. If it is necessary to give breathing exercises, the physiotherapist should stand behind the patient to avoid droplet infection as the patient coughs. Sputum must be disposed of very carefully so that cross-infection is prevented.

Bronchial and Lung Tumours

Key point
Tumours may be benign or malignant. The majority are malignant growths which may be primary or secondary.

Tumours arising within the lung (bronchial carcinomas) usually originate within the bronchi, whilst those that spread from other primary sites (e.g. breast, gastrointestinal tract) tend to develop in the lung tissue or the pleura.

In the United Kingdom, there are approximately 35,000 deaths from carcinoma of the bronchus each year. Men are more commonly affected than women, although the incidence is increasing in women. The peak incidence is amongst 65-year-olds.

Causative factors

People who smoke tobacco have a much greater risk of developing a malignant tumour than those who do not. The risk depends upon the number of cigarettes smoked, the age of starting to smoke and the timespan of smoking. The concept of pack-years is described at the beginning of this chapter.

The disease is more prevalent in urban dwellers than in rural dwellers. There is also evidence that exposure to carcinogens, either at work or leisure, can result in the development of the disease. Working with radioactive materials, nickel, uranium, chromates or industrial asbestos is associated with an increased risk of bronchial carcinoma.

Pathology

The majority of tumours originate in the large bronchi and spread by direct invasion of the lung, chest wall and mediastinal structures. The tumour grows to occlude the lumen of the bronchus and then atelectasis distal to the growth will occur. There are various types (Table 14.4).

Clinical features

Seventy per cent of patients present with local symptoms. The onset is insidious, and the clinical features may present in a variety of ways.

- *Cough.* This is the most common feature and is often ignored by the patient who may associate it with smoking. Initially the cough is dry and irritating but may become productive if infection occurs in accumulated secretions.
- *Haemoptysis.* There are recurrent small spots of blood in the sputum.

- *Dyspnoea.* This is highly variable and may be severe when there is pulmonary collapse or pleural effusion.
- *Pain.* Dull, deep-seated pain is common but it may be pleuritic in nature or intercostal when there is rib disease.
- *Malaise and weight loss.* These are associated with late stages of the disease.
- *Secondary concomitant disease.* Pneumonia or lung abscess may arise as a result of a tumour.
- *Hoarseness of the voice.* This is due to left recurrent laryngeal nerve involvement by tumour of the left hilum.
- *Stridor.* This is due to narrowing of the trachea or main bronchus.
- *Facial swelling.* This is due to superior vena caval obstruction following invasion of the mediastinum.
- *Arm and shoulder pain.* These are due to tumour at the apex of the lung (Pancoast tumour) invading the brachial plexus.

Metastases

Metastases are common in patients with bronchial carcinoma and may include the following.

- *Cerebral metastases.* These may cause stroke, headaches and epilepsy.
- *Bone metastases.* The patient may present with spinal cord compression, pathological fracture and bone pain.
- *Liver metastases.* The patient may present with jaundice and hepatomegaly (an enlarged liver).

Non-metastatic presentations include finger clubbing, and neuromuscular and endocrine abnormalities.

Table 14.4 Histology of bronchial tumours.

Histology	Proportion of bronchial cancers	Characteristics
Squamous cell	50%	Locally invasive, cavitation sometimes occurs
Oat/small cell	25%	Small lung primary, rapidly dividing, metastasise early
Large cell	12%	Intermediate between squamous and oat/small cell
Adenocarcinoma	12%	Slowly growing, metastasises late, often peripheral lung tumours
Miscellaneous	1%	For example, alveolar oat cell carcinoma

Investigations

- *Chest radiograph.* This is essential for any patient presenting with haemoptysis and will demonstrate over 90% of lung tumours. Small tumours or those close to the hilum may be missed.
- *CT scanning.* This may be used to identify smaller lesions. It may also be used to assess suitability for surgery by demonstrating metastatic spread.
- *Histopathology.* Sputum culture may have evidence of tumour cells. Three (early morning) samples should be obtained.
- *Bronchoscopy.* This is used to obtain tissue samples and may also be used to assess operability.
- *Percutaneous needle biopsy.* This may be useful for the histological assessment of a peripheral tumour.
- *Pleural aspiration and biopsy.* These may be used for the patient who presents with a pleural effusion.

Treatment

The appropriate treatment may be surgery, chemotherapy and/or radiotherapy. Drug therapy is essentially to relieve symptoms and includes analgesics, antibiotics and antiemetics.

- *Surgery.* This involves removing the lobe or lung. It is possible only whilst the tumour remains localised and in the absence of metastases. Stenting is another option for localised disease.
- *Chemotherapy.* Cytotoxic drugs are used with increasing regularity. Results are mixed but anaplastic tumours tend to respond to this type of treatment.
- *Radiotherapy.* This is used symptomatically particularly to relieve pain and obstruction.

Laser phototherapy or endobronchial radiotherapy can be used to treat persistent localised disease.

The prognosis depends on the type of tumour, but overall the average length of survival after diagnosis is around 1 year. Surgery can prolong the life of some patients.

In the terminal stages attention should be paid to the patient's general well-being and mental state. Some patients benefit from hospice care. Adequate opiate analgesia is essential for pain.

Physiotherapy for bronchial and lung tumours

Physiotherapy may be related to three aspects of management of the disease.

- Pre- and postoperative physiotherapy is essential for patients who have a lobectomy or pneumonectomy

- During and after radiotherapy, when the tumour begins to decrease in size, the patient will begin to expectorate sputum. Positioning and the active cycle of breathing technique (ACBT) should be used for sputum clearance. Percussion and vigorous shaking should not be used as there is a danger of pathological fractures in ribs or vertebrae in which metastases may be developing. Nor should shaking them be used in the presence of haemoptysis.
- During the terminal stage of the disease, where accumulation of secretions is causing distress, modified postural drainage and vibrations with breathing exercises may help to make the patient more comfortable. If coughing is ineffective, suction may have to be used. An active daily programme which fits the patient's requirements may need to be devised, in which case the physiotherapist works in close collaboration with the healthcare team.

Respiratory Failure

> **Definition**
> Respiratory failure denotes reduction of function of the lungs due to lung disease, or a skeletal or neuromuscular disorder. It is defined in terms of the gas tensions (pressures) in the arterial blood.

Normal arterial oxygen and carbon dioxide pressures (PaO_2 and $PaCO_2$) are 13.0 kPa (97 mmHg) and 6.1 kPa (46 mmHg) respectively. There are two types of respiratory failure:

- *Type 1*: A PaO_2 of less than 8.0 kPa (60 mmHg) is associated with a $PaCO_2$ which is either normal or below 6.7 kPa (50 mmHg).
- *Type 2*: A PaO_2 of less than 8.0 kPa (60 mmHg) is associated with a $PaCO_2$ raised above 6.7 kPa (50 mmHg).

Causes of type 1 respiratory failure

Lung disease results in hypoventilation of the alveoli leading to a ventilation/perfusion mismatch. The blood supply is normal but there is inadequate oxygen uptake from the affected alveoli. Diseases associated with this type are early chronic bronchitis and emphysema, pneumonia, asthma, acute pulmonary oedema, pulmonary embolism, pulmonary fibrosis and ARDS.

Causes of type 2 respiratory failure

Because of failure of the skeletal or neuromuscular components of the respiratory system there is loss of the pump mechanism essential for ventilation of the lungs as a whole. Therefore, there is a reduced tidal volume or a reduced respiratory rate, leading to a rise in $PaCO_2$ and a fall in PaO_2. Disorders associated with this type are head injuries, polyneuropathies, cervical cord injuries, advanced chronic bronchitis and emphysema, status asthmaticus, crushed chest, muscular dystrophy, myasthenia gravis and kyphoscoliosis.

Clinical features

- *Type 1 due to hypoxaemia*: There may be dyspnoea, restlessness, confusion, central cyanosis, tachycardia, renal failure, pulmonary hypertension.
- *Type 2 due to hypercapnia*: There may be flapping tremor of the hands, confusion, headache, warm peripheries, tachycardia. Dyspnoea occurs initially but the person may become drowsy and comatose if PaO_2 is allowed to rise.

Treatment

Key point

The diagnosis cannot be accurate until arterial blood gases have been measured. Treatment must be directed towards treating the cause.

In type 1 respiratory failure the main problem is the hypoxaemia, so it is important to raise the PaO_2 by giving oxygen therapy, which should be given in sufficient amounts to correct the hypoxaemia.

In type 2 respiratory failure there is a danger of reducing the respiratory drive which is dependent on the anoxic state of the blood stimulating the chemoreceptors in the carotid and aortic arteries. The danger then is that the patient's respiration slows or stops and the $PaCO_2$ rises, resulting in confusion and coma. A Ventimask giving 24% or 28% inspired oxygen may be applied (see the section on oxygen therapy in COPD).

Physiotherapy in respiratory failure

Type 1 failure

It is vital to clear the lung fields of secretions. If the patient is spontaneously breathing, positioning and the ACBT can be used with manual techniques to loosen secretions. If the patient is too weak to cough, suction has to be used. If bronchospasm is evident, a bronchodilator (e.g. salbutamol) may be given in combination with oxygen therapy. If intermittent positive pressure ventilation is applied, a bronchodilator may be

administered through the ventilator and shakings and vibrations should be performed with manual hyperinflation. Suction will be via the endotracheal tube. All treatment is monitored by regular blood gas analysis.

Type 2 failure

It is again necessary to raise the PaO_2 and this is achieved by oxygen therapy using a Ventimask delivering 24% oxygen. If this is not sufficient to raise the PaO_2 the Ventimask may be changed to one delivering 28% oxygen, provided the $PaCO_2$ is not rising from the already high level. If the $PaCO_2$ starts to rise this is indicative of hypoventilation, usually because the patient is becoming exhausted and NIPPV is indicated. Assisted ventilation may be necessary, although should be avoided if the patient has a chronic compensated respiratory acidosis. Physiotherapy follows similar principles to that for type 1 failure.

REFERENCES

Abman SH, Ogle JW, Harbeck RJ et al. 1991 Early bacteriologic, immunologic, and clinical courses of young infants with cystic fibrosis identified by neonatal screening. J Paediatr 119: 211–17

Adinoff AD, Hollester JR 1983 Steroid-induced fractures and bone loss in patients with asthma. N Engl J Med 309: 265–8

American Thoracic Society 1995 Standards for the diagnosis and care of patients with chronic obstructive pulmonary disease. Am J Respir Care Med 152 (Suppl): S77–S121

Armstrong P, Wilson AG, Dee P, Hansell DM 1995 Imaging of Diseases of the Chest. Chicago: Year Book Medical

Bell SC, Saunders MJ, Elborn JS, Shale DJ 1996 Resting energy expenditure and oxygen cost of breathing in patients with cystic fibrosis. Thorax 51: 126–31

Bellemare F, Grassino A 1982 Effect of pressure and timing of contraction on human diaphragmatic fatigue. J Appl Physiol 53: 1190–5

Bernard G, Artiglas A, Bringham K et al. 1994 Report on the American–European consensus conference on ARDS: definitions, mechanisms, relevant outcomes and clinical trial coordination. Inten Care Med 20: 225–32

Bollert FG, Paton JY, Marshall TG et al. 1999 Recombinant DNase in cystic fibrosis: a protocol for targeted introduction through n–of–1 trials. Scottish Cystic Fibrosis Group. Eur Respir J 13: 107–13

Bone RC 1996 Goals of asthma management: a step-care approach. Chest 4: 1056–65

British Thoracic Association 1982 Death from asthma in two regions of England. BMJ 285: 1251–5

British Thoracic Society 1997 The BTS guidelines on asthma management. Thorax 52 (Suppl 1): S1–S21

Brochard L, Manceebo J, Wysocki M 1995 Non-invasive ventilation for acute exacerbations of chronic obstructive pulmonary disease. N Engl J Med 333: 817–22

Brocklebank D, Ram F, Wright J et al. 2001 Comparison of the effectiveness of inhaler devices in asthma and chronic obstructive airway disease: a systematic review of the literature. Health Techn Assess 5(26): 1–149

Cerny F, Pullano T, Gerd J, Cropp A 1982 Cardiorespiratory adaptations to exercise in cystic fibrosis. Am Rev Respir Dis 126: 217–20

Chatham K, Baldwin J, Griffiths H et al. 1999 Inspiratory muscle training improves shuttle run performance in healthy subjects. Physiotherapy 85: 676–83

Chatwin M, Hart N, Nickol AH et al. 2000 Low frequency fatigue induced by a single inspiratory muscle training session. Thorax 55(Suppl 3): abstract

Christopher F, Chase D, Stein K, Milne R 1999 RhDNase therapy for the treatment of cystic fibrosis patients with mild to moderate lung disease. J Clin Pharm Ther 24: 415–26

Clanton TL, Diaz PT 1995 Focus on ventilatory muscle training: clinical assessment of the respiratory muscles. Phys Ther 75: 983–95

Clarke SW 1991 Chronic bronchitis in the 1990s. Respiration 58(Suppl): 43–6

Cobos N, Danes I, Gartner S et al. 2000 DNase use in the daily care of cystic fibrosis: who benefits from it and to what extent? Results of a cohort study of 199 patients in 13 centres. DNase National Study Group. Eur J Paediatr 159(3): 176–81

Cochrane GM, Webber BA, Clark SW 1977 Effects of sputum on pulmonary function. BMJ 2: 1181–3

Cochrane GM, Clark CJ 1990 Benefits and problems of a physical training programme for asthmatic patients. Thorax 1990: 345–51

Cole P 1995 Bronchiectasis. In Brewis RAL, Corrin B, Geddes DM, Gibson GJ (eds) Respiratory Medicine, 2nd edn. London: WB Saunders

COPD Guidelines Group of the Standards of Care Committee of the BTS. BTS guidelines for the management of chronic obstructive pulmonary disease. Thorax 52(Suppl 5): S1–32

Corless JA, Warburton CJ 2000 Surgery vs non-surgical treatment for bronchiectasis. Cochrane Database Systematic Review CD002180

Corraco WM, Braman SS, Erwin RS 1979 Chronic cough as the sole presenting manifestation of bronchial asthma. N Engl J Med 300: 633–7

Crossley DJ, McGuire GP, Barrow PM, Houston PL 1997 Influence of inspired oxygen concentration on deadspace, respiratory drive, and $Paco_2$ in intubated patients with chronic obstructive pulmonary disease. Crit Care Med 25: 1522–6

Currie DC 1997 Nebulisers for bronchiectasis. Thorax 52(Suppl 2): S72–S74

Davies DS 1973 Pharmokinetics of inhaled substances. Postgrad Med J 51(Supp 7): 69–75

Davis PB, Drumm M, Konstan MW 1996 Cystic fibrosis (State of the Art). Am J Respir Crit Care Med 154: 1229–56

Decramer M 1989 Effects of hyperinflation on the respiratory muscles. Eur Respir J 2: 299–302

Department of Health 1997 Health of the Nation Briefing Pack. Leeds: DoH

Donahoe M, Rogers RM, Wilson DO, Pennok BE 1989 Oxygen consumption of the respiratory muscles in normal and malnourished patients with chronic obstructive pulmonary disease. Am Rev Respir Dis 140: 385–91

de Jong W, Kaptein AA, Van der Shands 1997 Quality of life in patients with cystic fibrosis. Paediatr Pulmonol 23: 95–100

Driks M, Craven D, Celli C 1987 Nosocomial pneumonia in intubated patients given sucralfate as compared with antacids or histamine type 2 blockers: the role of gastric colonisation. N Engl J Med 317: 1376–82

Elborn JS, Johnston B, Allen F 1992 Inhaled steroids in patients with bronchiectasis. Respir Med 86: 121–4

Elborn JS, Cordon SM, Shale DJ 1993 Inflammatory responses prior to death in cystic fibrosis. Respir Med 87: 603–7

Elborn JS, Shale DJ, Britton JR 1991 Cystic fibrosis: current survival and population estimates to the year 2000. Thorax 46: 881–5

Elborn JS, Prescott RJ, Stack BH et al. 2000 Elective versus symptomatic antibiotic treatment in cystic fibrosis patients with chronic *Pseudomonas* infection of the lungs. Thorax 55: 355–8

Enright S, Chatham K, Baldwin J, Griffiths H 2000 The effect of fixed load incremental inspiratory muscle training in the elite athlete. Phys Ther Sport 1:1–5

Fleetham JA, Bradley CA, Kryger MH, Anthonisen NR 1980 The effect of low flow oxygen therapy on the chemical control of ventilation in patients with hypoxemic COPD. Am Rev Respir Dis 122: 833–40

Freitag L, Bremme J, Schroer M 1989 High frequency oscillation for respiratory physiotherapy. Br J Anaesth 63: 44S–46S

Fowler A, Goldman M 1990 Adult respiratory distress syndrome: prognosis after onset. Am Rev Respir Dis 132: 472–8

Goldstein RS 1993 Ventilatory muscle training: pulmonary rehabilitation in chronic respiratory insufficiency. Thorax 48: 1025–33

Green M, Moxham J 1993 Respiratory muscles in health and disease. In Barnes P (ed.) Respiratory Medicine: Recent Advances, pp. 252–275. Oxford: Butterworth–Heinemann

Gross NJ 1995 Airway inflammation in COPD: reality or myth? Chest 107(Suppl 5): S1–24

Hargreave FE, Dolovich J, Newhouse MT (eds) 1990 The assessment and treatment of asthma: a conference report. J Allergy Clin Immunol 85: 1098–2011

Haworth CS, Selby PL, Webb AK 1999 Low bone mineral density in adults with cystic fibrosis. Thorax 54: 961–7

Israel E, Rubin P, Kemp JP et al. 1993 The effect of inhibition of 5-lipoxygenase by Ziluteton in mild-to-moderate asthma. Ann Intern Med 119: 1059–66

Joint Health Surveys Unit 1996 Health Survey for England (1995). London: HMSO

Kaplan TA, ZeBranek JD, McKey RM 1991 Use of exercise in the management of cystic fibrosis. Paediatr Pulmonol 10: 205–7

Kearney CE, Wallis CE 2000 Deoxyribonuclease for cystic fibrosis. Cochrane Database Systematic Review CD001127

Kesten S, Chapman KR 1993 Physician perceptions and management of COPD. Chest 104: 254–8

Kikuchi Y, Okabe S, Tamura G et al. 1994 Chemosensitivity and perceptions of dyspnoea in patients with a history of near-fatal asthma. N Engl J Med 330: 1329–34

Konstan MW, Berger M 1993 Infection and inflammation of the lung in cystic fibrosis. In Davis PB (ed.) Lung Biology in Health and Disease. Vol. 64: Cystic Fibrosis, pp. 219–76. New York: Marcel Dekker

Konstan MW, Hillard KA, Norvell TM 1994 Bronchoalveolar lavage findings in cystic fibrosis patients with stable, clinically mild lung disease suggest ongoing infection and inflammation. Am J Respir Crit Care Med 150: 448–54

Lacasse Y, Wong E, Guyatt GH et al. 1996 Meta-analysis of respiratory rehabilitation in chronic obstructive pulmonary disease. Lancet 348: 1115–19

Levine S, Guillen M 1987 Diaphragmatic pressure waveform can predict EMG signs of diaphragmatic fatigue. J Appl Physiol 62: 1681–9

Ling SC, Wilkinson JD, Hollman AS et al. 1999 The evolution of liver disease in cystic fibrosis. Arch Dis Child 81: 129–32

Meecham-Jones DJ, Paul EA, Jones PW, Wedzicha JA 1995 Nasal pressure support ventilation plus oxygen compared with oxygen therapy alone in hypercapnic COPD. Am J Respir Crit Care Med 152: 538–44

Montgomery A, Stager M, Carrico C, Hudson L 1985 Causes of mortality in patients with adult respiratory distress syndrome. Am Rev Respir Dis 132: 485–9

Moxham J 1990 Respiratory muscle fatigue: mechanisms, evaluation and therapy. Br J Anaesth 65: 43–53

Murciano D, Auclair MH, Pariente R, Aubier M 1989 A randomised controlled trial of theophylline in patients with severe chronic obstructive pulmonary disease. N Engl J Med 320: 1521–5

Nebuliser Project Group of the British Thoracic Society Standards of Care Committee 1997 Current best practice for nebuliser treatment. Thorax 52(Suppl 2): S1–S3

Newman SP, Pavia D, Clark SW 1981 How should a pressurised beta-adrenergic bronchodilator be inhaled? Eur J Respir Dis 62: 3–21

Newman SP, Pavia D, Garland N, Clarke SW 1982 Effects of various inhalation modes on the deposition of radioactive pressurized aerosols. Eur J Respir Dis 63(Suppl): 57–65

Nicholson KG, Kent J, Ireland DC 1993 Respiratory viruses and exacerbations of asthma in adults. BMJ 307: 982–6

Nixon PA, Orenstein DM, Kelsey SF, Doershuk CF 1992 The prognostic value of exercise testing in patients with cystic fibrosis. N Engl J Med 327: 1785–8

O'Callahan C, Barry P 1997 Spacer devices in the treatment of asthma. Br Med J 314: 1061–2

Office for National Statistics 1997 Mortality Statistics for England and Wales (1996). London: HMSO

O'Neill PA, Dodd M, Phillips B 1987 Regular exercise and reduction of breathlessness in cystic fibrosis. Br J Dis Chest 81: 62–6

Oppenheimer EH, Esterly JR 1975 Pathology of cystic fibrosis: review of the literature and comparison with 146 autopsied cases. Persp Paediatr Pathol 2: 241–8

Patessio A, Iolo F, Donner CF 1993 Exercise prescription. In Casaburi R, Petty TL (eds) The Principles and Practice of Pulmonary Rehabilitation. Philadelphia: WB Saunders

Pearson MG, Calverley PMA 1995 Clinical and laboratory assessment. In Calverley PMA, Pride NB (eds). Chronic Obstructive Pulmonary Disease. London: Chapman & Hall

Pearson MG, Spence DPS, Ryland I, Harrison BD 1993 Value of pulsus paradoxus in assessing acute severe asthma. BMJ 307: 659

Polkey MI, Green M, Moxham J 1995 Measurement of respiratory muscle strength. Thorax 50: 1131–5

Prior JG, Cochrane GM 1980 Home monitoring of peak expiratory flow rate using a mini-Wright peak flow meter in diagnosis of asthma. J R Soc Med 73: 1329–34

Prior JG, Webber BA 1979 An evaluation of the forced expiration technique as an adjunct to postural drainage. Physiotherapy 65: 304–7

Quinton PM 1990 Cystic fibrosis: a disease of electrolyte transport. FASEB J 4: 2709–17

Ramsey BW, Farrell PM, Pencharz P 1992 Nutritional assessment and management in cystic fibrosis: a consensus report. Am J Clin Nutr 55: 108–16

Rees PJ, Clark TJH, Moren F 1982 The importance of particle size in response to inhaled bronchodilators. Eur J Respir Dis 119(Suppl): 73–8

Rimington LD, Davies DH, Low D, Pearson MG 2001 Relationship between anxiety, depression and morbidity in adult asthma patients. Thorax 56: 266–71

Roussos C, Zakynthinos S 1996 Fatigue of the respiratory muscles. Inten Care Med 22: 134–55

Rubinfeld AR, Pain MCF 1976 The perceptions of asthma. Lancet i: 882–4

Rudolf M, Riorden JF, Grant BJB et al. 1978 Bromhexine in severe asthma. Br J Dis Chest 72: 307–12

Sinuff T, Cook D, Randall J, Allen C 2000 Noninvasive positive-pressure ventilation: a utilisation review of use in a teaching hospital. Can Med Assoc J 163: 969–73

Smith K, Cook D, Guyatt GH, Madhaven J, Oxman AD 1992 Respiratory muscle training in chronic airflow limitation: a meta-analysis. Am Rev Respir Dis 145: 533–9

Smyth A, Walters S 2000 Prophylactic antibiotics for cystic fibrosis. Cochrane Database Systematic Review CD0011912

Solomon C, Christian D, Welch B, Balmes J 1996 Cellular pulmonary tract and pulmonary function responses to exercise and serial sputum inductions. Am J Respir Crit Care Med 153: A713

Speight AWP 1983 Is childhood asthma being underdiagnosed and undertreated? BMJ 286: 16–20

Tashkin DP, Ashutosh K, Bleeker ER 1986 Comparison of the anticholinergic bronchodilator ipratropium bromide with metaproterenol in chronic obstructive pulmonary disease: a 90-day multicenter study. Am J Med 81(Suppl 5a): 81–90

Thomas SH, O'Doherty MJ, Graham A et al. 1991 Pulmonary deposition of nebulised amiloride in cystic fibrosis: comparison of two nebulisers. Thorax 46: 717–21

Thurlbeck WM 1976 Chronic Airflow Obstruction in Lung Disease. Philadelphia: WB Saunders

Turpin SV, Knowles MR 1993 Treatment of pulmonary disease in patients with cystic fibrosis. In Davis PB (ed.) Lung Biology in Health and Disease, Vol. 64: Cystic Fibrosis, pp. 236–43. New York: Marcel Dekker

Vender RL 1994 Chronic hypoxic pulmonary hypertension. Chest 106: 236–43

Wark PA, McDonald V 2000 Nebulised hypertonic saline for cystic fibrosis. Cochrane Database Systematic Review CD001506

Webber BA, Hofmeyr JL, Morgan MDL, Hodson ME 1986 Effects of postural drainage, incorporating the forced expiration technique on pulmonary function in cystic fibrosis. Br J Dis Chest 80: 353–9

West JB 1995 Pulmonary Pathophysiology: the Essentials, 5th edn. Baltimore: Williams & Wilkins

Wilson GE, Baldwin AL, Walshaw MJ 1995 A comparison of traditional chest physiotherapy with the active cycle of breathing in patients with chronic suppurative lung disease. Eur Respir J 8: 1715

Zach MS, Oberwaldner B 1989 Chest physiotherapy: the mechanical approach to antiinfective therapy in cystic fibrosis. Infection 15: 381–4

Cardiac Disease

J. P. Moore

15

The primary aim of this chapter is to provide an introduction to the diseases and disorders of the heart and its circulation. An overview of the healthy heart is included. However, readers requiring more detail should refer to texts in the suggested further reading list at the end of this chapter.

Diseases of the heart and circulation claim more lives worldwide than any other condition. In the United Kingdom around 250,000 people die from a cardiovascular-related disease every year; this figure represents more than one in every three deaths. Similar mortality figures are reported in other technologically developed nations such as the USA and most European countries. The exact incidence of cardiovascular disease in the world population is difficult to determine because complete and adequate public health records are unavailable. However, it is clear that heart disease is also a common cause of death in other parts of the world including central African countries, Asia and the islands of the Pacific.

Key point

In clinical terms, cardiovascular diseases may be divided into those that affect the heart and those that affect the circulation. These are referred to as cardiac and vascular disease respectively.

STRUCTURE AND NORMAL FUNCTIONING OF THE HEART

Every organ of the body requires a relatively continuous supply of oxygen and other nutrients in order to function properly. In addition to this, unwanted carbon dioxide and other waste products must be transported away from the cells. These vitally important transport functions are fulfilled by the cardiovascular system. This system consists of a closed circuit of blood vessels through which the blood is continuously circulated by the repeated contraction of a muscular pump, the heart. Each day, the average heart contracts about 100,000 times and pumps around 7500 litres (5000 gallons) of blood.

Gross Anatomy of the Heart

The heart is a conical, hollow organ found in the mediastinum between the two lungs. It lies posterior to the sternum and superior to the diaphragm (Figure 15.1). The apex of the heart projects to the left of the midline and can be felt pulsating with each heartbeat.

The heart weighs between 200 and 425 grams when filled and is a little larger than the size of a clenched fist.

It consists of four muscular chambers that are specialised to carry out sequential filling and emptying of blood throughout life.

The superficial anatomy of the heart is shown in Figure 15.2. A pair of thin-walled *atria* lie behind and above a pair of thicker-walled *ventricles*. The atria act as receiving chambers for blood entering the heart and the more muscular ventricles pump blood out of the heart. Both atria and both ventricles lie side by side and the portions of their walls that separate them are called the *interatrial and interventricular septums*.

Although it is a single organ, the heart may be considered as a pair of functionally distinct pumps by hypothetically splitting it along its vertical midline into a left and a right heart. Consequently each side consists of an atrium and ventricle. The right heart receives deoxygenated blood from the great veins and distributes it into the low-pressure pulmonary circulation where it gives up carbon dioxide and takes up oxygen. Oxygen-enriched blood returns via the pulmonary veins to the left heart, which pumps it around the systemic circuit.

Structure of the Heart Wall

A membranous sac called the *pericardium* encloses the heart. This consists of two principal portions that are separated by a fluid-filled space called the *pericardial cavity*. An outer pericardial layer surrounds the origins of the great blood vessels and is attached by ligaments to the spinal column and diaphragm so that the heart is relatively fixed in the mediastinum. This layer is referred to as the *parietal pericardium* and it is composed of tough fibrous connective tissue lined with a more delicate serous membrane that secretes a small amount of fluid into the pericardial cavity.

The fibrous connective tissue of the parietal pericardium serves to protect the heart from excessive expansion due to overfilling with blood, whereas the pericardial fluid serves as a lubricant to allow friction-free movement of the heart within the pericardium as it contracts and relaxes.

The second inner pericardial portion, referred to as the *visceral pericardium*, adheres tightly to the surface of the heart. Also known as the *epicardium*, this represents the most superficial of three layers that comprise the heart wall. Underneath the epicardium is the *myocardium*, which is the predominant layer. The myocardium is the contractile element of the heart and is composed of specialised striated muscle fibres called *cardiac muscle*. The innermost layer, the *endocardium*, which comes into direct contact with the blood, lines all four heart chambers and covers the heart valves.

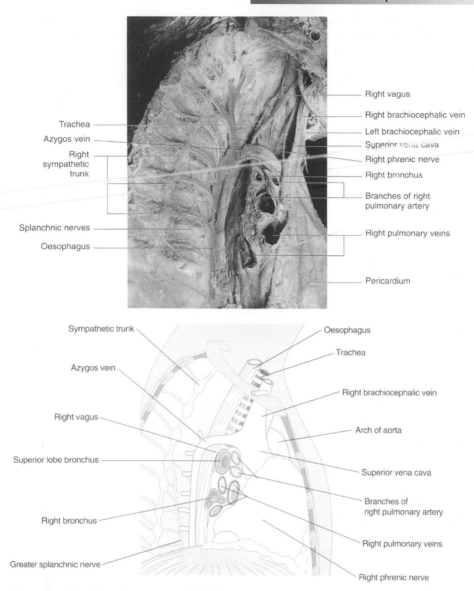

Figure 15.1   Position of the heart and associated structures in the mediastinum. (Reproduced from Jacob S 2002 Atlas of Human Anatomy. Edinburgh. Churchill Livingstone, with permission.)

Generation of the Heartbeat

Alternating contractions and relaxation of the myocardium facilitate the pumping action of the heart, commonly referred to as the 'heartbeat'. Like skeletal muscle, the myocardium contracts (i.e. shortens and thickens) when it becomes electrically stimulated, or depolarised. Unlike skeletal muscle contraction, however, myocardial depolarisation is initiated within the heart muscle itself (i.e. myocardial cells show an inherent or intrinsic rhythm that is independent of any extrinsic nerve supply). However, autonomic nerves that carry impulses to the heart, and chemical messen-gers in the blood, are also capable of influencing the rate of heart muscle depolarisation.

Although every individual myocardial cell is potentially capable of initiating its contraction, the heart possesses a specialised excitatory and conductive system that controls cardiac contraction (Figure 15.3).

The cardiac action potential begins in a group of cells referred to as the *sinoatrial* (SA) *node*. This small mass of specialised cells is located close to the point of entry of the great veins into the right atrium and is often referred to as the 'pacemaker node'. This region establishes its dominance because its cycle of electrical

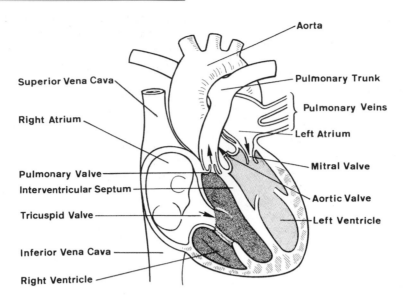

Figure 15.2   The structure of the heart.

depolarisation and repolarisation is more rapid than in other regions.

An electrical impulse emitted by the SA node disperses through the myocardium of the right atrium and then the left, leading to excitation and contraction of atrial muscle fibres as a single unit.

Since the atria are almost entirely separated from the ventricles by a band of connective tissue that does not conduct impulses, a conductive path from atria to ventricles is needed from a second group of specialised

cells located at the base of the interatrial septum. This second area of the conductive system is called the *atrioventricular* (AV) *node* and it consists of a narrow bundle of fibres through which conduction is relatively slow. Consequently the impulse originating in the SA node is delayed for about one-tenth of a second at the AV node. This ensures that the atria have time to contract before ventricular muscle is excited.

The depolarisation wave emerging from the AV node is quickly transmitted over a bundle of modified myocardial fibres – the *atrioventricular* (AV) *bundle* (also known as the 'bundle of His') – in the interventricular septum.

The bundle of His splits to form left and right bundle branches which carry the depolarisation wave at around one metre per second to the apex of the ventricles. The electrical impulse spreads out very quickly (at 3–5 m/s) from the base of the heart through an extensive network of branching fibres, called the *Purkinje fibres*. Consequently, the ventricular contraction radiates from the apex, forcing blood upwards out of the heart and into the large arteries.

Key point

The action potential of cardiac muscle is 100 times longer than that of skeletal muscle. The refractory period of cardiac muscle is also longer, preventing summation of repetitive stimuli and sustained cardiac contractions. Consequently cardiac contractions consist of relatively brief twitches.

Figure 15.3   The sinus node and the Purkinje system of the heart. (Reproduced from Guyton and Hall 2001, with permission.)

The electrocardiogram

Electrical activity arising from the sequential electrical depolarisation and repolarisation of the heart muscle is transmitted through the tissues by body fluids, which are rich in electrolytes that are good conductors of electricity. Voltage differences (around 1 mV) between pairs of electrodes (leads) placed on the skin surface on each side of the heart can be amplified and recorded as an electrocardiogram (ECG) trace.

The appearance of the ECG trace depends on the position of the electrodes with respect to the electrical activity of the heart. Standardised limb leads I, II or III or chest leads are used for this purpose.

A typical ECG trace is shown in Figure 15.4. The *P-wave* corresponds to atrial depolarisation, the *QRS complex* occurs as the impulse travels through the ventricles, and finally the *T-wave* corresponds to repolarisation of the ventricles.

Atrial repolarisation occurs during ventricular depolarisation and is masked by the QRS complex. The *P–R interval* is due to the delay in transmission through the atrioventricular (AV) node. *The ECG thus gives information about the normal and abnormal function of the ventricular myocardium.*

Regulation of Heart Rhythm

The rate at which the sinoatrial (SA) node discharges electrical impulses is referred to as *sinus rhythm*.

Sinoatrial nodal discharge frequency is influenced by cardiac autonomic nerves, metabolic factors and respiratory activity, and sinus rhythm may increase or decrease depending upon a variety of physiological conditions that bring about changes in these factors. For example during exercise, emotional excitement or fever, sinus rhythm will temporarily increase, and a heart rate in excess of 200 beats per minute is possible. This speeding up of heart rate is referred to as *sinus tachycardia*, and it is stimulated by increased activity in sympathetic nerves supplying the sinoatrial node and an increase in the circulating levels of the adrenal medullary catecholamines, *adrenaline* and *noradrenaline* (epinephrine and norepinephrine)

A reduction of sinus rhythm, referred to as *sinus bradycardia*, and which is caused by parasympathetic stimulation via the vagus nerve, is common under less stressful conditions and during sleep. Sinus rhythm during peaceful resting usually falls to give a resting heart rate of around 60–70 beats per minute. In certain physically fit individuals sinus rhythm can be slow enough to produce a heart rate of 40–50 beats per minute. Sinus rhythm is also affected by a variety of pathological conditions and abnormal heart rhythms may be symptomatic of underlying cardiac disease. Examples of electrocardiograms of sinus rhythms are shown in Figure 15.5.

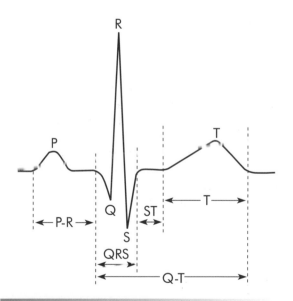

Figure 15.4 Configuration of a typical electrocardiogram or ECG. The P-wave signifies atrial depolarisation, the QRS complex signifies onset of ventricular depolarisation, and the T-wave signifies ventricular repolarisation. (Reproduced from Berne and Levy 2000, with permission.)

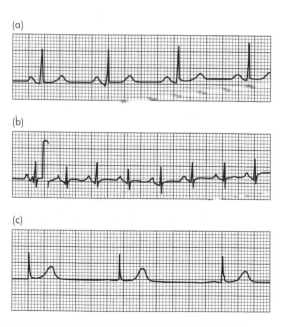

Figure 15.5 Sinus rhythms: (a) normal sinus rhythm; (b) sinus tachycardia; (c) sinus bradycardia. (Reproduced from Berne and Levy 2000, with permission.)

The Heart Valves

Two pairs of valves, the *atrioventricular* (AV) and *semilunar valves*, cover the inlets and outlets of both ventricles (Figures 15.6 and 15.7). Each valve consists of two or three flexible flaps, or cusps, of a yellowish brown connective membrane.

The atrioventricular valves – the *bicuspid mitral valve* on the left and the *tricuspid valve* on the right – lie between the atria and the ventricles and ensure that blood cannot move backwards into the atria during ventricular contraction.

The AV valves are planted in a ring of fibrous tissue that is continuous with that which separates the atria from the ventricles. Figure 15.8 shows a set of tendons, the *chordae tendineae*, that attach the free edges of each cusp of an AV valve to papillary muscles in the ventricles and prevent them from being pushed into the atria during systole.

At the ventricular outlets, the tricuspid *semilunar valves* – the *pulmonary valve* on the low-pressure pulmonary circuit and the *aortic valve* on the high-pressure systemic circuit – ensure that blood cannot flow back into the ventricles during ventricular relaxation. Unlike the AV valves, the semilunar valves are not supported by chordae tendineae.

Key point

Sequential opening and closing of the heart valves in response to pressure changes within the heart chambers is vital in the prevention of backflow of blood from the ventricles to the atria during contraction, and from the aorta and pulmonary arteries into the ventricles during relaxation. Consequently blood normally flows in one direction only through the heart during each heartbeat.

Circulation through the Heart

Figure 15.9 summarises the flow of blood through the heart chambers and great vessels.

Deoxygenated venous blood is carried to the right atrium via the *superior and inferior vena cavae*. This blood continues its passage through the tricuspid valve into the right ventricle, which propels it via the pulmonary valve into the pulmonary trunk and on to the left and right *pulmonary arteries*. As it passes through the pulmonary circulation, the blood comes into contact with inhaled air, picks up oxygen, and gives up carbon dioxide.

Oxygenated blood is returned to the left atrium through *pulmonary veins*, from where it flows to the left

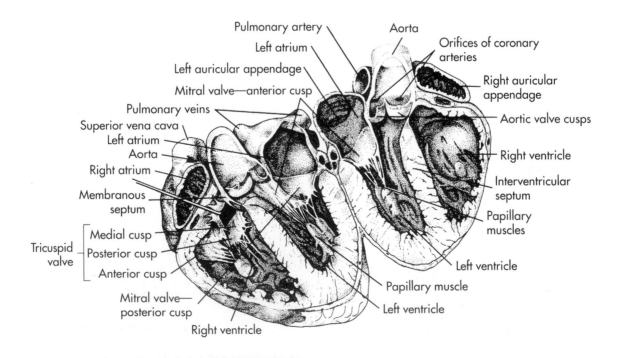

Figure 15.6   Section through the heart showing the anatomical relationships of the cardiac valves. (Reproduced from Berne and Levy 2000, with permission.)

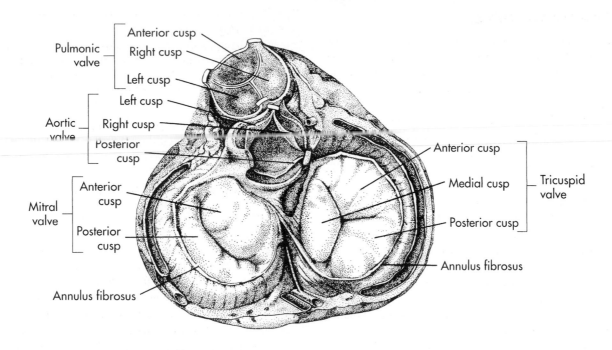

Figure 15.7   Four cardiac valves viewed from the base of the heart. (Reproduced from Berne and Levy 2000, with permission.)

ventricle via the mitral valve, and into the *aorta* through the aortic valve.

Passage of blood from the left ventricle, through the aorta and tissues of the body requires a considerable amount of driving force. Therefore, the left ventricle has the thickest walls of the four heart chambers as it has to generate the greatest pressure to propel blood.

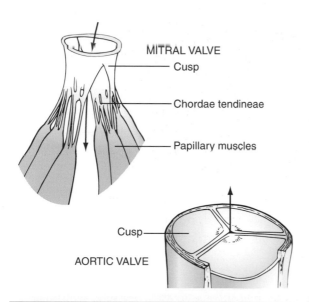

Figure 15.8   Mitral and aortic valves. (Reproduced from Guyton and Hall 2000, with permission.)

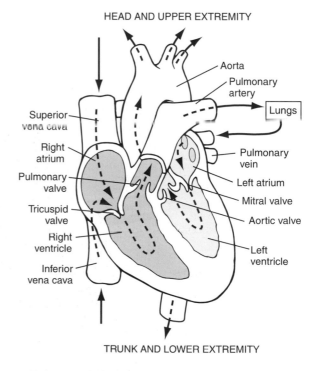

Figure 15.9   Direction of blood flow through the heart chambers. (Reproduced from Guyton and Hall 2000, with permission.)

The Cardiac Cycle

Alternating contraction and relaxation of the myocardium allows the heart to pump blood from the veins to the arteries, and the combined events of one contraction and the subsequent relaxation is known as the *cardiac cycle*. In a resting individual with a heart rate of around 70 beats per minute each cardiac cycle lasts approximately 0.8 seconds.

The contraction phase, known as *systole*, lasts around 0.3 seconds. The relaxation phase, known as *diastole*, lasts longer (around 0.5 seconds) and it is during this period that the heart chambers fill with returning blood. Each cycle is initiated by spontaneous generation of an action potential in the sinoatrial node. Figure 15.10 shows the relationship between the electrical events and mechanical events during the cardiac cycle.

Atrial systole, which coincides with the P-wave of the ECG and precedes ventricular systole, forces blood from the atria into the still-relaxed ventricles. The volume of blood (around 130 mL) present in each ventricle at the end of diastole is called the *ventricular end-diastolic volume* (EDV).

Ventricular contraction starts at the peak of the R-wave of the ECG (Figure 15.4) and forces blood from the right and left ventricles into the pulmonary artery and aorta respectively. The volume of blood (around 50–60 mL) remaining in each ventricle at the end of ventricular contraction is the ventricular end-systolic volume (ESV).

The amount of blood expelled from one ventricle during a single heartbeat (EDV minus ESV) is called the *stroke volume* and is about 70 mL in a resting human. The proportion of blood ejected during systole is called the *ejection fraction* (i.e. SV divided by EDV) and is normally around 60%.

The ability of the ventricles to fill with blood under low pressure and to squeeze this into the pulmonary and systemic circulations against high arterial pressures is critically dependent on the precise operation of the atrioventricular and semilunar valves. If ventricular relaxation is taken arbitrarily to be the start of the cycle, at this point in time the pressures in the atria are higher than those in the ventricles. Consequently the atrioventricular valves are open and venous blood is able to flow via the atria into the ventricles. This is known as the *ventricular filling phase* of the cardiac cycle. At the same time the pulmonary arterial and aortic pressures are greater than the ventricular pressures. Consequently the aortic and pulmonary valves are

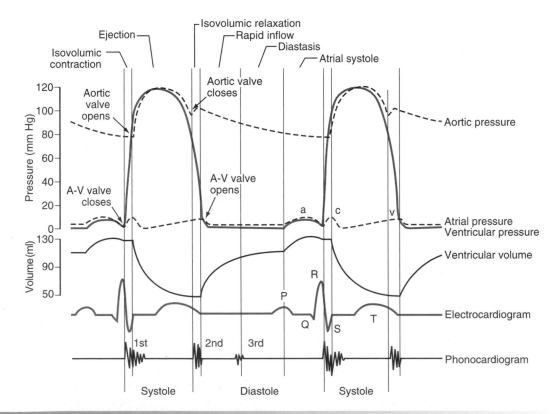

Figure 15.10   Events of the cardiac cycle for the left heart, showing changes in atrial pressure, ventricular pressure, aortic pressure, ventricular volume, the electrocardiogram, and heart sounds (phonocardiogram). (Reproduced from Guyton and Hall 2000, with permission.)

closed and there is no outflow of blood from either ventricle.

The volume of blood in the ventricles increases during this passive ventricular filling and the ventricular pressures begin to rise. Ventricular filling continues as long as atrioventricular valves remain open (i.e. while the atrial pressures exceed those in the ventricles).

Atrial pressures are elevated further by atrial contraction (denoted by *a* in the atrial pressure curve of Figure 15.10). This ensures that more blood is forced into the ventricles through the still-open valves. Atrial contraction contributes the final 20% of the blood filling the ventricles at the end of ventricular diastole.

With the onset of ventricular contraction, the ventricular pressure exceeds that of the atria and the atrioventricular valves snap shut. Closure of the AV valves prevents movement of blood in either direction between atria and ventricles. At the time of atrioventricular valve closure, both the aortic and pulmonary valves are still closed and each ventricle is in effect a sealed container. This phase of ventricular contraction is referred to as *isovolumetric ventricular systole* because there is no outlet for the blood contained within the ventricles and the intraventricular volumes remain unchanged even though the ventricles are contracting.

Compression of blood contained within the ventricles contributes to a rapid increase in ventricular pressures. At the same time, bulging of the AV valves backward toward the atria causes an elevation in atrial pressure referred to as the *c-wave*. As soon as the ventricular pressures exceed those in the great arteries, the semilunar valves are forced open and blood is now able to flow into the pulmonary and systemic circulations. This is the *ejection phase of ventricular systole*, which consists of a period of rapid ejection, followed by a period of rather slower emptying. Rapid ejection is characterised by increasing ventricular and arterial pressures as blood flows from the ventricles into the pulmonary and systemic circulations.

Throughout this phase of the cycle the semilunar valves remain closed and the blood leaving the ventricles is not being replaced by venous blood that is filling the atria. The combination of a reduction in ventricular volume and the onset of ventricular relaxation, however, rapidly results in ventricular pressures falling below those in the pulmonary artery and aorta. Consequently the semilunar valves snap shut preventing reflux of blood from the arterial system into the ventricles during diastole. Immediately before the aortic valve closes, there is a brief period of backward flow; this is followed by a brief surge in aortic pressure once the valve has closed. These aortic pressure changes are apparent as the 'notch' on a pressure trace recorded in a large systemic artery.

Once the semilunar valves have closed, another brief period during which all the heart valves are simultaneously closed ensues. During this isovolumetric relaxation phase, in which no blood can enter or leave the ventricles, relaxation of the ventricular myocardium accounts for a rapid decline of intraventricular pressures. Soon these fall below those pressures in the atria which have been filling with venous blood whilst the ventricles have been contracting, resulting in the *v pressure wave* in the atrial pressure curve of Figure 15.10. The mitral and tricuspid valves open and blood flows from the atria into the ventricles.

This restoration of the filling phase of ventricular diastole represents the completion of one complete cardiac cycle.

Normal Heart Sounds

The rhythmic closure of the heart valves during each cardiac cycle may be detected at the chest wall with a stethoscope, or by a technique known as phonocardiography that uses a low-frequency microphone connected to an amplifier and recording device.

Normally, closure of the mitral and tricuspid valves is characterised by a low, slightly prolonged 'lub' sound which identifies the onset of ventricular systole. This is referred to as the *first heart sound*. A *second heart sound*, a sharper, higher pitched 'dup', identifies closure of the semilunar valves and the end of systole. Occasionally a *third heart sound*, soft and low-pitched, is audible in normal hearts. This coincides with early diastole and is thought to be produced by vibrations of the ventricular wall.

Key point

Abnormal heart sounds – *heart murmurs* – may indicate the presence of a serious heart problem. These soft swishing or hissing sounds indicate that blood may be leaking through an imperfectly closing valve.

The Coronary Circulation

The heart muscle, like every other organ or tissue of the body, needs oxygen-rich blood to survive. Blood is supplied to the myocardium by its own special vascular system, called the *coronary circulation*.

Figure 15.11 shows how two main coronary arteries branch off from the aorta and divide into smaller arteries that supply the myocardial capillary network with oxygen-rich blood. The right coronary artery supplies blood mainly to the right side of the heart. The left coronary artery, which branches into the left anterior

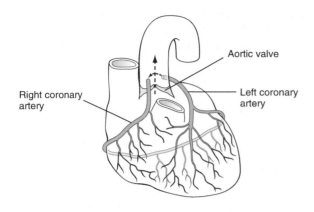

Figure 15.11   The coronary circulation.
(Reproduced from Guyton and Hall 2000, with permission.)

descending artery and the circumflex artery, supplies blood to the left side of the heart.

Veins accompany all the major arterial branches of the coronary circulation. Most eventually drain into the large *coronary sinus*, which lies on the atrioventricular groove on the posterior surface of the heart and opens into the right atrium.

The coronary arteries are composed of three layers. The outer layer, the *tunica adventitia*, is a loose fibrous tissue sheath that serves to anchor the blood vessel to the myocardium. A thick and elastic middle layer, the *tunica media*, is composed of smooth muscle that provides the mechanical strength of the blood vessel. Furthermore, contraction and relaxation of this muscular layer alters the radius of the coronary arteries– known as 'vasoconstriction' and 'vasodilatation' respectively – and changes the vascular resistance to coronary blood flow. The inner layer of the artery, the *tunica intima*, is made of smooth layer of endothelial cells overlying a thin layer of connective tissue.

Key point

At rest, around 225 mL per minute of blood flows through the coronary circulation, which accounts for about 4–5% of the output of the left ventricle.

An important feature of coronary blood flow is that it is intermittent. During systole, the external pressure exerted by the contracting myocardium compresses the coronary vessels – known as 'extravascular compression' – which impedes the free flow of blood through the coronary circulation. This is despite the fact that there is a high pressure driving blood out of the aortic root and into the coronary arteries during ventricular

systole. Consequently, flow to the myocardium is at its peak during early diastole when the mechanical compression of the coronary vessels is minimal.

Figure 15.12 shows the pattern of coronary blood flow in the left and right coronary arteries. The differences in flow may be attributed to the fact that the left ventricle has a greater muscle mass, and therefore larger blood supply, and the fact that myocardial contraction – and therefore coronary artery compression – is greatest in the walls of the left ventricle.

Despite the compression of coronary blood vessels that occurs during each cardiac cycle, coronary perfusion and myocardial metabolism are closely matched. Indeed, during maximal cardiac work the coronary blood flow can increase from a resting level of around 75 mL per minute to as much as 300–400 mL per minute for each 100 g of heart tissue. This increase in flow, known as 'hyperaemia', is mediated largely by local metabolic vasodilatation and takes place despite a reduction in the duration of diastole at high heart rates.

The precise nature of metabolic vasodilatation is largely unclear, but it is generally accepted that a decrease in the ratio of oxygen supply to oxygen demand releases some vasodilator substance(s) from the myocardium into the interstitial fluid, where it can

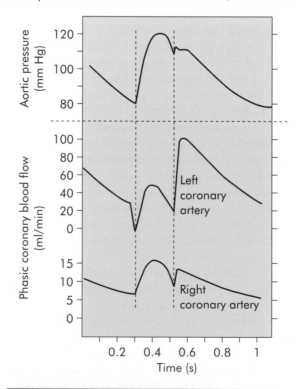

Figure 15.12   Comparison of phasic coronary blood flow in the left and right coronary arteries. (Reproduced from Berne and Levy 2000, with permission.)

relax the coronary resistance vessels. Among substances implicated are CO_2, O_2, hydrogen ions (liberated from dissociation of lactic acid produced by myocardial tissue), potassium ions and adenosine.

Normal Cardiac Function

The primary physiological function of the heart is to pump blood to vital organs and tissues to meet their metabolic requirements (i.e. delivery of oxygen and nutrients and removal of metabolic by-products). The volume of blood pumped out of the heart each minute, the *cardiac output*, is a measure of the total blood flow through the lungs and around the body and it is the product of heart rate and stroke volume.

> Cardiac output (litres per minute) = stroke volume (mL) × heart rate (beats/min)

Cardiac output is closely matched to the fluctuating demands of the body's organs and tissues for blood flow. Under steady-state conditions, the cardiac output of the right heart equals that of the left heart – i.e. flows in the pulmonary and systemic circulations are equal. In an adult human at rest, the cardiac output is between four and seven litres per minute. Normally this figure decreases during sleep, and is raised following a heavy meal or under conditions of stress. During periods of strenuous physical activity, cardiac output may be raised by as much as six-fold.

Since it is the product of heart rate and stroke volume, cardiac output is altered by changes in one or both of these variables. The influence of autonomic and humoral factors on heart rate, via the pacemaker cells of the SA node, has already been briefly discussed. Stroke volume is also influenced by autonomic and humoral factors, which alter the force of myocardial contraction. However, as stroke volume is equal to the end-diastolic volume minus the end-systolic volume, factors that influence these volumes also affect the stroke volume.

Myocardial muscle is similar to skeletal muscle in that it can generate a more forceful contraction when it has been prestretched or preloaded. This phenomenon is summarised by the *Frank–Starling relationship* which states that the greater the degree of tension in myocardial fibres at the end of diastole, the more forceful the subsequent myocardial contraction. The degree of tension in myocardial fibres at the end of diastole is determined by the end-diastolic volume, a phenomenon known as *preload*. Common examples of alterations to preload may be observed under conditions when the amount of blood returning to the heart, the *venous return*, is changing. This may occur during postural changes and in the transition from relative inactivity to moderate exercise. For example, if there is a transient increase in the venous return, the end-diastolic volume and therefore preload will be increased resulting in a more forceful myocardial contraction.

Another determinant of stroke volume is the resistive forces in the circulation that oppose ventricular ejection. The term *afterload* describes this resistance and an increase in this factor usually results in a transient reduction in stroke volume. However, stroke volume is normally able to recover within one or two heartbeats; reflex mechanisms ensure an unchanged venous return and this combined with the increased end-systolic volume result in ventricular distension and an increased preload. This results in a greater force of myocardial contraction and a more complete emptying of the ventricles, returning the stroke volume to normal. This feedback mechanism is known as *intrinsic regulation of myocardial contractility*.

Sympathetic nerve activity and circulating levels of various hormones, such as catecholamines, are also responsible for increasing the force of myocardial contraction. This extrinsic mechanism is particularly important when there has been an increase in heart rate, during exercise for example, which reduces the time available for ventricular filling. Under these conditions an increase in venous return plus increased sympathetic activity increase the force of contraction so that the ejection fraction increases.

Figure 15.13 summarises the four factors that determine cardiac output.

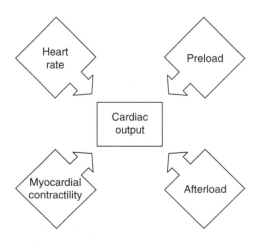

Figure 15.13   Factors that determine cardiac output.

HEART FAILURE

Definition

An abnormal pumping action is a principal component of almost all forms of heart disease. Consequently heart failure may be defined as the pathological state arising from some cardiac abnormality that is responsible for the heart's inability to pump enough blood to satisfy the demands of the body.

Introduction

The causes of heart failure are numerous because many conditions and diseases affect the heart, its valves and its blood supply. In most cases, the common denominator is severe myocardial damage leading to an extra workload being imposed on the heart.

This reduced capability to pump blood is often associated with a reduction in the *ejection fraction* that is accompanied by cardiac enlargement. There is a resultant fall in cardiac output and perception of a low blood pressure by neurohumoral reflexes. This results in a range of compensatory responses, including systemic vasoconstriction and blood volume expansion. The aim of these is to maintain perfusion to critical organs, notably the brain and the heart, which cannot survive a prolonged reduction in blood flow.

Whilst these compensations aid survival, they may become maladaptive over time and lead to further pump dysfunction. For example, the peripheral vasoconstriction that serves to maintain perfusion acutely causes an increase in afterload that when sustained becomes detrimental by exacerbating pump dysfunction.

Key point

Heart failure may be acute or chronic. Acute failure may be caused by toxic quantities of drugs or by certain pathologies, such as sudden coronary artery occlusion. Chronic heart failure may occur in conditions such as hypertension or ischaemic heart disease (IHD).

In the early stages of heart failure there may be no obvious circulatory impairment, though the heart may be dilated and enlarged on a chest X-ray. As the syndrome develops the symptoms are related predominantly to the retention of fluid and vascular congestion – oedema – throughout the body. Congestion can vary from the most minimal of symptoms to a sudden abnormal accumulation of fluid in the lungs. The term 'congestive heart failure' is often used to describe the clinical syndrome that results from central heart failure and the compensatory response of the peripheral organs and circulation.

Signs and Symptoms of Heart Failure

Fluid retention leading to vascular congestion is a prominent feature of early and untreated heart failure. A major cause of vascular congestion is an alteration in the person's ability to excrete sodium and water. Although the exact nature of these changes are unclear, they may be in some way related to a fall in renal blood flow.

It is well established that renin, a hormone released by the kidneys under conditions of decreased renal flow, initiates a sequence of events (involving angiotensin and aldosterone) that promotes the retention of salt and water. Accumulation of salt and water in the extracellular fluid can lead to clinical oedema. Whilst the person is in the upright position the fluid may gather around the ankles and feet, and in severe cases this peripheral oedema may extend to the lower legs, thighs and groin. Whilst lying down, fluid may accumulate in the back and around the abdomen, and is referred to as *ascites*.

Heart disease most frequently affects the left ventricle in some way or another. If the left ventricle fails to pump blood adequately around the systemic arteries, a rise in left ventricular end-diastolic pressure will cause an elevation of left atrial pressure that is transmitted to the pulmonary veins. The 'back pressure' resulting from an increase in pulmonary venous pressure can cause congestion of the pulmonary circulation and reduce the amount of space available in the lungs for air. Pulmonary congestion also tends to reduce lung compliance.

In extreme cases, pulmonary capillary pressure may reach a point at which there is transudation of fluid from the vascular space to the pulmonary interstitium and eventually the alveoli. Accumulation of fluid in the alveoli, referred to as *pulmonary oedema*, can result in breathing difficulties, and respiratory distress is the most dramatic symptom of pulmonary congestion. Less severe symptoms of pulmonary congestion include breathlessness (dyspnoea) during exercise or whilst lying flat at rest, or when asleep (paroxysmal nocturnal dyspnoea). The combination of left ventricular failure and pulmonary congestion is often called *left heart failure*.

Increased pulmonary venous pressure in left heart failure can also cause an increase in pulmonary arterial pressure, known as *pulmonary hypertension*. This often contributes to the development of right ventricular failure.

Under conditions of an elevated pulmonary arterial pressure, the right ventricular end-diastolic pressure becomes increased and is transmitted to the right atrium, causing back pressure in the veins all over the body. People with right heart failure often develop clinical signs of peripheral oedema, congestion of the liver and high pressure in the veins.

Key point

Other causes of pulmonary hypertension, which are independent of left heart failure, include tricuspid valve disease, and cor pulmonale, a condition that develops secondary to lung disease.

Detection and Treatment of Heart Failure

Detection

Throughout the various stages of heart failure it is rare for there to be any evidence that blood flow is insufficient to provide adequate tissue perfusion. One exception is the shock state that occurs in acute and severe cardiac failure and in which there is acute inadequacy of flow to some critical tissues.

In the early stages of heart failure the inadequacy of the heart may become apparent only under stressful situations. Symptoms such as fatigue and weakness are generally related to poor perfusion of active muscles during exercise following a decline of cardiac output. Difficulty in breathing during exertion may also occur, but pulmonary oedema is not usually present. Other manifestations of a reduced cardiac performance and low output state include sinus tachycardia, light-headedness or fainting (syncope), mental confusion, and cool pallid skin.

In moderate congestive heart failure, there is marked limitation of physical activity. Signs and symptoms may also become apparent at rest. Should the condition become severe, there will be increasing manifestations of left and right heart failure and the patient will become more disabled. Ultimately heart failure may become totally disabling, with severe respiratory distress and the inability to lie flat and to exercise. When such circumstances are prolonged, general ill-health may develop, with various secondary affects such as malnutrition or diarrhoea.

A degree of heart failure, from mild to severe, may occur following acute and severe cardiac damage (e.g. acute myocardial infarction). This can result in a rap-idly lethal shock-like state characterised in most cases by low blood pressure, a weak, rapid pulse, and cold sweaty skin. This is referred to as *cardiogenic shock* and it may or may not be accompanied by other symptoms of cardiac failure – peripheral oedema and pulmonary congestion – depending on the duration and severity of the shock state.

Treatment

Treatment of people with heart failure is generally aimed at:

* increasing the pumping function of the heart
* reducing the volume of blood that must be pumped
* reducing fluid retention
* controlling the vascular tone.

Digitalis drugs (also known as cardiac glycosides) increase the force of myocardial contraction without increasing heart rate and for many years these were the cornerstones of drug treatment for heart failure. One of these, digoxin, is still very useful in patients with arrhythmias that can lead to heart failure, but it is not often prescribed now for people with a normal rhythm. However, it retains a place in the treatment of heart failure in certain patients.

Blood volume reduction is achieved through the use of diuretics, which increase the amount of water excreted in the urine. This is a very effective way to reduce the amount of blood that must be pumped by the heart and to relieve any vascular congestion caused by heart failure. However, diuretic therapy sometimes causes excessive potassium loss through the urine. Low potassium can trigger abnormal heart rhythms, especially in those taking digitalis. The imbalance may be corrected using potassium supplements or by a potassium sparing antidiuretic.

Another group of drugs used to treat heart failure are vasodilators, which reverse the narrowing of blood vessels. This results in a reduction in resistive load, which is of major benefit to the heart as it reduces the amount of work that it must perform to pump the blood around the circulation. Several classes of drug are prescribed for their vasodilator effect: nitrates, angiotensin-converting enzyme (ACE) inhibitors, calcium-channel blockers, and sympatholytics.

Diagnosing Heart Disease

Electrocardiography, which was discussed earlier in the chapter, provides information on the passage of the cardiac action potential through the myocardium and is commonly used to detect heart rhythm disorders. Another common non-invasive diagnostic test during the initial evaluation of heart disease is a chest X-ray to determine if there is any cardiac enlargement.

In recent years, echocardiography, which produces an ultrasound picture of the heart and valves, has been more commonly used to provide a diagnosis of cardiac enlargement. By determining cardiac volumes during the cardiac cycle, echocardiography also provides an indication of the degree of myocardial dysfunction.

Cardiac catheterisation is an invasive procedure that enables a number of other tests to be performed. Catheterisation requires a fine tube to be introduced through a vein in the arm, or the femoral artery in the groin. The tube is advanced under X-ray guidance to the heart chambers. Once in place, the catheter may be used in a number of ways. A radio-opaque contrast medium may be injected through the catheter and its progress through the heart chambers followed by X-ray cinematography. This technique, known as angiocardiography, shows the movement of the heart walls, valve defects, and the extent of coronary artery occlusion by showing where and by how much the arteries are narrowed. The catheter may also be used to measure the rate of blood flow and blood pressures within the heart during the cardiac cycle. From the results of these tests it is possible to gain an idea of how well or poorly the heart is pumping.

Sometimes small pieces of heart muscle (biopsies) are also taken during the cardiac catheterisation for laboratory study. Such heart muscle biopsies are helpful in the evaluation of possible infections of the heart, as well as certain metabolic abnormalities of the heart.

DISTURBANCES OF HEART RHYTHM

Key point

The normal heartbeat is initiated by the pacemaking sinoatrial node and then passes along the conducting pathways so that the heart beats with a regular rhythm. If the conduction system fails, the heartbeat may be abnormal – either tachycardic, bradycardic, or irregular.

Arrhythmias

The general term for an irregular heart beat is *arrhythmia*, although the term *dysrhythmia* is also used. Occasional arrhythmias, such as an extra beat or skipped beat, can take place in a healthy heart and may be of minimal consequence. However, abnormal heart rhythms may also occur if there is a birth defect, coronary heart disease and other less common heart

disorder. Various systemic conditions including hyperthyroidism and certain drugs, caffeine for example, can disturb the heart rhythm.

A common manifestation of disordered heart rhythm is an uncomfortable awareness of a very rapid heartbeat, referred to as *palpitation*. However, exercise or anxieties are other possible causes of this.

Prolonged or chronic arrhythmias often lead to severe pump dysfunction and a reduction in cardiac output that lowers blood pressure and affects perfusion of vital organs like the brain and heart. Consequently arrhythmias may also be associated with shortness of breath, light-headedness, fatigue, blackout or syncope, and in extreme cases, sudden cardiac death. The presence of an arrhythmia usually represents a lack of normal communication between the atrial and ventricular conduction systems.

Atrial flutter and fibrillation

Atrial flutter is a term used to describe regular atrial activity so rapid – between 240 and 400 contractions per minute – that the conduction of impulses to the ventricles may be impaired so that only every other or every third impulse excites ventricular activity and a detectable pulse. This is characterised by the absence of a normal P-wave on the electrocardiogram and overall the pulse is around 150 beats per minute. Because the atria are electrically isolated from the ventricles except for the conduction system, the atria can enter tachycardia without the ventricle being affected.

Atrial fibrillation (AF) describes a common form of arrhythmia in which the atria beat rapidly and incompletely in a chaotic and irregular manner. Atrial fibrillation may be transient or persistent, and may contribute to ineffective pumping of blood by the heart. Figure 15.14 shows the electrocardiogram during atrial fibrillation.

Development of blood clots within the atrial walls is a complication of atrial fibrillation. If a formed clot fragments and passes into the circulation, it may precipitate a stroke or a pulmonary embolism.

Ventricular tachycardia and fibrillation

Ventricular tachycardia (VT) is a dysrhythmia characterised by a heart rate typically greater than 120 beats per minute and wide QRS complexes on the ECG (Figure 15.15). If a run of tachycardia lasts less than 30 seconds it is referred to as *unsustained VT*; a longer duration is considered *sustained VT*. Ventricular tachycardia is commonly associated with coronary heart disease and contributes to interference with normal cardiac filling and ejection. Consequently prolonged VT may result in congestive failure,

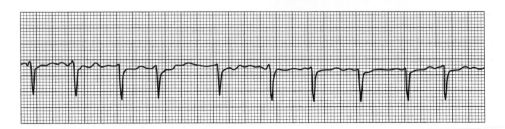

whereas severe and acute VT leads to the development of a shock state.

Ventricular fibrillation (VF) is a pulseless arrhythmia with irregular and chaotic electrical activity and ventricular contraction (Figure 15.16).

Consequences and treatment of arrhythmia

Fibrillating atria and/or ventricles lose the ability to function as a pump relatively quickly. During ventricular fibrillation in particular, a sudden loss of cardiac output, with subsequent lowering of tissue perfusion (hypoperfusion), creates global tissue ischaemia. The cells of the brain and myocardium are most susceptible to infarction.

Defibrillation

If treated in time, many atrial and ventricular arrhythmias can be converted into normal rhythm by applying an electrical shock that resets and restores the normal rhythm to the heart. This is referred to as *cardioversion* or *defibrillation* (Figure 15.17).

Drug treatments for arrhythmia include beta-blockers, calcium-channel blockers, digitalis drugs, and quinidine. These antiarrhythmic drugs work by altering the conduction rate of the cardiac action potential through the myocardium.

In patients who have had a life-threatening arrhythmia, or those with risk factors for such arrhythmias, surgically placed devices can deliver a small internal shock when abnormal rhythms occur. Such a device is called an 'automatic internal cardioverter/defibrillator' (AICD) and can prevent sudden death in high-risk patients.

Heart Block

Occasionally, malfunction of the conduction system results in the cardiac action potential impulse becoming delayed or interrupted. This results in a *bradycardia* or heart block. Also known as *atrioventricular* (AV) *block*, heart block is a condition characterised by a lack of synchronisation between atrial and ventricular contractions. This situation can be diagnosed on an electrocardiogram and is classified according to the severity of impairment. In *first-degree heart block* the conduction time from the atria to the ventricles is prolonged; this is characterised by a longer than normal (>0.2 seconds) interval between the P wave and QRS complex on an ECG (Figure 15.18a).

Electrophysiological studies have shown that first-degree heart block may be due to conduction delay in the AV node, in the His–Purkinje system, or both. This

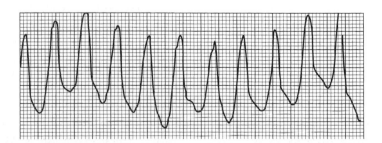

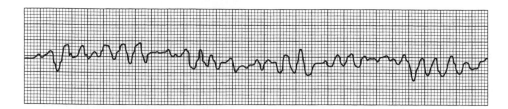

Figure 15.16   Ventricular fibrillation. (Reproduced from Berne and Levy 2000, with permission.)

condition does not normally result in clinical manifestation. Certain drugs used in the treatment of other heart conditions such as digitalis can cause first-degree heart block.

In *second-degree heart block* some action potentials that have travelled normally from the SA node to the AV node fail to induce ventricular contractions and a QRS complex on the ECG (Figure 15.18b). This results in missing or 'dropped' heartbeats. Since the conduction system below the AV node divides into two major branches, blockage of impulse transmission in either of these is termed *right- or left-bundle block*.

Third-degree (complete) heart block occurs when the cardiac action potential does not pass from the atria to the ventricles. In this situation, atrial contraction usually continues at a normal or higher than normal rate (Figure 15.18c). Ventricular contraction is established at a rate independent of atrial contraction. Consequently there is total dissociation of atrial and ventricular contraction, and third-degree heart block is characterised on the ECG by an abnormal relationship between the P and the QRS waves. If ventricular con-

traction is established at a rate close to normal, this condition may be without consequence to the circulation. However, if ventricular contraction is slower than normal, some degree of heart failure may ensue.

Complete heart block is often associated with heart disease or is a side-effect of drug toxicity. Other causes of heart block include congenital abnormalities of the conduction system or trauma caused during heart surgery. In these circumstances a pacemaker may be necessary to monitor the heart's rhythm and take over control if it becomes too slow.

PERICARDIAL DISEASE

Key point
Pericardial disease may occur as an isolated process or as a manifestation of disease elsewhere in the body.

Most commonly, pericardial disease involves inflammation of the pericardium – *pericarditis* – which is caused by a rubbing together of the visceral and parietal layers. Sometimes an outpouring of the pericardial contents (fluid, blood, pus, gas) – a pericardial effusion or hydropericardium – develops. The presence of excessive amounts of fluid in the pericardial space may be determined by abnormal findings on a chest X-ray or echocardiogram. Accumulation of large amounts of fluid can lead to an increase in the pressure within the pericardial sac and impaired diastolic filling of the ventricles. On rare occasions this can lead to cardiac tamponade, a form of heart failure that causes a fatal shock-like state.

Pericarditis has a number of causes. The pericardium may become inflamed due to an infection (bacterial, viral, fungal or protozoal) or as the result of a chemical or metabolic disturbance. Pericarditis can also develop during myocardial infarction and certain inflammatory or autoimmune diseases. In some cases pericarditis may have an idiopathic (unknown or non-

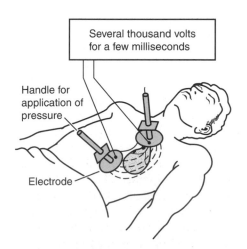

Figure 15.17   Application of electrical current to the chest to stop ventricular fibrillation. (Reproduced from Berne and Levy 2000, with permisison.)

Several thousand volts for a few milliseconds

Handle for application of pressure

Electrode

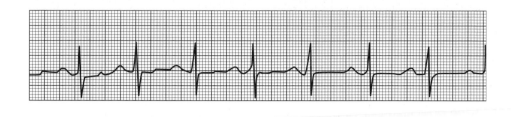

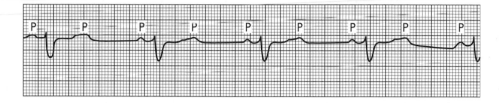

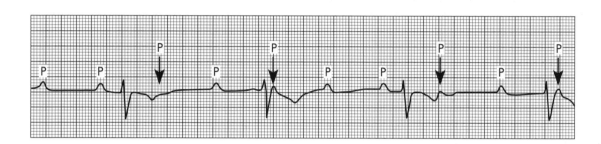

Figure 15.18 Heart block: (a) first-degree; (b) second-degree; (c) third-degree. (Reproduced from Berne and Levy 2000, with permission.)

specific) origin. Carcinoma, connective tissue disease and specific injury to the pericardium are also potential causes of pericardial disease. In constrictive pericarditis, thickening and fibrosis of the pericardium restricts diastolic expansion of the heart.

The most common symptom of pericarditis is chest pain, although it may exist without pain. A characteristic sound, called 'friction rub', can be heard on the left sternal border during examination with a stethoscope. Sometimes a person may get some relief from the pain by adopting a certain position, for example sitting up. There will also be symptoms related to the cause of the pericarditis (e.g. fever).

Treatment for pericarditis usually involves administering aspirin or other non-steroidal anti-inflammatory drugs. If there is evidence of cardiac tamponade, a needle is inserted just under the xyphoid process, to drain excess fluid. This is referred to a 'pericardiocentesis'. Sometimes treatment may involve surgical removal of thickened pericardium from around the heart, which permits normal filling and expansion of the ventricles and restores adequate cardiac output to the organs.

MYOCARDIAL DISEASE

Key point
Conditions that affect the myocardium and decrease the pumping ability of the heart are recognised as a major cause of morbidity and mortality worldwide.

Clinically, a number of diseases can cause damage to myocardial tissue. For example certain infections may occasionally affect the heart muscle to cause an inflammation known as *myocarditis*. Infections that can cause myocarditis include the coxsackie A and B viruses, the influenza virus, the diphtheria bacterium, the parasite *Trypanosomia*, and rheumatic fever. A number of systemic disorders can also affect the heart muscle; these include rheumatic disease, acromegaly, thyrotoxicosis, and myxoedema. Alcoholism and drug toxicity can also be a cause of myocarditis.

Myocarditis is a condition that can affect people of any age but young adults seem to be most susceptible. The patient usually experiences chest pains and there may be symptoms of heart failure and an abnormal ECG. Treatment includes rest and drug therapy to treat the cause. The majority of people who develop myocarditis recover after several weeks without permanent damage to the heart.

About 120,000 people in the United Kingdom have cardiomyopathy and no disease is responsible for more sudden deaths in the under-25s. Although it may be distinguished in general clinical terms from other forms of heart disease, cardiomyopathy is often misdiagnosed or not detected at all.

In general, the signs and symptoms of cardiomyopathy are similar to those of heart failure. The clinical and pathological features of cardiomyopathies are sufficiently different, however, so that they may be divided into three main classes: dilated, hypertrophic obstructive, and restrictive.

Definition

Cardiomyopathy is the term used to describe a syndrome of non-inflammatory heart muscle damage, or changes, which affect the heart's pumping performance (*myo* relates to muscles, and *pathy* refers to damage). Although other forms of heart disease (e.g. coronary heart disease) can eventually lead to cardiomyopathy, the term is generally reserved for myocardial changes that are independent of other forms of heart disease. Some clinicians use the terms 'primary' and 'secondary' to distinguish between the causes.

Dilated Cardiomyopathy (DCM)

Also known as *congestive cardiomyopathy*, DCM is most notable for an enlarged heart that contracts poorly. Stretching, or dilatation, of the heart walls causes them to become thin and flabby so that the heart becomes weak and is unable to pump as well as it should. This is indicated by a reduction in the ejection fraction.

DCM is not a common condition: it affects 35 in every 100,000 of the population, and twice as many men as women. Most cases of DCM are idiopathic (unknown cause). However, one known cause of DCM is myocarditis, possibly because of severe damage to the heart during the initial infection, or because the virus triggers an autoimmune reaction. In 20–40% of all cases there will be a family history of DCM, although the specific genetics are still not fully understood. Other causes of DCM are believed to be excessive alcohol consumption and exposure to toxic compounds.

Uncommonly, women in mid to late pregnancy, or soon after delivery, can develop DCM. This is termed *peripartum cardiomyopathy* and occurs in approximately one in 10,000 pregnancies. Some of these cases of DCM may be due to one of the other causes outlined above, but coincidence makes the disease first obvious during pregnancy, probably because of the extra demands placed on the heart. In around half the cases of genuine peripartum cardiomyopathy the condition resolves within 6–8 weeks of the delivery, but may recur in subsequent pregnancy. The cause of the occurrence or recurrence of peripartum cardiomyopathy is unknown. Women who have not completely recovered are advised to avoid further pregnancies.

DCM occurs with a spectrum of severity and outcomes. Depending on the cause and the degree of irreversible damage to the heart muscle following the acute illness, about one-third of patients have persistent very poor heart function, one-third improve but are left with some heart dysfunction, and one-third recover completely. It is difficult to predict into which category an individual patient will fall, so frequent cardiology follow-up is extremely important. Patients who do have irreversible damage and persistent poor function may go on to require a heart transplant. Sudden death as a culmination of chronic low-output heart failure is a feature of DCM.

Hypertrophic Cardiomyopathy (HCM)

The most notable sign of hypertrophic cardiomyopathy, also known as *hypertrophic obstructive cardiomyopathy* (HOCM), is an excessive thickening of the heart muscle. This wall thickening (hypertrophy) can result in problems with obstruction to outward flow and problems with relaxation of the ventricles, and can thereby affect the ability of the heart to fill.

The distribution of hypertrophy is variable. The left ventricle is almost always affected and in some individuals the muscle of the right ventricle also thickens. Typically, the septum is thicker than the free wall of the left ventricle, the left ventricular volume is reduced, and the diastolic pressure is raised.

It is important to note that heart muscle may also hypertrophy in normal individuals as a result of prolonged athletic training. In these athletic cases, the thickened muscle is healthy and usually contracts well and ejects most of the blood from the heart. In hypertrophic cardiomyopathy, however, the muscle is often stiff and relaxes poorly, requiring higher pressures than normal to expand with the inflow of blood. Ventricular end-diastolic volumes are therefore reduced and this will limit the amount of blood that can be ejected with the next contraction.

Typical presentations include dyspnoea and arrhythmia, but tragically sudden death is sometimes the first indication that something was wrong with the heart muscle. Although the incidence of sudden death is relatively rare (less than 1%), it is common in young people with HCM and for whom a keen interest in sport has exacerbated the condition. Risk factors for sudden death include episodes of sinus tachycardia, passing out and a family history of sudden death.

It is estimated that 1 in 500 people have HCM. The precise cause is unclear, although there is evidence for a familial connection in the majority of cases. In other cases of HCM there is either no evidence of inheritance or there is insufficient information about the individual's family to assess inheritance.

Restrictive Cardiomyopathy (RCM)

The hallmark feature of RCM is ventricles with normal or near-normal ventricular pumping function but abnormal filling due to fibrosis or scarring of the myocardium. Because a stiff rigid ventricle has difficulty in filling, damming of blood behind one or both AV valves ensues, and the atria become distended and enlarged. The ventricles remain normal or near-normal in size.

RCM is notable for increased work of breathing, often associated with a respiratory illness such as a cold, bronchitis or pneumonia. Other symptoms are those of left and right heart failure, including systemic and pulmonary congestion.

RCM is a very rare form of cardiomyopathy, accounting for around 5% of patients with cardiomyopathy. It may be idiopathic or may be secondary to another systemic disease. Endomyocardial fibrosis is common in tropical Africa. One cause of RCM in the UK is deposition of abnormal protein in the myocardium and endocardium. This condition is called amyloidosis. Other causes include scleroderma and sarcoidosis.

The prognosis for sufferers of DCM depends upon the underlying cause, but is generally poor.

Detection and Treatment of Cardiomyopathies

Key point
Signs and symptoms of congestive heart failure – such as rapid breathing, abnormal heart rhythms, abnormal lung and heart sounds and an enlarged liver – are common in patients with a cardiomyopathy. However, their absence does not rule out the diagnosis.

Although there is a long list of possible causes of cardiomyopathy, few of them are directly treatable and most therapy is aimed at treating the secondary effects on the heart.

Treatment is usually with drugs and is aimed at minimising symptoms and preventing the development of complications and progression of the disease. A combination of drugs used to treat heart failure may be prescribed. These include ACE inhibitors, beta-blockers, digoxin and diuretics. Patients with RCM are at high risk for blood clots within the heart, particularly the enlarged upper chambers, so use of an anticoagulant such as heparin is vital. Rhythm problems may develop from a dilated or hypertrophied myocardium; medication to treat this or implantation of a pacemaker or ICD may be necessary.

Some patients with cardiomyopathies do not respond to medical treatment and deteriorate to such an extent that their quality of life is very poor. At this stage the individual may be referred to a specialist hospital where an assessment will be made to see if heart transplantation is appropriate.

VALVE DISEASE AND ENDOCARDITIS

There are two ways in which a diseased or damaged valve can affect the flow of blood through the heart. If a valve becomes constricted or narrowed, the forward flow of blood is accelerated and turbulent, a condition called *valvular stenosis*. Alternatively, deformation of a valve may result in its incomplete opening and closure, allowing backward flow of blood, called *regurgitation*, during myocardial contraction. This situation is referred to as *valvular incompetence* or *insufficiency*.

Stenosis and incompetence interfere with normal flow of blood through the heart. In a case of stenosis, the heart must contract more forcefully to pump blood through the narrowed valve. With incompetence, the heart also has to work harder to pump the increased volume of blood forwards; however, some of this energy will be wasted as blood is going backwards also.

Key point
Stenosis and regurgitation often occur simultaneously in advanced disease. The heart becomes dilated in order to accommodate the greater than normal blood volume.

There are several causes of valvular disease, these include congenital abnormalities, and acquired diseases such as bacterial endocarditis or rheumatic fever.

In bacterial endocarditis, an infection becomes established on the endothelial lining of the heart chambers. Endocarditis may be acute or severe, or it may be chronic, often referred to as 'subacute endocarditis'. The endothelium becomes inflamed and frequently the location of the inflammation is at the line of valve closure. It may erode the valve structure, or it may produce nodules with the ulcerative surface of active infection. Subsequent fibrosis and scarring of the valves and chordae tendonae often results in deformity of one or more of the heart valves, which may cause valve malfunction.

Rheumatic fever is another example of an inflammatory condition that can cause endocarditis and valve malfunction. This involves a delayed hypersensitivity reaction in susceptible individuals, usually children and young adolescents, following an untreated streptococcal throat infection. The severity and incidence of the acute phase of rheumatic fever is decreasing, owing to improved social conditions and rapid and effective treatment or prevention of streptococcal infections. However, rheumatic fever is still a major cause of death from heart disease in 5–24 year olds of less developed countries of the third world. It is common for cardiac surgeons to perform operations to repair valves in middle-aged or older persons that were damaged years ago by the disease in childhood or young adulthood. Valve defects are also associated with a number of other diseases including ankylosing spondylitis, rheumatoid arthritis and systemic lupus erythematosus (SLE).

Abnormalities of the mitral valve apparatus are the most common valve defects caused by disease. Mitral stenosis is more common in women than men and the most frequent cause is rheumatic endocarditis. Scarring or fusion of the valve cusps, so that the valve opening becomes funnel-shaped, causes mitral stenosis and calcification of the valve in middle age makes it more narrow and non-compliant. Mitral regurgitation is the most common lesion of rheumatic heart disease. Changes in the chordae tendonae and papillary muscle of one or both cusps, or dilation of the valve ring, cause the valve to remain open during systole. Incomplete valve closure permits backflow of blood from the left ventricle to the left atrium during systole. Mitral stenosis and incompetence often coexist, but one or the other may be functionally predominant.

The tricuspid valve is subject to defects less frequently than either the mitral or aortic valves. These deformities almost always exist with mitral and aortic lesions and occur in approximately 10% of patients with chronic rheumatic heart disease. Pulmonary valve deformities are the most rare complication of rheumatic endocarditis.

Detection and Treatment of Valve Disease

The symptoms of valvular heart disease depend on which valve is affected, and the severity of the deformation. People with mild valvular heart disease may have few symptoms, although heart murmurs are a common feature. A murmur during ventricular diastole generally indicates an abnormal flow into the ventricle that is typical of a mitral stenosis. A murmur during ventricular systole, however, indicates an abnormal flow of blood back into the left atrium. This latter murmur is typical of mitral regurgitation. The presence of aortic stenosis may lead to a marked left ventricular hypertrophy. Over time there may be atrial dilation and ventricular hypertrophy that is typical of congestive heart failure, and increasing strain on the heart can cause tiredness or breathlessness on exercise. If the obstruction is severe, the onset of congestive heart failure may be relatively rapid.

Medical treatment for valvular heart disease involves medication to relieve the symptoms of heart failure and will depend on the severity of the condition. If the obstruction or leaking of valves is severe, then medicines alone may not be enough to maintain an adequate cardiac function. In these cases some form of remedial surgery is the only option to repair a defective valve or valves and prevent further damage to the heart muscle.

One relatively common procedure is valvuloplasty. This is carried out during cardiac catheterisation. A catheter with a small inflatable balloon at its tip is inserted into a vein in the groin and passed through to the orifice of the damaged valve. The balloon is gently inflated so that the deformed valve is stretched and widened. This is commonly used in the treatment of mitral stenosis. If a valve is damaged beyond repair it can be replaced with either an artificial valve made of stainless steel, or a valve from a deceased human or animal (usually pig) donor. The advantage a donor valve has over an artificial valve is the absence of clotting, which occurs occasionally using an artificial valve.

CORONARY HEART DISEASE

Definition
Coronary heart disease (CHD) is a nonspecific term used to describe a number of interdependent syndromes that are manifestations of a poor supply of oxygen-rich blood to the heart muscle. The main examples of CHD are angina pectoris, or chest pain, and acute myocardial infarction, or heart attack.

Complications of coronary heart disease are a leading cause of mortality worldwide. Although death rates from the disease have been falling since the early 1970s, CHD is still the most common cause of premature death in the United Kingdom. One in four men and one in six women die from the disease and in 2000 CHD caused around 125,000 deaths in the UK. Furthermore, illness and disability arising from CHD in older age groups is increasing. Thus, in addition to the human cost, CHD has major economic consequences. It is estimated that in the UK the combined CHD cost to the healthcare system and production losses from death and illness in those of working age represents a total of £10,000 million annually.

Pathogenesis

The pathological basis of CHD is partial or complete obstruction of one or more of the main coronary arteries. Under these conditions blood flow through the artery is decreased. Typically this results in an inadequate supply of oxygen and other nutrients to the heart muscle. The state in which the myocardial energy requirements exceed the energy supply is referred to as *myocardial ischaemia* (from the Greek *iskho*, to keep back, and *haima*, blood). Consequently the term *ischaemic heart disease* (IHD) may be used as a more precise alternative to CHD.

Initially the ischaemia may be mild or transient. Under conditions requiring an increase in the myocardial oxygen supply, for example during physical or emotional stress, the blood flow through a blocked or restricted artery may be insufficient to deliver the required amount of oxygen. Under these conditions the person often experiences chest pain that is symptomatic of an angina attack. With repeated angina attacks, or greater degrees of coronary blockage, or following a very sudden decrease in coronary blood supply, any area of myocardial tissue that is cut off from its oxygen supply for more than a few minutes will usually be irreversibly damaged and may even die. A region of dead cells is known as an *infarct*. The myocardial contractility of the affected area is severely compromised and this may precipitate abrupt loss of cardiac function, or cardiac arrest. It is estimated that around 275,000 people have a heart attack each year in the UK and that about 2.1 million people have or have had angina.

Coronary Atherosclerosis

Progressive changes to the wall and the inner lining of the coronary arteries are significant precursors of the syndromes of CHD. Known collectively as *coronary atherosclerosis* (*athero* is Greek for porridge, and *sclerosis* is hardening) or coronary artery disease, these changes include proliferation, or thickening, of the coronary arterial intima, and excessive deposition of fatty tissue, fibrous cellular debris and calcium salts in the endothelium. These deposits, referred to as *atherosclerotic plaques* or lesions, generally begin forming in childhood and clinical manifestations appear in middle to late adulthood.

Thickening of the intimal layer reduces the elasticity of the arterial walls, whereas plaques encroach into the lumen of the artery. The left coronary artery is more commonly affected than the right, and eventually this 'hardening' and 'narrowing' of the coronary vessels impedes blood flow to the left ventricle, apex, interventricular septum, and anterior surface of the atria; chronic occlusive syndromes of CHD may ensue.

However, it is worth noting that while coronary artery disease is responsible for almost all cases of CHD, many more individuals have plaques than those who have CHD. Furthermore, not all mechanisms that trigger coronary artery disease are the same as those that lead to CHD. For example, signs of CHD might never appear in an individual with a lesion of the left coronary artery, provided the area of heart muscle supplied by the artery is adequately supplied with oxygenated blood (e.g. from an alternative coronary artery circuit).

Plaque formation

The earliest lesions of the coronary arteries, fatty lipid streaks, may be found in children as young as 10 years of age. However, these areas of yellow discoloration may not be a precursor to atherosclerotic plaques in all cases. An advanced lesion, the fibrous atherosclerotic plaque, generally appears during early adulthood and progresses with age. Fibrous plaques are white in appearance and it is these that can increase in size leading to progressive arterial obstruction. Plaques can be complicated by ulceration, haemorrhage, thrombosis and calcification.

The pathogenesis underlying coronary artery disease is complex and incompletely understood. It is generally accepted, however, that there are three important components to consider in relation to advanced coronary atherosclerotic lesions: endothelial injury, lipid infiltration and platelet–fibrin deposition. Potential causes of injury to the delicate lining of the coronary arteries include mechanical trauma caused by (a) the coronary arterial pressure pulse, and (b) repeated compression of the arteries during heart contractions. Another possible source of endothelial injury is believed to be chronic exposure to a high level of cholesterol-carrying lipoproteins, referred to a *hyperlipi-*

daemia or *hypercholesterolaemia*. This is supported by a strong association between a high level of lipoproteins in the circulation and coronary atherosclerosis in human populations and experimental animals. Other potential causes of endothelial damage include immunological injury to the endothelium and exposure to certain vasoactive substances.

Lipid infiltration is an important feature of plaque formation inside the lumen of the coronary arteries. According to one hypothesis, white blood cells migrate into damaged arterial endothelium and become macrophages that accumulate lipid. In addition, macrophages synthesize and secrete a number of growth factors that are believed to stimulate thickening of the smooth muscle and connective tissue layers of the coronary arterial wall. The instability of cholesterol-rich low-density lipoproteins (LDLs) and LDL receptors on arterial walls has also been implicated in the lipid infiltration stage of plaque formation. As the plaques accumulate fat they enlarge and the arterial lumen becomes progressively occluded. Activation of the blood clotting system is an additional complication that can be seen, and the third and final stage of plaque formation involves the deposition of fibrous cellular debris and calcium salts in the plaques.

Several factors relating to the formation of advanced lesions may contribute to the involvement of thrombosis in coronary atherosclerosis. Cracks and fissures that appear in the advanced lesion may act as sites for platelet attachment and formation. Damage to the endothelium may be sufficient to cause a low-grade inflammation that leads to adherence of platelets and the formation of microthrombi (minute clots) in the vessel lining. A reduction of blood flow at the site of a lesion may activate clotting. Activation of the blood clotting system results in the formation of microthrombi consisting of cellular debris and calcium salts. These may become incorporated into existing advanced atherosclerotic plaques, from which unstable thrombi frequently break away. Alternatively a clot may become lodged in a coronary artery, a process described as a *coronary thrombosis*, causing severe occlusion that results in an *acute myocardial infarction* (MI).

Although the precise stages of plaque formation are unclear, it is obvious a number of synergistic processes are involved. Endothelial injury promotes:

- macrophage emigration and proliferation in the intima
- accumulation of lipid principally in the form of free cholesterol within the cell and surrounding connective tissue
- formation of platelet fibrinogen thrombi.

Growth factors released by platelets, macrophages and other formed elements stimulate proliferation of smooth muscle cells in the artery walls and formation of large amounts of connective tissue, including collagen and elastic fibres.

Key point

It is unclear whether plaques are reversible. Experimental evidence from studies in animal models and human femoral arteries suggest that lesions may undergo reversal. The extent to which it is possible to reduce advanced obstructive lesions in human coronary arteries is not yet understood.

Hypercholesterolaemia

It is widely acknowledged that individuals with elevated levels of total serum cholesterol (>5.2 mmol/L) have a higher than normal risk of developing plaques. However, it is the ratio of low-density lipoprotein (LDL) cholesterol to high-density lipoprotein (HDL) cholesterol, rather than the total serum cholesterol, which is thought to be the best indicator of the risk of developing coronary artery diseases.

LDL cholesterol is composed of about 20% protein and 80% lipid (around half of which is cholesterol) and this represents the main carrier of cholesterol to the tissues. Under most conditions it is incorporation of LDL cholesterol into plaques that determines whether or not the plaque progresses. Consequently this type of cholesterol is considered 'bad'. On the other hand, HDL cholesterol, which is being transported away from tissues to the liver, is considered 'good'. HDL cholesterol is around 50% protein and 50% lipid, of which around two-fifths is cholesterol.

There is accumulating experimental evidence to suggest that some defect of LDL receptors prevents the specific uptake of cholesterol into cells by receptor-mediated endocytosis, resulting in elevated levels of circulating cholesterol. It appears that this defect is inherited, although the influence of environmental factors cannot be ruled out. For example, it is reported that dietary fatty acids influence the relative proportions of LDL and HDL in the blood; unsaturated fatty acids increase the proportion of HDL, while saturated fatty acids increase the proportion of LDL. It is also believed that cigarette smoking is associated with a reduction in plasma HDL, whereas exercise causes an elevation of HDL. Finally, oestrogens cause an increase of HDL and a reduction of both total cholesterol and LDL. This may explain why the incidence of CHD is lower in pre-menopausal than post-menopausal women.

Symptoms of Coronary Heart Disease

An angina attack is characterised by the sensation of severe pain and heaviness or tightness behind the sternum. Pain radiating to the arms, neck, jaw, back or stomach is also common. One of the more common causes of angina is physical activity, particularly after a large meal. However, sufferers can also get an attack during other forms of stress, or even whilst resting or asleep.

Unlike a transient ischaemic attack (TIA), a myocardial infarction (MI) is a continuous process. Interruption of the myocardial blood supply is the first stage and the outstanding clinical feature is a heavy pain in the chest. This pain may also spread to the arms, neck, jaw, face, back or stomach, and in some cases may be mistaken for indigestion. There may also be sweating, nausea or vomiting, and often there is a shortness of breath and an impending sense of doom. The affected person may look ill and pale, and as the damaged heart may then lack the strength to circulate an adequate volume of blood, fainting (syncope) can occur.

The important difference between myocardial infarction and angina is that the MI pain lasts for a much longer period, at least 15–30 minutes, and sometimes for several hours or perhaps for a day. A heart attack may also be complicated by the appearance of one or more cardiac arrhythmias.

The severity of the symptoms of MI vary. Often there is severe pain and collapse, but sometimes a heart attack is 'silent' and produces very little or trivial discomfort. Signs of silent heart attack often remain undiscovered until the sufferer has a routine physical examination or undergoes a medical investigation for other symptoms.

Diagnosis of Coronary Heart Disease

As the symptoms of angina often occur during exertion, a resting ECG may be normal. Therefore a patient may be asked to perform a stress test on an exercise bicycle or treadmill. Even then some cases will show only transient changes with exercise.

Another test is a radionucleide scan, which is useful for people who cannot exercise, and for females, in whom it is sometimes difficult to make an accurate diagnosis with an exercise ECG. A very small amount of thallium, a radioisotope of potassium, is injected into the blood. A large camera, positioned close to the chest, picks up the gamma rays emitted by the isotope. This shows which parts of the heart muscle are short of blood and measures how severe the condition is.

Another common test for angina is cardiac angiography.

Diagnosis of MI may be confirmed by an elevation of cardiac enzymes in the blood, which indicate leakage from damaged heart muscle cells, or by ECG, which in most cases shows distinct abnormalities.

Treatment of Coronary Heart Disease

Drug treatments

Inhaled amyl nitrate or sublingual (under the tongue) glyceryl trinitrate (GTN) are good examples of drugs that can help to dilate the coronary vessels temporarily, as well as reduce the resistive load on the heart. Taken regularly, beta-blockers can help reduce the frequency of angina attacks by reducing the work of the heart so that it needs less oxygen, blood and nutrients. Beta-blockers are not usually suitable for people with asthma or bronchitis, and calcium-channel blockers may be used as an alternative. Potassium-channel activators are a new type of drug given to relieve angina. They have a similar effect to nitrates as they relax the walls of the coronary arteries and therefore improve blood flow. Unlike nitrates, they do not appear to become less effective with continued use. Nitrates and beta-blockers are often used together from the start of treatment. If they do not control the angina, a calcium-channel blocker may be used as well.

Key point

There are a number of alternative treatments for CHD and the one selected will depend upon the nature and the severity of the symptoms. One or more from a range of medications may be administered with the aim of increasing the coronary blood supply and reducing the myocardial workload.

Surgery

If the symptoms of angina cannot be stabilised using drug therapy alone, the sufferer may require varying degrees of surgical intervention.

Coronary angioplasty is often used in cases where obstructive lesions are relatively isolated and incomplete. A small inflatable balloon is gently inflated so that it squashes the fatty tissue responsible for the narrowing, and widens the artery. Coronary angioplasty is usually successful, but it can sometimes lead to a blockage of the artery; this will need immediate surgery. Sometimes the artery will become narrow again over the 4–6 months after the coronary angioplasty. The angioplasty can be repeated if necessary. Increasingly, specialists who carry out angioplasty place a short tube of stainless steel mesh, called a stent, inside the artery. The stent helps to hold the vessel open, reducing the chances of the artery narrowing again.

Revascularisation techniques, involving the use of a laser to drill small holes in the myocardium that allow blood to gain muscular access, are used in patients for whom angina cannot be eliminated by angioplasty. In cases where there is a more severe blockage in two or all three main coronary arteries, a more complicated surgical procedure – *a coronary artery bypass graft* (CABG) – may be necessary (see Figure 15.20 on p. 359).

Complications and sequelae of a heart attack

Complications of a heart attack include abnormal heart rhythms, heart failure, cardiogenic shock, and pericarditis. Around 20% of heart attack victims die before they reach hospital and most of these deaths are attributed to ventricular fibrillation. Therefore the sooner paramedics or an attending physician can monitor the ECG, the greater the chance of survival. Aspirin, a drug that helps to improve the anti-clotting effect of any subsequent treatments, is also administered as early as is possible. Ideally the patient should receive a thrombolytic drug, such as streptokinase or tissue plasminogen activator, within 90 minutes of the heart attack. Thrombolytics help to dissolve the clot that is blocking the artery and prevent the formation of any further clots. These drugs can be given later, but are less effective as time goes by.

A number of additional medications, such as anticoagulants, beta-blockers or antiarrhythmic drugs, may be administered to prevent further heart attacks. Diuretics or ACE inhibitors may be given to relieve heart failure and the associated breathlessness. The patient may also be prescribed other drugs used to relieve the symptoms of angina, and drugs that lower serum cholesterol.

The amount of myocardial damage after a heart attack is often relatively small, with the result that there is enough good muscle left for the heart to carry on its work satisfactorily. The area of the heart muscle that was damaged does not regenerate so the infarction is replaced by fibrous scar tissue; this takes from a few days to a few weeks. Within 2–3 months the hearts of many heart attack patients are functioning just as well as they were before the attack. These individuals do, however, have an increased potential for subsequent myocardial infarction. If a large area of tissue is involved there may be residual evidence of heart failure or other cardiac malfunction with the result that the pumping action of the heart is not as good as before. This can lead to symptoms of varying degrees associated with heart failure. Also, some people continue to experience angina symptoms because there is still narrowing of the coronary arteries.

Risk Factors for Coronary Heart Disease

A number of factors are identified as increasing the risk of an individual developing CHD. These are:

- hypercholesterolaemia
- physical inactivity
- blood pressure >140/90 mmHg (hypertension)
- tobacco smoking
- obesity.

Since the occurrence of CHD is undoubtedly due to many independent and interdependent influences, it is difficult to distinguish any one of these major risk factors over another. It is clear, however, that the coexistence of two or more risk factors can greatly increase the risk of developing CHD.

There is evidence that hypercholesterolaemia and hypertension may be inherited. Consequently the inherited nature of these factors may make them less susceptible to modification. Furthermore, familial (genetic) predisposition to CHD, whilst it is acknowledged, is not well understood. Research is ongoing with the aim of identifying rogue genes that contribute to coronary heart disease. However, it is worth noting that reducing human health to the activity of human genes ignores the fact that the surrounding environment in which those genes are operating has a profound influence upon the ways in which the effects are manifested.

Finally, a number of secondary factors – such as predisposition to develop thrombosis, metabolic disorders such as diabetes mellitus, and rarely oral contraceptives – increase the risk of CHD in susceptible persons.

Healthcare professionals recommend a number of lifestyle changes to reduce the risk of CHD. These include eating a healthy diet, increasing levels of physical activity, stopping smoking, and maintaining weight within normal limits. However, whilst there is impressive evidence from a wide range of sources supporting the effectiveness of these measures, much of this is circumstantial and not all of the recommendations have been shown to be as effective as expected or predicted.

Lowering high serum levels of cholesterol has a great impact on heart disease, particularly in people with familial hypercholesterolaemia. It has been estimated that reducing the intake of saturated fat by 10% is

Key point

It is reported that within a few years of stopping smoking, a risk factor for heart disease nearly equal to that of people who have never smoked is attainable.

linked with a reduction of 20–30% of deaths from coronary heart disease. However, conclusive evidence for this is yet to be presented.

Regular daily physical activity, such as brisk walking, swimming or cycling, can help improve serum cholesterol levels. Physical activity increases the level of HDL cholesterol (the protective cholesterol), but does not affect LDL cholesterol.

It is also reported that people at risk of CHD benefit from treatment with statin drugs to lower blood cholesterol levels, with the suggestion that use of statins reduces the risk of being hospitalised because of worsening angina and reduces heart attacks by around one-third.

SUDDEN CARDIAC DEATH SYNDROME

Definition

Sudden cardiac death syndrome results from cardiac arrest in a person who may or may not have diagnosed heart disease. Death occurs instantly or shortly after symptoms appear.

When the pumping ability of the heart is diminished, systolic blood pressure drops, and the sympathetic nervous system is activated, leading to peripheral vasoconstriction and tachycardia with the aim of maintaining arterial pressure and coronary and cerebral perfusion. The net effect increases the load on the heart and this may result in a fatal shock state.

All known heart diseases can lead to cardiac arrest and sudden death, but the most common underlying reason for a person to die suddenly from cardiac arrest is CHD. Other factors besides heart disease and heart attack can cause cardiac arrest. They include respiratory arrest, electrocution, drowning, choking or trauma.

Cardiac arrest can also occur without any known cause. One in 20 of all cases of sudden cardiac death in people aged under 65 years are unexplained, with no cardiac abnormalities ever found. Researchers feel that many people who have died suddenly may have inherited an undiagnosed tendency to an abnormal heart rhythm.

Simple clinical methods can be used to investigate and possibly identify some of the causes of unexplained sudden cardiac death in the population. These include resting or exercise ECG testing, 24-hour monitoring of ECG, and in some cases cardiac magnetic resonance image (MRI) screening to exclude certain forms of cardiomyopathy.

CONGENITAL HEART DISEASE

Types of Malformations

Fetal heart development is a complicated process that can sometimes go wrong. There are many different kinds of cardiac malformations and these are referred to as 'congenital abnormalities' or defects. Most occur because part of the heart, its valves or the adjoining vessels is missing or improperly formed. Other defects may arise from disturbance of the heart rhythm or if the pumping action of the heart does not work properly.

Most congenital heart defects have little effect before birth because the fetal circulation is adapted so that oxygenation of the blood is accomplished across the placenta. After birth, however, specific defects impair the normal circulation of blood through the heart, lungs and great vessels. Some infants are born with only one isolated abnormality, while others have two or more.

In around a half of the cases the defect is relatively minor and repairs itself without treatment. These are referred to as 'asymptomatic defects'. The remaining half are major defects and are repaired by medical or surgical procedures with varying degrees of success. Death is common in the most severe malformations.

Congenital heart defects may be categorised as *cyanotic* or *non-cyanotic*.

- In the cyanotic types the lungs are partially or completely bypassed and poorly oxygenated blood finds it way into the systemic circulation. This results in a bluish colouring of the skin, nail beds and lips (cyanosis comes from the Greek *cyan* for blue).
- In non-cyanotic defects, oxygenated blood is shunted from the left heart to the right side. This may increase the preload in the right heart and may also cause blood that has already been oxygenated to pass into the pulmonary circulation.

In severe non-cyanotic varieties of congenital heart disease, the infant may experience symptoms of congestive heart failure, a higher than normal risk of respiratory infection, and poor growth.

Fetal Circulation

Two shunts, the foramen ovale between the right and left atria, and the ductus arteriosus between the pulmonary artery and the first segment of the aortic arch, create a short-circuit in the fetal circulation so that most blood does not pass through the lungs. These organs do, however, receive enough blood to ensure their adequate development. Normally, functional closure of the foramen ovule and ductus arteriosus occurs spontaneously within a few hours of being exposed to atmospheric oxygen at birth. However, closure of either structure is sometimes delayed or does not occur at all, and some mixing of oxygenated and deoxygenated blood occurs.

Patent ductus arteriosus

Patent or persistent ductus arteriosus (PDA) describes the condition in which the ductus arteriosus remains open, or patent, following birth (Figure 15.19). While this condition is much more common in premature babies, it may also occur in term infants. If it is small the PDA may be asymptomatic, although it might be detected as a heart murmur.

Closure of a PDA in premature babies and young infants may be induced using a drug called indomethacin; alternatively a surgical intervention may be required in older infants and children. In cases when an infant is born with another cardiac abnormality, doctors may try to delay closure of the ductus, by administering prostaglandins, until corrective surgery or a heart transplant can be performed. Alone, this defect is often not too serious, and in some malformations of the heart is actually necessary for continued life.

Congenital valve abnormalities

Abnormal development within the womb often leads to infants being born with heart valves that are not well formed. The most common congenital valve defect is *pulmonary stenosis*, which is caused by thickening of the valve cusps and narrowing of the orifice. In some cases the valves are completely closed, a condition known as *atresia*.

Mild stenosis is usually compatible with normal activities and a normal life. More severe narrowing or complete atresia are often associated with the development of other heart abnormalities before or after birth.

Another problem of congenitally faulty valves is valvular incompetence. For example, a small percentage of the population (less than 2%) are born with fusion of the aortic valve, which is usually bicuspid rather than tricuspid. The valve is often obstructed and incompetent. Tricuspid atresia is an example of a valve defect that coexists with another congenital deformity; the pulmonary artery and valve also tend to be underdeveloped since a less than optimal volume of blood leaves the right ventricle.

Treatment of congenital valve defects depends upon the severity of the defect and whether or not the person has any symptoms. Surgery is sometimes required early in life. On the other hand, people may have a normal life expectancy.

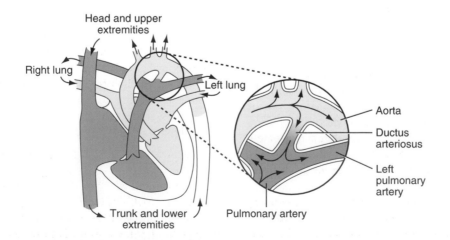

Figure 15.19 Patent ductus arteriosus. (Reproduced from Guyton and Hall 2000, with permission.)

Septal defects

Septal defects are a common example of non-cyanotic congenital heart disease. Holes of variable size in the interatrial, artrioventricular or inventricular septum enable blood to be shunted between the left and right sides of the heart.

A large right-to-left shunt at the level of the atria is a physiological condition in the fetus and atrial septal defects (ASDs) are commonly located in the area prenatally occupied by the foramen ovale. *Septum primum* refers to a hole in the portion of the septum below the site of the foramen ovale, whereas *septum secundum* refers to a hole above this site. Secundum atrial septal defects, which are the most common, are usually isolated, but may be related to other cardiac lesions (such as mitral, pulmonary, tricuspid or aortic atresia). In extreme cases, virtually no septum may exist between the atrial chambers.

Ventricular septal defects (VSDs) represent around 30% of all heart abnormalities and may be isolated or be part of a complex or multiple heart defect. A large proportion of these are relatively small and close spontaneously within the first year of life; this is not usually associated with serious disability. Larger, more severe defects allow a significant amount of blood to be shunted from the left to the right heart and infants with these defects normally present with manifestations of congestive heart failure at 2–8 weeks of life. Because many septal defects close spontaneously, they may be monitored for a short period before surgical closure is undertaken. Survival rates from surgery exceed 90% and survivors have a normal life expectancy and normal exercise tolerance.

Abnormalities of the great vessels

In complex forms of congenital heart disease, the origins of the aorta and pulmonary artery are malformed. For example, in a cyanotic condition known as *transposition of the great arteries*, the outflow tracts of the ventricles are reversed so that venous blood is pumped around the systemic circulation and oxygenated blood is circulated through the lungs. In some cases both the aorta and pulmonary artery may originate from the same ventricle; survival of infants born with this form of defect is dependent upon the coexistence of a patent ductus arteriosus or septal defect that allows oxygenated blood to enter the aorta. When there is no such shunt, it may be created surgically.

In *truncus arteriosus*, the aorta and pulmonary arteries arise from a common 'trunk', and blood from both ventricles mixes together as it all exits the heart through a single valve. *Coarction of the aorta* is a common abnormality that involves a narrowing of the aortic wall just distal to the origin of the left subclavian artery. Consequently there is a reduction in blood flow to the lower half of the body and an increase in upper body blood pressure. Cutting out the constriction and stitching the normal ends together can repair this defect.

Anomalous pulmonary venous return

One or more of the pulmonary veins may connect either directly or indirectly to the right, instead of the left, atrium. This is referred to as *anomalous pulmonary venous return* and is an example of a non-cyanotic congenital defect. Partial forms of anomalous pulmonary venous return, in which only one or two pulmonary veins are connected abnormally, may have few symptoms of vascular congestion, although surgical correction may be performed. Infants born with total anomalous pulmonary venous return (TAPR) usually develop problems related to cardiac failure within the first few weeks or months and thus require cardiac surgery.

Heart chamber abnormalities

Abnormalities of the heart chambers may be serious and potentially life-threatening. One of the most complex cardiac defects seen in a neonate is severe under-development, or hypoplasia, of one or more heart chambers. In *hypoplastic left heart syndrome* (HLHS) an infant may be born with a reduction in left ventricular/left atrial size and the mitral and aortic valves are either very small, or completely atretic. The initial part of the aorta is also very small, often only a few millimetres in diameter. This results in a situation where the left side of the heart is completely unable to support the circulation needed by the body's organs, though the right side of the heart is typically normally developed. Under these conditions, and provided that the ductus arteriosus remains patent, the right ventricle may be capable of performing a dual pumping role, distributing blood both to the lungs and out to the body. Children with HLHS rarely survive more than two or three days from their birth and cardiac transplantation can be considered.

Tetralogy of Fallot

This condition, which is a classic example of a cyanotic form of congenital heart disease, gets its name from the French physician who first described it. It is a relatively uncommon malformation consisting of a ventricular septal defect, pulmonary valve stenosis, right ventricular hypertrophy and a shift of the aorta from the left to the right side so that it receives blood from both sides of the heart (Figure 15.20). A child born with this con-

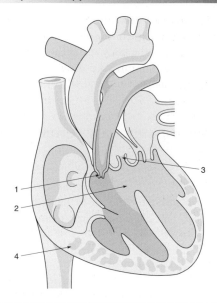

Figure 15.20   Tetralogy of Fallot. (1) = pulmonary stenosis; (2) = ventricular septal defect; (3) = dextra-position of aorta; (4) = hypotrophy of right ventricle. (Reproduced from Guyton and Hall 2000, with permission.)

genital disease can survive beyond infancy, but few survive to adulthood without surgery.

Causes of congenital heart disease

In most cases, the precise cause of a congenital heart defect is unknown. Certain chronic illnesses, such as diabetes and systemic lupus erythematous, may increase the risk of giving birth to an infant with a congenital heart defect. However, this does not imply that women with diabetes or epilepsy cannot have healthy children; they do however need to be carefully monitored during their pregnancies. Acute illness, such as the viral infection rubella, during pregnancy can also cause abnormalities before birth or interfere with an infant's heart as it develops. Finally, drugs taken in pregnancy, such as some of those prescribed for epilepsy, illegal drugs, or alcohol are also known to cause certain heart defects. Smoking is also thought to be a contributing factor.

In some cases, a genetic factor has been identified. This may be the result of a single mutant gene or it may be associated with a chromosomal abnormality. Down's syndrome is the most common example of chromosomal abnormality associated with congenital heart defects. Although the search for the causes of congenital heart diseases continues, it is generally accepted that in most cases it is probably caused by a variety of factors. Any inherited factor is usually unmasked only if it occurs together with an appropriate environmental hazard. The risk of a sibling of a child with congenital heart disease being similarly affected is 2–4%. The precise recurrence can vary for individual congenital cardiovascular defects. Between two and five babies in every 100 born to women with a defect have a similar abnormality. The risk is obviously greater in the unlikely event that the father also has a heart defect.

Detection and Treatment of Congenital Defects

Some abnormalities are diagnosed *in utero* (within the womb). Amniocentesis is an established method by which fetal chromosomes may be tested for abnormalities associated with congenital heart disease. A hollow needle introduced via the mother's abdomen into the womb is used to collect a small amount of amniotic fluid in order to study cells shed by the fetus. There is a small risk to the fetus with this test; about one in every 100 babies aborts after amniocentesis. A non-invasive ultrasound test, called a fetal echocardiogram, performed at about 16–20 weeks of pregnancy, is becoming increasingly effective at detecting some heart defects.

The presence of a congenital defect is not always detected at birth. Some are detected for the first time in older children when a heart murmur is heard. Furthermore, some defects do not become apparent or symptomatic until later in adult life. For example, a malformed bicuspid aortic valve may initially function near to normal, but can calcify and become stenotic and require replacement in middle age.

Some isolated defects, such as an atrial septal defect, a small ventricular septal defect, and patent ductus arteriosus, are not severe and the patient may live a normal life, because the shunt is not great. However, there is an increased predisposition to respiratory infections and endocarditis with these abnormalities. Other more complex defects, are survivable, but right heart failure eventually occurs. Modern heart surgery has advanced so much in recent years that it is now standard practice to operate on tiny babies. Severe defects such as hypoplastic left heart syndrome are generally not survivable and cardiac transplantation can be considered.

HEART SURGERY

Surgical treatment of heart disease may require the surgeon to make an incision into one or more of the heart chambers; this is referred to as 'open-heart surgery'.

Such a procedure is made possible by the use of a cardiopulmonary bypass device, which maintains circulation and oxygenation outside of the patient's body so that beating of the heart may be temporarily suspended. This means that the surgeon has a dry and motionless heart on which to work.

The most common open-heart procedures are those for correction of congenital heart defects, to repair diseased valves, and in the treatment of severe coronary heart disease. Cardiopulmonary bypass also enables surgery to repair damage to the great vessels that transport blood to and from the heart.

Other cardiac surgery can be performed without opening the heart. The main advantages that these have over open-heart procedures is that not all require cardiopulmonary bypass and they are less invasive, and consequently may be less traumatic.

Repair of diseased valves

For many years congenital and acquired disease of the heart valves was corrected using open-heart surgery. In the case of the mitral valve, an incision made into the wall of the left atrium gave access to the damaged valve. Replacement of the tricuspid valve, although less common than mitral valve surgery, may also be performed by open-heart procedures. Defects of the pulmonary valve usually can be repaired without opening the heart. The valve may be approached through the pulmonary artery and cut in three places to create a valve with three cusps. In older children and adults, pulmonary valvuloplasty represents a less invasive alternative to surgery. In the case of a malfunctioning aortic valve, the severity of the damage and whether or not the valve must be replaced will dictate whether a bypass is required.

Repair of congenital heart defects

Most congenital malformations can be repaired surgically and fall into two categories. The first consists of those that require cardiopulmonary bypass, such as intracardiac abnormalities. For example an incision into the heart enables the tissue on each side of a small septal defect to be sutured together; larger septal defects may require a patch of material to close the opening. The second category consists of procedures that do not need a bypass, such as ligation of a patent ductus arteriosus or removal of an aortic constriction.

Coronary artery bypass graft (CABG)

The aim of the operation is to restore adequate blood flow to the myocardium beyond severe ather-osclerotic obstructions of the coronary arteries. Cardiopulmonary bypass is used to support the circulation in most operations to replace these diseased arteries. Narrowed sections of the main coronary arteries are bypassed by grafting a blood vessel between the aorta and a point in the artery beyond the narrowed or blocked area. Multiple grafts are often used for multiple atheromatous lesions. For many years a section of vein removed from the leg was used for this, but increasingly the two internal mammary arteries (arteries that run down the inside of the chest wall) are also used. The internal mammary arteries are less likely than vein grafts to narrow over time. However, since there are only two internal mammary arteries many patients have a mixture of vein grafts and an internal mammary graft.

The principal uses of coronary artery bypass grafts may be to relieve angina that is resistant to other forms of treatment and/or to prolong a person's life (Figure 15.21).

Heart transplantation

In many cases of irreversible heart damage (by long-lasting disease or viral infection) that cannot be treated by any other medical or surgical means, heart transplantation is the only option. This procedure, which involves removing the diseased organ and replacing it with a healthy human heart, was first attempted in 1967 by surgeons in Cape Town, South Africa. On that pioneering occasion the recipient survived for 18 days before succumbing to a pulmonary infection caused in

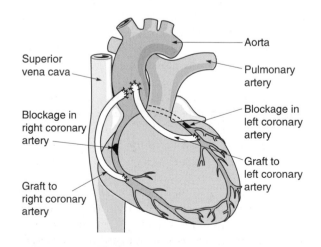

Figure 15.21   Coronary artery bypass.

part by immunosuppressive medication required to reduce the chance of donor organ rejection. Since then, however, long-term survival rates have improved and around 300 transplants are performed in the UK each year. A smaller number of combined heart and lung transplants are also performed each year in patients with lung disease, or heart disease that has caused secondary damage to the lungs. The number of available donor organs limits the number of transplants that may be attempted. Experimental artificial hearts have also been implanted, but these require an external power supply and long-term survival rates are unknown.

Perhaps the major factor affecting long-term survival in recipients of donor organs is the risk of rejection. Human beings have evolved a complex immune system that recognises and attacks foreign materials that enter the body. Unfortunately, this system cannot differentiate between disease-causing pathogens and the cells of a lifesaving transplant. Consequently, even before a transplant may be attempted, a number of tests must be undertaken to determine the compatibility of the tissue types of the potential recipient and the donor. This is referred to as 'histocompatibility', and the principles of tissue typing are similar to those for red blood cell typing. Unfortunately, a number of very sick patients may never have the opportunity to receive a donor heart as they die before a compatible organ becomes available.

If a compatible heart is found and transplanted, immunosuppresive drugs, such as azathioprene, cortisone, prednisolone, and cyclosporine, must be administered in the weeks and months following the operation to reduce the chance of acute transplant rejection. Unfortunately, this means that the patient has a greater risk of developing a postoperative infection. Another complication of chronic immunosupression is the higher risk of skin cancer and lymph gland tumours. Consequently the regimen of immunosup-pressants must be carefully monitored and after some months the dosage can often be reduced.

Acute rejection of the heart is rare after six months, although the body may continue to attack the coronary arteries of the donor heart, and symptoms of coronary heart disease may become a problem after several years.

Aside from the risk of rejection, recovery from heart transplantation is similar to that from other forms of cardiac surgery, although the patient may have been weaker than most before the procedure. Because the transplanted heart has no nerve supply, it will respond much more slowly to the demands of physical activity. However, most people who have undergone transplants are eventually able to undertake a normally active life.

The outlook for those people fortunate enough to receive a heart transplant is good. Between 85% and 90% of recipients survive for at least one year after the operation; 75% are still alive after 5 years; and 50–60% live for a further 5 years.

FURTHER READING

Braunwald E, Zipes DP, Libby P 2001 Heart Disease: a Textbook of Cardiovascular Medicine, 6th edn. London: WB Saunders

Berne RM, Levy MN 1986 Cardiovascular Physiology, 8th edn. London: Mosby

Guyton AC, Hall JE 2001 Textbook of Medical Physiology, 10th edn. London: WB Saunders

Julian DG, Camm AJ, Fox KM, Hall RJC, Poole-Wilson PA 1996 Disease of the Heart, 2nd edn. London: WB Saunders

Levick JR 2000 An Introduction to Cardiovascular Physiology, 3rd edn. London: Arnold

Petersen S, Rayner M, Press V 2000 Coronary Heart Disease Statistics. British Heart Foundation Statistics Database

Rang HP, Dale MM, Ritter JM 1999 Pharmacology, 3rd edn. Edinburgh: Churchill Livingstone

Thibodeau G, Patton K 1995 Anatomy and Physiology, 5th edn. London: Mosb

Physiotherapy in Thoracic Surgery

16

Anne Dyson

ANATOMY OF THE THORAX

The skeleton of the thorax is an osteocartilagenous framework within which lie the principal organs of respiration, the heart, major blood vessels, and the oesophagus. It is conical in shape, narrow apically, broad at its base and longer posteriorly. The bony structure consists of 12 thoracic vertebrae, 12 pairs of ribs and the sternum (Figure 16.1).

The musculature of the thoracic cage is in two layers. The outer layer consists of latissimus dorsi and trapezius, the inner layer of the rhomboids and serratus anterior muscles. Anteriorly the chest wall is covered by pectoralis major and minor. The intercostal muscles run obliquely between the ribs. The diaphragm forms the lower border of the thorax. It is convex upwards showing two cupolae, the right being slightly higher than the left. It is made up of muscle fibres peripherally and is tendinous centrally.

The Lungs

The two lungs are basically very similar (Figure 16.2). The right lung is made up of three lobes and the left of two lobes. The lingular segment of the left lung corresponds to the middle lobe on the right. Each lobe is divided into segments.

The thoracic cage is lined by the pleura. There are two layers, the parietal and visceral which are continuous with each other and enclose the pleural space. The parietal pleura is the outer layer and lines the thoracic cavity. The visceral pleura covers the surface of the lung, entering into the fissures and covering the interlobar surfaces. The two layers are lubricated by a thin layer of pleural fluid lying within the pleural space, which in health contains no other structure.

The Oesophagus

The oesophagus is a muscular tube stretching from the pharynx to the stomach. It is composed of mucosa and circular and longitudinal muscle layers. The oesophagus enters the stomach below the diaphragm at approximately the level of the eleventh thoracic vertebra.

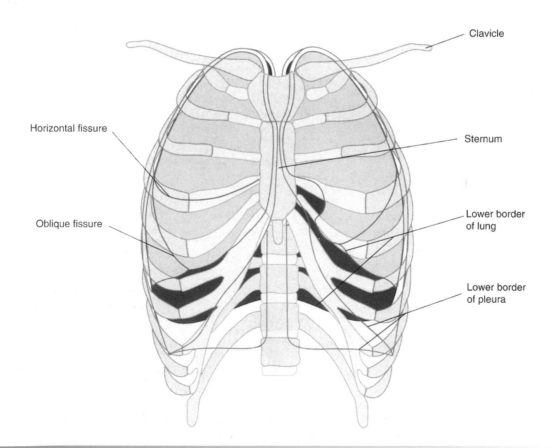

Clavicle

Horizontal fissure

Oblique fissure

Sternum

Lower border of lung

Lower border of pleura

Figure 16.1   Anatomy of the thorax. (Reproduced from Jacob 2000, with permission.)

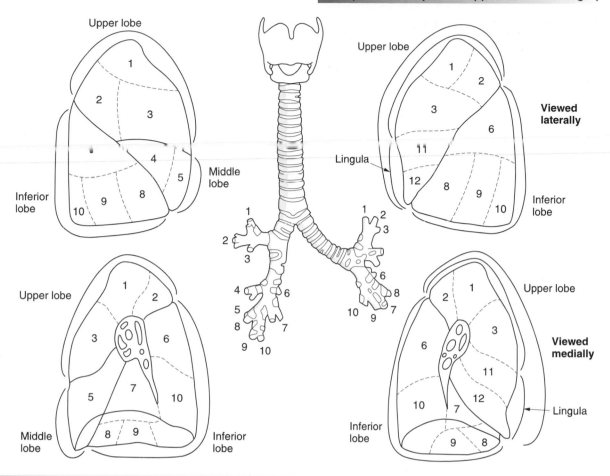

Figure 16.2 Anatomy of the lungs. Bronchopulmonary segments: 1 = apical, 2 = posterior, 3 = anterior, 4 = lateral, 5 = medial, 6 = apical basal, 7 = medial basal, 8 = anterior basal, 9 = lateral basal, 10 = posterior basal, 11 = superior, 12 = inferior. (Reproduced from Palastanga et al. 2002, with permission.)

THORACIC SURGERY

Indications for Surgery

Tumour

The most common reason for pulmonary and oeso-phageal resection is a malignant tumour (carcinoma). A small percentage of tumours can be benign.

> ### Lung and oesophageal cancer
> Lung cancer is the most common form of cancer in the UK. In 1998 there were 38,840 new cases of lung cancer diagnosed in the UK. This represents around 500 cases per million population. The male to female ratio is 7:4 (Cancer Research UK).
>
> Oesophageal cancer is the ninth most common form of cancer in the UK. There are approximately 7000 new cases of oesophageal cancer diagnosed in the UK every year. The male to female ratio is 4:3.

There are two histological types of lung cancer (World Health Organization):

- *non-small-cell*:
  squamous-cell type: 45–60%
  adenocarcinoma: 11–28%
  large-cell type: fewer than 1%
- *small-cell*: 35%.

Non-small-cell tumours are treated by resection if possible, if the tumour can be safely removed with clear margins and if metastatic disease is not in evidence. Small-cell cancer is virtually always widespread at diagnosis so surgery is usually not an option.

Malignant tumours of the oesophagus are generally adenocarcinoma, especially in the lower end. They may have arisen in the cardia of the stomach and spread proximally. In the middle and upper oesophagus squamous carcinomas predominate.

Benign tumours of the oesophagus and lungs are rare.

Pneumothorax

This is a collection of air in the pleural cavity. It usually occurs spontaneously and is due to rupture of the visceral pleura of an otherwise healthy lung. This is more common in men than women and more usual in the under-40s.

Patients with chronic obstructive pulmonary disease (COPD) can rupture a bulla resulting in a pneumothorax. Other much rarer causes include tumour, abscess and tuberculosis (TB). Traumatic pneumothoraces can occur with blunt trauma to the chest wall, such as following a car accident or heavy fall, or from a penetrating chest wound i.e. stabbing or gunshot. Iatrogenic (medical in origin) pneumothoraces can occur following intravenous line insertion, pacemaker insertion or in ventilated patients on high levels of PEEP (positive end expiratory pressure).

Empyema

Empyema is a collection of pus in the pleural cavity. The cause is commonly pneumonia, lung carcinoma or abscess, bronchiectasis or more rarely tuberculosis. It can occur in patients with septicaemia or osteomyelitis of the spine or ribs. Most empyemas are located basally but they can occur between two lobes.

Bronchiectasis

Bronchiectasis is a chronic lung condition in which abnormal dilatation of the bronchi occurs associated with obstruction and infection. Patients present with excessive production of purulent secretions, which become chronically infected. Bronchiectasis is generally managed medically with a physiotherapy regime and antibiotics. In some severe cases where the condition is localised to one area of the lung, lobectomy can offer some relief of symptoms.

Oesophageal perforation

Trauma and perforation to the oesophagus may result from the accidental swallowing of a foreign body (such as a dental plate). The oesophagus can rupture in cases of severe vomiting especially if the patient tries to suppress the vomiting action. Iatrogenic perforation can occur following oesophagoscopy or surgery associated with the pharynx.

Preoperative Investigations

Patients are assessed preoperatively in order to establish the nature of the lesion, and whether they are fit for operation. The following investigations are commonly done.

Chest X-ray

A standard chest X-ray will be done on all patients to establish preoperative lung status.

CT scan

In patients with cancer a CT scan is done universally. The scan will locate the lesion accurately and show if there is invasion into surrounding structures, which determines operability. The presence of metastases in distant organs is a contraindication to surgery.

Bronchoscopy/oesophagoscopy

This will establish the site of the lesion and allow biopsy or bronchial washings to be sent for histology. It can be carried out under sedation or general anaesthetic.

Pulmonary function tests (PTFs)

Respiratory function tests will help the surgeon decide whether the patient can withstand lung resection. It will also provide the anaesthetist with valuable information to assess suitability for general anaesthesia.

Arterial blood gases (ABGs)

Blood gases may be analysed routinely at some hospitals or on high-risk patients such as those with a pre-existing lung condition.

Types of Thoracic Incision

Posterolateral thoracotomy

This incision is most commonly used for operations on the lung. It is a curved incision, which starts at the level of the third thoracic vertebra and follows the vertebral border of the scapula and the line of the rib extending forward to the anterior angle or costal margin. An incision through the bed of the fifth or sixth rib is used for pneumonectomy or lobectomy.

The muscles cut are trapezius, latissimus dorsi, rhomboids, serratus anterior and the corresponding intercostal. A small piece of rib, approximately 1 cm, may be removed to allow easier retraction and avoid a painful fracture.

Anterolateral thoracotomy

This incision is used primarily for cardiac surgery but can be used to perform pleurectomy.

The incision starts at the level of the fifth costal cartilage. At the sternal edge it follows the rib line below the breast to the posterior axillary line. The muscles cut are pectoralis major and minor, serratus anterior, and the corresponding intercostal (Figure 16.4).

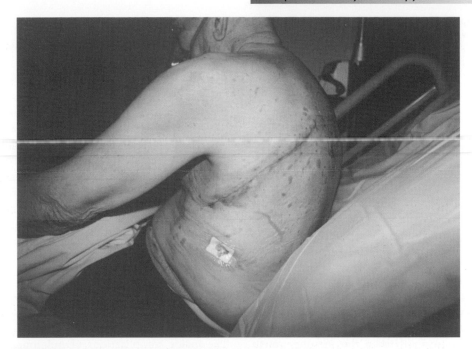

Figure 16.3   The incision for a posterolateral thoracotomy.

Median sternotomy

This incision is used for lung volume reduction surgery and bilateral pleurectomy. It is a vertical incision that involves splitting the sternum.

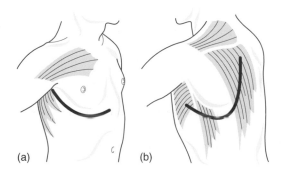

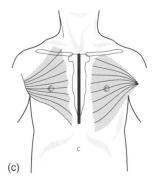

Figure 16.4   Sternotomy. Common incisions. (a) Anterolateral thoracotomy; (b) posterolateral thoracotomy; (c) median sternotomy.

The incision extends from just above the suprasternal notch to a point about 3 cm below the xiphisternum. No muscle is cut except the aponeuroses of pectoralis major (see Figure 16.4c).

Left thoraco-laparotomy

This incision is used for surgery on the lower oesophagus and stomach. The thoracotomy incision follows the curve of the seventh rib and extends anteriorly over the costal margin towards the umbilicus. The muscles involved are lattisimus dorsi, serratus anterior, the corresponding intercostal and the abdominal muscles.

Video-assisted thoracoscopic incisions

This relatively new technique aims to carry out conventional thoracic operations through several very small (1–2 cm) incisions, as opposed to a posterolateral thoracotomy. Instead of the surgeon seeing inside the patient directly, an endoscope with video camera attachment is introduced into the chest through one of the small incisions – the surgeon sees the image produced on television monitors in theatre. Specialised instruments are inserted via the other incisions so the operation can be completed. Advantages are reduced pain and less impact on respiratory mechanics in the postoperative period, and much smaller scars.

If an oesophageal tumour is involving the middle third of the oesophagus, surgical access may be easier through a right thoracotomy and a separate abdominal incision. If the tumour is in the upper third, then a cervical incision will also be required.

OPERATIONS ON THE LUNG

Figure 16.5 shows resection margins in lung surgery.

Pneumonectomy

Extrapericardial pneumonectomy is carried out for tumours involving a main bronchus. The whole lung is removed and the resulting cavity will fill with protein-rich fluid and fibrin over a period of weeks.

Lateral shift of the mediastinum, upward shift of the diaphragm, and reduction of the intercostal spacing on the operated side reduce the size of the cavity.

Intrapericardial pneumonectomy is a more radical procedure involving the removal of part of the pericardium. This is required when the tumour growth involves the pericardium.

Lobectomy

This means removal of a complete lobe with its lobar bronchus. On the right side, two lobes can be removed together – the upper and middle or middle and lower. Removal of the upper lobe on the right can sometimes include a section of right main bronchus – known as a 'sleeve resection'.

Segmental resection

A segment of a lobe along with its segmental artery and bronchus are removed.

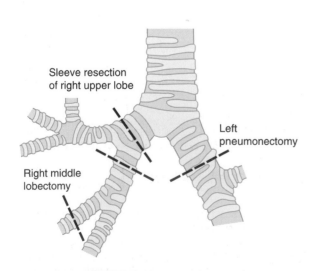

Sleeve resection of right upper lobe

Left pneumonectomy

Right middle lobectomy

Figure 16.5   Resection margins in lung surgery.

Wedge resection

This is a small local resection of lung tissue.

Lung volume-reduction surgery (LVRS)

LVRS is a procedure designed to improve respiratory function in patients with severe bullous emphysema. These patients present with hyperinflated lungs and a flattened diaphragm. By excising the bullous tissue and shaping the remaining lung, expansion of the healthy lung and doming of the diaphragm can be achieved. This will result in improved respiratory mechanics and symptomatic relief of dyspnoea (breathlessness). Patients should undergo a period of pulmonary rehabilitation preoperatively to maximise their respiratory function.

Complications of Pulmonary Surgery

The major complications of pulmonary surgery are listed in Table 16.1.

OPERATIONS ON THE PLEURA

Pleurectomy

Recurrent pneumothoraces will require surgical treatment. In young patients this is usually on the second or third occasion. In a small number of patients, bilateral pleurectomy will be required. In the older patient presenting with pneumothorax as a complication of COPD, surgery may be required on the first occasion.

The procedure involves removing the parietal layer of pleura from the chest wall in the area adjacent to the lung injury. This leaves a raw area to which the lung becomes adherent and thus unable to 'collapse' again. At the same time any bullous lung tissue can be either ligated or excised.

Decortication

Decortication is carried out following chronic empyema. The procedure involves the removal of the thickened, fibrous layer of visceral pleura from the surface of the lung. This allows the lung to re-expand into the space previously occupied by the empyema.

OPERATIONS ON THE OESOPHAGUS

Oesophageal resection

Tumours in the lower third of the oesophagus are resected via a left thoracolaparotomy. The upper third of the stomach is removed and the oesophagus from

Table 16.1 Complications of pulmonary surgery.

Respiratory
- Sputum retention +/– infection
- Atelectasis/lobar collapse
- Persistent air leak/pneumothorax
- Bronchopleural fistula (breakdown of the bronchus from which the lung tissue has been resected, more likely to occur following pneumonectomy and generally occurs about 8–10 days after surgery)
- Pleural effusion
- Surgical emphysema
- Respiratory failure

Circulatory
- Haemorrhage
- Cardiac arrhythmia: atrial fibrillation will occur in approximately 30% of lung resection patients
- Deep vein thrombosis
- Pulmonary embolus
- Myocardial infarction

Wound
- Infection
- Chronic wound pain
- Failure to heal

Neurological
- Stroke
- Recurrent laryngeal nerve (RLN) damage (the RLN supplies the vocal chords and trauma during surgery will impair the patients' ability to cough)
- Phrenic nerve damage, resulting in paralysis of the hemi-diaphragm

Loss of joint range
- Loss of shoulder range on operated side
- Postural changes

about 10 cm above the tumour margins. The remaining stomach is passed through the hiatus of the diaphragm into the posterior pleural cavity and a circular anastamosis created between the distal oesophagus and tip of the gastric tube.

Tumours in the middle third are more easily dealt with via a right thoracotomy and separate laparotomy. This is known as an Ivor–Lewis procedure. The stomach is passed into the right pleural cavity and the anastamosis constructed above the level of the aortic arch.

Tumours of the upper third will require resection of virtually all the oesophagus and the anastamosis will be made via an incision in the neck. The stomach is placed as with the previous procedures.

Repair of oesophageal perforations

Oesophageal perforations are treated surgically by direct repair. The site of the perforation will decide the nature of the operation. Some perforations can be treated conservatively and allow natural healing of the perforation without operative intervention.

Complications of Oesophageal Surgery

All the complications of pulmonary surgery apply to oesophageal operations. In addition there may be chylothorax, a pleural effusion resulting from the severing of the thoracic chyle duct. The effusion when drained will appear milky and on testing contain fat-staining globules. Occasionally surgical repair will be required but usually an intercostal drain (see below) will suffice until the leak stops.

There may also be anastamosis breakdown, usually due to variable degree of gastric tubes necrosis.

INTERCOSTAL DRAINS

Key point

When thoracotomy has been performed and the pleura opened, it is necessary to insert chest drains. These will commonly be referred to as intercostal drains.

Most patients will require two intercostal drains, one sited in the apex of the pleural cavity to drain air and allow the lung to re-expand, and a second drain in the basal area to drain postoperative bleeding. Patients undergoing pneumonectomy need only a single drain.

The drainage tubes are introduced through stab incisions, in an intercostal space below the level of the thoracotomy and positioned within the chest before closure. They are secured with a purse-string suture which will allow a tight seal to be achieved whilst the drain is in situ and on its removal. The apical drain is generally sited anteriorly and the basal posteriorly, It is always wise to check this in the operation notes.

The drainage tube passes from inside the pleural cavity down to a bottle containing sterile water, and attaches to a tube that continues to below the level of the water (Figure 16.6). Above water level is a second tube that is open to the atmosphere. This maintains atmospheric pressure within the bottle. This is known as 'an underwater sealed drain' and provides a simple one-way valve allowing air and blood to drain from the pleural cavity. Suction can be applied to the short tube to reduce the pressure in the bottle to below atmospheric and therefore encourage the evacuation of air and blood.

On free drainage the fluid level in the tubing will rise and fall. On inspiration the negative pressure in the thorax pulls water up the tube and on expiration there is less negative pressure in the thorax and the water level falls. If the level ceases to swing then the lung is either fully expanded or the drain is blocked. There will be no swing if the drain is connected to suction.

Drainage bottles must be kept below the level of insertion to prevent the siphoning of fluid back into the pleural cavity (Figure 16.7).

Amount and type of drainage

The amount of drainage is measured on a calibrated scale on the side of the bottle. Initially this will be

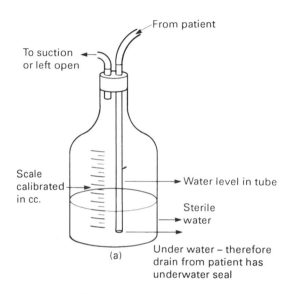

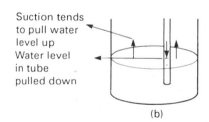

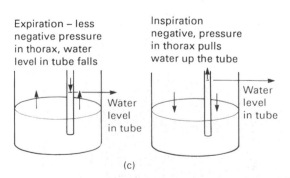

Figure 16.6 Effects of suction on water level: (a) the drainage bottle; (b) the effect of suction on water level; (c) the effect of the patient's breathing.

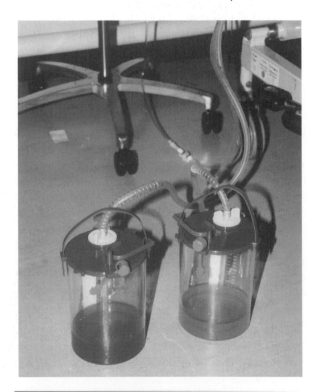

Figure 16.7 Underwater seal drainage in use.

bloodstained but progress to serous fluid and then stop. Air drainage can be seen as bubbles in the water, especially after coughing. Persistent air leaks are the result of a hole in the lung tissue or at the resection site. Bubbling may continue for many days and an apical drain cannot be removed until this stops. The basal drain will be taken out 24–48 hours postoperatively, the apical drain after 48–72 hours unless there is continued drainage.

PAIN CONTROL IN THORACIC SURGERY

> For all the happiness man can gain is not in pleasure but rest from pain.
> John Dryden (1631–1700)

Postoperative pain relief is not solely for the relief of an unpleasant sensation. Disturbances of pulmonary function are common after any form of intrathoracic operation. A decrease in functional residual capacity (FRC) with minimal change in closing volume leads to atelectasis (Sabanathan et al. 1990). Patients also experience an inability to cough effectively, thus becoming prone to sputum retention leading to infection and arterial hypoxaemia (Ali et al. 1974). Pain from the incision site and drains can be severe for up to three days (Kaplan et al. 1975) and abnormal patterns of breathing due to pain will only worsen these problems.

Good postoperative pain control is essential in order to carry out effective physiotherapy. This can be delivered in several ways; epidural anaesthesia, paravertebral block, patient-controlled analgesia (PCA), transcutaneous nerve stimulation (TENS) and oral analgesia are the most commonly used.

Epidural anaesthesia (Figure 16.8)

An epidural provides delivery of a local anaesthetic agent such as bupivicaine, and an opiate such as fentanyl, directly into the small space just outside the dura mater – the 'epidural space'. The local agent will provide dermatomal relief over the incision site and the opiate a more central effect.

Epidurals can provide profound analgesia in considerably smaller doses of opiate drug than if used systemically (Chaney 1995). This will minimise the

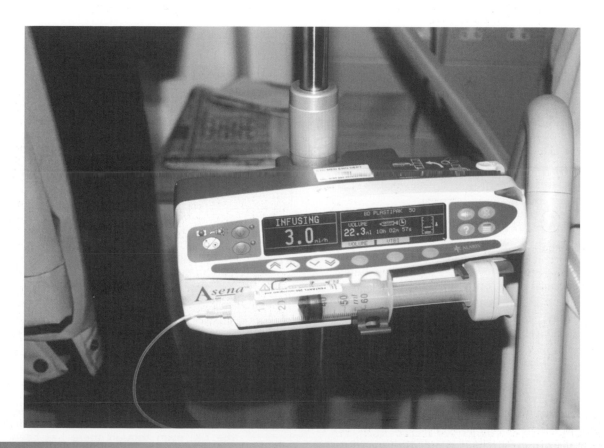

Figure 16.8   An epidural used to provide pain relief after surgery.

unwanted side-effect of respiratory depression commonly seen in opiate use. Lui et al. (1995) demonstrated improved analgesia with physiotherapy in thoracotomy patients using bupivicaine epidurals. An epidural will be inserted by an anaesthetist before the operation begins.

Paravertebral block

If it is not possible to insert an epidural, continuous delivery of a local anaesthetic agent can be achieved using a paravertebral catheter positioned in the paravertebral groove. This can provide safe and effective pain relief after thoracotomy (Inderbitzi et al. 1992). The catheter will be sited by the surgeon prior to closure of the chest.

Patient-controlled analgesia (PCA)

Patient-controlled analgesia allows the administration of small doses of intravenous opioids on demand by the patient. The patient must be awake, co-operative and have had adequate instruction preoperatively on how to use the system. The dose delivered is dependent upon patient weight. A 'lock-out' interval is set to allow time for the opiate to work, and this will also prevent overdosing.

Transcutaneous nerve stimulation

TENS can be useful if it is initiated postoperatively to relieve referred shoulder pain. The phrenic nerve supplies the diaphragm and if irritated during operation patients can experience ipsilateral referred shoulder pain (Scawn et al. 2001). TENS can also be of benefit in patients with persistent wound pain when an epidural or paravertebral has been removed.

Oral analgesia

Epidurals, paravertebrals and PCAs will continue, on average, for 72 hours, but analgesia will still be required for many days. The pain experience is individual and oral analgesia required will vary from patient to patient. Simple analgesia such as paracetamol or ibuprofen may be adequate, but some patients require stronger medication such as dihydrocodeine or diclofenac. Oral medication can be prescribed on regular or an 'as required' (p.r.n.) basis.

Most hospitals will have a specialist nurse for pain control. The nurse will be very helpful in the care of patients with severe pain that is difficult to control on standard analgesia.

THE PHYSIOTHERAPIST AND THORACIC SURGERY

Key point

Chest physiotherapy has a place in the prevention as well as the treatment of postoperative pulmonary complications.

Preoperative Care

The provision of preoperative chest physiotherapy is not routine, but it has been shown to be of benefit in high-risk patients. For example, Nagasaki et al. (1982) demonstrated that preoperative physiotherapy for elderly patients and those with COPD reduced postoperative pulmonary morbidity.

Patients with pre-existing COPD are prone to increased bronchial secretions (Massard and Wihlm 1998) and may require chest clearance prior to surgery. Physiotherapy may be requested by the patient's medical team following bronchoscopic findings (i.e. sputum retention).

The preoperative care may vary from simple education in postoperative techniques to more intensive chest clearance.

Key point

Communication is of great importance in the successful treatment of thoracic patients. The physiotherapist must communicate with nursing and medical staff in order to monitor the patient's progress. Medical notes and chest X-rays should be monitored on a daily basis. Effective communication skills will result in improved patient compliance and make treatment more effective.

Postoperative Care

Postoperative complications commonly present as a restrictive pattern with reduced inspiratory capacity, reduced vital capacity (VC) and reduced functional residual capacity (FRC) (Craig 1981). There are changes in defence mechanisms due to anaesthesia and reduced cough effort (Scuderi and Olsen 1989) that can lead to retention of secretions.

Key point

The provision of chest physiotherapy after thoracic surgery is fairly routine in the UK, even though there has been little research specifically on the subject.

Postoperative physiotherapy aims to minimise the risk of non-infectious and infectious pulmonary complications (Scuderi and Olsen 1989), the most common being atelectasis and pneumonia. Other common problems are loss of joint range in the shoulder on the incision side and reduced mobility. So the main aims of physiotherapy are:

- patient education
- maximisation of lung volume
- prevention of sputum retention
- sputum clearance
- maintenance of shoulder range of movement
- early mobilisation.

Patient Assessment

The initial assessment of the patient leads to identification of specific problems. Without an accurate assessment an appropriate treatment plan cannot be initiated (Pryor et al. 1998). Re-assessment is then an ongoing process to judge the effectiveness of treatment, to identify new problems and to modify a treatment plan. Table 16.2 lists what the initial patient assessment should include.

Following assessment, the problems identified will commonly include:

- reduced lung volume
- retention of secretions
- increased work of breathing
- poor breathing control/pattern
- ineffective cough
- pain.

MODALITIES OF PHYSIOTHERAPY

From the initial assessment and problem identification a treatment plan can be formulated.

Key point

A particular treatment modality can be used to address more than one problem. For example, the active cycle of breathing technique (ACBT – see below) will be effective in treating reduced lung volume and sputum retention.

The amount of chest physiotherapy required will vary from patient to patient. The patient's individual requirements will primarily dictate how often and for how long treatment is needed. Consultant preference

Table 16.2 The intial patient assessment notes.

Database: obtained from medical notes

- Preoperative information: PFTs/ABGs (pulmonary function tests and arterial blood gases respectively)
- Surgical procedure and incision
- Concise relevant history of present condition
- Relevant past medical history including previous surgery
- Social history
- Drug history, specific note of respiratory medicines; e.g. inhalers

Subjective: information the patient tells you

- Ask open-ended questions: how do you feel?
- Ask about pain control: can the person cough?

Objective: information based on examination of the patient and tests carried out

- Cardiovascular status (CVS): blood pressure, heart rate and rhythm
- Oxygen delivery system and FIV1
- Blood gases or O2 saturation
- Respiratory rate
- CXR
- Method of pain control
- Number and type of drains
- Auscultation
- Ability to cough
- Range of movement of shoulder on incision side

and hospital protocols may also influence this (Stiller et al. 1992).

Breathing Exercises

The active cycle of breathing technique (ACBT) used in sitting may be sufficient to maintain effective airway clearance (Webber and Pryor 1998). ACBT consists of cycles of breathing control and thoracic expansion exercises followed by the forced expiratory technique (FET) – see Figure 16.9. The thoracic expansion exercises can be combined with inspiratory hold and vibrations. In patients with reduced breath sounds, atelectasis and/or sputum retention positioning in conjunction with ACBT may be indicated.

The whole cycle should be repeated 2–3 times or until the patient becomes non-productive. In early postoperative patients, fatigue may be an issue and treatment should be terminated at this point.

The thoracic expansions should be slow deep breaths in through the nose and sigh out through the mouth. The end-inspiratory hold can improve air flow to poorly ventilated regions (Hough 2001); the breath hold should be encouraged at the height of the inspiratory effort for 2–3 seconds.

Patients should be encouraged to carry out at least two full cycles every waking hour in order to maintain improvements gained in lung function.

Forced Expiration

The forced expiratory technique (FET) is used to help in the clearance of excess bronchial secretions.

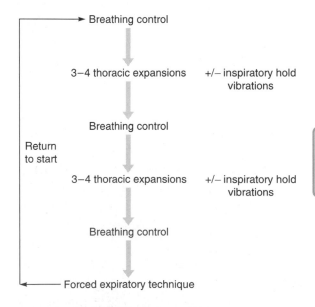

Figure 16.9   The active cycle of breathing technique (ACBT). (Adapted from Pryor and Webber et al. 1998.)

The forced expiratory technique
The technique was defined by Webber and Pryor in 1979. FET is one or two forced expirations from mid-lung to low-lung volumes (Partridge et al. 1989).

An effective FET should sound like a forced sigh. It is dependent on:

- mouth open
- glottis open
- abdominal wall contracted
- chest wall contracted.

Crackles may be heard if secretions are present.

FET performed to low lung volumes will aid removal of secretions peripherally situated. High lung volumes will clear secretions from proximal airways (Webber and Pryor 1998).

Supported Cough

A cough is created by forced expiration against a closed glottis. This causes a rise in intrathoracic pressure. As the glottis opens there is rapid, outward airflow and shearing of secretions from the airway walls.

Improved coughing and FET can be achieved if the wound is supported (Figure 16.10). This can be done by the physiotherapist during treatment sessions or by the patient. The arm on the unoperated side is placed across the front of the thorax and over the incision and drain sites. Firm overpressure is applied during coughing/FET. A towel, folded lengthways, passed around the back of the patient and pulled across the front of the thorax can also be useful to support coughing.

Positioning

Key point
The major function of positioning postoperatively is to improve FRC. A good sitting position either in or out of bed, as opposed to slumped in the bed, can achieve this (Jenkins et al. 1988).

There are recognised positions for segmental drainage (Thoracic Society 1950) and these may be utilised if there is a segmental or lobar-specific problem. It is much more likely, however, that modified positions only will be required, especially in view of the changed anatomy of the area.

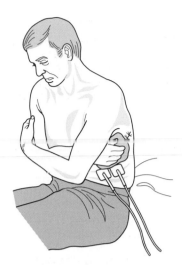

Figure 16.10   Coughing: patient supporting wound.

Positioning can also be used to improve gas exchange. Improvement in oxygenation can be achieved in side-lying with the affected lung uppermost; the ventilation/perfusion match is improved, resulting in increased oxygen uptake (Winslow et al. 1990).

Pneumonectomy patients should *not* be positioned on their unoperated side. This can result in bronchopleural fistula due to space fluid washing over the bronchial stump. Patients undergoing intrapericardial pneumonectomy should be treated in sitting for the first 4 days unless advised otherwise by the medical team.

Early Mobilisation

Mobilisation should commence as soon as is safely possible as functional residual capacity is maximally improved in standing (Jenkins et al. 1988). Dull et al (1983) proposed that early mobilisation in uncomplicated patients could render breathing exercises unnecessary. Patients must be cardiovascularly stable and not requiring high concentrations of oxygen before mobilisation can begin. If intercostal drains are on suction, mobility will be restricted to standing and spot-marching at the bedside. Some anaesthetic departments restrict mobility when an epidural is *in situ*, owing to the risk of profound hypotension on mobilising. Hospital protocols should be noted.

Shoulder Exercises

The shoulder on the operated side should be checked for range of movement. The patient should practice elevation and abduction of the shoulder at least three

times a day. Auto-assisted exercises may be necessary to begin with. Any limitation of range should be more formally assessed and treated.

Adjuncts to Physiotherapy

Physiotherapy is a 'hands on' practice. There are several adjuncts that can be used to augment the basic breathing exercise regimen.

Incentive spirometer

Incentive spirometry is a feedback system to encourage patients to take a deep breath and produce a sustained maximal inspiration in order to open atelectatic areas of lung (Su et al. 1991). It is cheap to provide, non-invasive and when taught well needs minimal supervision.

Bastin et al. (1997) deduced that deterioration in incentive spirometer performance could be used as a warning of pulmonary deterioration.

Mini-tracheostomy

Sputum retention is a frequent complication in patients recovering from thoracic surgery (Busch et al. 1994). It

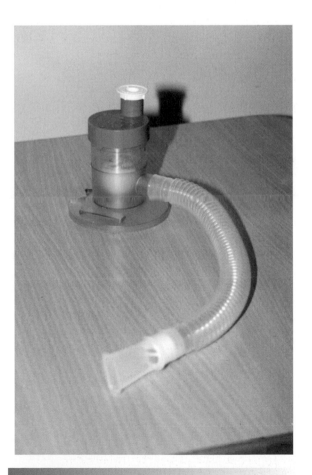

Figure 16.11   The incentive spirometer.

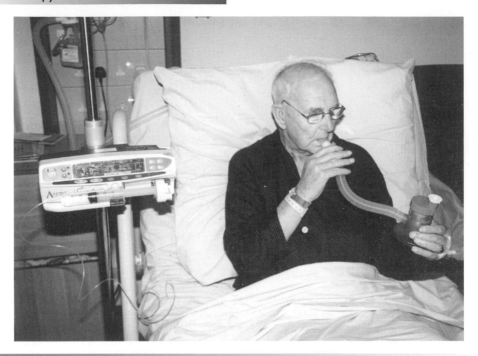

Figure 16.12   The incentive spirometer in use.

can be a result of sputum tenacity or a weak ineffective cough. Mini-tracheostomy can be an invaluable tool in the postoperative patient to aid removal of secretions in conjunction with a physiotherapy regimen.

Quidaciolu et al. (1994) concluded that mini-tracheostomy was safe and effective in reducing respiratory morbidity in high-risk patients following pulmonary surgery.

Heated humidification

Pulmonary secretions can become tenacious following surgery. This may be due to anaesthesia, infection, or dehydration – especially in the oesophageal patients who are 'nil by mouth'. Improving humidification to the airways by heating the oxygen/air delivery can help in mucous clearance.

Continuous positive airways pressure (CPAP)

Patients with poor arterial blood gases and reduced lung volume can be supported by the use of CPAP. It can be used continuously or intermittently. When used continuously it must be humidified.

CPAP is effective in improving FRC and arterial oxygen in patients with acute respiratory failure. It can also reduce the work of breathing (Keilty et al. 1992). Care must be taken in thoracic patients because of the anastamosis, and medical opinion should be sought.

Intermittent positive pressure breathing (IPPB)

There is little literature to support the use of IPPB, but with good teaching and in the right patient it can be effective. It is of particular use in patients who have loss of lung volume and are tiring. It works to improve lung volume and reduces the work of breathing.

Extreme care must be used when considering IPPB on lung resection patients as the anastamosis may be vulnerable to positive pressure. The physiotherapist should discuss the use of IPPB with the patient's medical team.

DISCHARGE

Patients will reach discharge from treatment at varying points in their recovery. A low-risk patient with no postoperative complications may only need 3–4 days of physiotherapy. High-risk patients and those experiencing pulmonary complications will need considerably more. FRC and VC can be regained even in lung resection patients. The time for full recovery of FRC is about 2 weeks and for vital capacity it can be in excess of 3 weeks (Craig 1981). Once discharged the patient should be advised to continue with regular breathing exercises and gradually increase their mobility.

Acknowledgements

The author and editor would like to thank Mr Richard Page (consultant thoracic surgeon), Mary Kilcoyne (physiotherapist) and all physiotherapy staff at The Cardiothoracic Centre, Liverpool and Jo Sharp (lecturer) at the University of Liverpool.

FURTHER READING

Hough A 2001 Physiotherapy in Respiratory Care, 3rd edn. London: Nelson Thornes

Pryor A, Webber J, Barbara A et al. 1998 Physiotherapy for Respiratory and Cardiac Problems. Edinburgh: Churchill Livingstone

REFERENCES

Ali J, Weisel RD, Layug AB, Kripke BJ, Hechtman HB 1974 Consequences of postoperative alterations in respiratory mechanics. Am J Surg 128: 376–82

Bastin R, Moraine J-J, Bardocsky G, Kalm R-J, Melot C 1997 Incentive spirometry performance: a reliable indicator of pulmonary function in the early postoperative period after lobectomy? Chest 111: 559–63

Busch E, Verazin G, Antkowiak VG, Driscoll D, Takita H 1994 Pulmonary complications in patients undergoing thoracotomy for lung carcinoma. Chest 105: 760–6

Chaney MA 1995 Side-effects of intrathecal and epidural opiods. Can J Aanaesth 42: 891–903

Craig D 1981 Postoperative recovery of pulmonary function. Anaesth Analg 60(1): 46–52

Dull JL, Dull WL 1983 Are maximal inspiratory breathing exercises or incentive spirometry better than early mobilisation after cardio pulmonary bypass? Phys Ther 63: 655–9

Hough A 2001 Physiotherapy in Respiratory Care, 3rd edn. London: Nelson Thornes

Inderbitzi R, Fleveckiger K, Ris HB 1992 Pain relief and respiratory mechanics during continuous intrapleural bupivicaine administration after thoracotomy. Thorac Cardiovasc Surg 40(2): 87–9

Jacob S 2001 Atlas of Human Anatomy, Edinburgh: Churchill Livingstone

Jenkins SC, Soutar SA, Moxham J 1988 The effects of posture on lung volumes in normal subjects and in pre- and post-coronary artery surgery. Physiotherapy 74: 492–6

Kaplan JA, Miller ED, Gallagher EG 1975 Postoperative analgesia for thoracotomy patients. Anaesth Analg 54: 773

Keilty SE, Bott J 1992 Continuous positive airways pressure. Physiotherapy 78(2): 90–2

Lui S, Angel JM, Owens BD, Carpenter RL, Isabel L 1995 Effects of epidural bupivicaine after thoracotomy. Reg Anaesth 20: 303–10

Massard G, Wihlm JM 1998 Postoperative atalectasis. Chest Surg Clin N Am 8: 281–90

Nagasaki F, Flehinger BJ, Martini N 1982 Complications of surgery in the treatment of carcinoma of the lung. Chest 82(1): 25–9

Palastanga M, Field D, Soames R 2002 Anatomy and Human Movement, 4th edn. Butterworth–Heinemann: Oxford

Partridge C, Pryor J, Webber B 1989 Characteristics of the forced expiratory technique. Physiotherapy 75(3): 193–4

Pryor A, Webber J et al. 1998 Physiotherapy for Respiratory and Cardiac Problems. Edinburgh: Churchill Livingstone

Quidaciolu F, Gausone F, Pastorino G et al. 1994 Use of mini-tracheostomy in high risk pulmonary resection surgery: results of a comparative study. Minerva Chir 49: 315–18

Sabanathan S, Eng J, Mearns AJ 1990 Alterations in respiratory mechanics following thoracotomy. J R Coll Surg Edinb 35(3): 144–50

Scawn ND, Pennefather SH, Soorae A, Wang JY, Russell GN 2001 Ipsilateral shoulder pain after thoracotomy with epidural and the influence of phrenic nerve infiltration with lidocaine. Anesth Analg 93: 260–4

Scuderi J, Olsen GN 1989 Respiratory therapy in the management of post operative complications. Respiratory Care 34: 281–90

Stiller KR, Munday RM 1992 Chest Physiotherapy for the surgical patient. Br J Surg 79: 745–9

Su M, Chiang CD, Huang WL et al. 1991 A new device of incentive spirometry. Zhonghua Yi Xue Za Zhi (Taibei) 48(4): 274–7

Thoracic Society 1950 The nomenclature of broncho-pulmonary anatomy. Thorax 5: 222–8

Winslow EH, Clark AP, White KM et al. 1990 Effects of a lateral turn on mixed venous oxygen saturation and heart rate. Heart Lung 19: 551–61

The Research Process

Lynne Goodacre

17

INTRODUCTION

The word 'research' causes fear and panic in some students. This should not be so, because we all undertake research every day. You probably undertook research when deciding which textbook to buy for your course. You had a question in mind: 'Which book is the most suitable to help my studies?' You then set about the research process and, by asking colleagues, looking on the Internet, speaking to your lecturers, or looking in the library you came to your conclusion.

Physiotherapy students are now usually required to undertake a research project or a critical evaluation of a research paper as part of their course of undergraduate study. This chapter discusses the research process, taking you through some of the parts of the research process that students often find confusing and hard to comprehend.

The research process comprises a sequence of steps that are designed to increase the sum of what is known about a certain phenomenon (Hockey 1996). A scan through academic journals will be testament to the different approaches taken to research. However, the steps encompassed within the research process apply to all research whether conducted by healthcare professionals within the clinical setting of a hospital, or by scientists undertaking research within a laboratory. The aim of this chapter is to introduce readers to this systematic process with a focus on the completion of a research project appropriate for an undergraduate dissertation.

The chapter starts by focusing on the development of a research question and moves on to explore the relationship between the question asked, the methodological approach taken, and the specific methods used to collect data. The chapter then addresses the issue of how all of the stages in planning a project are brought together within the context of a research proposal.

Note

It is not within the scope of a single chapter to provide in-depth information about specific methods of data collection and data analysis. However, an introduction is provided to some of the main methods used in undergraduate research projects. To enable readers to access more detailed information, a further reading list is provided at the end of the chapter. The appendices on pages 513–538 contain points on how to critically evaluate a research paper and a glossary on research terms.

It is likely that students approaching their dissertation will have preconceived ideas about what it means 'to do research' and the nature of quantitative and qualitative methods. For many these preconceptions may centre around notions of research being undertaken by academics within a university environment and the distinction between data that are expressed by numbers (quantitative) and data that are expressed by words (qualitative). You may also have opinions about which approach you wish to adopt in your own work, or perceive one methodological approach to be 'better' than another.

The approach taken in this chapter is to advocate that in undergraduate research it is important to develop an understanding of the relationship between the research question, the methodological approach and the methods used, and not to develop a blinkered approach about the perceived supremacy of one approach over another. Research skills, like any clinical skill, are learnt and developed over time. The focus of learning at undergraduate level should be to develop an understanding of the strengths and weaknesses of different approaches and the way in which different methods produce different kinds of data. There should be no such thing as the quantitative versus qualitative debate; the real issue should be 'How can I best answer the research question?'

An undergraduate dissertation provides an opportunity to develop an understanding of the research process and the main theories and methodological issues, the experience of conducting a small study and of using one or two methods of data collection. It provides a platform from which research skills can be developed and built upon in a clinical setting.

Key point

Research is not just a pursuit of academics within universities but should be viewed as a central component of clinical practice, whether related to the critical appraisal of evidence to inform clinical practice or the conduct of research to develop the evidence base of the work of physiotherapists.

DEVELOPING A RESEARCH QUESTION

Getting Started

The first issue confronting the majority of students is the decision regarding the area in which they wish to develop their research. This decision should be the result of careful consideration rather than last minute panic. For most new researchers the identification of a research area and the development of a research question is the result of a process that can take several weeks of refinement. It is therefore unwise to leave this decision until a day or two before a supervisory meeting in which you are expected to have your research question defined.

The area chosen should be one which is personally stimulating and hopefully exciting as this is a piece of work with which you will be living for a considerable amount of time and which will be demanding in terms of time, intellect and energy. The research process is rarely smooth and the chosen topic should be of enough interest and importance to sustain you through times when your work may not be going well and your enthusiasm might be waning. Many factors can influence the choice of an area of research (Figure 17.1).

> ### *Key point*
> Before undertaking a great deal of work on a proposal it is important to discuss potential areas of research with your supervisor to ensure that he or she feels the chosen area to be relevant and one in which a research project can be conducted and completed within the time and resources available.

Having identified a topic of research, the next stage is to develop a specific research question. Many students when asked about the research they are undertaking answer with a description of the area of research rather than the research question itself. To move from a research area to a research question there is a need to become more focused in your thinking to be able to answer specifically what it is that you are trying to address in your research.

To help define your research question it is helpful to undertake a broad review of the literature within your chosen topic. This means identifying, within current publications, the main research questions being addressed, different theoretical positions being adopted and the main arguments/positions being taken. Familiarising yourself with the literature in this way will also help you to identify key papers that are referenced or referred to consistently, the main methodological approaches being taken and the different methods being used. This type of literature search can often be done by hand-searching journals within the library and identifying key textbooks, if appropriate.

Whilst you are reading around your intended area of research it will be helpful to start drawing up a list of potential research questions. At this stage do not worry too much about the specificity of the questions but write down all the possible research questions you think of. When you feel you have developed a broad understanding of your chosen area you can then start to work on the development of your research question by returning to your list and starting to refine the general questions you have noted. It is often helpful to do this in conjunction with other students as the process of verbalising and explaining helps to clarify your thinking and focus more clearly on exactly what the aim of your work is. Over time the list of potential questions should be refined to identify what you feel may be two or three potential research questions. These can be used to inform discussion with your supervisor to identify a single research question that will become the focus of your investigation.

What Makes a Good Research Question?

Developing a research question is a process of becoming more and more focused on the specific issue you are trying to address. This means being very clear in your own mind about exactly what it is that you are trying to measure or understand. Most new researchers need help and guidance with this process, as some questions are not amenable to research. This is usually because the question posed relates to philosophical or ethical questions, which can be debated extensively but not answered. A good research question therefore is one that is clear, novel and *answerable*. This is achieved by developing an understanding of your research area and thinking very carefully about the exact focus of your project. Whilst there may be a temptation to ask a complex question, success at undergraduate level will be achieved by being very clear about a simple question.

As well as focusing on the question it is also important to think about the amount of time and the kind of resources that will be needed to complete the project. If, for example, you want to evaluate the impact of a

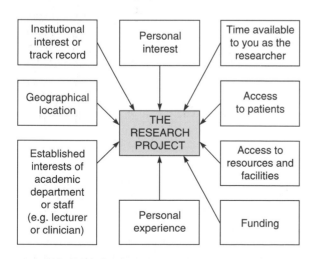

Figure 17.1   Factors that can influence the choice of area of research.

specific intervention but you do not have access to a clinical setting or participants, no matter how good your question is it is unlikely that you will be able to conduct the research. Trying to assess the amount of time taken to conduct a project is difficult if you have no previous research experience, but your supervisor will guide you on the feasibility of completing the project within the time available and the resources that you are able to access within your department.

THE METHODOLOGICAL APPROACH

Many students undertaking research for the first time want to move quickly on to learning about methods, to enable data collection to start. Within the context of research methods textbooks, the temptation is to skip over the first few chapters containing what at times can seem to be complex philosophical debates about the nature of truth and different ways of gaining knowledge. However, at undergraduate level it is important to demonstrate an understanding of these issues and to be able to explain how they have influenced your research – rather than getting too embroiled in heavy methodological and philosophical debates. It is important, therefore, to understand the different methodological approaches and the link between a research question, methodological approach and methods, in order to explain the rationale for the decisions you made in your research.

Methodology can be a difficult concept to understand as it is used to describe a philosophical position being taken by a researcher that guides their approach to research. Methodological approaches are often presented as being founded upon a person's beliefs about the nature of truth and ways of knowing and, in the past, this has led to researchers being described as either 'positivists' or 'naturalists'. Whilst some researchers always work within either a positivist or naturalist paradigm, others are more willing to adapt their approach depending on the specific question being addressed.

The Positivist Paradigm

A positivist paradigm is perhaps best understood by reflecting upon the kind of philosophical assumptions that underpin the scientific or experimental method. This kind of research is guided by the belief that knowledge can be gained by the measurement and quantification of a phenomena in a way that can be replicated by an independent observer. Within this paradigm, research questions are usually framed as hypotheses. It focuses on the discovery of a single 'truth', which is generalisable and is achieved by breaking a phenomenon

down into its constituent parts and understanding them and their relationships to each other. For this reason it is sometimes described as *reductionist* in approach. Central to this approach are the notions of objectivity and control which lead to researchers being seen as detached from the research process and their influence being eliminated as far as is possible.

The Naturalistic Paradigm

Within this paradigm the approach to research is based on the belief that human experience is affected by the interpretation placed on it by individuals, and influenced by such things as previous experience and personal beliefs. The focus of research is therefore on describing or understanding the meanings people attach to these experiences and how they make sense of the social world.

Key point
Owing to the emphasis on how human experience is interpreted, it should be possible to see that within naturalistic research the notion of a single truth that is generalisable to a whole population is not relevant. There may be a number of realities or truths.

The notion of objective value-free research is contested strongly. In contrast to conducting research in a controlled environment researchers emphasise the relevance of the wider social context, and research often takes place within this wider context rather than being removed from it. The notion of a detached researcher is also challenged. The researcher is seen as central to, not detached from, the research process; he or she seeks to become involved in the world of the participants, sometimes, in the case of observational studies, literally in order to gain as much insight as possible into the lived experiences of participants.

Given the different focus of positivist and naturalist methodologies it should seem logical that different methods are used within each paradigm to generate data. The term *method* is used to refer to data-genera-

Note
The next section will familiarise you with some of the techniques of data collection used frequently in undergraduate dissertations. More in-depth information about these and other methods can be found in the references provided at the end of the chapter.

tion techniques and procedures, the selection of data 'sources' and sampling (Mason 1996).

QUANTITATIVE RESEARCH

Hypothesis Testing

It is usual for the research question in an experimental design to be expressed in terms of a *hypothesis*. A hypothesis has been described as 'a predicted answer to a research question' (Punch 1998) in which the predicted effect of the factor (or intervention) to be tested is defined. The wording of a hypothesis may be a general statement of an effect using words like 'influence' (a two-tailed hypothesis), or it may be more specific and indicate the direction of the effect using words like 'increase' or 'decrease' (a one-tailed hypothesis).

An alternative way of expressing a hypothesis is as a *null hypothesis*. This acknowledges the important philosophical premise that it is never possible to obtain absolute proof that a biological factor or a clinical intervention is having a significant effect in a given experiment. A null hypothesis embodies the notion that, strictly speaking, the results of an experiment can be interpreted only in terms of the likelihood that an intervention has *no* effect on the outcome under study.

In this sense, for example, if the effect of a particular intervention were being tested in a clinical situation, the null hypothesis would state that there will be no difference between the test group and the control group. The analysis of the data would enable the likelihood of this to be calculated, thereby providing an expression of the level of certainty with which the null hypothesis could be rejected.

Key point
In clinical research, most hypotheses are structured as null hypotheses, and the statistical methods used for data analysis are designed to test null hypotheses.

Clinical Trials

Whilst different experimental designs exist, the focus of this section will be on the basic experimental design of a study comprising two groups, one of which (the *experimental* group) is exposed to the intervention being researched and the other (the *control* group) which is not. The experiment is based on comparisons between the groups achieved by the collection of data prior to the intervention taking place (*pre-test*), which provides baseline data, and after the intervention has taken place (*post-test*) which provides data on differences in effect between the groups. The effect of an intervention is determined by comparisons of the data between the pre-test and post-test data measurements and comparisons of data between the two groups.

Randomisation

Two concepts central to clinical trials are those of randomisation and control. *Randomisation* refers to the way in which participants are allocated to either the experimental or control group in order to create groups that are as similar as possible. This is necessary to ensure that the results of the experiment are attributable to the intervention rather than to some other variable such as age, disease duration or socio-economic status.

There are many different methods of randomisation. Two methods encountered commonly in health research are the use of computer-generated numbers and stratification.

Computer-generated numbers randomly allocate participants to either treatment or control group on the basis of, for example, all odd numbers being allocated to the treatment group and all even numbers to the control group.

In *stratification*, participants are divided into groups according to a baseline variable such as gender and then allocated from each group. A group stratified by gender would ensure that the experimental and control groups had equal numbers of men and women in them. This method is used to ensure that groups are equally balanced in relation to variables that have been identified as having a potential impact on the results – such as gender, disease duration or age. Such balance would not be achieved by using computer-generated numbers.

Controls

The concept of control has several applications. As has already been described it can refer to a group of participants who do not receive an intervention. But there are other factors that a researcher may seek to control – they are known as confounding variables as they have the potential to confound (confuse) the results. Here are some examples:

- *Variables relating to the therapist.* If the outcome measure used is assessment of joint range of movement and several therapists took measurements, there could be variability in the measurements arising from the different ways in which the therapists assess range of movement.
- *Variables relating to treatment method.* If a research question focuses on the impact of a treatment and

several different pieces of equipment can be used to produce measurements, it will be important to make sure that all the equipment is measuring with the same degree of accuracy and all departments taking part in the research are using the same equipment.

- *Variables relating to the environment.* If people recruited to a study are from different hospitals, one hospital might be in an area of social deprivation, have a higher proportion of people from different cultural groups, or the GPs might have different approaches to referring patients to the hospital.

The ability to create an environment in which all confounding variables can be controlled is very difficult in most clinical settings. It is important, however, for researchers to demonstrate that they have identified the potential confounding variables and taken steps to minimise their effects.

Measurements and data analysis

As the aim of an experiment is to explore the effect of an intervention, a method of measuring the effect is required. The method used to measure the effect will be influenced by the variable being measured but may include assessment of range of movement, physiological measures such as cardiovascular output and respiration, or standardised measures assessing symptoms such as pain or fatigue and measures used to assess psychological factors such as anxiety and depression.

Once the experiment has taken place and data have been collected, statistical tests are then conducted to describe and summarise the results and make inferences about them and the degree of confidence with which the results obtained from a sample can be generalised to a whole population.

Surveys

Surveys can be used to describe certain phenomena (*descriptive surveys*) within a population of interest, or to investigate causal associations between variables (*longitudinal surveys*) (Bowling 1997). The sample used for descriptive studies is called 'cross-sectional', meaning it describes a population at one point in time. Longitudinal surveys are used to analyse the phenomenon of interest at more than one point in time, so each participant will complete the survey on more than one occasion, sometimes over a period of years.

Key point
The time and resource constraints of most undergraduate projects dictate that the most likely survey method used will be descriptive.

Prospective Cohort Studies and Case–Control Studies

These are two further methods used within health research.

- A prospective cohort study is used to examine the likelihood of developing an impairment when people are exposed to a risk factor. A group of people will be followed over a period of time with measurements being taken at regular intervals.
- Case–control studies are used to look *back* over time at a group of people all of whom have been exposed to a risk factor but only some of whom have developed an impairment. Comparisons are made between the two groups.

Questionnaires

Key point
Questionnaires are a common method of data collection used by undergraduates in both experimental designs and surveys.

Before embarking upon the development of a new questionnaire it is sensible to check whether an existing questionnaire can be used. An immense amount of time is invested in the development of reliable and valid questionnaires and, once validated, they enable you to conduct a more sophisticated statistical analysis than a questionnaire you have developed yourself for the purpose of your study.

In choosing a questionnaire it is important to understand the concepts of reliability and validity.

- A *reliable* measure is one that is consistent. When used with the same group of people under the same conditions it should produce the same score. If different scores are obtained, that is an indication that the measure in not reliable.
- A *valid* measure is one that measures what it is supposed to measure.

A word of caution is necessary about the reliability and validity of questionnaires published in journal articles. Not all questionnaires described in research papers have been tested for reliability and validity. Some questionnaires will have been developed by the researchers for their own study without undertaking testing of the questionnaire. Just because someone has used it and published results from it does *not* mean it is reliable and valid. In choosing to use a measure that has been standardised you should be able to identify papers describing the development of the measure and the degree of reliability and validity obtained.

A frequent reason given for not using existing measures is that they do not address all of the issues of relevance. However, it is permissible to include additional questions either at the start or the end of a standardised questionnaire. It is important to understand, though, that you should not change the wording, ordering or formatting of an existing questionnaire or omit questions – if you do that you will be changing the established reliability and validity of the questionnaire. It is also important to realise that any questions added would need to be analysed separately.

The questions

Note

If you are unable to find a relevant questionnaire the following subsections introduce you to some basic principles of questionnaire design.

Use simple and unambiguous language and avoid technical language and jargon. Every question should have a purpose to ensure that the questionnaire remains focused on the research question. The two types of questions used in questionnaires are open and closed.

1 *Open questions* enable a respondent to provide his or her own answer. Whilst this is an advantage in finding out the person's experience of the phenomena being assessed, it is more demanding for the person completing the questionnaire. This should be borne in mind, especially if conducting a postal survey, where people are less likely to provide lengthy written explanations. However, if the questionnaire is being administered face to face this is less of a problem if the researcher is writing down the response.

2 *Closed questions* provide a predefined list of responses and ask the respondent to choose one, or in some instances, more than one answer (e.g. questions asking respondents to rank a number of choices). They impose a structure for the respondents who have to choose a response that best reflects their experiences.

The most common response options used in closed questions are:

- *dichotomous* – which enable a respondent to choose between two answers (e.g. yes/no)
- *multiple-choice* – which provide respondents with a number of options from which to select an answer

(e.g. a Likert scale asks people to rate agreement with a statement usually on a scale of 1 to 5).

Some questionnaires use a mixture of open and closed questionnaires (e.g. starting with a closed question and then asking the respondent to explain the answer).

Key point

Whichever form of questionnaire you choose, think carefully about the questions included and make sure that they are all focused on answering an aspect of your research question. It is usual to produce several drafts of a questionnaire before you think about piloting it.

Formatting your questionnaire

The appearance of the questionnaire is important, especially if it is being sent by post, as this is one of the factors that will influence a person's decision as to whether or not to complete it. If it is very long, full of spelling mistakes and muddled in appearance people will be deterred from filling it in! The tools available on modern word-processing packages permit attractive results to be obtained in relation to layout and print quality.

Whilst trying to keep the length of the questionnaire to a minimum, do not be tempted to compromise on the font size at the expense of excluding people who may have a visual impairment.

Once you feel you have produced a questionnaire that addresses the issues, seek the opinions of your supervisor and (if possible) other people who have knowledge of your research area.

Piloting your questionnaire

Piloting a questionnaire involves far more than asking a couple of people to complete the questionnaire and looking at the answers they have written. As with all stages in the research process, a structured approach should be taken which requires both forethought and preparation.

When piloting the questionnaire with members of the proposed study group it is usual to adopt a semi-structured interview approach to the discussion. It is important to explain what you are trying to achieve to ensure that participants feel free to provide constructive feedback.

The issues you are seeking to address at this stage of the study are:

- the clarity and understanding of the questions
- the clarity of instructions

- identification of questions that may be left consistently unanswered or for which respondents ask for advice before answering
- the respondents' views on the content of the questionnaire (e.g. whether anything has been omitted, views on the length and time taken to complete, whether enough response categories have been provided).

Feedback from these discussions should inform revisions of the questionnaire.

Methods of questionnaire administration

The three main methods of administering questionnaires are by post, face-to-face and over the phone. The method of administration will be influenced by issues such as the geographical area within which participants live, access to participants, your time and resources.

If, for example, you want to obtain data from a patient group who meet on a regular basis in an accessible location, it may be feasible to attend the group and administer the questionnaire face-to-face. If you are trying to elicit the views of a group of therapists on a specific issue and recruiting them via a national database, either a postal or phone-based method of administration will be more appropriate.

Preparing questionnaire data for analysis

The first step in analysing questionnaire data is the allocation of numeric values to answers or coding.

If closed questions are used it is possible to develop the coding framework whilst the questionnaire is being developed. Dichotomous questions may be coded with 1 being given to all 'yes' answers and 2 to all 'no' responses. In information questions all men may be coded as 1 and women as 2. In scale questions a 1–5 code may be needed where 1 = extremely satisfied, 2 = moderately satisfied etc.

Key point

It is usual to analyse statistical data using a software package such as Statistical Package for the Social Sciences (SPSS) or Minitab. The coded data are entered into such a package in preparation for analysis.

If open questions have been included a coding framework is needed for each of the themes. The approach to this will depend on whether data are being analysed within a quantitative or qualitative paradigm. This will involve firstly grouping together all of the answers for the same question and identifying the core themes contained within the answers. If a quantitative paradigm is being used categories are given numbers.

ANALYSING QUANTITATIVE DATA

Within the context of research, statistics have two main functions.

- *Descriptive statistics* are used to convey information about and interpret large sets of numbers in an efficient way (Clegg 1990).
- *Inferential statistics* are used to make inferences from the data you have collected and express the confidence with which we can generalise from a sample to a whole population (Howitt and Cramer 1997).

Explanations of specific statistical tests can be obtained from the further reading list provided at the end of the chapter.

Descriptive statistics

Commonly used examples of descriptive statistics relevant to undergraduate research are measures of central tendency, dispersion and frequencies.

Measures of central tendency include calculating the mean (adding together all the values and dividing by the number of values), the median (ordering all the numbers and identifying the number which falls in the middle), and the mode (identifying the number which is the most popular). They provide an indication of where the mid point of a set of numbers lies but do not tell you how wide the range of numbers is. For example if describing the age of a group of patients they will not tell you how old the youngest or oldest people are.

Measures of spread or dispersion describe over how many numbers the data are spread and how much variation there is in the scores. Two measures of dispersion encountered frequently are the range and standard deviation.

- The *range* describes the difference between the smallest and largest number and is calculated by subtracting the smallest number from the largest.
- The *standard deviation* describes the variability of the scores about the mean.

Frequencies are another way of summarising and describing data. Individual scores are tabulated to show how many participants have, for example, given a particular response to a question or fall within a specific category. Frequencies are often expressed in terms of percentages and, if used, should always be used in conjunction with the actual value to give people an idea of what, for example, 28% means in the context of your sample.

Distribution

Measures of central tendency and dispersion enable you to examine the distribution of data. Plotting all the scores on a graph will illustrate the kind of curve they produce. If data are *normally distributed* they will be symmetrical and form a bell-shaped curve. For normally distributed data, the mean, the mode and the median all have the same or similar values. Some scores, however, may not be evenly distributed and the scores may fall predominantly above or below the mean. When scores fall mainly below the mean they are described as *positively skewed* and when they fall mainly above they are known as *negatively skewed*.

The relevance of understanding the concept of the normal distribution is that many statistical methods can only be applied reliably to normally distributed data.

Inferential statistics

The aim of conducting an experiment, as discussed earlier, is to examine the relationship between two variables. If your data indicate that an intervention has had an effect and the statistical tests conducted indicate a difference, there are two questions you will probably like answered:

1 How likely is it that the results can be attributed to the intervention rather than that they happened by chance?
2 With what degree of confidence can I generalise the results I obtained from my sample to the population as a whole?

These two questions are addressed in terms of significance testing and confidence intervals.

Significance

Significance is expressed as a '*p*-value' and is the one thing that most people, however limited their statistical knowledge, will know to look for when reading a research paper.

Key point
The significance level indicates the probability of an effect happening by chance.

One of the things that can be confusing is that there is more than one *p*-value. The lowest level of confidence that is acceptable is a *p*-value of 0.05, indicating that there is a 5% likelihood of the result occurring by chance (5 times in a 100). Other *p*-values seen frequently are 0.01 (1% or 1 in 100) and 0.001 (0.1% or 1 in 1000).

Confidence

If it were possible to conduct an experiment on a whole population the results achieved would not be the same as those achieved from conducting the same experiment on a sample of the population. *Confidence intervals* are used to express the values between which a researcher is 'confident' that the true value for a population can be found. As well as the range, an indication of the level of confidence is given – usually 95%.

Levels of measurement

There are various ways in which numbers are used to measure things. The main types of measurement encountered in health research are classified as:

* nominal
* ordinal
* interval
* ratio.

It is important to understand the difference between these levels of measurement as the degree of precision varies from category to category and influences the type of statistical analysis you can conduct on your data.

Nominal data are used to classify things and can be binary (with only two possible choices, such as alive/dead) or have several values (e.g. ethnic origin). The numbers given to each category are arbitrary and could just as easily be letters. When coding your data you could use 1/2 or A/B to represent alive/dead – it would make no difference.

Ordinal data refers to scales where the numbers are ordered or ranked but there is no assumption that the distance between the numbers is equal. An example is a question relating to pain: the respondent is asked to tick one box on a linear scale that is marked from 1 to 5, where 1 = severe, 2 = moderate etc, in answer to the invitation 'Please rate your pain over the last week'. 1 = severe, 2 = moderate, 3 = mild etc.

Interval data refer to scales where the numbers are ordered, as in an ordinal scale, but the intervals between the numbers are known to be equal. For example, in the question above we do not know whether the distance between 'severe' and 'moderate' pain is the same as between 'moderate' and 'mild'. Each person answering the question may have a different perception of this. However, in an interval scale we know that the distance is always the same (e.g. the distance between 1 cm and 2 cm is always the same as between 2 cm and 3 cm).

Ratio scales are the same as interval scales in that the numbers have an order and the distance between them is the same, but ratio scales also have an absolute zero. Examples of ratio scales include weight and height.

The importance of data type

The importance of being able to identify the kind of data you are using and the distribution of the data are that these factors will influence the kind of analysis you can conduct.

A distinction is made in statistical tests between parametric and non-parametric statistics.

- *Non-parametric statistics* refer to statistical tests that can be conducted on data for which no assumptions are made regarding the Normal distribution of the data. Examples of non-parametric tests include the Mann–Whitney U test and the Wilcoxon signed-rank test.
- The use of *parametric statistics* is based on the assumption that the data have a Normal distribution, that they are derived from interval or ratio scales, and that the variance within the data is approximately the same. Parametric statistics are more powerful statistically than non-parametric tests.

Key point

It is not possible to enter into discussion here about specific statistical tests, but further references are supplied at the end of the chapter. It is important to stress that discussing your proposal with a statistician at an early stage will help to identify the kind of data you will generate from your work and the tests that will be relevant.

QUALITATIVE RESEARCH

Qualitative methods are used to understand the interpretations and motivations of people, and this aim is reflected in the methods adopted within this approach. The focus of the research may be a group of people who have a shared experience or it may be gaining insight into the culture of a group or an organisation. Qualitative research does not set out to test a hypothesis but to explore and interpret the area being studied based on the descriptions and explanations provided by participants.

Interviews

An interview is a guided conversation between a researcher and a participant the aim of which is to create an environment in which the participant can tell a story in his or her own words.

Interview structure

The extent to which an interview is structured varies. A highly structured interview follows a predefined list of questions asked in a systematic way. In an unstructured interview the researcher introduces the topic and facilitates the discussion within minimum guidance.

Highly structured interviews are usually associated with survey questionnaires in which the questionnaire is being administered face-to-face. The approach used most commonly in qualitative research is described as 'semi-structured'. Such interviews are guided by an interview schedule (a predefined list of questions) but encourage flexibility so that the researcher can follow lines of enquiry raised by the participant.

Three characteristics described as being shared by all types of qualitative interviews are that (Rubin and Rubin 1995):

- Interviews are modifications of ordinary conversations.
- Interviewers are more interested in people's understanding, knowledge and insights than in categorising people and events into academic theories.
- The content of interviews as well as the flow of discussion and choice of topics changes to match the experiences of the interviewee.

Whilst interviews are similar to conversations, several distinctions should be made. It would be wrong to approach an interview by feeling that you are going to visit a person at home to have a chat about the individual's experiences of, for example, using a wheelchair. The researcher usually guides the conversation to focus on the area of interest. This requires careful preparation, thinking about the questions that will be asked, ways of asking what might be perceived as sensitive questions, the order in which questions will be asked etc. In seeking to gain insight into a person's experiences or understanding, the researcher needs to spend time clarifying the experiences being described. This requires checking during the discussion that you both have the same understanding of what is being described. The researcher needs to listen carefully to make sure that important points are not missed or that points raised by the interviewee that are not on the schedule but are important are followed up.

The potential to vary questions within the interview is something new researchers often worry about in qualitative interviewing. If a highly structured approach is being used this is not possible, but if a semi-structured approach is adopted it would be normal to change the questions as the research progresses. After conducting several interviews your understanding of the area of interest will have changed. People may have identified issues that you had not thought about and introduced new lines of enquiry, so these need to be included in subsequent interviews. It would be unusual if this did not happen.

Key point

If you have not prepared well for the interview it is likely that you will be so focused on remembering the questions or checking the tape machine that you will not actually listen to what is being said.

The interview questions

In preparing for an interview it is important to think carefully about the types of questions that will be asked and the order in which they will be asked. Whilst it is tempting to include as many questions as possible, the conversational element of the interview must be borne in mind. If a person is faced with a long stream of questions it is likely that they will give short answers and feel that they are being subjected to an interrogation. A fundamental task for the interviewer is to develop the skill of listening rather than talking.

Three kinds of question have been described (Rubin and Rubin 1995):

- main questions
- probing questions
- follow-up questions.

Main questions identify the main focus of the area of study. Having identified your research question the topic is broken down into a series of main questions. The wording of these questions should encourage discussion.

Probing questions are a way of increasing the depth of a person's explanation and finding out more; for example: 'Could you tell me a little more about that?' They can also be used to clarify a point made that you are unsure about: 'Could you explain that please? I don't quite understand what you mean by....'

Follow-up questions are used to follow-up themes that emerge during the interview. A person may make a comment that throws a new light on the area you are interested in and you will want to explore this new line of thought with other people you are interviewing; for example: 'Another person mentioned that .... Was this your experience?'

Question order

Most people participating in an interview are keen to help but are nervous at the start of the discussion. It is helpful to start the interview by asking the person to talk about something with which they are familiar. This gives the individual the opportunity to talk for a little while to get used to being in a situation where personal experience is the focus of attention and is to be recorded. Some researchers send their questions to participants prior to the interview to enable them to think about the questions in advance and prepare their thoughts.

As the interview develops the interviewee's confidence may increase to the point where more sensitive or probing questions can be introduced.

It is important also to think about how to end an interview. Interviews can be an emotionally draining experience for the interviewee. If a person has become upset or emotional during an interview or has been asked to discuss a personally challenging topic, the interview needs to end on a lighter note. Therefore it is important to think about what questions can be asked to bring the discussion to an end leaving the person feeling in a positive frame of mind.

Before conducting an interview you should be very clear in your own mind about the content of your interview schedule to enable you to steer a smooth course through the discussion without having to keep referring to notes to remind yourself of the next question.

Recording the interview

Interviews are usually tape-recorded to enable a full transcript of the discussion to be made. In some instances a researcher may choose to take notes instead, but this requires skill to ensure that all the relevant points are recorded whilst maintaining the flow of the conversation.

Key point

If a recorder is being used it is wise to practise using it before any interviews take place. The production of a tape-recorder at the start of an interview can make people nervous, and if you are nervous about using it and need to keep checking that it is switched on and working you will constantly draw attention to the fact that a recording is being made.

It is important to check as soon as possible that you have actually recorded the discussion. If something has gone wrong this will enable you to make as many notes as possible about the discussion whilst it is fresh in your memory. Once completed, interviews are then transcribed – which entails typing the interview verbatim. Transcription is a lengthy process. A rough guide to the time required is four or five hours of typing for one hour of discussion. Access to a transcription machine can significantly reduce the time required to produce a transcript.

Focus Groups

Focus groups have been described as carefully planned discussions designed to obtain participants' perceptions of a predefined area of interest. The group setting provides an environment in which the group members influence each other as they respond to ideas and points raised during the discussion (Krueger 1994). The group setting is used to encourage interaction between participants so that they discuss and exchange experiences and points of view and ask questions of each other.

Conducting a focus group

As with interviews, it is necessary to prepare for the group both in terms of practical arrangements like the organisation of time, venue, transport and refreshments and developing the questions to be asked during the session.

Focus groups should be held in an environment that is accessible and comfortable and creates a relaxed and welcoming feel. Most sessions last between one and two hours. Groups usually comprise between four and eight people to ensure that everyone has an opportunity to be actively involved in the discussion. Larger groups tend to put some people off talking and also provide the opportunity for some people to take a more passive role.

Given the emphasis on the group discussion, the role of the researcher should be limited to asking a few questions and facilitating discussion. Four or five questions should really be the maximum number of main questions posed in a group. Probing questions may also be used to explore a point further.

The researcher usually introduces the session by explaining what the purpose of the group is, emphasising that it is the discussion between participants that is important and establishing any ground rules for the group such as a no-smoking policy and issues of confidentiality regarding what is said. It is helpful to explain that the aim of the group is to obtain different views and that if a person disagrees with what is being said to say so. To stimulate discussion some researchers use group activities such as sorting a set of statements into piles labelled agree and disagree or using pictures or photographs.

It can be difficult for one person to both facilitate the discussion and keep a track of all of the group dynamics taking place. Therefore it is usual for groups to be facilitated by two people, one to facilitate the discussion the other to make notes about the group dynamics and interactions.

As with interviews, focus groups are usually tape recorded, given that all participants consent to this happening, and transcribed in preparation for analysis.

Observational Studies

A number of approaches can be taken in observational studies, one factor being the level of participation of the researcher.

- Participant observation involves the researcher in the activity or group being observed.
- In non-participative studies the researcher observes rather than participates.

Another distinction is whether the participation of the researcher is known about by other members of the group or is concealed. The setting of such studies can vary. A psychologist may choose to undertake an observational study in a clinical or laboratory setting, whereas a sociologist is more likely to observe the phenomenon of interest in the context in which it occurs. Within the social sciences, observational studies are usually called 'ethnography' and are closely associated with anthropology. Both are built upon the premise that to understand a group of people a researcher needs to observe their daily lives, usually by living with them or like them.

The term 'observation' can be misleading as data collection in observational studies tends to derive from a number of methods, including interviews and documentary research. The processes involved in observational studies include: negotiating access to the area of study, determining methods of collecting observational data, watching, recording events taking place, and analysing data.

The Delphi technique

The Delphi technique uses a group of people identified as experts in the field of interest and comprises a number of stages. A group of experts are invited to give their opinions on a specific issue using a postal questionnaire comprising open and closed questions. The questionnaires are analysed and data are then grouped into a series of statements. The statements are then sent back to the participants who are asked to indicate their level of agreement with each statement. These are returned to the researcher who, based on all the responses, provides an overall ranking of the statements; the ranking is then re-circulated. Participants are given the opportunity to review the ranking they gave each statement and these responses are returned to the researcher. These data are then re-analysed to assess the level of consensus. If at this stage consensus is reached the process stops and the results are fed back to the participants. If consensus is not reached then the process is repeated.

Nominal groups

This consensus method brings together a group of 'experts' in a setting, which is highly structured in content. Participants may have been asked to prepare for the meeting by being given the topic of interest in advance or may spend time writing down key points about a given topic at the start of the group. Each person is then asked to contribute one point that is written on a flip chart by the researcher and this continues until all points have been covered. Each person is asked to rank the points on the flip chart privately to ensure that the views of other group members do not influence the ranking. The researcher collects these rankings and calculates the overall ranking of issues for the group. This ranking is then discussed. Following a group discussion participants are asked to re-rank the issues and once again an overall group ranking is worked out and fed back to the group.

Case Studies

This method of research focuses on one case (a single case study) or a small number of cases (multiple case studies). A 'case' may be a person or an environment such as a place of work or an institution. The numbers are usually small owing to the amount of detail that is required in such studies. This method may be used to explore an issue retrospectively or at a single point in time, it may be used also to explore something over time, e.g. the impact of a new management structure on an organisation. A variety of methods are often used to collect data about each case and may include conducting interviews, analysis of documents and observations. Such studies are often undertaken to understand complex social situations and in relation to healthcare or to develop understanding about something like a disease.

ANALYSIS OF QUALITATIVE DATA

Whilst in quantitative research analysis happens when the data have been collected, in qualitative research the processes of data collection and analysis are often inter-

Key point

A qualitative study can produce a large amount of data from which sense needs to be made. There are a number of ways in which qualitative data can be analysed.

twined and a more interactive approach is adopted. This approach to data analysis provides the researcher with the opportunity to explore new insights as they occur during data collection and follow leads that emerge during the course of the interviews. It is likely, therefore, that by the end of the process of data collection the researcher will have a good level of familiarity with the data.

It is important to understand that there are a number of ways in which qualitative data are analysed and the approach taken will be dependent on the theoretical approach taken in the research. For example, if a 'grounded theory' approach has been adopted, specific steps in the analysis include open coding, axial coding and selective coding (Glaser and Strauss 1967; Strauss and Corbin 1990). This approach also supports the use of diagrams and memos to lead to the development of theory that is derived from the data.

Transcribing and Coding

Before detailed analysis can begin, the recordings from interviews or discussions need to be transcribed. A transcript usually refers to a verbatim (exact word by word) reproduction of the taped conversation. Whilst time-consuming to produce, transcripts enable a researcher to locate a segment of text within the wider context of the conversation and help to ensure that coding reflects the meaning derived from participants.

When transcripts have been produced, the first stage of analysis is to, in effect, reduce and reorganise the data. This involves coding, the allocation of descriptive labels to segments of text. Segments of text will vary in size and can be given more than one code. The codes used at this stage may describe or summarise what is being said; this is sometimes referred to as 'first-level coding'.

Once all of the text has been coded the data are reorganised and merged to bring together data for each code. When all the segments for each theme are brought together it is then possible to conduct a more focused analysis of each theme, looking for similarities and differences in what has been said. It is important to compare discourse and to question whether there are themes common to everyone or differences in what is being said. If apparent differences emerge, thought must be given as to why this is the case. If, for example, your sample comprises men and women, do they have different perspectives? The same questions should be asked of people from different background or of different ages. It may be that a contradictory view represents the view of just one person.

Computer-Assisted Coding

The use of dedicated software packages in qualitative analysis has increased significantly in recent years. However, the use of such software to aid analysis is a source of debate amongst qualitative researchers.

Software packages such as ATLAS.ti and QSR NVivo have been developed to facilitate analysis, but it must be stressed that they do not analyse data for you. Such packages enable you to code segments of text on the screen and then sort data automatically into themes. They also enable you to set up enquiries about data; for example, to ask for all the discourse relating to a specific issue derived from men living in London or women over 40. These comparisons can be made far more easily than if doing the same process manually. The software also includes tools to build diagrammatic representations of relationships between themes to help build theory, to write and organise memos whilst you are conducting your analysis.

These packages require a significant investment of time to learn how to use them. Given the quantity of data generated from an undergraduate project, it is likely to be more efficient to analyse the data using the cut and paste options of a word processor, unless someone in your department is familiar with the use of such packages and willing to provide advice and assistance. With many software packages it is easy to get carried away with the tools and facilities they offer and the speed at which they produce outputs without really understanding the rationale for what you are doing or the meaning and relevance of the outputs you have obtained. Developing and understanding the processes involved in analysis and *then* using software to facilitate the process is perhaps a more meaningful use of software packages.

Consensus Methods

These methods are used to assess the extent of agreement or resolve disagreement where there may be contradictory evidence on an issue. Two commonly used methods are the *Delphi technique* and the *nominal group technique*. Both seek to estimate the degree of consensus on a given issue and data are derived from panels of 'experts'.

Within normal group discussion a very persuasive individual or group of individuals with a strong point of view or vested interest can dominate the group and influence the outcome of a decision. These techniques have been developed to overcome that problem. However, caution is needed in relation to these techniques as there are questions relating to how representative the views of such panels are and of the reliability and validity of these methods.

USING MULTIPLE METHODS

More than one method can be used within a single project, for several reasons. For example the use of different methods can increase the validity of the findings by demonstrating that the same conclusions can be drawn when a number of methods are used to observe the same phenomena. Using more than one method can also provide the opportunity to 'throw light on different phenomena relevant to the research question by providing different versions or levels of answer' (Mason 1996). Common examples of the use of multiple methods are a combination of interviews and focus groups, and survey questionnaires and interviews.

Key point

If you decide to use more than one method within your project it is important to think about how the methods will be combined both in terms of the research design and the data analysis.

RECRUITMENT AND SAMPLING

Having identified a research question and the relevant methods to collect data, the next stage of the research process focuses on deciding the number and type of people to involve in the study and how they will be identified.

Sampling Strategies

Sampling strategies are divided into:

- random sampling whereby every person in a population of interest has an equal chance of being chosen for the study
- non-probability sampling in which the selection is not random.

The main methods of random sampling include 'simple' random sampling using computer-generated numbers, and 'stratified' sampling, which have been described previously in relation to the experimental method. Another form of random sampling is 'cluster' sampling which focuses on sampling from clusters of the population.

Non-probability sampling is used often in qualitative research. 'Convenience' sampling means sampling from people who are easy to access or most likely to respond. 'Purposive' sampling is derived from people who were selected on purpose for the experience of the phenomena being investigated. 'Quota' sampling is used by market researchers who have specific targets for their study population (e.g. numbers of people required from different socio-demographic or age groups. 'Snowballing' means the researcher may have identified a small group of participants and then asks them to recruit others they know who would be in the target group. They are contacted to ask if they would be willing to take part in the project and are likewise asked for potential contacts.

Sample Size

'How many people do I need to recruit for my research?' is an obvious question to ask, but the answer is not at all straightforward. The statistical approach to calculating sample size is a *power calculation*. This method is used to calculate the number of people needed in a study to detect a true difference between two groups. However, it is unlikely that the size of an undergraduate project would warrant such an approach. Given the diversity of methods it would be wise to obtain guidance on determining the sample size once you have identified your question and methods.

Key point
In the written account of your work you will need to describe and justify the sampling strategy you used, the size of the sample, and how it was selected.

In relation to qualitative research the guidance given most often is to carry on with the project until your data reach saturation – when the interviews or focus groups you are conducting are not coming up with any new insights. This means that it can be difficult to specify a definite number of participants at the start of the project. At undergraduate level, however, a more pragmatic approach will probably be needed with the decision being based on the time and resources available as well as factors like access to participants.

PREPARATORY WORK

Students can be keen to embark upon the actual process of 'doing the research', but time should be allocated at the start of a project to do some preparatory work. This might seem to be an unnecessary distraction from the excitement of 'getting started', but it is

guaranteed to be time well spent. Experienced researchers will testify to the frustration of loosing a crucial reference or of not having made careful note of the source of a key quotation as the submission deadline looms. The 'eureka' moment you had – and thought you would never forget – fades rapidly as the focus of a project moves through the various stages and the research develops.

Keeping a Research Diary

Key point
Research or fieldwork diaries are closely associated with qualitative research but are of equal value in quantitative research.

The aim of keeping a diary is to provide a record of the development of a research project from inception to completion. It provides a way of keeping what could be described as personal memos about your research in one place that is easy to reference as the project develops. The diary usually takes the form of handwritten or word-processed notes. The structure varies from researcher to researcher: some people choose to keep notes in chronological order as in a personal diary, whilst others organise their diary under headings such as 'literature', 'methods', 'data collection' and 'personal thoughts'.

The diary provides a place in which to keep track of how the research question has evolved. You can note methodological issues arising throughout the data collection process, such as your thoughts on the different kinds of standardised measures that could be used and why you choose one measure over another. You can record particular papers or discussions that may have stimulated a specific train of thought. Once the process of data collection begins the diary may be used to record personal profiles of the participants. If you are conducting interviews you may note information about the actual process of the interview – questions which elicited a good discussion or those which people found hard to understand or engage with, or issues which have been raised by a participant which you thought were really important.

Research is a reflective process and a research diary provides a place in which this reflection can be recorded.

Keeping Track of References

The development of a systematic method of recording and referencing is as much a research skill as that of conducting an interview or undertaking an experiment. At the start of a project it is easy to underestimate the time taken to compile the reference section of a dissertation, and the benefits of developing a systematic method of recording and filing references from day one. Doing this will save an immense amount of effort towards the end of the dissertation, when time, energy and resources will be challenged considerably.

Note

It is a common experience to have a memory of reading a crucial piece of information or writing down a quotation but not being able to locate the exact source!

There are several methods of managing references, the most common being the use of a card index system or dedicated computer software such as Reference Manager or Endnote. Whichever system is used, the minimum amount of information recorded should be as follows:

For a journal or magazine:

- author (or authors) including surname and initials
- name of the journal or magazine
- title of the article
- date of publication
- volume number, and issue number if relevant
- the pages of the article (e.g. 331–338).

For a book or report:

- author (or authors) including surname and initials
- title of the book
- date of publication
- name of publisher
- place of publication.

For a chapter in an edited book:

- editor (or editors) including surname and initials
- author (or authors) including surname and initials
- title of the book
- title of the chapter
- page numbers of the chapter
- date of publication
- name of publisher
- place of publication.

It is helpful also to write a short summary of the relevant points of the paper or chapter and to note, carefully, any quotations which you feel you may wish to use in the dissertation. If you are noting direct quotations, keep a record of the page on which the quotation can be found – to save having to check through the whole publication to find, for example, a two sentence quotation.

If a card index system is used, separate cards should be used for each publication and a filing system developed to help with retrieval. Software packages have several advantages over card indexes, as they offer a number of tools helpful in the management of references, including:

- a mechanism for importing full reference details and abstracts from literature searches conducted without having to enter individual references
- scope to input summaries and key words alongside the reference details
- the incorporation of references into text whilst word-processing
- automatic formatting of reference sections in a specified style (e.g. Harvard, Vancouver).

A filing system is needed for storage and retrieval of papers. These may be stored alphabetically or under subject headings.

Regulations

The regulations for dissertations vary from college to college, so make sure you are familiar with and understand the regulations that apply to your dissertation before starting work. They will detail the format of your dissertation and procedures for issues such as gaining ethical approval for your project. The regulations will have been produced for a reason and must be followed. At undergraduate level, ignoring such guidance can result in the need to revise and resubmit the work. In the context of proposals written for funding applications, failure to follow the regulations and guidance can result in the application being rejected. It is therefore worth getting used, at an early stage in your research career, to reading and following any guidance or regulations provided.

As well as understanding the regulations of your college you may also need to give careful consideration to other regulations such as the Data Protection Act, Codes of Professional Conduct and Codes of Research for your college. Your supervisor will be able to advise you on the regulations that apply to your chosen project, including the issue of research governance.

Supervision

An important component of conducting any research project is the quality of supervision provided throughout the work and the relationship between the student and supervisor. The supervisory process is two-way, there being an onus on both parties to create an informative, discursive and supportive environment. The supervisor does not tell a student what to do next.

Your supervisor may not have in-depth knowledge and clinical expertise in your chosen area of study but is likely to have extensive experience in the supervision and successful completion of dissertations, and experience of the methodological approach and methods being used.

Here are some key points to remember:

1 Plan ahead for your supervision. Prior to your meetings make a list of the issues you wish to discuss with the supervisor and make sure that at the start of supervision you agree on the issues you both wish to discuss.

2 If the aim of a session is to discuss work that needs to be submitted prior to the meeting, make sure you give the supervisor plenty of time to read the work. It is not uncommon for students to push deadlines to the limit, leading to work being handed in a day or two before supervision, or being brought to the meeting. Such an approach is unlikely to generate high-quality discussion about your work as supervisors need to have time to read and reflect on the work and prepare for the meeting in the same way that you do.

3 Keep notes of the key issues discussed during supervision. These notes can form part of the fieldwork diary. Either write notes during the meeting or straight afterwards. It is easy to forget key issues discussed or lines of enquiry recommended as supervisory meetings can cover several topics in one session.

4 At the end of the meeting make sure you are clear about the next stage of your work and expectations regarding work that needs to be completed before the next meeting.

5 If you are encountering problems with your research bring them to the attention of the supervisor as soon as possible. Research is rarely a process that is smooth and problem-free. Things not going to plan should be seen as part of the process rather than a failing on your part.

Key point
Completing your dissertation on time requires planning – based not only on your own time but taking into consideration the time of others involved in the project.

Time Management

The reality of many research projects is that completion is often dependent on the time commitments of other people over which you will have no control. These will include research and ethics committees, people or groups involved in the recruitment of participants, participants themselves, and your supervisor. Whilst your project may be your number one priority it will not be given the same priority by others. You therefore need to develop an understanding of the time constraints within which other people are operating, and to be prepared to give people realistic timescales for the things you are asking them to do.

At the start of the project draw up a calendar divided into weeks and also a list of the key milestones in your research process. Then start marking on the calendar the time required for each task. Be realistic, and if you are not sure how long some things will take discuss it with your supervisor. Allow time for slippage in the plan as this is bound to occur. As your project progresses keep going back to your time frame and make revisions if necessary. This will also help when you are asking other people to be involved in the project as you will be able to give them an indication of when things need to be done. For example, if someone is sending out questionnaires on your behalf you will know when this has to be done by rather than plucking a date out of the air.

Personal Presentation

It is as important to think about how you are going to present yourself in a research setting as it is in a clinical setting. This will be done either in person or in writing. Which ever form it may take you need to convey your professionalism and communicate the importance of your work. The manner in which you approach people will have a direct impact upon their willingness to engage with your study.

If you are approaching potential participants in person, think about your appearance, plan the way in which you will present your project and allow time to give a proper explanation of who you are, what you are wanting to do and why. These may seem obvious points, but the successful completion of your project will in some instances be influenced by your ability to present yourself and communicate your work. You will usually have only one opportunity with each person to do this.

If you are contacting potential participants by post, spend time working on the letter you intend to send, not only in relation to content but also in terms of format. Try to keep to a minimum the amount of medical terminology used, if writing to potential participants, and explain the relevance of the project and the exact implications for a person taking part in the study. A useful tool in checking the language you have used in your letter is the readability tool provided in some software packages. Readability scores provide an indication of the reading level of the document and can assess the ease of reading, rated on a 100-point scale, and also indicate the school grade level in relation to reading level.

Note

The issues outlined so far in this chapter should help in the planning and implementation of a research project. The focus will now move on to consider how all of the different components discussed in this chapter are brought together within the context of writing a research proposal.

WRITING A RESEARCH PROPOSAL

The role of the proposal is to 'describe what the research is about, what specifically it is trying to achieve, how you will go about doing this, what will be learnt from the research, and the contribution it will make to existing knowledge' (Punch 2000). The components of a proposal are fairly standard but it is essential to check the specific regulations governing your dissertation.

Writing a research proposal will provide a clear plan of action for conducting your project as well as the structure for your dissertation, with the addition of a results section.

Components of the Proposal

A research proposal should have the following elements:

- title
- abstract
- introduction
- planned literature review
- statement of the research question
- methods to be used
- analysis intended
- initial references
- appendices.

The title and abstract

Think carefully about the title of your proposal. Try to convey the key points of your project in a clear and concise manner. An abstract provides a summary of the project and is usually the last section of the proposal written. It is normally limited to around 250 words. At the proposal stage the abstract should enable the reader to understand the context of the research, the research question and the methods being used to address the question. Once the research has been completed the revised abstract will also need to include the main results and conclusions. Whilst the word length of an abstract is small, the skill required to write it should not be underestimated – considerable effort is required to summarise a project in 250 words.

The introduction

A distinction needs to be made between an introduction and a literature review as they perform two different functions. An introduction should provide the reader with an understanding of how the study fits into what is already know about the research topic and provides a justification as to why this particular piece of research is important. Introductions need not be lengthy. A structure used frequently is to start with the broad context of the topic and move towards the specific area of the proposed research, culminating with a statement of the research question.

The literature review

Key point

The literature review has been described as 'a systematic, explicit, and reproducible method for identifying, evaluating and interpreting the existing body of recorded work produced by researchers, scholars and practitioners (Fink 1998).

The function of a literature review is to locate your work within the context of the work already conducted in the chosen area. It should demonstrate that you have an understanding of your area of research by providing the reader with an overview of the state of knowledge in the field and the major questions being asked.

The definition provided by Fink provides insight into the core elements of conducting a comprehensive literature review. It requires two very different skills:

- searching the literature, and
- appraising the literature.

The literature review should also identify the theoretical base of the project and, if you are studying an area where several theoretical positions exist, should justify the particular perspective you have chosen to adopt. The methods used to undertake the review should be made explicit by detailing the major databases or information sources used. The literature reviewed can take many forms and may include journal articles, books, reports and government circulars.

The main focus of searching for most undergraduate dissertations will be via computer-based systems, primarily accessed via a college network (e.g. Medline or CINAHL (Cumulative Index of Nursing and Allied Health Literature). The process of conducting a search begins with the identification of key words. Most databases contain a thesaurus that enables you to check that the key word or terms you have chosen actually appear in the database. You need to put time and effort into planning the literature search before starting to use the databases. Keep a record of the key words you have used, the searches that you have carried out and the results of each search. It is likely that this process will take place over a number of sessions and it may be difficult to remember exactly what you have done and how you refined the searches.

Having identified key words you may find that one of two things occurs:

1 You are presented with a list of hundreds of references, which probably indicates that the terms you have used are too general
2 You are presented with only a few references, which may indicate that your search was too narrow.

The majority of databases make use of what are known as 'Boolean operators' to enable you to refine or expand your search by combining words by using the keyword AND or excluding words by using the keyword OR.

The results of your search will be a list of articles of potential relevance to your project. It is likely that not all references listed will be relevant, so you need to read the abstracts to check on the relevance before locating the articles within the library or requesting them via inter-library loans. Photocopying and requesting articles is expensive for you and the college, so you should be convinced of the relevance of an article before obtaining the full text. Most databases enable you to move back and forth between the reference list and abstracts marking the references of interest and thus refining your initial search further.

Not all of the literature you review will come from journal publications – a large amount of information is to be found from books, government departments and professional organisations as well as voluntary organisations and websites. Conducting an Internet search requires a systematic approach similar to that used to search databases as the potential to identify sources of information is immense. It is important to remember that you will also need to develop and demonstrate an

understanding of literature to support your methodology and methods.

Key point

An important distinction to understand is the difference between describing the literature and evaluating and appraising it. Many students conducting a literature review for the first time present a description of the papers they have obtained rather than an evaluation and appraisal of them.

Evaluating and appraising literature is a skill that needs to be developed. Being able to critique research papers when you are developing your own understanding of the research process is difficult, but further reading has been provided at the end of the chapter to provide you with guidance. Understanding the criteria used to critique literature will also provide insight into the criteria that will be used to judge your own work once it is completed.

Whilst the literature review is normally one of the first tasks in developing your research proposal, it should not be viewed as complete until the project has been completed. The majority of undergraduate dissertations are typically conducted over a 12 month period during which time new papers of relevance are published. Having conducted a systematic review you will develop an understanding of the specific journals in which new papers are likely to be published. During the period of your research you should keep up to date and, where appropriate, incorporate new papers into your review. This can be difficult to achieve once you have embarked upon the process of data collection as time and resources will be focused elsewhere. However, if you have access to the Internet it is worth setting up journal alerts for key publications. This will ensure that each time a journal issue is published the contents page will be e-mailed to you.

The research question

Whilst the research question may have been introduced at the end of the introduction it is worth restating it before the methods section to refocus the readers' attention on the specific question being addressed.

Methods to be used

The methods section should explain both the methodological approach and the specific methods. It is usual to begin with an explanation of the relevance of the methodological approach to the question being asked. Is a quantitative or qualitative approach appropriate to address the specified question? Or has a mixed approach been chosen incorporating both quantitative and qualitative approaches? What is it about your research question that makes your chosen approach appropriate?

The methods section should set out the way in which you are going to address your research question. It should include details of the ethical considerations of the project, whether or not ethical committee approval will be obtained, and details of how you will obtain informed consent, if appropriate. The method of recruitment you intend to use should be described and your sample and sample size provided and justified along with the sampling strategy you intend to use. You should describe any inclusion or exclusion criteria you have determined for the study.

The methods section should provide a detailed account of the specific methods of data collection being used. If you have chosen to use standardised measures or treatment interventions they should be explained and referenced and details of their validity and reliability provided. If you have chosen to develop your own method of measurement you need to explain the steps you plan to take to develop your measure.

The intended analysis

In this section you should demonstrate that you have considered the analysis of data and provide insight into the techniques you are going to use. For a quantitative study you will need to specify any statistical package you intend to use (e.g. SPSS or Minitab) as well as the statistical tests. For a qualitative study, again you need to detail the process of analysis you will be using and whether or not you will use software such as ALTAS.ti or NVivo.

It may be helpful to include at the end of this section a time plan which identifies key milestones for the project and a target for completion.

The references

Your college regulations may specify the format in which the reference section is to be compiled. Make sure that you check this and comply with the relevant requirements.

Appendices

One or more appendix sections can provide additional information of relevance to the study. Things included might be examples of standardised questionnaires, and a copy of the interview schedule which will guide qualitative interviews.

The Dissertation

When the project has been completed and you start writing it up, the structure of your dissertation will be very similar to that of the proposal. There will, of course, be additional sections: one for the results, which is placed after the analysis, and one for the discussion and conclusions, which comes after the results section.

CONCLUSION

By the time you are preparing to start writing your dissertation you will already have been introduced to the importance of research in informing the evidence base of clinical practice in physiotherapy. For a newly qualified therapist, the grounding you will have developed in understanding the research process should not be underestimated. Many senior therapists have not had this opportunity and find the concept of understanding and undertaking research immensely challenging. As a new member of a department, with research experience, you have a great deal to offer to help demystify research and facilitate its integration into clinical practice.

If you are stimulated by the practice of research, do not underestimate the potential of your first dissertation. Unfortunately many dissertations collect dust in cupboards or on shelves, even though they could possibly form the basis of a journal article or a presentation at a seminar – so do explore this prospect with your supervisor.

To end where we started: many people are overwhelmed by the prospect of research and tend to diminish what they have achieved in dissertations. Your dissertation could be the first building block of a research career.

FURTHER READING

General

Bell J 1999 Doing Your Research Project: a Guide for First-Time Researchers in Education and Social Science, 3rd edn. Buckingham: Open University Press

Blaxter L, Hughes C, Tight M 2001 How to Research, 2nd edn. Buckingham: Open University Press.

Bowling A 1997 Research Methods in Health: Investigating Health and Health Services. Buckingham: Open University Press

Burns RB 2000 Introduction to Research Methods, 4th edn. London: Sage

Punch KF 1998 Introduction to Social Research: Quantitative and Qualitative Approaches. London: Sage

Punch KF 2000 Developing Effective Research Proposals. London: Sage

Literature reviews

Fink A 1998 Conducting Research Literature Reviews: From Paper to the Internet. Thousand Oaks, CA: Sage

Hart C 1998 Doing a Literature Review: Releasing the Social Science Research Imagination. London: Sage

Questionnaires and measurement scales

Bowling A 1991 Measuring Health: a Review of Quality of Life Measurement Scales. Buckingham: Open University Press

Bowling A 1995 Measuring Disease: a Review of Disease-Specific Quality of Life Measurement Scales. Buckingham: Open University Press

Oppenheim AN 1992 Questionnaire Design, Interviewing and Attitude Measurement, 2nd edn. London: Pinter

Streiner D, Norman G 1995 Health Measurement Scales: a Practical Guide to their Development and Use, 2nd edn. Oxford: Oxford University Press

Statistics

Altman D 1991 Practical Statistics for Medical Research. Chapman & Hall: London

Clegg F 1990 Simple Statistics: a Course Book for the Social Sciences. Cambridge: Cambridge University Press

Hart A 2001 Making Sense of Statistics in Healthcare. Oxford: Abingdon Radcliffe Medical Press

Howitt D, Cramer D 2000 An Introduction to Statistics in Psychology: a Complete Guide for Students, 2nd edn. Harlow: Pearson Education

Qualitative methods

Hammersley M, Atkinson P 1995 Ethnography: Principles in Practice, 2nd edn. London: Routledge

Hart E, Bond M 1995 Action Research for Health and Social Care. Buckingham: Open University Press

Krueger RK 1994 Focus Groups: a Practical Guide for Applied Research, 2nd edn. Thousand Oaks, CA: Sage

Mason J 1996 Qualitative Researching. London: Sage

Morgan D 1993 Successful Focus Groups: Advancing the State of the Art. London: Sage

Morgan D 1998 The Focus Group Guidebook. London: Sage

Renzetti CM, Lee RM (eds) 1993 Researching Sensitive Topics. London: Sage

Rubin H, Rubin I 1995 Qualitative Interviewing: the Art of Hearing Data. Thousand Oaks, CA: Sage

Strauss A, Corbin J 1998 Basics of Qualitative Research, 2nd edn. London: Sage

REFERENCES

Bowling A 1997 Research Methods in Health: Investigating Health and Health Services. Buckingham: Open University Press

Clegg F 1990 Simple Statistics: a Course book for the Social Sciences. Cambridge: Cambridge University Press

Fink A 1998 Conducting Research Literature Reviews: From Paper to the Internet. Thousand Oaks, CA: Sage

Glaser B, Strauss A 1967 The Discovery of Grounded Theory: Strategies for Qualitative Research. Chicago: Aldine

Hockey L 1996 The nature and purpose of research. In Cormack DF (ed.) The Research Process in Nursing, 3rd edn. Oxford: Blackwell Science

Howitt D, Cramer D 2000 An Introduction to Statistics in Psychology: a Complete Guide for Students, 2nd edn. Harlow: Pearson Education

Krueger RK 1994 Focus Groups: a Practical Guide for Applied Research, 2nd edn. Thousand Oaks, CA: Sage

Mason J 1996 Qualitative Researching. London: Sage

Punch KF 1998 Introduction to Social Research: Quantitative and Qualitative Approaches. London: Sage

Punch KF 2000 Developing Effective Research Proposals. London: Sage

Rubin H, Rubin I 1995 Qualitative Interviewing: the Art of Hearing Data. Thousand Oaks, CA: Sage

Strauss A, Corbin J 1998 Basics of Qualitative Research, 2nd edn. London: Sage

18

Upper and Lower Limb Joint Arthroplasty

Ann Birch and Ann Price

INTRODUCTION

There is no 'typical' patient who is appropriate for a joint arthroplasty. As with all modern medicine, a decision has to be made which balances the risks of surgery against the potential improvements.

Patient age per se is no longer an acceptable clinical decision-making tool (Brander et al. 1997). Generally, the surgical team will wait until pain or disability is severe enough to cause a significant impact on the person's quality of life, where surgery would make things significantly better or prevent a major deterioration. It is quite feasible for example, to replace the hips of a 16-year-old with severe rheumatoid arthritis. An artificial joint is not as efficient as its organic counterpart. If a synthetic joint becomes worn or damaged, it does not repair itself as a normal joint does. It will also not be as efficient at absorbing the stresses and strains of daily life as an organic joint. The field of joint prosthetics is making remarkable improvements, however.

PART I: UPPER LIMB ARTHROPLASTY

There are prostheses available for every joint in the upper limb. Elbow, wrist and finger arthroplasties are mainly performed for patients with rheumatoid arthritis, although metacarpophalangeal (MCP) and proximal interphalangeal (PIP) joints are now being developed for patients with osteoarthritis and following trauma. The carpometacarpal joint of the thumb is the most common joint replacement for osteoarthritis. There are also prostheses available to replace the ulnar head and the radial head; these are normally used for reconstruction following difficult forearm and elbow fractures.

Part I of this chapter will look at the two most common upper limb joint arthroplasties in some detail (shoulder and MCP joints). The chapter also includes a selection of illustrations of other upper limb arthroplasties.

SHOULDER ARTHROPLASTY

Developments

The first shoulder arthroplasty is thought to have been carried out in 1894 (Hamblen 1984) but it was in 1951 that the modern story of shoulder replacement began.

In 1951 Charles Neer developed a hemi-arthroplasty, primarily for the reconstruction of severe proximal humerus fractures. However, it was also used for people suffering from osteoarthritis, with surprisingly good results. In 1973 Neer redesigned the humeral component and added a glenoid to make the first unconstrained Total shoulder arthroplasty (TSR) – known as

the Neer II. The basis of the design was to produce as near to an anatomical replacement as possible. Neer published his early results in 1982 (Neer et al. 1982). This principle is followed in most modern prostheses.

A single-piece prosthesis such as the Neer would require a huge number of sizes to be kept in stock, in order to cater for the variety of dimensions encountered in the population. To attempt to address this problem, modular systems such as the 'global shoulder' have been developed, in which different sizes of shaft, head and glenoid can be interchanged (Figures 18.1 and 18.2).

Key point

There are currently 20 different prosthetic systems in use in the UK (Mackay et al. 2001). A survey carried out by Mackay and Williams (1999) suggested that around 2800 shoulder replacements were carried out in the UK in 1998.

Factors Influencing Outcome of Shoulder Arthroplasty

There are many factors influencing the outcome of shoulder arthroplasty (Iannotti and Williams 1998; see Table 18.1). It is mainly in the last section, that of the rehabilitation programme, that physiotherapists have influence, but practitioners need to know as much about the other factors as possible so that realistic goals can be set. We do not want patients to be given unrealistic expectations, but neither do we want them to fail to achieve their full potential. Good communication with the surgical team is therefore very important.

Key point

There are three main situations in which a shoulder arthroplasty operation is performed: in osteoarthritis, in rheumatoid arthritis, and following a complex fracture.

Primary Osteoarthritis (OA)

This is the indication for TSR from which the best results can be expected. Godenèche et al. (2002) reviewed a series of 267 operations for osteoarthritis and found that 77% of them had results which were classed as good or excellent. They found that the result was dependent on the severity of the degenerative changes that had taken place prior to surgery. It seems, therefore, that for patients who have primary

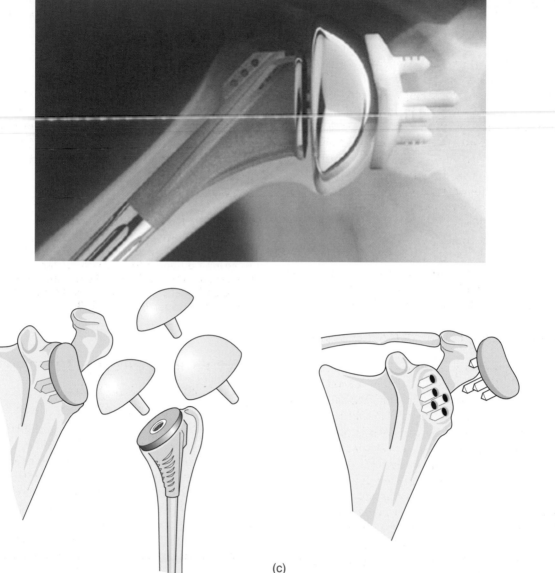

(a)

(b)

(c)

Figure 18.1 (a) The global shoulder implant. (b) Sketch to demonstrate the different heights of humeral head available. (c) Sketch to show how the glenoid component is attached to the glenoid fossa. (Reproduced by kind permission of De Puy Orthopaedics Inc., IN, USA.)

osteoarthritis without gross soft-tissue damage or loss of bone, we can expect to achieve near-normal range of movement and strength. Patients who start off with rotator cuff disease or glenoid erosion should have less high expectations.

Procedure

The most common surgical approach is known as the 'deltopectoral approach'. The incision passes between the deltoid and pectoralis major, and access to the shoulder joint is via the subscapularis muscle and the anterior part of the capsule. Thus the subscapularis muscle is the only active structure which will need to be protected in the early postoperative period.

Table 18.2 shows a typical postoperative protocol. Details will vary depending on surgeon preference. As always, the postoperative regimen must be agreed between the surgeon and the physiotherapy team.

Rheumatoid Arthritis (RA)

People with RA who undergo shoulder arthroplasty are likely to have a number of the adverse pathological fac-

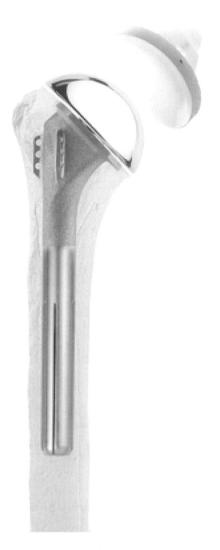

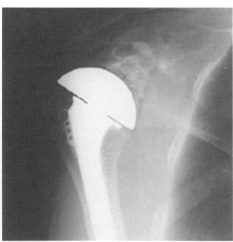

Figure 18.2   Shoulder replacement showing humeral and glenoid components and the appearance on X-ray. (Reproduced by kind permission of Adam C. Gaines.)

Table 18.1 Factors affecting outcome of prosthetic shoulder reconstruction.

Pathology
Rotator cuff disease
Glenoid erosion bone loss
Humeral bone loss
Bone loss
Bone density

Surgical technique
Prosthetic placement
Prosthetic–cement–bone interface
Soft-tissue balancing

Prosthetic design
Size selection
 Glenoid
 Humeral head
 Humeral stem
Offsets
Material properties

Rehabilitation programme
Range of motion
Strength
Stability

tors listed in Table 18.1. The expected results will depend on how many and how severe they are. People with rheumatoid arthritis do not tend to be referred for replacement arthroplasty until these factors are fairly advanced, so the results are generally not as good as in osteoarthritic patients. The surgical approach and basic postoperative management are the same.

In advanced disease of either the OA or RA type it is not always possible to insert a glenoid component. If there is gross bone loss around the glenoid fossa, it is not possible to attach the implant securely enough. Also the lack of rotator cuff function causes the humeral head to 'rock' the glenoid component, causing loosening. The problem of glenoid fixation is one of the ongoing dilemmas in shoulder arthroplasty.

Complex Fracture

Following a complex fracture it is normally a hemi-arthroplasty that is performed as the glenoid is intact.

The operation can be performed either acutely as the primary treatment for the fracture or later as a secondary procedure. The results are better if it is performed acutely. This is a different operation from the one performed as an elective procedure as there is disruption of the tuberosities to which the rotator cuff muscles are attached. The challenge to the surgeon is to restore the anatomy to as close to normal as possible

Table 18.2 Example of postoperative routine following primary total shoulder arthroplasty for osteoarthritis.

Day 1
Usual post-op check, maintenance of range of movement in hand and wrist.

Day 2
Assisted active flexion and abduction, first by physiotherapist followed by teaching patient-assisted active of same movements using pulleys and exercise stick.

Patient is taught to do exercises x 4 daily.

Day 3 to 3 weeks
Continue with exercises as above and add extension, internal rotation and lateral rotation to 30 degrees, with the arm by the side. Abduction should always be with the arm in neutral as the combined movement of abduction and lateral rotation should not be attempted until 6 weeks post-op.

The patient can progress from assisted active to active movement as they are able. Once the person is comfortable he or she may begin to use the arm for self-care activities within the limits of pain and strength.

3 weeks to 6 weeks
The patient should now have discarded the sling completely during the day and should be progressing from assisted active to active movement. The physiotherapist will be showing appropriate ways to do this.

Active external rotation can be progressed beyond 30 degrees but stretching should still be avoided.

6 weeks to 3 months
Progressive strengthening exercises in all ranges should be encouraged according to the patient's individual capabilities. Rotator cuff strengthening should be emphasised, using a progressive system such as Theraband.

3 months onwards
Many patients are discharged from treatment but should be encouraged to continue with strengthening exercises until optimum function has been achieved.

and attach the tuberosities securely enough so that mobilisation can be commenced early.

The trauma that caused the fracture will also have caused soft-tissue damage, so the physiotherapy regimen must take this into account as well. Once again details may vary from surgeon to surgeon and individual patients will have different concurrent injuries, so the regimen will have to be personalised to take account of these.

METACARPOPHALANGEAL JOINT REPLACEMENT

Rheumatoid arthritis can affect any joint in the body, but it is particularly devastating to the complex collection of joints and intricate soft tissues that make up the hand. The most obvious aspect of the deformity shown in Figure 18.3 is the ulnar deviation of the fingers,

Key point
A principal role of the upper limb is to allow for maximum use of the hand. Without a functioning hand the rest of the upper limb becomes mainly a component of balance.

referred to by the French as 'coup de vent' or windswept; but the more functionally debilitating deformity is the volar subluxation of the metacarpal heads as this robs the flexor tendons of a proportion of their power, thus weakening grip.

The factors influencing the development of the deformities at the MCP joint are complex. They have been well described in rheumatology and hand therapy textbooks.

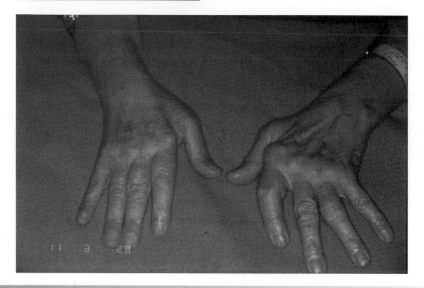

Figure 18.3   The hands of a person with rheumatoid arthritis showing the common deformities of ulnar drift and subluxation of the MCP joints.

Surgical Procedures

There are many reconstructive and preventative procedures that can be performed for this condition, but by far the most common is the replacement of the metacarpophalangeal (MCP) joint by a silastic flexible hinge (Figure 18.4). Swanson developed this in the 1960s when he saw that the results of simple resection arthroplasty were unsatisfactory (Swanson et al. 2000). There have been other attempts at designing MCP joint replacements, but none so far has stood the test of time like the Swanson version.

Key point

Swanson devised an equation to explain the process: bone resection + implant + encapsulation = new joint (Swanson et al. 1978).

A flexible implant arthroplasty is different in principle from other joint arthroplasties in that the implant acts as an inert flexible spacer, which is quickly surrounded by a layer of synovial tissue. The new tissue

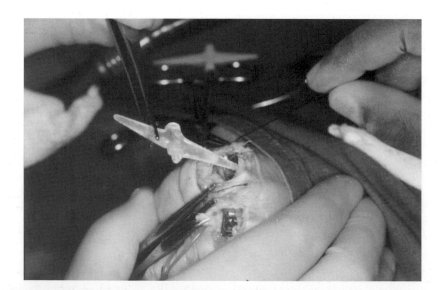

Figure 18.4   Insertion of a Swanson silastic MCP flexible implant. (Reproduced courtesy of Wright Medical Inc.)

remains in contact with the implant and surrounding this a stronger capsule develops.

As well as excising the destroyed joint surfaces and inserting the flexible hinge, the surgeon must release and rebalance the soft tissues crossing the joint if function is to be restored.

Postoperative Management

The short-term aims are:

- to achieve a functional arc of movement
- to protect soft tissue repairs.

The long-term aims are:

- to strengthen weak muscles
- to re-educate function
- to teach specific joint protection techniques.

The short-term aims are achieved by early controlled movement, which stimulates the formation of a strong but flexible capsule around the implant. The pattern of collagen formation is influenced by the forces applied to it. The dynamic splint allows movement to take place only in a flexion extension arc, which influences the collagen to be laid down in straight parallel lines rather than in a haphazard manner (Swanson et al. 1978).

The most common way of controlling the movement is by the use of a dynamic extension splint, often referred to as an 'outrigger' (Figure 18.5a). This provides proprioceptive input for the patient to carry out flexion at the MCP joints and provides assistance for the weak extensor muscles.

Longer-term aims are achieved by strengthening exercises, re-education of pulp–pulp pinch, and education in joint protection techniques. When the outrigger is first removed patients are fitted with a splint to wear when doing heavier functional activities, to protect against the ulnar deviation forces which are inherent in strong gripping (Figure 18.6).

An example of a postoperative regimen is given in Table 18.3. This is just an example because details will vary greatly from unit to unit, and some protocols are now being developed that do not include the use of a dynamic splint. Studies examining their efficacy are few and at present only short-term results are available.

> ### Individual patient regimens
> When treating rheumatoid patients following surgery, always remember that they have a systemic disease, and often postoperative regimens need to be individually tailored to take account of other deformities.

Expected Outcome

The patient normally attends the department for treatment and education until 3 months after surgery. By that time it is hoped that the person will have gained:

- a functional grip
- the ability to open the hand wide enough to grasp jars and glasses
- the ability to manipulate small objects such as coins or buttons with pulp-to-pulp pinch.

Delaney and Stanley (2000) have shown that the range of movement, particularly into extension, can continue to increase for up to 12 months following surgery. The average range of movement from this study was from 20 degrees of flexion to 70 degrees of flexion, although the enhanced stability of the joints and the functional factors listed above are far more important than the actual range of movement.

EXAMPLES OF OTHER UPPER LIMB ARTHROPLASTIES

Figures 18.7–18.10 show photographs of radial head, wrist, finger and trapezium arthoplasty photographs and X-rays.

PART II: LOWER LIMB ARTHROPLASTY

Modern successful joint replacements are based on appropriate patient selection, selection of the appropriate implant, specific surgical technique and expertise, and multidisciplinary patient preparation and rehabilitation.

> ### Key point
> Lower limb joint replacement began in the 1950s: Sir John Charnley refined and researched the low-friction hip arthroplasty that today is the gold standard against which all other joint arthroplasty is compared. Bizot et al. (2000) claim 90.4% 10-year survival rates for certain types of hip prostheses.

The aims of lower limb joint replacement are:

- to relieve pain
- to improve the range of motion at the joint
- to improve the functional ability of the individual
- to improve the person's quality of life
- to prevent further deformity.

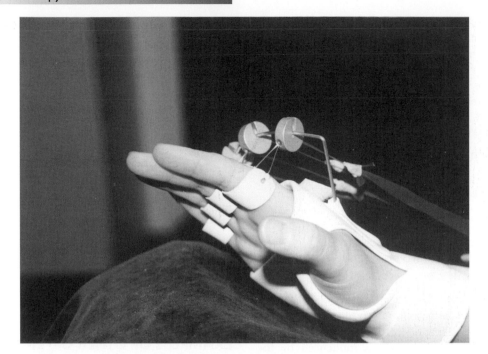

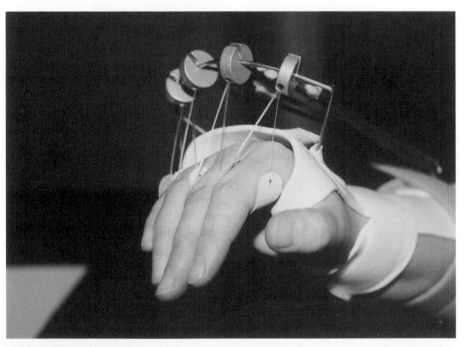

Figure 18.5 (a) Dynamic extension splint (outrigger) in the resting position. (b) Flexion at the MCP joints against the resistance of the elastic bands.

Indications for Lower Limb Joint Replacement

Hip joint replacement is a major yet commonplace orthopaedic procedure. The two main pathologies that lead to replacement surgery are osteoarthritis (primary and secondary) and rheumatoid arthritis, although other indications include congenital dislocation of the hip (CDH), trauma, necrosis of the femoral head, and infection. Specialist centres offer more complex procedures including arthrodesis to implant conversions. Previously the majority of these patients would be in marked pain with encroaching severe disability.

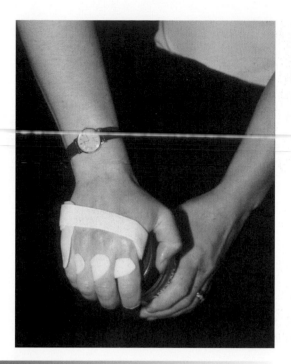

Figure 18.6 Splint to protect against recurrence of ulnar drift. Protection is particularly important in strong gripping activities.

These pathologies and their respective drug therapies can lead to varying bone structure that the surgeon has to allow for at operation. For example, in the rheumatoid joint the bone tends to be 'soft', whereas if the patient has had previous surgery (e.g. upper tibial osteotomy) then the bone is more 'hard'.

An increasing number of patients are requiring revision surgery owing to implant failure from wear. The minimum life of a joint replacement should be 10 years, and many hip replacements can last over 20 years. The main factors determining implant life are surgical skill, bodyweight, life demands (working/not working) and levels of high-impact stress. There are many functional replacement hip joints that have been in place for up to 30 years. Hip replacements are now being used which have ceramic components, which do not wear as quickly.

General Principles

Patient selection

Many objective assessments have been devised, particularly for the hip and knee, to quantify the severity of a patient's problem. None is used universally or routinely, but they are valid tools for research purposes.

To manage their condition, most patients will have had drug therapy, minor procedures where indicated

Table 18.3 Metacarpophalangeal (MCP) joint replacement postoperative regimen.

Day 0–1
Elevation, antibiotics, pain relief.

Day 2
Immediate post-op dressing removed, wound inspection, drain removed.
POP slab replaced by thermoplastic night resting splint.

Day 3–5
Patient maintains elevation of the hand, pain relief as appropriate.

Day 5
Construction of dynamic extension splint.
Commencement of exercise programme

Day 6
Supervision of exercise regimen.
Arrangements for discharge, including ADL assessment.
Patient discharged home when needs have been met.

Day 14
Removal of sutures, splint check and adjustment if necessary, exercises checked.

Day 21
Attendance at therapy as outpatient.
Commence scar massage.
Teach new exercises:
■ Active flexion/extension with forearm mid-prone, hand resting on the table.
■ Radial abduction of fingers one by one with hand resting palm down on table (finger walking).

3–6 weeks
Patient attends minimum of once weekly to check/ progress exercise, carry out adjustments on splint, addition of extra splints to aid flexion range if necessary.

6 weeks
Cease use of dynamic splint if joints stable.
Commence light function
Provision of ulnar drift protection splint
Joint protection advice.

Source: Wrightington Hospital Hand and Upper Limb Surgery Unit.

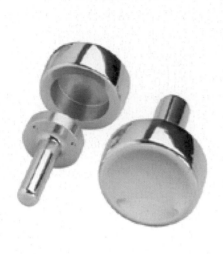
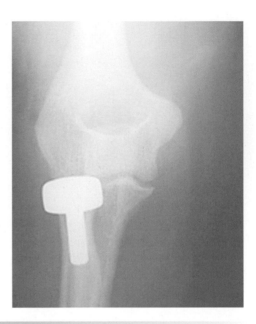

Figure 18.7 Radial head arthroplasty and the appearance on X-ray. (Reproduced by kind permission of Adam C. Gaines, Wright Medical Technology, TN, USA.)

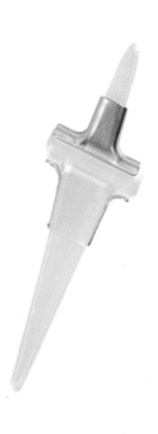
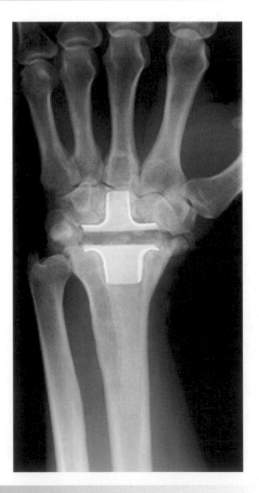

Figure 18.8 Wrist joint arthroplasty and the appearance on X-ray. (Reproduced by kind permission of Adam C. Gaines, Wright Medical Technology, TN, USA.)

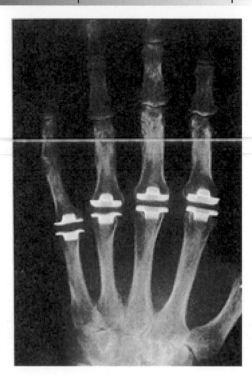

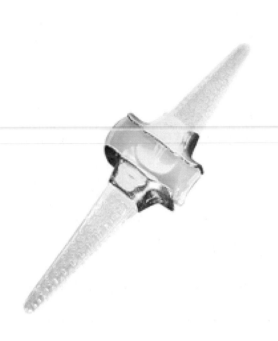

Figure 18.9   Swanson finger replacement and the appearance on X-ray. (Reproduced by kind permission of Adam C. Gaines, Wright Medical Technology, TN, USA.)

(particularly in the knee) and physiotherapy, including self-management programmes. Joint replacement is then the only option that will allow a return to an improved quality of life that is on the whole pain-free with good function.

Factors taken into account by the surgeon when listing a patient for surgery include:

- severity of disease – onset, progress, other joints affected, investigations

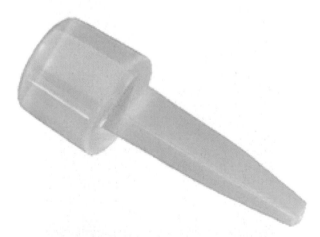

Figure 18.10   Trapezium replacement. (Reproduced by kind permission of Adam C. Gaines, Wright Medical Technology, TN, USA.)

- pain and sleep disturbance
- disability – effect on work and lifestyle
- age – given the life expectancy of the implants
- weight – keeping the implant stresses as low as possible
- emotional stability – less successful after shock or bereavement
- cognitive function.

Cognitive function needs to be assessed in relation to the pain relief gained by surgery set against the significant problem of potential failure.

Preoperative patient preparation

Any underlying medical condition must be stabilised prior to surgery. The GP is informed so that the appropriate steps can be taken, such as referral to a specialist for cardiac pathology.

The anaesthetist will review patients with significant medical history, decide the level of anaesthetic risk and, if possible, plan appropriate anaesthesia for the given procedure. Frequently spinal anaesthesia with peripheral blocks is used instead of a general anaesthetic and this does facilitate postoperative mobilisation, as the patient usually feels less unwell in the first couple of postoperative days.

As the date for surgery approaches, the patient is again reviewed by the preoperative staff to ascertain fitness for surgery. The physiotherapist assesses the patient for rehabilitation needs and walking aids, and gives instruction in movement procedures and exercises to practise. The occupational therapist will assess the patient for managing at home following discharge and can start the liaison with other agencies that can provide equipment and home help if required.

In specialist centres where the volume of patients is high, the multidisciplinary team may invite patients and their relatives to group information and preparation sessions that are more informal. The less medical environment reduces anxiety and facilitates learning. This preparation allows for speedy successful rehabilitation.

Biomechanical Considerations

Modern implants aim as far as possible to replicate the surfaces of the joint to be replaced. Experience has shown that failure to fully understand joint motion and to engineer components capable of tolerating the complex interplay of forces generated by muscle pull (a three-dimensional effect), ligaments, acceleration, deceleration, weight and gravity, will result in implant failure, pain and disability.

There has been much research into materials that are biologically inert, hard-wearing, with minimum coefficient of friction. This has led to the use today of components manufactured from metal alloys and high-density polyethylene.

Fixation of the components within the bone is again a complex issue, but most success is through pressurised cementing techniques or the use of hydroxyapatite-coated implants that enable a fibro-osseous fixation to develop as part of the bone healing process.

Complications of Surgery

Complications of joint replacement can be divided postoperatively into short-term (up to 8 weeks) and long-term (up to 18 months).

In the short term the complications are likely to be secondary to having a surgical intervention: deep-vein thrombosis (DVT), pulmonary embolism, chest infection, wound infection, heart dysfunction, paralytic ileus, and bleeding. Specific early orthopaedic complications include dislocation, deep infection, neuropraxia, and haematoma.

In the long term the complications include dislocation, joint infection, and procedure failure.

TOTAL HIP REPLACEMENT (THR)

The hip is the largest and deepest joint in the body. It takes the form of a multiaxial spheroidal joint with three degrees of freedom of movement with high levels of congruency (stability and surface area for stress transmission) and extensive range of movement.

The implant

The modern hip implant is a metal-alloy femoral head and stem (e.g. stainless steel, chromium cobalt) with a high-molecular-weight (high-density) polyethylene cup (Figure 18.11). Where the small head of the Charnley prosthesis is used the procedure is known as the 'low-friction arthroplasty' (LFA).

The Operation

The surgical approach to the hip joint depends on the surgeon's preference and impacts upon postoperative rehabilitation. Commonly used approaches include the lateral transtrochanteric division, necessitating trochanteric rewiring at closure, and posterolateral intermuscular division. The femoral neck is divided, the joint dislocated (where possible) and the head removed.

The femoral canal and acetabulum are reamed down to fresh bleeding bone and prepared for component implantation. Cavity size depends on the fixation technique.

If the components are to be cemented *in situ*, trial components are inserted and size/fit determined. These are then removed and quick-setting cement, available impregnated with antibiotics, is pushed into the cavities. The implants (with their surfaces protected) are pushed into the cement – a complete cement mantle between the implant and the bone is essential for even distribution of forces and therefore implant life/procedure success. Significant pressure is applied to ensure this.

The joint is then relocated and tested for stability. Once the surgeon is satisfied, the joint is adducted, flexed and medially rotated to dislocate the joint. The surface protection is removed from the implant, the joint relocated and closure commenced.

If the greater trochanter was sawn off for access, then it is rewired back on to the femur with specialised wiring techniques, developed to resist breaking.

Soft tissues are repaired in their layers, and deep and superficial drains may or may not be used. The patient is usually catheterised for fluid balance measurement in the early days. The patient has IV fluids and possibly patient-controlled analgesia (PCA) through a Venflon inserted into a hand or forearm vein. The operating time is usually about 90 minutes.

After the patient has been roused in the recovery room, heart and respiratory monitoring is continued

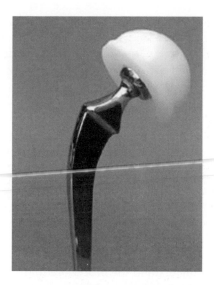

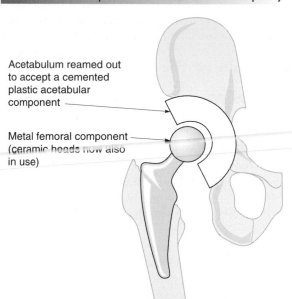

Acetabulum reamed out to accept a cemented plastic acetabular component

Metal femoral component (ceramic heads now also in use)

Figure 18.11   Total hip replacement. (Reproduced by kind permission of Medical Models Ltd, UK.)

for several hours. The patient is returned to the ward as soon as medically stable.

Figure 18.12 shows an X-ray of a total hip replacement.

Complications of Hip Replacement

No surgery can be totally effective and joint arthroplasty is no exception. In particular an artificial pros-

thesis has a finite lifespan. Hozack and Rothman (1990) examined causes of failure in a study of 1151 Charnley low-friction total hip arthroplasties performed as primary procedures. The figures below relate to 15-year failure probabilities:

- hip revision 13%
- cup revision 8%
- femoral revision 12%
- radiographic femoral loosening 13%
- radiographic cup loosening 49%.

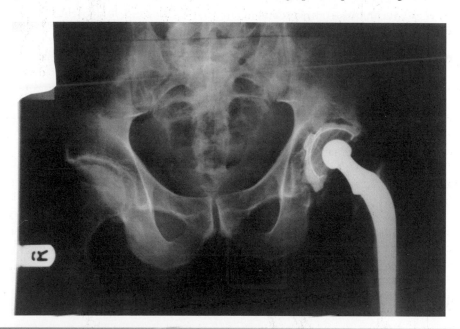

Figure 18.12   X-ray of a hip replacement.

Table 18.4 lists other complications and their possible solutions.

The Role of the Physiotherapist

The preoperative visit

The preoperative period is a busy time for all staff involved in patient care and a stressful time for the patient. Nevertheless there are many benefits to seeing the person before surgery, and even a brief visit will often be enough to allay the fears of the patient.

Hip replacement is now very commonplace and most people who come for the operation will know or will have spoken to someone who has already had a hip replaced. However, the fact that it is commonplace does not detract from the fact that it is still a major orthopaedic operation. People often have unrealistically high or unrealistically low expectations of the surgery. It is useful to provide the patient with written information sheets, and essential to avoid making unrealistic claims about the person's subsequent rehabilitation.

The preoperative visit allows the therapist to evaluate the person's current state of physical ability, including gait, aids used, activities of daily living, muscle strength, preoperative range of movement, housing, hobbies, function and so on.

Explain the operation only if necessary. Some people want to know a lot of detail about what is to follow, but others would rather not – you must respect their wishes in this respect.

Key point
It is vital for the physiotherapist to understand the procedure that the person is about to undergo, and the likely routine to be followed. Watching the operation at least once is useful.

Table 18.4 Complications of hip arthroplasty.

Complication	Caused by	Solution
Anaesthetic risk (chest, heart)	General anaesthetic	Careful preoperative anaesthetic assessment, spinal anaesthetic/epidural if necessary Appropriate respiratory physiotherapy
Infection	Open surgery	Prophylactic antibiotics post op. Operate in a Charnley tent
Dislocation	Difficult surgery, poor surgical technique, complex case, inherently unstable, e.g. if patient has had a CVA the risk of subsequent dislocation may be higher owing to decreased muscular stability at the hip joint	Abduction wedge, no adduction/flex beyond 90 degrees, special restraining acetabulum may be used in cases of previous dislocation
DVT/PE	Pelvic surgery, immobility Damage to the blood vessels during surgery	Prophylactic anticoagulants, early mobilisation by physiotherapists, release leg periodically during surgery to restore blood flow
Anaemia	Blood loss during/post surgery	Transfuse if haemoglobin (Hb) below 10
Swollen ankle	Ineffective muscle pump	Reassure, walk little and often, frequent rest in bed, compression stockings may help
Back pain	Unequal leg length or perceived by pelvis as unequal leg length	Reassure
Arm pain	Crutch walking	Time
Neck pain	Neck trauma due to neck being held in an extended position during the intubation	Time
Stiffness after immobility	Inflammatory exudate builds at rest	Reassure, walk little and often

Also at this stage, if there is time, practice walking with crutches or the appropriate walking aids, and show the person how to get in and out of bed properly (always on the operation side with no adduction of the limb). Other tasks may include preoperative respiratory physiotherapy as necessary.

Common questions asked by people about to undergo surgery

Will it hurt me?

Take care when answering this question. Although most people mobilise remarkably quickly, a hip or knee joint replacement is major orthopaedic surgery and it is unreasonable to say that the person will have no pain at all. A suggested answer is: 'You will probably experience some discomfort after your operation but your pain will be closely monitored by all staff, and you should not be afraid to call for attention if your pain does become severe.'

Typically a person who has undergone a joint replacement will not experience pain until the physiotherapist appears at the bedside! It is therefore in the best interests of patient, physiotherapist and other members of the healthcare team that the person's pain be controlled adequately. The timing of analgesia should be such that maximum pain relief occurs during mobilisation by the physiotherapist, and this requires close liaison between nursing staff and the physiotherapist.

Will it come out of its socket?

There is a small risk that a dislocation will occur following hip replacement. (Knee replacements do not carry the same potential problems of dislocation.) Reassure the person that you are aware of the risks and that you will take all appropriate steps to minimise them.

How long will I be in hospital?

The average stay for a first total hip replacement is probably between a week and 10 days. A person who is on bedrest following a revision (redo) will not fall into this category.

How will I manage to walk again?

Patients are understandably very anxious about how they are going to manage, especially after the first time out of bed when they might not do as well as they had hoped, or as well as the patient in the next bed. Encouragement is vital. Set realistic goals and explain the psychological benefits of walking slightly further each time. It may be necessary to explain that the person in the next bed had different surgery, or that it was performed earlier.

Do not underestimate the psychological benefit to the patient of a positive attitude on the part of the physiotherapist. Patients watch their therapist very closely for signs of impatience or disatisfaction with progress.

Can I put my weight on it?

This depends on the operation, the prosthesis, and the surgeon's instructions. The physiotherapist must know the routine for the unit, and certainly not guess.

Will the physio hurt me?

The nature of physiotherapy means that what we do often causes some discomfort. An important skill is to gain the confidence of the patient, and strike a balance between pushing the patient and being compassionate.

Will they let me use my frame?

If a person has used a frame for many years and only feels comfortable with it, then he or she should be allowed to use it as long as it is not contraindicated.

The immediate postoperative period

The patient usually returns from the theatre to the recovery ward until medically stable. The patients will have a drip *in situ* for a day or so, and this is usually removed once the patient is drinking properly. The patient sometimes has drainage tubes coming away from the operation site which are connected to vacuum drainage bottles; the purpose of these is to remove any haematoma from the area. These usually stay in for 48 hours and are simply pulled out with no need for anaesthetic.

The patient will have an abduction pillow in place to encourage the tissues to heal in the most stable position. Gallay et al. (1997) advocate use of anticoagulation therapy and this can be given up to 30 days post-op. However, use of pneumatic compression devices may rival the effectiveness of pharmacological prophylaxis (Hooker et al. 1999). The thromboprophylaxis debate continues.

There will be skin sutures which stay in place for 12–14 days. Fat sutures or tension sutures are deep and

Key point

After a few years in clinical practice, physiotherapists and allied health professionals may become blasé about procedures such as hip replacement. Never forget that most patients are very apprehensive.

connect to deep fascia and fatty layers; they usually remain in place for up to 7 days.

Physiotherapy includes active exercises for feet and ankles, isometric hip and knee contractions of all muscle groups, chest physiotherapy as necessary, advice on positioning, and mobility in the bed.

Patient mobilisation usually commences 24–48 hours postoperatively. Initially the patient will stand out of bed and take a few steps with crutches or another appropriate aid (usually partial weight-bearing). Walking distance is progressed daily until the patient is walking independently with crutches or a frame.

Routines vary, but patients usually commence sitting at 2–7 days (no adduction or flexion beyond 90 degrees), with stair practice before discharge if needed. Usually patients remain on crutches for 6 weeks, at which time they progress to sticks, then full weight-bearing.

Dos and dont's must be stressed to the patient (Table 18.5), and an educational booklet provided as a reminder. It is also important that occupational therapists and other members of the multidisciplinary team (MDT) see the patient.

Rehabilitation Protocol Following THR

Key point

All activity should be documented to the CSP documentation standards. MDT care pathways can also be completed – these aid effective communication between all staff, ensure all goals are met and allow for ease of service audit.

Day 1

There should be assessment by the physiotherapist of neurovasculomotor and respiratory systems. Active exercises for circulation and static exercises for muscle tone around the hip can be started, along with deep breathing exercises. Notes and X-rays should be studied as soon as available. Note the surgical approach and any non-standard procedure.

Day 2

Provided the surgeon is satisfied, mobilisation starts with the physiotherapist and assistant. The routine protocol can be followed.

The assistant prepares the environment and the patient and assists the patient from behind in bed transfers with the physiotherapist. A sliding sheet may be used in accordance with the moving and handling policy where the patient is heavy and/or has difficulty with transfers. Drains, catheters and drips are dealt with appropriately according to nursing policy.

The physiotherapist assists with the operated leg and ensures hip protection at all times. The patient is taught and reminded throughout the procedure of the hip protection measures required:

- partial weight-bearing
- limited flexion
- maintenance of some abduction
- no rotation.

Perch-sitting balance and standing balance are assessed. Mobilisation starts with three-point gait on elbow crutches, using a walking frame only if necessary initially. Distance is not important, patients being taken as far as their ability allows. Constant monitoring

Table 18.5 Dos and don'ts following total hip replacement.

DON'T
- Do not pick up any objects from the floor or reach into low cupboards. Use a reaching aid if possible
- Do not cross your legs.
- Do not force your hip to less than a right angle (knee towards chest).
- Do not sit on low chairs, low stools, or low toilets.
- Avoid sitting on chairs without arms. You may need to use the arms of the chair to help you to rise.
- When sitting, standing or lying down, do not allow your hip to rotate, keep your leg in a neutral position – toes pointing forwards.
- Move to the edge of the chair before you stand up (keep your operated leg straight at the knee).
- Do not lie on your side without a pillow placed between your legs.

DO
- Take your time when you get home.
- Rotate your activities, i.e. lie for short periods if you are very tired, walk little and often, sit for short periods.
- Set yourself small achievable targets with your walking.
- Pace yourself.
- Remember that you will get good days and bad days.
- It may be useful for you to keep a progress diary so that you can reflect back on your progress.

of the patient by observation and questioning is essential, as faintness is common and hazardous. The patient is returned to bed. This is done at least once per day, twice ideally.

Functional activities such as toilet procedure and sitting are taught in accordance with the surgeon's routine, usually from day 2 or 3. Advice as to length of time in sitting is given – no more than an hour at a time, perhaps at mealtimes – to try to limit leg swelling and subsequent discomfort in the initial weeks of recovery. Techniques to safely manage stairs, steps and ramps are taught according to the individual home circumstances.

Day 3 onwards

Mobility is progressed on a daily basis. The patient may be walked and instructed by two assistants, if his or her condition allows, then with one assistant until the patient is safe to mobilise unsupervised – i.e. has good dynamic balance, correct gait with walking aids, and is competent at hip protection. Advice as to amount of activity/rest is given up to walking hourly/bedrest morning and afternoon – the usual level for discharge.

Advice is given prior to discharge concerning expected levels of activity until clinic review. No other specific exercises are recommended during this period. Regular and gradually extended walking practice is necessary in/outdoors. Emphasis is on hip protection and recovery (effective capsular scarring). There are simply three golden rules:

1 Do not overbend the hip (flex beyond a right-angle).
2 Do not cross the leg over the mid line (adduct beyond neutral).
3 Do not twist in either standing or sitting.

These rules apply for 6 weeks in all cases. If the trochanter is to be protected then the rules apply for longer and it is generally accepted that the patient can return to normal activities at 3 months.

After discharge

If the soft-tissue approach was used the patient may be issued with sticks and advised to gradually increase weight-bearing over the next 6 weeks. If the transtrochanteric approach was used then the site of bony union must be protected for 12 weeks. The patient remains on elbow crutches for a minimum of 6 weeks but then can start to gradually increase weight-bearing until ready for full weight-bearing at 12 weeks, weaning from crutches to sticks/stick over that time. If the surgeon has used a cementless implantation then the patient is non weight-bearing (toe touch with elbow crutches – hopping is not safe) for 6 weeks, then partial weight-bearing for at least another 6 weeks. This allows for the ingrowth of fibroblasts into the hydroxyapatite coating.

A long-term rule is to avoid high-impact activities as sudden high pressures cause the most wear to the plastic. Plastic particulates have an exponential wear action that involves the alloy head and the cement mantle/bone interface. This process eventually means the patient needs a new hip arthroplasty – a revision procedure.

The patient may ring with queries following discharge but must contact the GP with any sudden significant pain or swelling.

Further physiotherapy/exercise may be required following clinic review and the appropriate referral can be made. Some centres offer outpatient rehabilitation programmes.

Rehabilitation following revision surgery

Depending on the reason for revision (commonly wear and loosening, fracture, infection, dislocation) and the complexity of the procedure, the physiotherapy as outlined above is modified appropriately in the light of the surgeon's instructions.

There is frequently augmentation of the bone required on the acetabular side – by bone grafting and in some cases the use of screws to hold the graft in place. The graft acts as scaffolding for migrating osteocytes which then lay down new bone.

Following any procedure that subsequently requires bony healing or union, the patient is mobilised following the non-weight-bearing protocol outlined above. It is common for the revision patient to need longer bedrest prior to mobilisation, and a slower rate of progression.

TOTAL KNEE REPLACEMENT (TKR)

The knee is a complex joint whose stability is dependent on extra-articular ligaments and muscular control. Knee problems usually present with gross biomechanical deformity requiring soft tissue release at operation in order to regain biomechanical alignment and normal soft-tissue lengths.

In the case of a severely deformed joint, physical constraint to movement can be incorporated by use of a moulded tibial implant. This will give increased inherent stability. The risk of failure secondary to its inability to move freely is less likely in the patient with low functional demand.

The implant

The implant uses metal-alloy components over the distal femur and proximal tibia. A high-molecular-weight (high-density) polyethylene bearing is inserted between (Figure 18.13). The patella may be resurfaced with a metal-alloy articulating button if necessary.

The Operation

Commonly a tourniquet is applied, the leg is exsanguinated and the tourniquet tightened for a timed period.

With the knee in flexion the surgical approach is on the whole by anterior skin incision followed by medial parapatellar incision through quadriceps expansion. The patella is reflected laterally and the joint exposed. Very rarely (and seen more in revision surgery) the tibial tuberosity has to be sawn off with a large piece of anterior tibial bone. This allows better access to the joint.

The femoral component is held in place by two short pegs cemented into each condyle and the tibial component by a large single peg into the tibia. The pressurised cementing technique as described previously for the hip replacement operation is used. Bone cuts and preparation followed by component trial is carried out. Closure of the joint is in layers.

The patient may or may not have drains inserted. A wool and crêpe bandage is applied to control oedema and a backsplint applied to maintain the knee in extension until quadriceps function is regained. The operating time is about 90 minutes.

Figure 18.14 shows an X-ray of a total knee replacement.

Rehabilitation Protocol Following TKR

The general postoperative physiotherapy is as previously described for hip replacement, except that the emphasis is on regaining quadriceps control. If the patient has had a femoral block for pain relief, active quadriceps function may take up to 24 hours to return.

Mobilisation and the start of the exercise programme commences on day 2. The patient starts to walk with two crutches, partial weight-bearing for 6 weeks. Transfer on to sticks is possible at any point during this time. It is a weaning process to full weight-bearing depending on the level of pain, bruising, swelling, muscle function and range of movement.

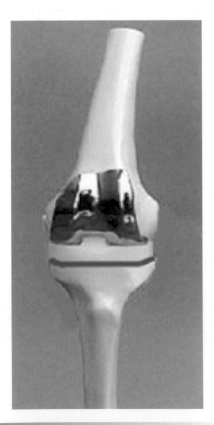

Figure 18.13 Total knee replacement. (Reproduced courtesy of Medical Models Ltd.)

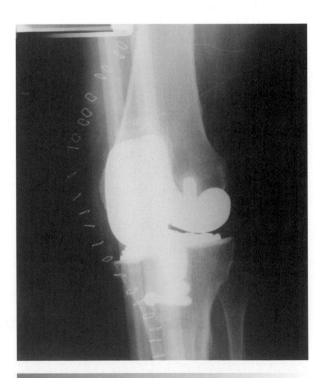

Figure 18.14 X-ray of a knee replacement.

Exercises are prescribed according to the surgeon's routine and the physiotherapeutic assessment of the patient. The splint and bandage must be removed prior to physiotherapy. It is vital that exercises be practised very regularly – little and often, almost hourly at first, progressing to several times per day of more differing exercises. It is paramount that quadriceps function be regained and therefore the control and protection of the joint established.

Common in the early phase is the use of simple equipment: closed-chain quadriceps over a sponge ball or in prone with toes tucked under, progressing to open-chain quadriceps over a wedge, and sliding boards for hamstrings. It is useful to provide the patient with a written exercise programme tailored to the individual's needs that can be adjusted and reviewed as progress continues.

Flexion is usually hampered by pain, fear, bruising and swelling. Physiotherapy should therefore include help in the control of these symptoms by reassurance, coordination with analgesia, cryotherapy and careful massage leading into assisted flexion. The patient can be instructed in the safe application of ice and massage at home. Do not forget that full extension is a vital component of knee joint function.

Length of hospital stay is usually 7–8 days, by which time the patient should be functionally independent and progressing with rehabilitation. Ideally the range of movement should be 0–90 degrees with active quadriceps – SLR with minimal lag.

On discharge most patients are referred for outpatient physiotherapy to review progress, continue with assisted exercises or start more advanced strengthening and mobilising workouts.

TOTAL ANKLE REPLACEMENT (TAR)

Total ankle replacement is the 'youngest' of the lower limb joint replacements. Attempts were made in the 1970s but were unsuccessful. There is now a semi-constrained implant that is working very successfully, although as yet there are insufficient numbers to compare outcomes with the knee or hip replacements.

Hind foot function and pain is closely related to both the function of the ankle joint and the subtalar joint. The success of a TAR will depend on the health of the subtalar joint below it. Often, particularly in people with rheumatoid arthritis, the diseased subtalar joint is fused (no replacement is currently available) prior to the TAR to give the optimum outcome.

The ankle joint is an anatomically constrained hinge joint. Particularly in this region the integrity of the circulation is vital and great care is taken in the selection of a patient in whom both circulation and skin can withstand the stress of operation and support the demands of the healing process.

The articular surfaces of the tibia and the talus are replaced with metal-alloy implants. The talar implant is centrally ridged forward to back to accommodate the sulcus on the inferior surface of the polyethylene bearing inserted between them (Figure 18.15). This allows for flexion and extension and decreases the risk of malleolar fracture by medial slip of the bearing.

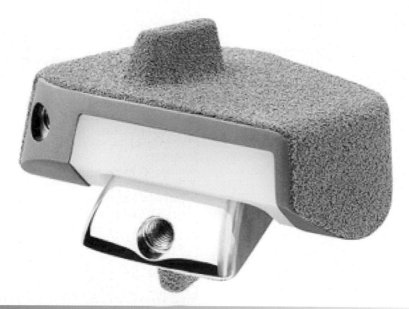

Figure 18.15   Ankle joint replacement. (Reproduced by kind permission of De Puy Orthopaedics Inc., IN, USA.)

The Operation

Approach to the joint is via a 10 cm anterior incision. Care is taken to avoid the anterior tibial neurovascular bundle. The bones are cut and prepared as previously described. The implant is usually uncemented; the components being hammered into place. The tissues are closed in layers and compression dressing applied.

The patient is roused and nursed as previously described, the limb maintained in elevation.

Rehabilitation Protocol Following TAR

Postoperative physiotherapy is as previously described for hip and knee replacements, except that routine ankle exercises are avoided and toe exercises substituted. It is necessary for the physiotherapist to ensure dorsiflexion to a right-angle (plantigrade) and where this is difficult to show the patient an appropriate stretch exercise with a strap.

Mobilisation is usually on day 3 or 4 when the swelling is controlled and the compression dressings removed, according to the surgeon's instructions. A protective knee-length plastic boot that can be removed for wound inspection can be fitted and the patient mobilised in partial weight-bearing with elbow crutches for functional requirements only (the leg is rested in elevation otherwise). Techniques to manage stairs/steps/ramps are taught.

The length of stay is usually 5–6 days. The patient is reviewed in clinic at 3 weeks for removal of sutures and the plastic boot. Exercises can be started at this point to facilitate rehabilitation, including Achilles tendon stretches, muscle strengthening and balance function. Specific moilisation of the ankle is avoided.

FURTHER READING

Atkinson K, Coutts F, Hassenkamp A-M 1999 Physiotherapy in Orthopaedics: a Problem Solving Approach. Edinburgh: Churchill Livingstone

Birch A, Gwillian L 2000 Rheumatoid arthritis and its effects on the hand. In Salter M, Cheshire L (eds) Hand Therapy Principle and Practice. Oxford: Butterworth–Heinemann

Mackin JM, Callahan AD, Skirven TM Schneider LH, Osterman AL (eds) Rehabilitation of the Hand and Upper Extremity, 5th edn. St Louis: CV Mosby

Simmen BR, Allieu Y, Luch A, Stanley J (eds) 2001 Hand Arthroplasties. London: Martin Dunitz

REFERENCES

Bizot P, Banallec L et al. 2000 Alumina-on-alumina total hip prostheses in patients 40 years of age or younger. Clin Orthop 379: 68–76

Brander VA, Malhotra S et al. 1997 Outcome of hip and knee arthroplasty in persons aged 80 years and older. Clin Orthop 345: 67–78

Delaney R, Stanley JK 2000 A prospective study of range of movement following metacarpophalangeal joint replacements: optimum time of recovery. Br H Hand Ther 5(3): 85–7

Gallay S, Waddell JP et al. 1997 A short course of low-molecular-weight heparin to prevent deep venous thrombosis after elective total hip replacement. Can J Surg 40(2): 119–23

Godenèche A, Boileau P, Favard L et al. 2002 Prosthetic replacement in the treatment of osteoarthritis of the shoulder: early results of 268 cases. J Should Elbow Surg 11(1): 11–18

Hamblen DL 1984 History of Shoulder Replacement. University of Glasgow Department of Orthopaedics Study Day, 13th January 1984, printed by 3M Healthcare, Bracknell

Hooker JA, Lachiewicz PF et al. 1999 Efficacy of prophylaxis against thromboembolism with intermittent pneumatic compression after primary and revision total hip arthroplasty. J Bone Joint Surg Am 81: 690–6

Hozack WJ, Rothman RH 1990 Long-term survival of the Charnley low-friction total hip arthroplasty. Semin Arthroplasty 1(1): 3–6

Iannotti JP, Williams GR 1998 Total shoulder arthroplasty: factors influencing prosthetic design. Ortho Clinics N Am 29: 377–91

Mackay DC, Hudson B, Williams JR 2001 Which primary shoulder and elbow replacement? A review of the results of prostheses available in the UK. Ann R Coll Surg Engl 83: 258–65

Mackay DC, Williams J 1999 A Survey of Elbow and Shoulder Surgeons in the UK. Sheffield: British Elbow & Shoulder Society

Neer CS, Watson KC, Stanto FJ 1982 Recent experience in total shoulder replacement. J Bone Joint Surg 64A: 319–37

Swanson AB, Swanson G de G, Leonard J 1978 Postoperative rehabilitation program in flexible implant arthroplasty of the digits. In Hunter JM, Schneider LH, Mackin EJ, Bell JA (eds) Rehabilitation of the Hand, pp 477–81. St Louis: CV Mosby

Swanson AB, Swanson G de G, DeHeer DH 2000 Small joint implant arthroplasty: 38 years of research experience. In Simmen BR, Allieu Y, Luch A, Stanley J (eds) Hand Arthroplasties. London: Martin Dunitz

Tissue Inflammation and Repair

Elaine N. Court and Robert W. Lea

19

INTRODUCTION

Physiotherapists encounter inflammation or its consequences daily, and it can be considered as both a blessing and a curse. Without it, sprained ankles would never resolve and wounds would never heal. But if the inflammatory response is prolonged or out of proportion to the original injury or disease, that poses problems. It could result in excessive scar tissue, adhesions, prolonged pain and loss of function.

Key point

Inflammation is not relevant only to the sphere of musculoskeletal physiotherapy. A person who has sustained a head injury or has chronic bronchitis, or has had a heart transplant, will also experience the inflammatory process.

Knowledge of the process and clinical features of inflammation is vital for a physiotherapist to effectively evaluate the degree or stage of a disease. If a reasoned treatment plan is to be constructed it must take into account the severity, nature and irritability of an injury (see Chapter 2 on musculoskeletal assessment). It is also useful for the physiotherapist to be able to confidently reassure patients that the symptoms they are experiencing are part of the normal healing process (for example that all surgical scars will show some signs of inflammation).

Our knowledge of inflammation goes back thousands of years. Certainly the condition was well recognized by the ancient Greeks and Romans. In fact, four components of inflammation described by Cornelius Celsius, a Roman physician as early as the first century AD, are still regarded as forming the classical clinical signs. These comprise 'calor', indicating heat (relevant primarily to inflammation of the skin); 'rubor', redness; 'dolor', pain; and 'tumor', swelling (Figure 19.1). These signs are indicative of the extravasation of plasma and infiltration of leucocytes at the site of inflammation. Later a fifth sign described by Virchow as 'Functio laesa', relating to loss of function was added.

If humans are to survive it is necessary for our bodies to maintain a constant internal environment, a process known as *homeostasis*. The environment, however, contains a multitude of potential dangers, biological, chemical and physical, which are likely to disrupt this delicate balance. As a result, by the process of evolution we have had to develop a complex defence mechanism against these potential insults, which is able to become activated and effective within seconds. A key component of this response is known by the term 'inflammation'.

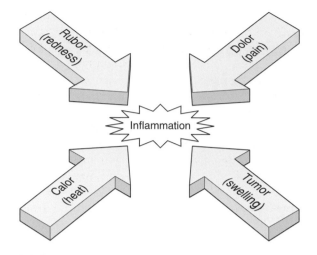

Figure 19.1   Components of inflammation.

Inflammation is the immune system's response to tissue damage. The processes involved will occur whether the damage is due to an exogenous source such as a cut or burn or to endogenous failures such as a bone fracture. The principal aim behind inflammation is to repair the tissue and bring it back to its original state.

Inflammation occurs in response to tissue damage whatever that damage may be, so it is wrong to equate it with 'infection'. This is illustrated by the situations of stress or trauma where there is no infection, yet still inflammation occurs. Similarly there are numerous situations where an infectious agent does not produce inflammation – for example in Creutzfeldt–Jacob disease (CJD).

Inflammation has often been described as a complex stereotypical reaction of vascularised living tissue to local trauma. In those regions of the body that do not receive a full blood supply, such as the cornea, a true inflammatory response does not occur, though few would deny that inflammation can be present.

This chapter will describe the process involved in an inflammatory response and how it impacts upon the body. Bear in mind that when it occurs for only a short period of time inflammation is a very beneficial sequence of events for the body. Inflammation is an attempt to eliminate antigens and damaged tissue; indeed in most instances it will probably be occurring without you having any real awareness of the situation. If, however, your body encounters an unusually large amount of antigen or that antigen is either difficult to digest or is sited within an awkward location, or alternatively if the inflammatory process fails to terminate, then clinical inflammation can be observed.

These symptoms are easy to visualise if for example you have just damaged a finger. There are situations, however, where damage is less obvious and so the clinician will need to recognise a number of characteristic symptoms that indicate the patient has inflammation. The pulse rate is increased, with an associated fever and feeling of general tiredness, and often there is the sensation of pain which is localised in the affected area. For example, in appendicitis the sufferer will experience pain in the right iliac fossa. Upon further investigation, blood tests will reveal a raised neutrophil cell count together with an increase in the concentration of acute-phase proteins (discussed later in the chapter).

TYPES OF INFLAMMATION

Key point
Inflammation is usually subdivided into two types, acute and chronic. The terms relate to the duration of the inflammation and to the nature of the inflammatory response.

Acute inflammation usually lasts for only a few hours to a few days. By the end of this time the accumulated fluid and degraded proteins in the extracellular spaces will have been drained by the lymphatic system, the phagocytic cells will have removed the exudates, debris and fibrin, and the inflammatory cells themselves will undergo cell death or 'apoptosis'. In this way the tissues return to normal. Acute inflammation may be seen, for example, following a surgical incision.

Chronic inflammation is characterised by a persistence of the inflammation usually beyond 10–14 days and is accompanied in most instances by fibrosis (the accumulation of synthesised collagen in the tissue). Chronic inflammation can occur, for instance, when the described resolution to the acute inflammatory process is not achieved, possibly through the causative agent not being removed; hence the inflammation becomes prolonged. Chronic inflammation can, however, arise as a low-grade inflammatory process without a preceding acute phase. Rheumatoid arthritis is an example of a chronic inflammatory condition.

ACUTE INFLAMMATION: THE MECHANISMS

Phases of Acute Inflammation

Three processes are responsible for giving the previously described symptoms involved in acute inflammation.

Firstly there is a *vascular component* where there is a significant change in blood flow due to dilation of blood vessels and consequently the amount of blood constituents reaching the affected site. The changes making up this vascular component were described in 1927 by Lewis and are known as the *Lewis triple response*. This flush, flare and wheal effect can be demonstrated by drawing a blunt instrument firmly across the skin (for convenience the forearm is often used) and watching the following sequence of events, which are similar irrespective of the type of injury:

1 Instantly a white line forms following the 'injury'. This is due to vasoconstriction of the underlying arterioles as a direct response to the injury and is only transient. This vasoconstriction is not considered to be fully part of the inflammatory process.
2 There rapidly follows a flush, seen as a dull red line which occurs as the capillaries dilate. To the naked eye, the vasodilation can give the impression that the affected tissue actually contains a greater number of blood vessels. This dilation may last for as long as the inflammatory process persists.
3 An irregular red zone develops called the flare. This occurs owing to the response of the surrounding arterioles, which have been affected by both nervous and chemical mediators.
4 A 'wheal' (a raised area of skin) develops owing to the fluid passing out of the blood vessels and into the extravascular space, so leading to oedema.

Secondly (though it occurs at the same time as the above process) the endothelial cells which form the internal wall of the blood vessels retract such that they no longer form a completely continuous lining of the vessel. Consequently, the vessels become 'leaky' to the extent that fluid – namely water and some of the salts and smaller proteins (one of these is fibrinogen) contained in plasma – may pass out directly into the extracellular spaces of the damaged area.

Thirdly, the fluid exudate becomes transformed into a cellular exudate. This is achieved through circulating neutrophils leaving the blood vessels and entering the extracellular spaces in the area of tissue damage. In the first 6–24 hours of an inflammatory response it is the neutrophils which predominate. After 24–48 hours they are superseded by monocytes and lymphocytes acting in a similar way.

Detailed Consideration of Acute Inflammation

Initiating events

The tissue becomes physically damaged and may in addition become exposed to micro-organisms as a result of that damage. A complex sequence of events then occurs in which various mediators are released in order to orchestrate the inflammatory response.

At the site of the tissue damage, three cytokines IL-1α, TNFα and IL-6 are released. These in turn cause the generation of the lipid mediator PGE_2 which is believed to act on the hypothalamus so leading to the rise in body temperature that is often seen with inflammation. This rise in body temperature inhibits the growth of many pathogens and appears to enhance the immune response to the pathogen.

Among the other chemical mediators released in response to tissue damage are various serum proteins known as *acute-phase proteins*. The concentrations of these proteins can increase from between 50% to several-fold over normal levels when there are tissue-damaging infections present. Acute-phase proteins have a wide range of activities; they can neutralise inflammatory cells, help to minimise the extent of local tissue damage and participate in tissue repair and regeneration.

A major acute-phase protein produced by the liver is C-reactive protein. C-reactive protein binds to the C-polysaccharide cell-wall component found on a variety of bacteria and fungi. This binding will activate the complement system (a series of inactive proteins normally present within the blood), which leads to an increased clearance of the pathogen. Other acute-phase proteins include components of the complement cascade, and fibrinogen along with some metal-binding proteins which act to prevent iron loss during infection and injury and additionally minimise the level of haem iron available for uptake by bacteria.

Events at the site of damage

The initial response of the arterioles is vaso*constriction*, but this is transient and the major influence on the circulation is that of vaso*dilation*. Vasodilation can be induced by the activation of complement so leading to the production of the anaphylatoxins C3a and C5a (Figure 19.2).

As mentioned earlier, IL-1α, TNFα and IL-6 are released from the damaged tissue. These, along with released histamine and other mediators, induce vasodilation and increased capillary permeability.

Vasodilation

The vasodilation resulting from injury will depend on the level of damage, and it may last from 15 minutes to many hours. This vasodilation can increase blood flow to the area by up to 10-fold, so providing the appropriate cells and chemicals to the area ready to assist in the inflammatory response.

Increased capillary permeability

Fluid normally passes out of small blood vessels by a process of microfiltration, because of the high hydrostatic pressure at the arteriolar end of the capillaries. Owing to the loss of the fluid, but not large molecules and cells, the colloid osmotic pressure within the capillaries increases. This, coupled with the reduction of hydrostatic pressure at the venous ends of the capillaries, results in the fluid originally removed being returned from the extravascular space into the venous ends of the capillaries (Figure 19.3).

In an inflammatory situation, it is not just fluid that is lost from the vasculature. The retraction of endothelial cells causes intracellular gaps through which larger molecules can pass into the extravascular space. The loss of proteins such as complement factors and immunoglobulins not only assists in the destruction of invading micro-organisms, but also results in the colloid osmotic pressure not being increased as much as normally. Consequently there is no 'driving force' to ensure the re-entry of fluid back into the vasculature, so fluid will remain at the inflammatory site leading to oedema (swelling).

The exudate produced does not just remain at the inflammatory focus. It is drained by the lymphatic channels but is replaced by new exudate. Hence the oedema persists.

Cell migration

In the normal situation for any blood vessels larger than capillaries, blood cells (including the leucocytes) are kept away from the vessel walls by circulating within the central region of the blood vessel. The area around the vessel wall is in contact with mainly plasma. When there is vasodilation (and increased capillary permeability) the rate of blood flow decreases, so allowing the blood cells to begin to flow nearer to the endothelium. As a result of this, granulocytes (e.g. neutrophils) come into contact with the endothelium.

The initial events leading to the production of mediators (e.g. activated complement fragments or cytokines that activate the leucocyte and/or endothelial cells) cause specific complementary molecules to be produced on both the granulocytes (particularly phagocytes) and endothelium, so allowing them to adhere. As a consequence of activation, one or both cell types become adhesive, leading initially to transient adherence and rolling of the granulocytes along the endothelium (Figure 19.4). This is known as *margination*. With the production of further molecules the granulocytes will become more firmly attached (stick-

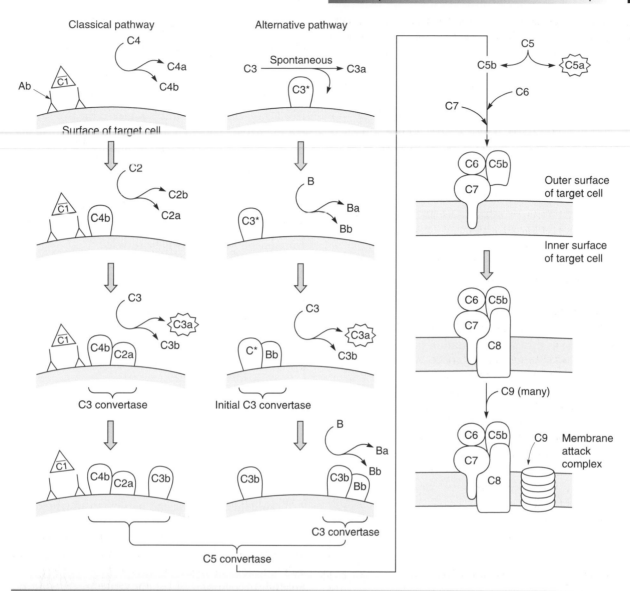

Figure 19.2   Activation of complement. This can be achieved through the activation of the classical pathway (where Ab, either one immunoglobulin (Ig) M is bound, or two IgG molecules are bound in close proximity to one another), as shown on the left-hand side of the figure. This leads to the production of the activated complement factor 1 complex C1 (⌂). The alternative pathway (which is initiated by spontaneous decay of C3 but which is unable to continue unless there are specific sites for C* – a C3b-like molecule – to bind with on the target cell) is shown on the right.

Whichever pathway is used, a cascade of events occurs such that the activation of one complement protein leads to the activation of the next, and so it continues. Once the C5 convertase complex has been formed, the production of the membrane attack complex (where a hole is inserted through the target cell) occurs through the same process, whichever was the initiating pathway.

C3a and C5a are anaphylatoxins, small molecules which can diffuse away from the area. Anaphylatoxins have the ability to cause aggregation of platelets, extravasion and chemotaxis of neutrophils and monocytes, and degranulation of eosinophils, mast cells and basophils – which in turn leads to the release of many mediators including histamine. The released histamine will induce contraction of smooth muscle and an increased vascular permeability. All these are powerful events in the inflammatory process.

ing) to the adhesion molecules produced by the endothelium, and in this 'fixed' position the granulocytes will produce pseudopodia which enable them to pass through the wall of the endothelium (through the junctions between the cells) – a process known as *emigration*. In this way the cells are able to gain access to the damaged tissue and any 'invaders' which have occupied the tissue.

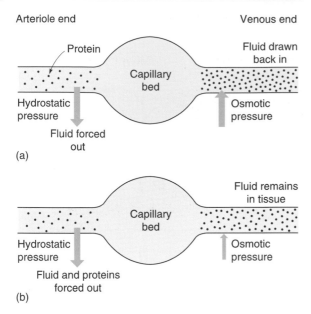

Figure 19.3 Generation of oedema in inflamed tissue. (a) In the normal situation the removal of fluid into the extravascular space at the arteriole end of the capillary bed is balanced by its return to the vasculature at the venule end of the bed. (b) When inflamed, the removal of proteins as well as fluid at the arteriole end of the vascular bed means the driving force for the return of the fluid is not generated, so fluid remains within the tissue.

Phagocytosis

Definitions

Phagocytosis is the ingestion and destruction by certain cells (phagocytic cells) of other cellular or particulate material.

Chemotaxis is the process through which phagocytic cells are attracted to a substance and then follow the concentration gradient from an area of low concentration moving towards a high concentration.

Once the phagocytic cells have migrated across the blood vessel wall, chemotactic signals direct the movement of the cells to their required site of action.

A number of chemical factors are known to stimulate leucocyte chemotaxis; examples are the anaphylatoxin C5a (see Figure 19.2), platelet-activating factor (PAF) and leukotriene B_4 (LTB_4). All of these agents act through G-protein coupled receptors and cause the movement of the phagocytic cells towards the target area.

On reaching the site of action, the granulocytes (particularly neutrophils) may encounter, for example, damaged tissue or bacteria, either of which will need to

be removed. This is achieved by the process of phagocytosis or, for material that is large or difficult to engulf, the release of substances from the phagocytic cell so leading to extracellular killing. Phagocytosis is achieved by the phagocyte using amoeboid-like movements of its plasma membrane to encircle the foreign material (see Figure 19.4). Once this is achieved the two sides of the membrane combine to form a phagocytic *vacuole* (also known as *phagosome*). The phagosome then fuses with a lysosome within the cell to form a *phagolysosome*. The lysosome contains powerful enzymes which, coupled with the various reactive oxygen species generated, will now come into contact with the unwanted material, causing it to be broken down. Any usable components produced will be recycled.

In order to assist phagocytosis it is common for opsonisation of the particles to take place.

Definition

Opsonisation is the process whereby a particle becomes coated in another substance, so making it more open to phagocytosis.

One example of an opsonin is generated due to the presence of lipopolysaccharides in the cell wall which activate the alternative complement pathway. As a result of this activation C3b is generated and binds to the surface of the bacteria (see Figure 19.2). The phagocyte contains receptors which will bind to the C3b; this will cause the phagocyte and particle to adhere to one another, so assisting the engulfment process.

A second example of an opsonin is the binding of antibody (immunoglobulin G, IgG) to the particle. The IgG binds owing to the presence of its variable regions enabling recognition of specific structures present on the bacterium (known as *antigenic determinants*). Once bound by the variable regions (Fab) of the IgG, this effectively labels the bacterium hence the exposed constant region of the antibody (Fc) is able to bind to complementary receptors on the phagocyte, again allowing adherence between the phagocyte and bacterium which will assist engulfment. These two systems can work in concert, as the binding of two IgG molecules in close proximity with one another will enable the activation of the classical complement pathway, which in turn causes the generation of C3b (see Figure 19.2) which binds to the cell, so aiding opsonisation.

For particles unsuitable for ingestion, possibly because they are too large, the phagocyte will use extracellular killing to remove the agent from the system. In this situation the contents of the lysosome are released into the vicinity of the unwanted agent. Whilst this can be an effective means of killing unwanted bacteria, the

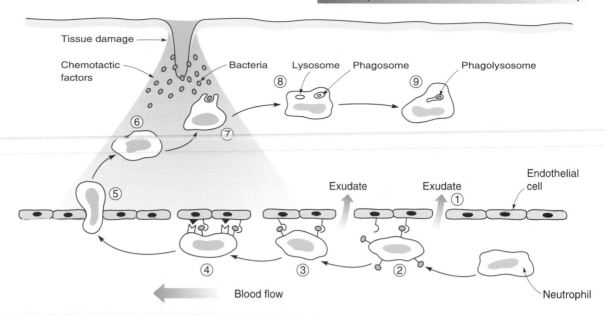

Figure 19.4 Schematic illustrating neutrophil margination, emigration, chemotactic attraction and phagocytosis in an inflammatory response. [1] Increased vascular permeability causes fluid to leave the blood vessel. [2] The neutrophils now circulate closer to the endothelium, where the release of TNFα will have caused the production of P- and E-selectins (adhesion molecules) to be synthesised and placed on the surface of endothelial cells. At the same time a complementary adhesion molecule will be generated by the neutrophil. [3] With the aid of the adhesion molecules the neutrophil will start to roll along the endothelium. [4] With the addition of further adhesion molecules, IL-8 receptor on the neutrophil and ICAM-1 on the endothelium, the neutrophil will become firmly fixed. [5] Diapedesis enables the neutrophil to leave the blood vessel. [6] Following the concentration gradient of the chemotactic factors, the neutrophil will approach the site of tissue damage. [7] On encountering material (e.g. bacteria) to be engulfed, the neutrophil produces pseudopodia to encircle the substance. [8] A vacuole is formed within the phagocyte containing the bacteria. [9] A lysosome will fuse with the phagosome so enabling the engulfed material to be broken down.

environment is not as controlled as in the phagolysosome and consequently the agents released can act on surrounding healthy tissue.

To illustrate this, consider two enzymes which are released, elastase and collagenases, which will hydrolyse proteins in bacterial cell envelopes so leading to death of the bacterium. The elastases can also use collagen cross-linkages and proteoglycans as substrates along with elastin components of blood vessels, ligaments and cartilage. Collagenases are active in cleaving type I and, to a lesser degree, type III collagen from bone, cartilage and tendon. Thus although the body does have some defence mechanisms in place to help protect it from the damaging effects of the agents released from the phagocytes, these mechanisms can become overwhelmed, leading to damage of otherwise healthy tissue.

Benefits and Drawbacks of the Inflammatory Response

Benefits

The initial passage of fluid exudate into the surrounding damaged tissue immediately delivers further nutrients and oxygen to the damaged site. This extra energy will be vital for any of the body's immune cells which will arrive later. The fluid exudate also has the action of diluting any possible toxins, such as may be produced by certain bacteria, and allows them to be disposed of through the lymphatic system. The exudate may also contain certain specific immunoglobulins that are able to bind with and neutralise potentially harmful pathogens and toxins.

The fibrinogen, which is also contained within this exudate, will initiate fibrin formation. Such an action helps to block the possible movement of micro-organisms and helps to facilitate the chances of these organisms being phagocytosed on the arrival of the body's immune cells.

Drawbacks

The consequent cellular exudate is primarily composed of neutrophils. This cell type is relatively short-lived, perhaps lasting for about only two weeks, so they must be constantly replaced. Neutrophils are designed chiefly for the phagocytosis of invading micro-organisms and any associated cell debris, and for this reason they contain a number of lysosomal enzymes (as described earlier). In the inflammatory situation, either as a deliberate release process (as described earlier) or perhaps following the death of the neutrophil, these cells may release these lysosomal enzymes. A beneficial consequence of this would be assistance in the digestion of the inflammatory exudate. However, such a release can be harmful in that some of the enzymes may digest normal tissue and result in considerable 'collateral' tissue damage.

In certain situations, swelling of the tissue can cause serious restriction of some of the body's vital actions. One example of this is in *Haemophilus influenzae* infection. Particularly in children, this bacterium can cause epiglottitis (considerable swelling of the epiglottis), which can result in obstruction of the airway.

Inflammatory swelling is very serious whenever it occurs in an otherwise restricted area, such as the skull. For this reason acute meningitis (perhaps again caused by *H. influenzae*) may lead to increased intracranial pressure, impairment of the blood flow to the brain, and so ischaemic damage to the brain.

FORMS OF ACUTE INFLAMMATION

Although the term 'inflammation' applies to the processes involved, as outlined in the previous section, the clinical appearance of acute inflammation will vary according to the type of tissue involved. Consequently a number of terms are employed to describe these different forms of inflammation.

Serous inflammation

Perhaps the most commonly observed instance of serous inflammation is a blister caused by a burn, or by the rubbing of an ill-fitting shoe. This form of inflammation is typically characterised by the production of copious exudate, which upon analysis is relatively scarce in cells but which contains comparatively high concentrations of protein.

The source of this fluid may be either plasma (as in the above examples), or the mesothelial cells which line the peritoneal, pleural and pericardial cavities and synovial tissue. Inflammation of this type may be seen, for example, in cases such as acute synovitis, in which the synovial joint is affected, or in peritonitis. In some situations such as conjunctivitis occurring as a response to either a viral or allergic assault (leading to the production of a serous exudate), the typical inflammatory vasodilation is clearly visible in the form of 'bloodshot' eyes.

Catarrhal inflammation

Acute inflammation of mucous membranes results in the production of a large amount of mucinous (mucus) secretion, the condition being classified as 'catarrhal'. Examples of areas affected are the nasopharynx, lungs, gastrointestinal tract or mucus-secreting glands elsewhere. In tissues it can be seen as large amounts of amorphous stringy material containing some white blood cells, whilst the underlying mucosa shows distension of glands. Probably the best example of such a condition is the common cold.

Fibrinous inflammation

As previously described, the formation of a plasma protein-rich fluid exudate is common in inflammation. When the predominant protein present is fibrinogen then fibrinous inflammation can occur. Fibrinogen is a large molecule so it requires more severe inflammation if it is to leave the vasculature.

Upon activation of the coagulation process, fibrinogen has the ability to polymerise to form sticky, solid fibrin. This rubbery fibrin may be visible as a variable number of yellow–white strands, or even as thick sheets, which stick out from the surface of the affected site with an irregular (shaggy-like) surface. Fibrinous inflammation is commonly associated with mucosal and serosal membranes and particularly with the pleura and pericardium.

This type of inflammation can be characteristically present in pericarditis, which may for example occur as a result of rheumatic fever. In this instance the heart is affected and the parietal and visceral pericardium take on a peculiar appearance often described as 'bread and butter'. Another common situation where this type of inflammation is usually present in pneumococcal pneumonias.

Haemorrhagic inflammation

In situations where, for some reason, there is a deficiency in those compounds in the plasma responsible for coagulation, or perhaps where vascular damage is very severe, red blood cells may leave the vessels either through the damaged area or by a process of passive diapedesis, so resulting in haemorrhagic inflammation. Examples of where this might be observed are in meningococcal septicaemia and acute pancreatitis.

This type of inflammation is commonly found mixed with another form, usually either suppurative or fibrinous, or indeed both.

Suppurative inflammation

Suppurative inflammation is also referred to as 'purulent' inflammation, and occurs when there is evidence of copious amounts of pus (or purulent exudate) present. Pus can vary in appearance from yellow–white to grey and from watery to viscous in consistency. Essentially, however, pus consists of some of the damaged tissues, which have become liquefied by the actions of proteolytic enzymes, together with those cells, particularly neutrophils, which had invaded the area and are now dead or dying themselves along with the inflammatory exudate. Such inflammation may occur following infection by a pyogenic organism such as *Staphylococcus*, *Pneumococcus* or *Escherichia coli*.

When a localized collection of pus occurs in a tissue or organ where it has been contained in a membrane of fibrous tissue, then an abscess may be formed. Certain chemicals such as turpentine, and micro-organisms such as *Staphylococcus*, tend to elicit abscesses. Usually as the abscess progresses the pressure from the pus will advance in the line of least resistance, so forming a 'point' (fortunately this tracking is usually towards the surface of the body). This 'point' will then burst, allowing the cavity to empty and allowing scar formation in a healing process. On occasion surgical intervention is necessary – the abscess (or boil) is lanced and the pus drained.

If the abscess is deep-seated, pus may also form inside a hollow viscus, such as those found in the appendix or gallbladder. Alternatively a lung infection can spread and lead to the accumulation of pus within the pleural space. Such a condition is described as *empyema* and it can even arise in the subdural cavity in the brain where it is a significant cause of neurological morbidity and mortality.

Occasionally the pointing of the abscess does not result in tracking towards the surface of the body. When this happens, so-called 'sinus tracts' are sometimes formed which may, for example, spread along the course of veins or in subcutaneous structures. When formed between bone and periosteum, the 'pointing' of the abscess can clearly be hindered and so it tends to result in direct pressure being exerted on the resisting tissue or may result in the blood supply being cut off to the area. This then allows for sloughing of the parts covering the abscess, and so the pus eventually makes its way through sinus tracts to another cavity. An example of this type of situation is in *Neisseria gonorrhoeae* infection, when it is possible for the abscess to arise in the endometrial cavity and discharge into the peritoneal cavity.

Abscesses will also occasionally form deep in striated muscles, as in the condition *pyromyositis*. In this case the muscle has become infected by pus-producing bacteria, by the bacteria spreading either from a nearby infection in a bone or other tissue or through the bloodstream from a distant part of the body. Pyomyositis is more common among people in the tropics but it can also occur in immunocompromised individuals, especially those with AIDS. The muscles most commonly affected are in the thighs, buttocks, upper arms and around the shoulders. Symptoms include cramping pain followed by swelling, mild fever, and increasing discomfort, especially when the infected muscle is moved.

Pseudomembranous inflammation

If an inflamed mucosal surface becomes covered by a layer of fibrin, inflammatory cells and necrotic debris, then it can appear as if this has formed a membrane over the affected area – hence the term pseudomembranous inflammation. It occurs on mucosal surfaces such as the pharynx, larynx and other respiratory passages, as well as in the digestive tract. Pseudomembranous inflammation could occur, for instance, following heavy antibiotic therapy which destroys normal flora in the patient's bowels, so allowing colonisation by *Clostridium difficile* – in this case it is known as *pseudomembraneous colitis*.

Gangrenous or necrotising inflammation

In this situation the exudate is dominated by the accumulation or induction of tissue necrosis without appreciable fluid or cell exudation. Necrotising inflammation can be observed in many toxic injuries to the gastrointestinal tract or in diseases that induce arterial thrombosis. Oedema produces pressure increases in the surrounding tissues which in certain situations may lead to closure (occlusion) of the associated blood vessels. This lack of blood supply (and consequently the lack of nutrients which it would normally supply) inevitably leads to widespread necrosis of the tissue. This, together with bacterial invasion, can result in tissue putrefaction, which materialises as gangrene. The above situation arises when the necrotising inflammatory reaction occurs on an epithelial surface; hence it may produce a defect in the epithelium to the level of the basement membrane.

Key point

When epithelial defects occur to levels below the basement membrane, they are referred to as *ulcers*, and the corresponding inflammatory reaction is referred to as *ulcerative*. Ulcers are local defects on the surface of an organ or tissue that have been produced by the sloughing of inflammatory necrotic tissue.

CHRONIC INFLAMMATION

Whereas acute inflammation is characterised by changes in the vasculature and the production of exudate (both fluid and cellular), in chronic inflammation this exudation is less obvious. Chronic inflammation is characterised more by changes in cell and connective tissue proliferation.

Forms of Chronic Inflammation

Key point
Chronic inflammation is usually subdivided into two forms, *diffuse interstitial* and *granulomatous*.

Diffuse interstitial inflammation has no particularly characteristic pattern of tissue reaction. The cells involved are monocytes, lymphocytes, plasma cells and fibroblasts (connective tissue cells).

In *granulomatous inflammation* there is an attempt to wall-off and so isolate the affected site. The cells involved here are the reticuloendothelial cells and their derivatives (largely macrophages).

Granulomas occur in relatively few diseases, in for example tuberculosis, syphilis, rheumatic fever, rheumatoid arthritis (as subcutaneous nodules) and in foreign-body inflammation. A granuloma is a focal area of granulomatous inflammation which consists of a spherical accumulation of activated macrophages (epithelioid histiocytes) surrounded by lymphocytes and occasional plasma cells and giant cells and usually connective tissue. Giant cells have been formed in this situation by the fusion of several (10–20) activated monocytes/macrophages; hence the cell contains many nuclei. When the nuclei of the giant cells are sited around the rim of the cell these giant cells are known as *Langhans cells*.

Causes of Chronic Inflammation

Chronic inflammation is associated with a large heterogeneous group of diseases, lasting from weeks to months or longer, either as a development of acute inflammation or as a low-grade inflammatory process without a preceding acute phase. This section looks at four causes.

Persistence of infection with micro-organisms

The type of micro-organisms which might be causative of chronic inflammation are essentially of low virulence, such as those associated with tuberculosis or syphilis along with numerous fungi, protozoa and metazoal parasites.

Autoimmunity

Autoimmune-derived chronic inflammation is characterised by macrophages, lymphocytes and plasma cells such as is observed in rheumatoid arthritis or systemic lupus erythematosus (SLE). In this case there is a 'normal' tissue component, which the immune system is now recognising as foreign; thus inflammation occurs in an attempt to remove the self tissue.

Prolonged exposure to either exogenous or endogenous toxins

When irritant non-living material becomes implanted into wounds, either accidentally (grit, or splinters of wood, metal or plastic) or deliberately (sutures, surgical prosthesis), then chronic inflammation may begin. The situation may also arise in disease conditions such as osteomyelitis where a fragment of dead bone (sequestrum) has become detached from sound bone during the process of necrosis.

The morphology of chronic inflammation arising from prolonged exposure to an environmental toxin will depend on the toxin involved. In a case of inhaled silica, for example, there is chronic lung fibrosis. Alternatively, high levels of plasma lipid would lead to atherosclerosis of the arteries.

Persistence of acute inflammation

Chronic inflammation developing from acute inflammation occurs, for example, in alcoholic cirrhosis and gastric peptic ulcers. Commonly, the morphology includes the presence of inflammatory cells more characteristic of chronic inflammation than that of acute, such as macrophages, lymphocytes and fibrosis. This type of chronic inflammation can occur where infectious organisms are protected from the host's defence mechanisms and so are able to persist in damaged regions. Such a situation can arise in an undrained abscess cavity where bacteria are continuing to grow in the pus.

SYSTEMIC EFFECTS OF INFLAMMATION

In addition to the localised symptoms of inflammation described in the earlier sections, there are systemic effects that may also have important consequences.

Constitutional symptoms

This term covers a whole range of feelings experienced by the patient. He or she often will feel tired and restless (malaise) often accompanied by nausea. Consequently, during occasions of long-term chronic inflammation, significant weight loss is common. In the nineteenth century when tuberculosis was relatively common, these symptoms were recognised as being closely associated with such a disorder and given the general term 'consumption'.

Haematological changes

Leucocytosis (an abnormal elevation of the white blood cell count) and lymphocytosis (a high number of normal lymphocytes) occur in chronic infection such as whooping cough. Neutrophilia (increased numbers of neutrophils) occurs in pyogenic infections. Eosinophilia (increased numbers of eosinophils) is found in parasitic infections and allergies. Monocytosis (an abnormal increase in the number of monocytes in the circulating blood) often accompanies bacterial infections.

Anaemia may result from blood lost in the formation of exudates. This is particularly significant in situations such as ulcerative colitis, but anaemia may also be a result of the chronic inflammation actually causing a depression in bone marrow function.

Pyrexia

When activated through the action of phagocytosis, such as occurs during an inflammatory reaction, white blood cells such as macrophages are able to produce so-called 'endogenous pyrogens' which can act upon the hypothalamus to affect the thermoregulatory mechanisms for which this area of the brain is responsible for. As a consequence the general body temperature is increased.

Reactive hyperplasia of the reticulo-endothelial system

This can be seen as lymph node enlargement and is a result of the rapid cell division occurring in these tissues as a consequence of the adaptive immune response's involvement in the inflammatory response. In certain infections such as malaria where blood-borne antigens are involved, a similar effect may be observed in the spleen, a condition known as *splenomegaly*.

Amyloidosis

In situations of long-term chronic inflammation such as that observed in rheumatoid arthritis, leprosy, tuberculosis and SLE, the elevated levels of the acute-phase protein serum amyloid A (SAA) often results in the glycoprotein amyloid being deposited extracellularly in various tissues around the body. This in turn can lead to secondary (reactive) amyloidosis which is charac-

terised by the ultimately fatal deposition of insoluble fibrils in a number of tissues, including the spleen, liver and kidney.

FACTORS AFFECTING HEALING

Many factors affect the healing of an individual, from their own hormonal status through to the use of deliberate interventions such as the use of a cold compress, ultrasound or drugs.

> **Key point**
> Whilst it would appear that hormones can have wide-ranging effects on the functioning of the immune system, as yet there is still uncertainty about their actions. Consequently differing studies can demonstrate apparently opposing actions, some indicating an increased activity of the immune system, others demonstrating decreased responsiveness.

It has been found that under situations of acute stress, the time taken for recovery of inflammation from bacterial origin is improved. This is possibly achieved through alterations in leucocyte trafficking such that the leucocytes will be targeted towards the relevant organs. For example, an increase in the leucocyte trafficking to the skin is accompanied by a significant enhancement of skin immunity. As a consequence of this the immune response is more effective and so less damage is potentially done; hence recovery time is reduced.

In contrast to the potential benefits of acute stress, chronic stress will induce the adrenal gland to create additional quantities of cortisol (an endogenous corticosteroid). Cortisol has wide-ranging actions, including controlling blood glucose and lipid levels and influencing blood pressure (too much results in hypertension). In addition to these effects, cortisol will act as a suppressant on the immune system. The mechanism through which this immunosuppression takes place is the same as that initiated by synthetic corticosteroids and is described later under drug therapies.

Sex hormones have also been suggested as influencing inflammation. A study looking at the prevention of systemic inflammation resulting from external perfusion of the blood during corrective cardiac surgery in infants indicated that girls were less likely than boys to develop inflammation. It was suggested that this might be due to the higher levels of progesterone within the girls, which in turn led to raised levels of IL-10 (an anti-inflammatory cytokine).

It has been proposed that the repair process may take longer and be less effective in postmenopausal women owing to the detrimental effects of oestrogen and/or progesterone deficiency in the early stages of healing. The exact relationship between the hormone levels and the phases of inflammation and repair remain unclear owing to the conflicting findings from various studies.

TREATMENT OF INFLAMMATION

Successful healing results in scar formation and the removal of necrotic debris. Many therapeutic approaches used to facilitate the healing process aim to reduce the key component – inflammation. This section looks at some of the current approaches.

> ### Key point
> Despite a mass of anecdotal evidence, convincing properly controlled studies are still needed to give guidance as to which treatments should be recommended. Furthermore, the actual mechanism of action of the treatments is often poorly understood.

Temperature Therapy

Cold therapy (cryotherapy)

Many physiotherapists use ice packs (or packs of frozen peas) as an initial treatment for injury. The coolant should be wrapped sufficiently to avoid contact burns. The person should be encouraged to persist with the ice pack until the initial discomfort is replaced with the anaesthetic effect. Cold application for 15–20 minutes has been shown to significantly reduce pain in sufferers of acute gouty arthritis.

Reducing the local temperature has the effect of decreasing blood flow in the area and consequently will reduce the symptoms of inflammation associated with changes in blood flow, such as swelling. In addition, recent electrophysiological studies have demonstrated that reducing the temperature from 31°C to 14°C inhibited the activity of spinal neurons. This helps to explain both the pain relief and reduction in inflammation caused by strong cooling of the skin. Another consequence of a decrease in temperature is the localised decrease in metabolic demands, a useful effect which limits the hypoxic effects of vasoconstriction and oedema.

Recent animal studies have examined the effects of cold water stress upon the inflammatory response of various infections. Interestingly it appears that the application of cold water can decrease the expression of certain cytokines, such as IFNγ, TNFα and IL-2, which

are normally released as part of the inflammatory response.

Heat Therapy

There is still uncertainty and disagreement about the physiological effects of adding heat to the body. In 1949, Horvarth and Hollander demonstrated a *decrease* in intra-articular temperature upon applying superficial heat over that joint. Yet, in 1989, Weinberger and associates found small *increases* in intra-articular temperature.

One thing is certain: when heat is applied to the body it is distributed to adjacent parts according to heat flow and blood flow. The distribution of heat depends on:

- the size of the heated area
- the depth of absorption of specific radiation
- the duration and intensity of heating
- the method by which it is applied.

What physiotherapists do is often aimed at speeding up or slowing down the metabolism within a cell or group of cells. Metabolic rate increases by 13% for every 1 degree Celsius rise in temperature. This means that the cells require more oxygen and nutrients, and accordingly there is an increased production of metabolites or waste products. This is one of the reasons for the development of fever when a person is fighting an infection such as a influenza or the common cold; the body is trying to kill the bugs more effectively. The same logic accounts for the fact that a boil or spot is red.

When an injured ligament becomes chronically inflamed, the inflammatory response almost grinds to a halt and healing ceases. By applying a treatment such as ultrasound, the metabolism to the area can be selectively increased, the inflammation changed to an acute response, and the healing process recommenced.

There is, however, a limit to how far the temperature of tissues can be raised effectively. Proteins coagulate above a certain temperature (that is what happens to the white of an egg when it is cooked). Generally speaking, irreversible tissue damage occurs at approximately 45°C.

Essentially, the application of heat will cause the local blood vessels to dilate, in part due to local spinal

> ### Key point
> In many situations a warm moist towel giving a wet heat, as opposed to a dry heat, is preferred, giving soothing penetrating warmth which can provide comfort and pain relief.

cord reflexes, causing the relaxation of smooth muscle. This in turn results in an increased blood flow, so enhancing the oxygen and nutrient supply to the area. The effect of topical heat application may penetrate to a depth of 2 cm depending on the temperature of the appliance and duration.

A recent study examined the possible anti-inflammatory mechanism of action of the application of a hot mud pack. The elevation in temperature to about 47°C for 20 minutes appeared to inhibit the expression of one of the plasma cytokines, IL-6, which is often associated with inflammation.

Mechanical Manipulation

All organisms are constantly exposed to external forces of mechanical stress, including those of gravity and movement, and internal forces arising from muscular action. It has also been recognised for many years that exposure to such forces is essential for tissue homeostasis and, importantly, for the healing of damaged areas. Numerous studies have indicated how the application of mechanical stress is vital to the differentiation of certain cell types involved in the healing process. For example tension is essential for the formation and differentiation of cell types such as tendon fibroblasts and skeletal muscle fibres. It is also known that following a fracture, the healing of long bones can be significantly influenced by the form of local stresses applied.

Research is continuing into whether cells respond differently to externally applied as opposed to internally applied forces. Meanwhile, some form of mechanical manipulation is often used successfully by physiotherapists to advance the healing process. A number of techniques have been developed relevant to the particular organ, structure or tissue to be treated. An example is deep transverse friction (DTF).

Electrotherapy

Various methods of applying small amounts of electrical current to an affected area have been advocated to reduce inflammation and facilitate the healing process. This, like many aspects of physiotherapy, has its advocates and opponents. The application of electrotherapy for wound healing has been found to increase the rate of healing by more than 50%. However, despite a number of clinical studies demonstrating the beneficial impact of electrotherapy, the optimal delivery techniques have yet to be fully determined.

A number of closely controlled scientific studies have been performed recently, in a number of clinical situations, in order to demonstrate the significance of this form of treatment and to increase our understanding of the underlying mechanism of action. In one study in pigs, the effect of the application of alternating current or direct current stimulation on experimental pressure-ulcer healing was examined. Both forms of electrical stimulation reduced the healing time and increased the perfusion in the damaged areas.

Ultrasound Therapy

Ultrasound (US) consists of sound waves above the frequency range that we can hear. It is usually applied to the person's body from the 'head' of an ultrasound machine (a solid crystal applicator). A gel is used to aid the passage of the waves into the body. Application can be achieved in two ways: either pulsed, in which the waves go in short pulses to prevent the tissues heating; or continuous, when heat will be transferred into the body tissues.

US has been used to treat a wide range of injuries and disorders. Despite its widespread use, relatively little is understood in detail about the actual beneficial effects of US. The thermal effects as a result of the production of continuous waves are proportional to the amount of collagen in the tissue, so maximal effects may be seen at the junctions of bone with tendons. Additional effects may be increased blood flow, cell permeability and protein synthesis.

Pulsed US has been shown to act on some cellular reactions involved in each phase of the healing process, such as the inflammatory reaction, angiogenesis, chondrogenesis, intramembranous ossification, endochondral ossification, and bone remodelling.

Together, stable cavitation and cellular streaming are thought to provide the means whereby the activity at the cell membrane is altered (Williams 1983). Thermal doses of US are thought to promote soft-tissue healing by enhancing cell metabolism (Dyson 1995). As well as increasing the amount of collagen secretion, US appears to encourage alignment of collagen into stronger bundles than haphazard strands that can sometimes occur – in other words, US can make scar tissue stronger. Da Cunha et al. (2001) showed increased organisation and aggregation of collagen bundles within the Achilles tendon of the rat following application of pulsed US (Figure 19.5).

US may also interact with mast cells, platelets and macrophages to accelerate tissue repair. Acoustic streaming causes release of serotonin from platelets. US causes mast cells to release histamine into the surrounding tissues (probably by increasing permeability of the mast cell membrane to calcium ions). US also reduces sodium/potassium ATP-ase pump activity which may decrease neural transmission – accounting possibly for the analgesic properties of US.

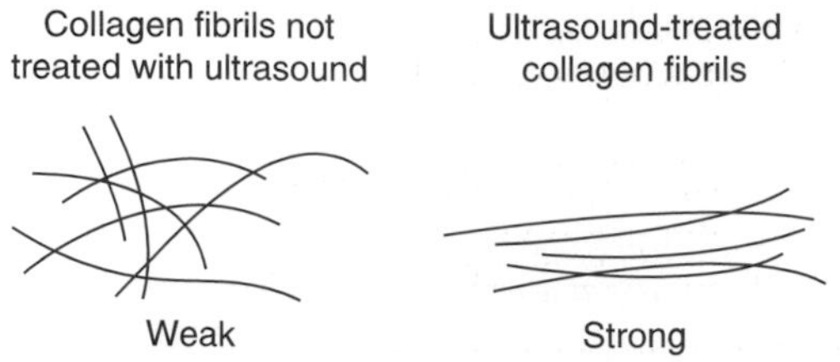

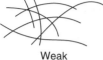

Collagen fibrils not treated with ultrasound — Weak

Ultrasound-treated collagen fibrils — Strong

Figure 19.5   The effect of ultrasound on scar tissue.

The most common uses of US are in the management of soft-tissue injuries, rheumatic complaints, and lesions of tendons and ligaments. There is still a need for thorough adequately controlled studies and, indeed, some recent studies have indicated that low-intensity US may facilitate fracture healing, particularly during the late phases.

Drug Therapy

Non-steroidal anti-inflammatory drugs (NSAIDs)

NSAIDs are among the most commonly used medicines, being prescribed largely for their anti-inflammatory, antipyretic and analgesic properties. The classic example of this type of agent is aspirin (acetylsalicylic acid) which acts to prevent the production of prostaglandins and thromboxanes, which are powerful pro-inflammatory lipid mediators. There are, however, a multitude of other agents which act in the same way: ibuprofen, naproxen, mefenamic acid, flufenamic acid, piroxicam, and others.

NSAIDs work by irreversibly acetylating cyclo-oxygenase, thereby blocking the conversion of arachidonic acid to prostanoids (Figure 19.6). These mediators are then not available to act to enhance the inflammatory response, so the inflammation decreases.

An unfortunate side-effect of NSAIDs arises from their intrinsic toxicity to the gastrointestinal mucosa. They can cause complications ranging from dyspepsia (chronic indigestion) to life-threatening gastrointestinal ulcers. This limits their use, although some (e.g. ibuprofen) carry considerably less risk of these complications than others (e.g. azapropazone).

It has been discovered that there are different isoforms of cyclo-oxygenase, now known as COX-1 and COX-2. COX-1 is the constitutive form of the enzyme. Its concentration remains relatively stable, although small increases can occur when stimulated with hormones or growth factors. COX-2, however, is virtually undetectable in resting cells. Following stimulation by cytokines, endotoxins, growth factors or tumour promoters, COX-2 is induced and can thus be found in, for example, macrophages, fibroblasts, vascular endothelial and smooth muscle cells. Consequently it is believed that in inflammation it is COX-2 dependent prostaglandin production which is the most important of the two isoforms of the enzyme. This has important implications for the use of selective COX-2 inhibitors in the treatment of inflammation, as, in principle, their use should significantly reduce the incidence of gastrointestinal side-effects (as the prostanoids in this case are believed to be synthesized via COX-1). Agents within this class are celecoxib and rofecoxib.

Corticosteroids

Physiotherapists encounter the use of steroids in both local and systemic administrations (e.g. injections and inhalers, respectively). Synthetic glucocorticoids are among the most effective anti-inflammatory drugs available; examples include prednisolone, dexamethasone, methylcortisone and methylprednisolone. They are able to affect the immune system in a number of ways which help to contribute to their powerful anti-inflammatory action.

Corticosteroids induce cells to synthesise the protein lipocortin-1. This lipocortin then acts to inhibit the enzyme phospholipase A_2 (PLA_2). As a result of this inhibition the mediators formed following PLA_2 activation are not produced (see Figure 19.6). By preventing the formation of prostanoids, leukotrienes and PAF these mediators will no longer contribute to the inflammatory response; hence the inflammation is reduced.

In addition to this action, corticosteroids have a number of other actions which will contribute to their anti-inflammatory effectiveness. These actions are not fully clear but may include:

- reducing the production of adhesion molecules (so preventing cells from leaving the circulation and entering the target area)
- suppressing activated macrophages
- stabilising membranes (so decreasing the ability of cells to present antigen)
- slowing down cell division (so possibly influencing the overall size of the lymphocyte pool)
- altering the distribution of T lymphocytes (such that the number circulating around the body have been considerably decreased).

These actions can prevent the production of antibodies and lymphocyte-mediated destruction of agents recognised as foreign, and consequently prevent an effective mounting of an immune response.

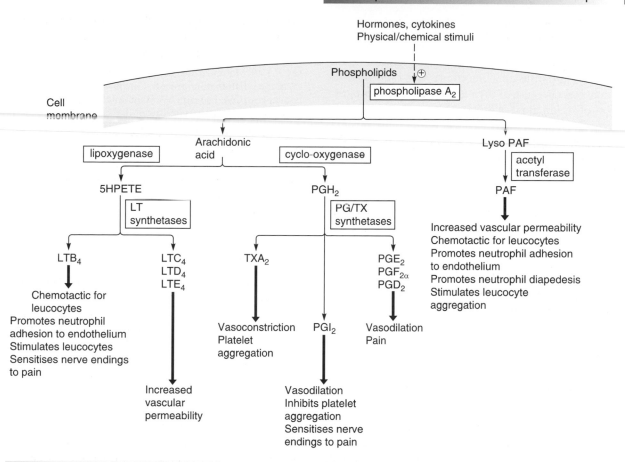

Figure 19.6   Production of eicosanoids and platelet-activating factor (PAF). Both eicosanoids and PAF are autocoids (local hormones) which are released from membrane phospholipids. Eicosanoids is the name given to a group of compounds which are formed from polyunsaturated fatty acids (principally arachidonic acid) and includes prostaglandins (PG), thromboxane A2 (TXA2) and leukotrienes (LT). PAF is a modified phospholipid which is often coupled with arachidonic acid such that the release of lyso-PAF from the membrane will also release free arachidonic acid.

Anti-histamines

Key point

There are a number of different sub-types of receptor which histamine can act upon. So, although the term 'anti-histamine' is commonly used, it is more accurate to use the term 'histamine H_1 receptor antagonist' when referring to this class of agent.

Examples of agents within this category are diphenhydramine, tripelenamine and promethazine. All these are known as first-generation H_1 antagonists and they have the side-effect of causing decreased alertness, slowed reaction times and sleepiness. Second-generation H_1 antagonists such as terfenadine, astemizole and loratadine have the advantage that they are not sedating as they do not cross the blood–brain barrier.

The principle behind the use of these agents is that, although they do not prevent the release of histamine in an inflammatory response, they will prevent that histamine from being able to act. To achieve this the histamine H_1 receptor antagonist will combine with the H_1 receptors and, although it will not produce a response in its own right, it will prevent histamine from being able to bind to those receptors. Thus the inflammatory effects mediated through histamine – namely, vasodilation, increased capillary permeability (hence oedema formation as seen in a weal), increased exocrine secretions (particularly salivary, nasal and lacrimal) and stimulation of nerve endings (which when released into the epidermis is experienced as an itch, or if released into the dermis as pain possibly accompanied by an itch) – can be blocked.

Gold

Gold-based therapies such as auranofin (oral administration), aurothiomalate and aurothioglucose (both given by intramuscular injection) have been used for many years because of their ability to slow the progression of rheumatoid arthritis, along with reducing the symptoms and possibly also decreasing bone/articular cartilage destruction.

Its mechanism of action remains unclear. It is known that gold is accumulated in lysosomes of macrophages and that it reduces the activity of lysosomal enzymes. Gold compounds will also suppress phagocytosis by polymorphonuclear leucocytes and decrease the release of histamine from mast cells.

FURTHER READING

Belanger Alain-Yvan 2002 Evidence-based Guide to Therapeutic Physical Agents. Philadelphia: Lippincott Williams & Wilkins

Burg ND, Pillinger MH 2001 The neutrophil: function and regulation in innate and humoral immunity. Clin Immunol 99(1): 7–17

Calvin M 2000 Oestrogens and wound healing. Maturitas 34: 195–210

Cook SD, Salkeld SL, Patron LP, Ryaby JP, Whitecloud TS 2001 Low-intensity ultrasound improves spinal fusion. Spine J 1: 246–54

Gardner TN, Stoll T, Marks L, Mishra S, Knothe Tate M 2000 The influence of mechanical stimulus on the pattern of tissue differentiation in a long bone fracture: an FEM study. J Biomech 33: 415–25

Ley K 1996 Molecular mechanisms of leukocyte recruitment in the inflammatory process. Cardiovasc Res 32: 733–42

Lundeberg TCM, Eriksson SV, Malm M 1992 Electrical nerve stimulation improves healing of diabetic ulcers. Ann Plast Surg 29: 328–31

Reger SI, Hyodo A, Negami S, Kambic HE, Sahgal V 1999 Experimental wound healing with electrical stimulation. Artificial Org 23: 460–2

Sluka KA, Christy MR, Peterson WL, Rudd SL, Troy SM 1999 Reduction of pain-related behaviors with either cold or heat treatment in an animal model of acute arthritis. Arch Phys Med Rehabil 80(3): 313–17

Speed CA 2001 Therapeutic ultrasound in soft tissue lesions. Rheumatology 40: 1331–6

REFERENCES

Da Cunha A, Parizotto NA, Vidal Bde C 2001 The effect of therapeutic ultrasound on repair of the Achilles tendon (tendo calcaneus) of the rat. Ultras Med Biol 27: 1691–6

Dyson M 1995 Role of ultrasound in wound healing. In McCulloch JM, Kloth LC, Feeder JA (eds) Wound Healing: Alternatives in Management, 2nd edn, pp. 318–45. Philadelphia: FA Davies Co.

Williams AR 1983 Ultrasound: Biological Effects and Potential Hazards. London: Academic Press

Neurological Physiotherapy

Alison Chambers and Christine Smith

INTRODUCTION

The challenges facing physiotherapists working in the clinical field of neurology are many and varied. The complex nature of the human nervous system and the vast array of neurological conditions found in clinical practice place heavy demands on physiotherapists. The onset of a neurological condition, as a result of disease or trauma, has a devastating effect not only on the patient but also on families. It is essential that any approach to management encompasses the needs of the patient and significant others. Many neurological conditions are progressive and longstanding and result in some element of residual impairment. There are many challenges in the rehabilitation process from diagnosis to discharge. The longstanding nature of many neurological conditions, means that professionals are involved in management and rehabilitation over many years.

Historically, there has been a lack of research in the field of rehabilitation and in particular the role of the physiotherapist. There is now a growing evidence base that supports a variety of approaches to the rehabilitation of the neurologically impaired patient. The role and function of the physiotherapist is contextualised within a team approach, to the treatment and rehabilitation of neurologically impaired adults. The importance of a collaborative approach to rehabilitation is widely found within the literature (Edwards 2002; Plum and Morissey 2002; Fawcus 2000; Stokes 1998). Neurological dysfunction can result in the disruption of normal physical, psychological, cognitive and social functions. Consequently this demands the collaboration and coordination of a number of rehabilitation professionals. No one professional group can offer all the expertise required to enable patients to reach their maximum level of recovery. It is vital that a truly holistic approach to the management and treatment of patients and their families be adopted, with clinical reasoning and problem-solving at its centre.

This chapter begins by outlining the principal causes of neurological dysfunction and then describes some of the commonly occurring clinical features. Some of the general principles of physiotherapy assessment and treatment are discussed in relation to present-day clinical practice. The variations in approaches to rehabilitation add to the complexity and challenges facing the physiotherapist working in neurology. The section on the general principles of physiotherapy offers the reader an eclectic approach to rehabilitation and is not intended to promote any one approach over another.

Measurement of outcome is an important aspect of neurological rehabilitation. The chapter provides a sec-

Further reading
It is outside the scope of this chapter to provide the reader with details of each different approach, or to advocate the use of or extol the strengths of any specific approach. Readers are directed to Edwards (2002), Partridge (2002), and Stokes (1998) for more comprehensive information on the different approaches.

tion on outcome measurement and goal-setting in relation to the International Classification of Function framework set out by the World Health Organization (WHO) in 2001.

The chapter concludes with an overview of the more commonly known neurological conditions, namely Stroke, Parkinson's Disease, Multiple Sclerosis, Motor Neurone Disease and Traumatic Brain Injury. These sections are not intended to be exhaustive, and readers can consult the lists of further recommended reading at the end of the chapter.

Background knowledge
Readers are also advised to refer to appropriate literature for details of the anatomy of the central nervous system (CNS) in relation to its function. A thorough understanding of the structure and function of the CNS and the neural control of movement will be needed to effectively manage patients with complex neurological dysfunction.

Glossary
Towards the end of this chapter is a glossary of some of the terms used.

NEUROLOGICAL DYSFUNCTION: BASIC ISSUES

Principal Causes of Neurological Dysfunction

Causes of neurological dysfunction include trauma, as in head injury or spinal injury, where direct or indirect trauma results in temporary or (if there has been destruction of nerve tissue) permanent damage. Diseases can affect the nervous system and some seem to have an affinity for a particular part of the system. Examples of diseases that can affect the nervous system are Meningitis, Syphilis and (less commonly) Tuberculosis and Poliomyelitis. Diseases of unknown origin that affect the central nervous system include Multiple Sclerosis, Motor Neurone Disease and Guillain-Barré. Multiple Sclerosis and Motor Neurone Disease are discussed later in the chapter.

Other causes of deficits within the nervous system include circulatory conditions, the most common of which is stroke (again detailed more fully later). Congenital defects such as spina bifida, inherited conditions such as Huntington's chorea, vitamin B deficiency, neoplasms and toxic substances such as lead, arsenic and mercury can all also have a detrimental effect on the nervous system.

Clinical Features of Damage to the CNS

The clinical features of disruption to the central nervous system are determined partly by the site(s) and the severity of the damage. However, the CNS is integrative in nature and so damage to one part will result in a disruption in function of other parts. The site of damage alone is not necessarily a predictor of the clinical features that patients will present with. No two patients' nervous systems are the same and how each patient responds to any given damage will also be different. Despite the fact that patients do not present exactly the same, there are common clinical features that arise. Some of the main features are covered below.

Cognitive/emotional changes

Occasionally patients may present with altered cognitive function. Damage to the frontal lobes tends to predispose patients to these types of change. Examples include altered levels of arousal, reduced attention span, and memory impairment. Changes in behaviour can include agitated states, disinhibition and reduced

Key point

Care must be taken to distinguish emotional changes that occur as a direct result of the pathology and those that are the person's reaction to the newly acquired or diagnosed condition.

motivation. Emotional changes can present in the form of emotional lability, depression or euphoria.

Physical dysfunction

Smooth and efficient movement is reliant upon intact sensory and motor pathways. Any disruption to these pathways will lead to movement disorders.

Incoordination of movement

Weakness or paralysis of muscle groups will result in an imbalance of activity and therefore incoordination of movement.

Ataxia

Movements are jerky and patients have difficulty grading or controlling movements. Sometimes this can be due to a loss of postural control and an inability to produce co-contraction within muscle groups. The type of ataxia is determined by the system affected. The various forms of ataxia are listed in Table 20.1.

Involuntary movements (dyskinesia)
Dystonia (previously known as athetosis)

Movements produced are writhing and slow and are often brought on by attempts to move. Generalised dystonia may produce gross movements of the arms and legs. Focal dystonias usually involve the eyes, neck

Table 20.1 Types of ataxia and associated motor disorder.

Sensory ataxia	A 'high stepping' gait pattern More reliance on visual or auditory information about leg or foot position
Vestibular ataxia	Disturbed equilibrium in standing and walking Loss of equilibrium reactions A wide-based, staggering gait pattern
Cerebellar ataxia	Disturbance in the rate, regularity and force of movement Loss of movement coordination Overshooting of target (dysmetria) Decomposition of movement (dyssynergia) Loss of speed and rhythm of alternating movement (dysdiadochokinesia) Incoordination of agonist–antagonist muscles and loss of the continuity of muscle contraction (tremor, e.g. intention tremor)

From Stokes M 1998 Neurological Physiotherapy. New York: Mosby International.

or upper limbs. They are thought to occur as a consequence of damage to the basal ganglia. There may also be disruption in facial and tongue movements. It is thought that these movements may be due to a disturbance in reciprocal inhibition.

Chorea

Although patients with chorea also present with jerky movements, these movements tend to occur more randomly throughout the body. The absence of sustained abnormal posturing distinguishes this condition from dystonia.

Ballismus

The movements are large and sudden and can affect one side of the body (hemiballismus).

Tremor

These are fine, rapidly oscillating, unwanted movements. Tremors are often classified in relation to the circumstances in which they occur. For example an intention tremor is made worse by voluntary movement of the limb, particularly at the end of a movement. The precise mechanisms related to tremors are continuing to be explored.

Disturbances in muscle tone

Tone can be defined as 'a state of readiness'. Each person has his or her own particular state of readiness that changes according to the circumstances. Muscle tone consists of both neural and non-neural components. Both tonic reflex activity and the viscoelastic components of the muscle are important to consider. In clinical practice muscle tone may be abnormally increased (hypertonia) or decreased (hypotonia).

> **Further reading**
> Readers are referred to Edwards (2002) for a detailed account of abnormal muscle tone.

Sensory disturbances

Disturbances in cutaneous sensation result from a disruption in afferent information. This can be classified as *paraesthesia* or *anaesthesia* where there is diminished or absent afferent information. An increase in cutaneous sensitivity is termed *hyperaesthesia* and can be an equally troublesome feature. The presentation depends on the site of the lesion and the severity of the damage.

Pain is a common feature of many neurological conditions. The source of the pain can vary ranging from disturbances in nerve endings and/or pathways, to pain caused by secondary complications such as malalignment of joints. It is important to carry out a comprehensive assessment to identify the cause of pain. Effective management of the pain is essential, as patients who present with pain will report that this is the symptom they are most concerned with.

Perceptual disturbances

This is a non-specific term that describes the way in which the individual perceives sensory information. Perception requires the interaction of visual and spatial components. Types of perceptual disturbance include disruption in figure–ground differentiation, spatial awareness, inattention or neglect, disturbances in constructional abilities, and many other forms.

Visual disturbances

Many neurological conditions affect visual pathways. Examples include hemianopia where the patient loses vision in half the visual field of each eye, diplopia (double vision), nystagmus (incoordination of eye movements), and optic neuritis (lesions of the optic nerve).

Auditory disturbances

Deafness directly related to neurological conditions is relatively uncommon in neurological patients. When it occurs it is usually due to trauma to the structures of the auditory system.

Communication disturbances

These can be particularly frustrating and disturbing for patients, particularly those who have a good insight into their difficulties. Communication involves both receptive and expressive components. Examples of communication disorders are dysarthria (motor disturbance), dysphasia (receptive and expressive language disorder), and dyspraxia.

Autonomic disturbances

Dysfunctions may be due to damage affecting autonomic areas or pathways. Following spinal cord injury, some patients can present with autonomic dysreflexia. This is a sympathetic nervous system discharge producing hypertension, bradycardia, sweating, skin vasoconstriction, headache, pilo-erection and capillary dilation. This response is often triggered by impaired bladder or bowel function or other noxious stimulus.

APPROACH TO PHYSIOTHERAPY

Rehabilitation and Team Working

The patient's main goal is usually to achieve as great a degree of independence and quality of life as possible. This will depend on many factors:

- the extent of damage to the central nervous system
- the patient's motivation to achieve his or her goals
- the rehabilitation programme
- the environment in which the person will be functioning.

Physiotherapists need to employ a problem-solving approach to the rehabilitation of a patient with neurological damage, wherever possible engaging the patient in this process. Many different approaches to the rehabilitation of patients are emerging and an eclectic approach to neurological rehabilitation is becoming increasingly accepted. Emerging approaches to neurological rehabilitation include:

- constraint-induced movement therapy
- robot-assisted therapy
- virtual-reality based therapy
- locomotion training using devices for automating bodyweight support.

Key point
The increasing amount of research in the field of neurological rehabilitation and the growing acceptance and knowledge of the mechanisms of neuroplasticity are informing modern therapies. Physiotherapists need to stay abreast of new developments and the emerging evidence base on which to base their practice.

Physiotherapists need to be able to make a comprehensive assessment of the patient's neurological deficit and remaining abilities in order to formulate an appropriate programme of rehabilitation. This can only come from a sound understanding of the control of human movement, the likely implications of damage to areas of the nervous system, and knowledge of the types of treatment approaches available and when best to apply them. Advantages and disadvantages of the various types of interventions need to be considered.

There is increasing acceptance that the nervous system and the musculoskeletal system cannot be separated, as they work harmoniously together to meet the demands placed upon them. Hence many concepts previously utilised exclusively within each of these fields are becoming commonly used in both areas.

Physiotherapists have a key role in all aspects of patients' management. This might be selecting the most appropriate treatment programmes for patients, implementing review programmes to maintain patients at their optimum level of functioning, or delaying deterioration in the case of progressive neurological conditions. Realistic goals that are measured, time-framed and that consider the whole person and their family/carers need to be negotiated.

Therapy programmes should be carried out in the environment that is most appropriate for the patient, taking into account the stage of the rehabilitation process, the facilities available and the intended goals. This might mean that treatment is implemented in the hospital setting or in the community. The shift of programmes towards community settings allows therapists to choose the most appropriate location for treatment, be it the patient's home, the gymnasium or the supermarket!

Key point
Using a team approach within rehabilitation is considered standard practice these days. However, the composition of the team and the model of team working adopted can vary.

Assessment of Neurological Patients

Irrespective of changes in approaches to rehabilitation, one factor that remains consistent is the need to carry out a comprehensive assessment of the patient and the environment in which he or she is likely to be functioning. Many members of the healthcare team will carry out assessments. Wherever possible, joint assessments with sharing of information, sometimes in shared case notes, will be carried out.

Assessment is an on-going process that, in reality, is an integral part of treatment. Assessment of neurological patients is complex, multifaceted and contains many interrelated elements. Often assessment occurs over a number of sessions with the patient, because carrying out a full assessment in one attempt can frequently be too tiring for the patient. Gathering the necessary information over a longer period of time often gives a much more accurate picture of the patient's strengths and difficulties.

A basic assessment format has been included as an appendix to this chapter.

Clinical interview

As in all assessments, obtaining a thorough subjective history is very important. This can come from a variety of sources: the medical notes, nursing notes, the patient, relatives and carers. Initial interviews can be very important, not just for gathering information, but also because this is where establishing a rapport with the patient and carers begins.

Physiotherapists need to draw on all aspects of their communication skills to allow the patient and family to be at ease. Increasingly, in appropriate cases, initial interviews take place in the patient's home. This not only ensures the person is more relaxed, but allows assessment of the patient's functional environment. Later when home programmes are being devised, knowledge of the patient's home can be invaluable.

When assessing patients with communication disorders, it is important to find alternative or supplementary methods of communicating with the patient. Collaboration with the Speech and Language Therapist is invaluable at such times.

Whilst interviewing the patient, important clues can be observed with regard to communication, cognition, emotion, hearing, vision and attention span. It should also be noted by how much the patient changes position, attends to posture and so on. Assessment thus begins the minute contact is made with the patient.

Clinical examination

The main purpose of the clinical examination is to gather information about the patient's movement disorder and level of functional ability (Freeman 2002).

Initially, observe the patient and try to draw conclusions about what he or she is able to do unaided. Then assistance can be given to ascertain what the person can achieve in this way. This is where assessment and treatment begin to merge into one and the same thing. By conducting an assessment in this manner, it is possible to see how the patient responds to handling, all be it in the short term. It is not uncommon for physiotherapists' eyes to tell them one story and their hands to tell them something quite different!

It is prudent to begin the assessment wherever the person happens to be when the initial contact is made. For instance, observing the person's gait when he or she walks into the room often gives a more accurate picture of functional gait pattern than when the person is asked to walk whilst being watched.

Wherever possible, observations should be backed up by clinical or other forms of measurement. In this way, baseline information on which to base interventions and evaluation of effectiveness is made more reliable.

OUTCOME MEASURES AND GOAL-SETTING

Once the assessment is complete, key problems need to be identified by using clinical reasoning processes. Goals of treatment, with appropriate timescales, can be formulated with the patient and the family. Goals need to be negotiated and discussed with all parties, including the rehabilitation team, so that there is a clear understanding of the processes involved. Failure to go through this process and to keep re-visiting it can lead to frustration and misunderstanding, particularly by the patient and the family.

Note on Terminology

The World Health Organization's (WHO) model of illness provides a useful framework and common terminology for describing and measuring the consequences of disease and the impact that rehabilitation may have on them (Edwards 2002).

The original WHO International Classification of Impairments, Disabilities and Handicap from 1980 has been replaced by the International Classification of Functioning (ICF). This change has led to a move away from the emphasis on impairment, handicap and disability to a more positive emphasis on activity and participation. Table 20.2 compares the old and new terminologies.

Key point
Readers are reminded that the change to the international terminology is relatively new and therefore the old terminology will be seen in documents and articles prior to 2002. This does not detract from the usefulness of such texts but might lead to confusion in the unwary.

- 'Body function' refers to physical as well as psychological functions.
- 'Activity' refers to the execution of a task or action; it can refer to the individual's capacity to carry out

Table 20.2 Comparison of the old and new WHO terminologies.

Terminology prior to 2002	Terminology after 2002
Impairment	Body function
Disability	Activity
Handicap	Participation

the task as well as the actual performance of the task.

- 'Participation' is described as the involvement in a life situation.

Activity limitations can be described as the difficulties an individual may have in carrying out activities. Participation restrictions can be described as the problems an individual may experience whilst engaged in life situations.

This classification provides the background against which healthcare interventions can be determined and outcome measures developed.

The Principle of Measurement of Outcome

The responsibilities of healthcare professionals to provide evidence of the effectiveness of their treatment and management is of increasing importance. The introduction of the clinical governance framework within the National Health Service (NHS) and the implications this has with regard to accountability and clinical effectiveness has resulted in the growth and interest in outcome measurement.

Measurement implies the quantification of data in either absolute or relative terms. Determining the effectiveness of an intervention by measuring its effect on outcome provides the basis for evidence-based healthcare (Edwards 2002). Outcome measures take the guesswork and subjectivity out of evaluation and can assist the physiotherapist in proving clinical effectiveness.

Outcome measures also provide a method of communication. The importance of a language of universal use among clinicians cannot be over-emphasised. The focus on multidisciplinary care and the blurring of traditional professional boundaries requires at the very least a system of measurement that can be understood by and utilised by the whole multidisciplinary team.

There are a wide range of outcome measures available and care is required when deciding which outcome measure to use, and when. The general principles to follow when developing and/or considering the use of outcome measures are:

- clinical utility (does it measure what you want it to measure?)
- selection of the outcome to be measured
- selection of an appropriate outcome measure
- ease of use on a day-to-day basis.

CSP website
The Chartered Society of Physiotherapy (CSP) has provided a summary of the outcome measures currently available which have relevance to physiotherapy care interventions. It can be found on the CSP website at www.csp.org.uk.

Outcome measures should be sensitive enough to allow for measurement of changes over time. The use of a suitable outcome measure for all physiotherapy interventions is an essential part of the treatment and management process, and the clinical area of neurology is no exception.

Outcome Measures in Context

Physiotherapy outcome measures should be considered in the wider context of rehabilitation. Rehabilitation can be defined as a problem-solving and educational process aimed at reducing disability and enhancing function in people who are affected by disease (Wade 1992). Rehabilitation principles are based upon the enhancement of activity by restoring skills and capabilities through functional retraining and environmental adaptation. They promote independence and facilitate the fullest potential physically, psychologically, socially and vocationally. Rehabilitation involves the recovery or improvement of function as well as prevention of disability and the maintenance of social role.

Irrespective of the approach taken towards rehabilitation, the ability to quantify the function is the key to successful treatment. The process involves assessment, treatment planning, goal-setting and evaluation of outcome. The WHO ICF classification and the process of rehabilitation together provide the context against which outcome measurement is used in physiotherapy.

Table 20.3 provides a summary of the outcome measures commonly used within neurology. It is not meant to be comprehensive and the reader is directed to the recommended reading list at the end of the chapter.

The types of measures available include functional, technical and quality-of-life measures.

- *Functional measures* are concerned with the level of disability or dependency. It is the change in the

Table 20.3 Outcome measures frequently used within the clinical setting.

Dimension	Outcome measure	References
IMPAIRMENTS		
Muscle strength	Hand-held dynamometer	Bohannon et al. (1995)
	MRC grades	Medical Research Council (1976)
Range of motion	Goniometry	Norkin and White (1975)
Tone	Modified Ashworth scale	Bohannon and Smith (1987)
Sensation	Stereognosis	Lincoln and Edmans (1989)
Fatigue	Fatigue severity scale	Petajan et al. (1996)
DISABILITY		
Global disability		
Generic	Barthel Index	Mahoney and Barthel (1965)
	Functional independence measure	Granger et al. (1993)
Disease-specific	Motor assessment scale for stroke	Carr et al. (1985)
Focal disability		
Gait	10-metre timed walking test	Wade (1992)
	Hauser Ambulatory Index	Hauser et al. (1983)
Mobility	Rivermead Motor Assessment Scale	Lincoln and Leadbitter (1979)
Balance	Functional reach test	Duncan et al. (1990)
	Timed get-up-and-go test	Podsialo and Richardson (1991)
Upper-limb function	Nine-hole peg test	Mathiowetz et al. (1985)
	Action Research Arm Test	Crow et al. (1989)
	Frenchay Arm Test	Sunderland et al. (1989)
HANDICAP	London Handicap Scale	Harwood et al. (1987)
	Environmental status scale	Mellerup et al. (1981)
QUALITY OF LIFE		
Generic	36-item Short Form Health Survey	Ware et al. (1993)
	Nottingham Health Profile	Hunt et al. (1981)
Disease-specific	39-item Parkinson's Disease Questionnaire	Peto et al. (1995)
	Functional assessment of multiple sclerosis	Cella et al. (1996)

From Edwards S (ed.) 2002 Neurological Physiotherapy, 2nd edn. London: Churchill Livingstone.

functional status of the patient and in the amount of caring and assistance required by the patient that tends to be the aim of neurological rehabilitation (Stokes 1998). At this time there is no standard outcome measurement available. Examples of the outcome measures currently used are Barthel Index, FIM, Gross Motor Function Measurement (GMFM) and the Motor Assessment Scale (MAS).

- *Technical measures* are concerned with the level of impairment. Examples of these are muscle tone measurement, range of movement and muscle performance measurement.
- *Quality-of-life measures* are concerned with the level of handicap and the patient's ability to function in the community and interact with society. Examples of these are the Nottingham Health Profile and the Short Form 36 (Stokes 1998).

Goal-Setting

Definition

Goal-setting refers to the identification and agreement of targets that the patient, therapist and team will work towards over a specified period of time (Wade 1999a,b).

The planning of goals is necessary to ensure that the rehabilitation effort is as effective and efficient as possible (Elsworth et al. 1999). Outcome is better if the goals are challenging, involve the patient and are set at different levels.

The evidence relating to goal-setting is limited, but there is a general trend towards the inclusion of goal-setting in the rehabilitation process (Wade 1999c). With the emphasis on patient-centred care and inclusion of the patient in the decision-making processes, a formal process of goal planning will help to improve the coordination and cooperation of all those people involved. Cooperative goal-setting makes the process of rehabilitation more patient-focused and helps to motivate the patient through the long period of rehabilitation, and beyond. In other words the effects of treatment will be long-lasting and continue to be evident when treatment has ceased.

Good rehabilitation practice should involve SMART goals (specific, measurable, achievable, realistic, time-framed):

1 Set meaningful and challenging but achievable goals.
2 Involve the patient and carers.
3 Include short-term and long-term goals.
4 Set goals both at a team and an individual professional level.

Key point
Patients may or may not be present at the goal planning meeting but it is obviously important that the patient's wishes be represented. Being present at the actual meeting may be too stressful for the patient.

It is common practice to set goals for the long, medium and short term. In summary the terms commonly used to document goals are:

- long-term goals = aims
- medium-term goals = objectives
- short-term goals = targets.

Wade (1999a) defines these terms as in Table 20.4.

In summary, goal-setting allows for the alignment of patient and professional goals. It is is a method of

ensuring that the rehabilitation team focuses on the needs of an individual patient and can help to motivate patients. It should lead to an overall improvement in treatment effectiveness and provide a method of measuring the effectiveness of treatment interventions (Edwards 2002; McGrath and Adams 1999).

STROKE (CEREBROVASCULAR ACCIDENT)

Introduction

Each year in England and Wales 110,000 people have their first stroke and 30,000 go on to have further strokes (Department of Health 2002). Stroke is the single biggest cause of severe disability and the third most common cause of death in the UK. A substantial proportion of health and social care resources are devoted to the immediate and continuing care of people who have had a stroke (DoH 2002) and approximately 5% of all hospital costs can be attributed to stroke care (Fawcus 2000). Stroke accounts for 10–12% of all deaths in industrialised countries, and 88% of stroke deaths occur in patients over the age of 65 years (Bonita 1992).

A stroke has a major impact on a person's life. It can lead to long-term disability and necessitate long-term care. Patients who have suffered a stroke (cerebrovascular accident) present healthcare professionals with a variety of complex physical, psychological and social problems. The sudden loss of any capacity causes severe stress not only to the patient but also to the family. The resultant neurological deficit can have a devastating outcome.

The signs and symptoms associated with a stroke are dependent upon the size and location of the lesion.

A stroke usually results in hemiplegia (paralysis of one side of the body). This hemiplegia is contralateral to the side of the brain in which the lesion occurs. An

Table 20.4 Aims, objectives and targets.

Aim	Describes a state Is for the patient and family Is in terms of a social role or functioning or well-being
Objective	Is set within the medium term Involves direction of change as much as achieving a specific state Is framed in terms of patient behaviour and environment
Target	Is set within the short term Is specific and often involves only one named person/profession May be set at any level or in terms of the rehabilitation process

From Wade DT 1999b Goal planning in stroke rehabilitation: what? Top Stroke Rehabil 6(2): 8–15.

Definition

Stroke can be defined as an interruption of blood flow (of vascular origin) to the brain resulting in a range of focal neurological deficits that last longer than 24 hours (Lundy-Ekman 1998). The World Health Organization (WHO) defines stroke as 'a condition with rapidly developing clinical signs of focal loss of cerebral function, with symptoms lasting longer than 24 hours or leading to death, with no apparent cause other than that of vascular origin' (Fawcus 2000).

interruption of blood flow to the brain leaves the patient with a focal loss of function of varying severity. The most common deficit is a motor deficit. Other neurological deficits can include:

- visual
- perceptual
- sensory
- communication
- swallowing.

These can be seen in isolation or in any combination and vary widely between patients. Disorders of balance and posture are a commonly occurring feature (Fawcus 2000).

The neurological deficit ranges from a temporary loss of function followed by complete recovery, to permanent life-altering impairment and disability, to death. It is generally referred to as a *non-progressive lesion* – the severity of signs and symptoms is worse initially and declines with time and treatment intervention.

Key point

Eighty-four per cent of strokes are ischaemic in origin, 16% result from a haemorrhage. The prevalence is 2 per 1000 of the population. Forty per cent of sufferers have a residual neurological deficit, 30% die, and 30% make a full recovery.

Transient ischaemic attack (TIA)

A number of people suffer from a brief focal loss of function with full recovery occurring in 24 hours. This is known as a *transient ischaemic attack*. This may lead to a major stroke and is sometimes seen as a warning event. Approximately 5–10% of people who have a TIA will go on to have a major stroke. Some people have a mild residual deficit which persists for days or weeks. This is referred to as a *minor stroke* or a *reversible*

ischaemic neurological deficit (RIND; Hume-Adams and Graham 1998).

Risk factors

Strokes can occur at any age but are more common in the elderly. There are several risk factors associated with cerebrovascular disease, listed in Table 20.5.

Pathology

Strokes are non-progressive in nature and are caused by ischaemia or haemorrhage. A small number of strokes are caused by congenital abnormalities of the blood vessels and can result in spontaneous intercranial haemorrhage. These defects of the blood vessels are known as arteriovenous malformations (AVMs). They are liable to subsequent bleeding and surgical intervention is the treatment of choice (Stokes 1998; Fawcus 2000).

Ischaemic stroke

Ischaemic stroke occurs when an embolus (a migrating clot) or thrombus (a fixed clot) lodges itself in a blood vessel, obstructing the blood flow to the area distal to the blockage. This causes an abrupt interruption to blood flow and leads rapidly to cell death and focal neurological deficit. The thrombus is usually due to atherosclerosis and often associated with hypertension, diabetes mellitus, and coronary or peripheral vascular disease. The symptoms of ischaemia develop over a few minutes.

The area affected by the stroke will depend upon the distribution of the artery and the degree of anastomosis by other cerebral arteries. The addition of oedema at the site of the lesion will add to the focal deficit. Once the oedema has reduced the residual deficit will become apparent. Patients will complain of headache with hemiplegia, and there may be a disruption of speech. The hemiplegia is initially hypotonic but may develop into hypertonicity within a few days of the stroke.

Table 20.5 Risk factors for stroke.

Major risk factors	Minor risk factors
Hypertension	Contraceptive pill
Raised cholesterol	Excessive alcohol
Atherosclerosis	consumption
Diabetes mellitus	Physical inactivity
Cardiac disease	Obesity
Smoking	

From Weiner WJ, Goetz CG 1994 Neurology for the Non-neurologist, 3rd edn. Philadelphia: Lippincott.

Haemorrhagic stroke

A haemorrhagic stroke occurs when there is a rupture of a blood vessel into the brain tissue. This can occur as a result of hypertension that causes lipohyalinosis to occur in the small arteries of the brain causing micro-aneurysms to form. These then rupture. The onset is dramatic, with severe headache, vomiting and loss of consciousness.

Subarachnoid haemorrhage

This occurs when there is bleeding into the subarachnoid space following the rupture of a berry aneurysm near the circle of Willis. There is a sudden intense headache associated with vomiting and neck stiffness. Loss of consciousness may occur. Ten per cent of people will die within a few hours, 40% within 2 weeks (Stokes 1998). Surgical intervention is the best hope of recovery, followed by intensive rehabilitation.

Clinical Features

The clinical manifestations of occlusion of the cerebral arteries are shown in Table 20.6.

Further reading

The range and severity of clinical features is extremely varied. The recommended reading at the end of the chapter provides readers with texts that deal with these signs more comprehensively.

The clinical features depend on the size and severity of the lesion. Generally there will be a mixture of the features listed in Table 20.7. These features will affect the motor, sensory, proprioceptive and cognitive functions. The list is not exhaustive and it is beyond the scope of this text to cover every possibility. It is important to note that no two patients are alike.

Management

There are three stages of management: medical management, rehabilitation and prevention (Fawcus 2000). The increase in chronic disease generally has led to an increased importance of health promotion strategies.

Medical management

It is important to establish the type of stroke that has occurred because the medical management will depend on whether it is an ischaemic, haemorragic or a subarachnoid stroke. The national clinical guidelines for stroke published by the Royal College of Physicians (2000) outline the recommended treatments and management (Table 20.8).

The diagnosis of stroke is primarily dependent upon the clinical presentation. Medical management usually consists of the treatment of any underlying pathology (e.g. hypertension) and the prevention of secondary complications.

In the UK there are recommendations for the type of service provision stroke sufferers can expect. Research suggests that stroke patients do better when treated in a specialised stroke unit that has a coordinated multidisciplinary stroke team (Fawcus 2000; Edwards 2002). This type of service should be expected within the first 6 months; after that time patients can be cared for equally well in a community or general hospital setting.

Physiotherapy management

Table 20.9 outlines the typical management of stroke patients.

Table 20.6 Arteries involved in cerebral vascular occlusion.

Middle cerebral artery (supplies most of the convexity of the cerebral hemispheres)	Dense contralateral hemiplegia Contralateral homonymous hemianopia Cortical type of sensory loss Speech problems in left hemisphere lesions, with neglect of contralateral side Lesions in the right hemisphere result in parietal damage, visuospatial disturbances and left-sided neglect
Posterior cerebral artery	Visual disturbance Contralateral homonymous field defect Memory disturbance and contralateral sensory loss
Anterior cerebral artery	Contralateral monoplegia Cortical sensory loss Sometimes behavioural abnormalities associated with frontal lobe damage

From Stokes M 1998 Neurological Physiotherapy. New York: Mosby International.

Table 20.7 Clinical features of common neurological deficits.

Dysfunction	Clinical feature
Motor deficit	Abnormal tone:* • hypotonus: decreased muscle tone with little or no resistance to passive movement • hypertonus: increased muscle tone with increased resistance to passive movement Movement disorders: • ataxia • rigidity Balance/posture abnormality
Sensory deficit	Anaesthesia Parasthesia Proprioceptive: • joint position sense • stereognosis • somatognosia
Visual deficit	Double vision Homogonous hemianopea
Speech deficit	Aphasia – expressive and receptive Dysphasia – expressive and receptive Dysarthria
Cognitive deficit	Dyspraxia Unilateral neglect Memory loss Attention deficit
Affective deficit	Emotional lability Inappropriate behaviour

* The initial presentation is one of hypotonus. Hypertonus may develop over time.

Physiotherapy management follows a problem-solving approach and involves the following elements:

• rehabilitation of movement
• maximisation of function
• prevention of secondary complications
• treatment of social/psychological factors.

Many physiotherapists adopt an eclectic approach to rehabilitation, rather than adhering to rigid rules of intervention as indicated by models of therapy.

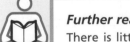

Further reading

There is little evidence to support the superiority of one treatment approach over another in terms of outcome. Historically research into the numerous treatment approaches has been sparse. Readers are directed to Edwards (1998), Carr and Shepherd (1998), Partridge (2002) and Bobath (1999) to provide details of specific treatment approaches.

The physiotherapy-specific national guidelines for stroke are depicted in Table 20.10 (Royal College of Physicians/Chartered Society of Physiotherapy 2000). The guidelines should be viewed as a framework to guide clinical decisions rather than as rigid rules. The guidelines are continually updated in the light of new evidence. The national clinical guidelines should be referred to for guidance on the involvement of carers and families, discharge planning, long-term management and service evaluation.

The following key factors have been identified by Ashburn (1997) as important features of physical recovery following stroke:

1 Recovery is the most rapid in the first few months and movement patterns recur in similar hierarchal patterns in most patients.
2 The timing and achievement of independent sitting balance are key indicators of functional independence.
3 The initial level of motor dysfunction and the time interval between paralysis and return of movement are important indicators of movement recovery.
4 Studies have shown a link between unilateral neglect and poor function.

Table 20.8 National guidelines for treatment of stroke.

Section	Recommendation
Diagnosis	• Essentially clinical • Brain imaging will be required if there are any unusual features, if there is a deterioration in the patient's condition, if subarachnoid haemorrhage is suspected, if trauma is suspected, if the patient is on anticoagulant treatment, or if hydrocephalus is suspected secondary to cerebral haemorrhage • Brain imaging should be done within 48 hours of diagnosis • A neurologist or physician with a special interest in stroke should always review the diagnosis
Acute treatment	• Aspirin 300 mg should be given as soon as possible (if haemorrhagic stroke is unlikely) • Neurosurgical opinion should be sought if hydrocephalus is suspected • Thrombolytic treatment should be given only in a specialist centre within 3 hours of the onset • Local policies should be in place to manage hypertension, hyperglycaemia, hydration and pyrexia • Long leg compression stockings should be given to those patients with paralysis or weakness of the legs
Secondary prevention	• Blood pressure should be checked and hypertension treated if persisting for more than 1 month. Systolic pressure should be lower than 140 mmHg and diastolic should be lower than 85 mmHg • All patients should be taking aspirin. Those patients who are unable to take aspirin should be given other antiplatelet treatment • Those with a carotid artery stroke should be considered for carotid endarterectomy • All patients will be assessed for other vascular risk factors and advised about lifestyle • Therapy with a statin (antithrombolytic) should be considered for all patients with a past history of myocardial infarction and cholesterol greater than 5 mmol/L
Rehabilitation	*Core principles* • Exercise therapy be provided within a neurological framework to improve function • Treatment approach should be multidisciplinary • Valid outcome measures should be utilised *Multidisciplinary assessment* • Protocols should be used and documented within 48 hours of admission • Assessment should include consciousness level, swallowing, pressure sore risk, nutritional status, cognitive impairment, communication, moving and handling assessment *Management* • Goal-setting to include the patient • Patient assessed for depressive illness • Speech and language and neurological physiotherapists and occupational therapists to be involved in rehabilitation • All necessary equipment should be provided to the carer

5 There is a paucity of evidence with regard to the extremes of motor function. Why do some patients do very well and others don't?

6 The description of active selected movement recovery has so far been neglected.

7 Knowledge of long-term movement patterns is limited.

Summary

Physiotherapy management is based upon a holistic problem-solving multi-disciplinary approach aimed at the promotion of independence, improved function, maximisation of activity, ameliorisation of symptoms and prevention of abnormality.

Table 20.9 Typical time history for stroke rehabilitation.

Stage	Definition	Typical management
Acute	Immediate period following the stroke	Initial assessment of basic systems Physiotherapy intervention for respiratory system Initial dialogue with patient and carers about the nature of stroke Assessment of patient's environment and social milieu
Intermediate	Period that commences once the patient is medically stable, conscious and actively engaged in the rehabilitation process	Regular identification and assessment of agreed rehabilitation objectives Active engagement in physiotherapy intervention programme Formulation and adherence to self-treatment strategies
Discharge and transfer	Period immediately prior to and following discharge from formal rehabilitation	Assessment of residual disability Physiotherapy intervention for agreed discharge objectives Modifications to the patient's environment Management of transfer of skills between environments Review and monitoring of self-treatment strategies Determine the pattern of rehabilitation once the patient has returned home or when community physiotherapy stops
Long-term		May include: Regular review of patient status Task-specific treatment sessions Review and modification of self-treatment strategies

From Stokes M 1998 Neurological Physiotherapy. New York: Mosby International.

Table 20.10 National clinical guidelines for stroke physiotherapy.

Approaches to rehabilitation	Examples
Use of valid and reliable assessment and measures Appropriate re-assessment	A multidisciplinary assessment using a formal protocol should be used and documented in the notes within 5 working days of admission This should include a manual handling risk assessment
Team work	Patients need to be assessed for the most suitable position and posture to facilitate feeding and involve all the relevant therapists in the assessment
Multidisciplinary goal-setting	Prevention of complications should be instigated This includes positioning, mobilisation, hydration and bowel and bladder management
Underlying approach to therapy should include improvement of function A task-specific rather than impairment focus should be used	Patients should be given time to practice activities of daily living (ADLs)
Intensity/ duration of therapy	Daily treatment should be the norm

PARKINSON'S DISEASE AND PARKINSONISM

Introduction

Parkinson's disease (PD) is a progressive, primary neurodegenerative disorder first described by James Parkinson in 1817; it was named 'the shaking palsy'. Parkinson's disease and parkinsonism comprise a group of disorders called *motor system disorders*. There are four primary symptoms:

- tremor
- rigidity
- bradykinesia (slowness of movement)
- postural instability.

Parkinsonism is the collective term for a group of conditions that includes PD (the most common manifestation) as well as several other degenerative brain disorders. The signs and symptoms of parkinsonism include the four cardinal signs of PD. The causes include the secondary effects of a primary neurological condition and those that result from trauma, for example boxing (Stokes 1998).

The aetiology of these diseases is unknown, but different theories continue to emerge. The list below provides an example of these theories, *which have not been proven and remain speculative*.

- Free radicals contribute to cell death via a process of oxidation?
- External or internal toxins selectively destroy dopaminergic neurons (e.g. exposure to pesticides)?
- There is a genetic predisposition?
- There is acceleration of the degeneration of the dopamine producing cells (accelerated ageing)?
- There is a combination of oxidative damage, environmental toxins, genetic predisposition and accelerated ageing?

PD affects men and women in equal numbers and there are no known social, economic or geographic variations. It is a disease of late middle age – usually affecting people over the age of 50. The average age of onset is 60 years, but one in seven patients with PD are diagnosed under the age of 50 (Caird 1991).

Diagnosis can sometimes be difficult because other conditions can mimic the signs and symptoms usually associated with PD. Early signs of the disease are subtle and develop gradually. Classically, it is the tremor that is the first sign patients present to their doctor and it often interferes with activities of daily living. Friends and families may notice the changes first. These minor changes can be:

- tiredness and general malaise
- shaking
- a soft voice
- spidery handwriting
- forgetfulness
- irritability/depressed mood.

Pathology

PD is a slowly degenerating disorder of the central nervous system. It specifically affects the substantia nigra and the corpus striatum (caudate nucleus and putamen) of the basal ganglia. The substantia nigra are two darkly pigmented dopamine-producing nuclei found in the midbrain. It is the most common basal ganglia disorder.

Death of the dopamine-producing cells of the substantia nigra and the corpus striatum occur long before clinical features are present. This results in a loss of the production of dopamine.

Key point

Dopamine is an inhibitory chemical neurotransmitter responsible for the transmission of impulses between the substantia nigra and the corpus striatum. The action of dopamine acts as a counterbalance to the excitatory neurotransmitter acetylcholine.

Neurotransmitters transmit electrical impulses across a synapse from one neurone to another. The depletion of dopamine results in a lack of inhibition on the cholinergic neurones, leading to unapposed excitation. The normal balance between excitatory and inhibitory neurotransmitters acting on the neurones is lost. In the normal state this balance between excitation and inhibition of the motor cortex via the basal ganglia results in the production of smooth, purposeful muscle activity. In addition, the loss of dopamine results in a reactive increase in the production of acetylcholine in the basal ganglia. This loss of dopamine-producing ability, the reactive increase in acetylcholine and the subsequent degeneration of the pigmented neurones in the substantia nigra result in the lack of normal movement control. Patients are unable to direct or control their movements. Approximately 80% of dopamine-producing cells are estimated to be lost before clinical signs of the disease manifest themselves.

The lack of inhibition of the reticulospinal and vestibulospinal pathways results in excessive contraction of postural muscles. The disturbance of inhibition and excitation results in the classical clinical features outlined below.

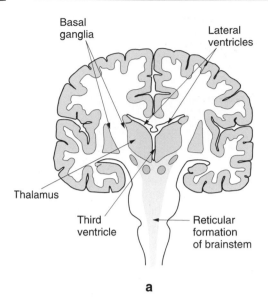

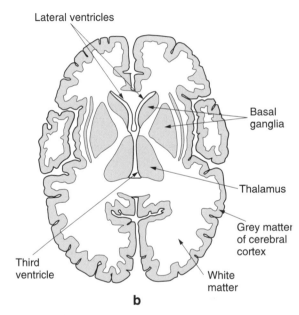

Figure 20.1   Internal appearance of the brain and brainstem. (Reproduced from Palastanga et al. 2002, with permission.)

Clinical Features

Onset of the disease is usually slow with the rate of progression varying between patients. Some patients become severely affected whilst others develop only minor symptoms. Improvements in the treatment of PD means that life expectancy is usually not shortened.

There are currently no diagnostic tests for Parkinson's disease. Diagnosis is usually made on the presentation of the characteristic signs of the disease: tremor, rigidity, bradykinesia and postural instability.

Tremor

The tremor associated with Parkinson's disease is a resting tremor and disappears on movement. It is described as a *pill-rolling tremor* and is highly characteristic. It resembles the action of a pill being rolled between the thumb and the tips of the fingers. It is usually unilateral and tends to characteristically be observed in the hand but can affect the arm and the leg. It is often seen under conditions of stress.

Rigidity

Rigidity is defined as an increased resistance to stretch and the inability to achieve complete muscle relaxation (Wichmann and DeLong 1993). There is a disruption of normal reciprocal inhibition. It is difficult to move the patient's limbs passively, and active movement is difficult.

Two types of rigidity are seen in people with PD:

- *Lead pipe rigidity* manifests as a uniform resistance to movement throughout the range of movement.
- *Cogwheel rigidity* presents as an intermittent on/off resistance throughout the range of movement, making the movements jerky.

The rigidity is a result of an increase in muscle tone. It contributes to the pain associated with PD and to the impoverished movement found in this disease.

Bradykinesia

Bradykinesia is the term used to describe slowness in the execution of movement. There is a slowing down and a loss of spontaneity of movement. This contributes to problems with posture and balance. It affects the patient's ability to carry out activities of daily living. The unpredictability of the bradykinesia can be very frustrating to patients.

Bradykinesia occurs as a result of loss of normal basal ganglia function. All movements become slow and are reduced in speed velocity and range. Steps are small when walking. Speech is slow and quiet. Handwriting is small and untidy. Repetitive movements are difficult (Stokes 1998; Hume-Adams 1998; Wiener and Goetz 1994). Automatic movements are affected. Blinking and facial expression is reduced resulting in the typical mask-like expression. Swallowing can be affected, and patients tend to dribble.

Postural instability

The clinical features listed above have a detrimental effect on the movement, posture balance and gait of Parkinson's disease sufferers. Patients tend to either lean backwards or forwards. Posture is generally flexed and is described as 'simian'.

Posture in PD

Simian posture results in knees and hips that are slightly flexed, rounded shoulders, and a flexed head. In standing, patients have a tendency to fall forwards and appear to be chasing their centre of gravity.

There is a lack of ability to make quick compensatory movements and so patients tend to fall over. Classically, the gait consists of small shuffling steps as the person is unable to shift his or her centre of gravity during walking. Patients may lean too far forward – this is called 'festination' (so the typical Parkinson's gait is called a 'festinating gait'). In addition to this there are characteristic difficulties with freezing during the gait cycle, particularly when coming across obstacles, doorways or a change in walking surface.

Other associated symptoms can include depression, emotional changes, difficulty in swallowing and chewing, speech changes, urinary, bowel, skin and sleep problems. Pain can be a significant symptom.

Management

The general approach to the management of PD and parkinsonism is multidisciplinary in emphasis. The coordinated approach to management means that the best care is provided at the best time and provided by the most appropriate healthcare professional. The general principles are to:

* improve function
* improve safety
* delay the loss of independence.

Assessment involves determining the underlying impairments, functional limitations and abilities. Multidisciplinary goal-setting is integral to the success of management interventions. Intervention strategies are both *compensatory* and *preventative*. Management includes management of the musculoskeletal, cardiopulmonary and neurological systems.

Medical management

The medical management of PD is primarily the prescription of drugs which aim to replace the lost dopamine or reduce the signs and symptoms associated with a loss of dopamine.

Because the disease manifests itself differently in different patients, it can take time before the most appropriate drug regimen is established. The main drug used in PD is the dopamine precursor *levadopa*, but in the early stages of the disease less powerful drugs may be used.

Levadopa is considered to be the gold standard of treatment. It is usually given with caridopa, which has the action of delaying the conversion of levadopa into dopamine, thus reducing the possible side-effects of the drug. Levadopa is especially effective against the bradykinesia and the impoverished voluntary movement (Cutson et al. 1995).

Other drugs used to treat PD are:

* bromocriptine, which mimics the role of dopamine
* selegiline, which delays the breakdown of dopamine and enhances and prolongs the effects of levadopa
* anticholinergics, which help to control tremor and rigidity by blocking the action of acetylcholine
* amantadine, which reduces other symptoms.

Physiotherapy management

The normal model of delivery of treatment for patients with PD is a combination of individual treatment sessions and group work. Treatment may be specifically targeted towards the different stages of the disease.

* In the *early stages* emphasis is placed on prevention and education.
* In the *middle stages* emphasis is placed on compensatory strategies to help overcome the difficulties being experienced by the patient.
* In the *later stages* emphasis is placed on respiratory status, functional aids and adaptations and palliation of the signs and symptoms (Turnbull 1992; Banks and Caird 1982; Kamsma 1995).

Assessment

The assessment should include both background history but also components specific to physiotherapy. Background history should include demographic details, past medical history, time since diagnosis of PD, presenting problems, medication, social factors (housing, family, lifestyle, care issues) and details of the involvement of other healthcare professionals (Table 20.11).

The assessment specific to physiotherapy concentrates on movement and function. Ideally the assessment should take place in the patient's usual surroundings. Motor impairments such as tremor, bradykinesia, hypokinesia, akinesia, rigidity and postural instability should be assessed in relation to the functional abilities of the patient. The physiotherapist should assess the patient performing a variety of activities, including walking, turning, sitting, standing, up and down stairs, and upper limb activities. Assessment of pain, muscle strength, range of movement, respiratory function and posture should be included as appropriate.

Table 20.11 Assessment guidelines for Parkinson's disease.

Background history	Demographic details, past medical history, years since onset of symptoms, years since diagnosis, presenting problems
Motor impairment	Tremor, bradykinesia, akinesia, dyskinesia, rigidity
Functional status	Walking, sit to stand, turning, change in direction, bed mobility, stairs, car transfers, upper-limb function (e.g. reaching, grasping, writing, manipulation of objects), postural instability, use of mobility aids
Specific tests	Muscle strength, range of movement, posture, pain, respiratory status

Treatment approaches

Physiotherapists draw upon a wide range of approaches when managing patients with PD. For example, theories of learning, neurophysiological and biomechanical approaches are utilised. The dominant treatment concept has been termed METERS (movement enablement through exercise regimes and strategies; Plant 2000).

Treatment techniques include the use of general exercise regimens and specific exercise programmes (Table 20.12). General exercises help to maintain overall fitness to maintain functional ability and support an active lifestyle. Specific exercise regimens help to improve individual problems and can promote increased flexibility which will help to prevent secondary problems associated with a loss of flexibility (Partridge 2002). Specific exercises have also been shown to promote psychological well-being (Palmer et al. 1986).

Degeneration of the basal ganglia results in the inability to perform complex motor sequences and therefore produce skilled movement. Treatment approaches include the use of compensatory strategies. These strategies involve breaking down complex movement sequences into smaller component parts. These

components are then arranged sequentially and are performed at a conscious level.

Key point
It is important to avoid simultaneous motor and cognitive tasks.

Physiotherapists also use mental rehearsal techniques and cueing strategies to help the client function more effectively within the limits of the disease. The cues used are visual, auditory, proprioceptive and cognitive (Table 20.13). External and internal cues utilise cortical mechanisms to activate and sustain movement (Morris 2000).

A range of other techniques can be used as appropriate if the patient is presenting with pain or pulmonary problems. General physiotherapy techniques can be used to alleviate these symptoms. Examples are massage, electrotherapy modalities, and mobilisation techniques.

To provide a comprehensive service, which supports patients with PD, a multidisciplinary approach is essential. The service needs to span primary, secondary and intermediate health and social care settings. A wide

Table 20.12 Exercise guidelines for Parkinson's disease.

General exercises	Specific exercises
For the trunk, upper and lower limbs and face	Individual home exercise programmes aimed at specific functional problems
Speech and breathing exercises	Strengthening exercises for the trunk with aerobic exercise to improve stability
Gait re-education	Individual programmes to improve flexibility to improve overall function
Balance training and re-education	Balance and lower limb strengthening to prevent falls
Transfer practice and training	Slow stretching regimes
Relaxation techniques	

Table 20.13 Cueing strategies for Parkinson's disease.

Cues	Examples
Visual	Strips of card on the floor can assist step length and initiation problems Strategically placed cue cards containing a key word helps to activate movement
Auditory	A musical beat or voice can help with gait
Proprioceptive	Rocking from side to side or taking a step backwards before walking can help to overcome freezing
Cognitive	Memorising the separate parts of a movement and rehearsing them mentally can be helpful

range of healthcare professionals will be involved in the management in a variety of settings. Multidisciplinary goal-setting is recommended and the use of appropriate outcome measures is essential. Table 20.14 provides examples of the outcome measures that may be used when managing clients with Parkinson's disease.

MULTIPLE SCLEROSIS

Introduction

Multiple (disseminated) sclerosis is a progressively degenerative disease of the central nervous system (CNS), of unknown cause, whose pathological trademarks are inflammation and demyelination. The presenting clinical features can be very varied, resulting in a complex combination of physical, psychological and cognitive problems. This highly variable presentation (and often unpredictable condition) poses a major challenge to therapists if they are to assist individuals in managing the condition as effectively as possible.

The prevalence of MS varies worldwide, with the lowest amongst populations living nearest to the equator. The condition appears to be most common in temperate climates. People who emigrate before the age of 15 years exhibit the rate of incidence of their adopted country (Dean and Kurtze 1971). These facts seem to suggest that there may be an environmental trigger that

Table 20.14 Outcome measures in Parkinson's disease.

Measurement of:	Outcome measure
Function	Parkinson's Activity Scale Rivermead Mobility Index Timed up-and-go test
Balance	Berg balance test Functional reach test
Gait	Clinical gait assessment 10-metre walk test

allows the disease to develop through a genetic or immunological susceptibility in children below age about 15 that is no longer present in adults.

Approximately 15% of individuals with MS have an affected relative. This risk rises to 1:50 for offspring and 1:20 for siblings of affected persons (Sadovnick et al. 1988).

Another possible contributing factor to the onset of MS could be gender. MS is more common in women than men in a ratio of approximately 2:1. Race appears to have an influence, with black and Asian populations having a lower incidence. Other suggested factors are diet and socioeconomic status, with the higher the standard of living the higher the risk of developing MS.

Key point

In the UK, an estimated 80,000 people have been diagnosed with MS. This makes it the second highest cause of neurological disability in young adults. Approximately 1 per 800–1000 of the population is affected, with the average onset of the condition being at 30 years of age (Sadovnik and Ebers 1993). The range of onset is extremely broad, from 10 years to 59 years.

Pathology

Acute stage

Breach of the blood–brain barrier is one of the first significant events to occur at this stage. T-lymphocytes in particular are targeted against the vascular wall. They are responsible for the secretion of cytokines, which then recruit other cells including macrophages. The lymphocyte makes a hole in the endothelium and enters the CNS. This results in a perivascular inflammatory lesion that leads to tissue damage, particularly of myelin.

This inflammatory stage can vary in its duration from days to a month. The intensity and duration of the attack will determine the overall extent of the damage. This phase is associated with vasogenic oedema that ultimately resolves over a matter of weeks, with repair of the blood–brain barrier. A residual fibrous scar is then left on the myelin sheath, termed a *plaque* or *sclerosis*.

Later stages

In the early stages of the condition, demyelination is not the main cause of any symptoms but rather the inflammation itself. However, as the condition progresses, repeated onset of the attacks results in more permanent damage. Over a period of time the CNS combats this damage by a number of compensatory mechanisms, but eventually the amount it can compensate for the deficits is superseded by the structural damage. Permanent deficits are the final outcome of this run of events.

Forms of MS and Diagnosis

About 45% of sufferers initially present with a *relapsing–remitting* form of the condition (RRMS). An acute flare-up, lasting from a few days to a few weeks, is followed by a period of remission where no symptoms are displayed. The periods of relapse and remission can vary in themselves, with an acute relapse being followed by a period of remission lasting weeks to months.

About 40% of the people who initially presented with RRMS will go on to develop a secondary stage of progression with or without superimposed relapses – known as *secondary progressive MS* (SPMS). The person appears to exhibit a steady deterioration, without any noticeable acute periods to account for this.

The third main form of the condition, known as *primary progressive MS* (PPMS), presents as a steadily deteriorating condition from the onset, with no identifiable relapses or remissions. The rate of deterioration can be fairly rapid in some cases. About 10–15% of cases are in this category.

Two further categories need to be included for completeness: *benign* (10–20% of cases), with no significant disability due to MS 10 years after onset; and *malignant* (Marburg's disease).

In spite of the increasing reliance on magnetic resonance imaging (MRI) as a diagnostic tool, clinical evaluation continues to be the main method of diagnosing MS. Other investigations used are evoked potentials and, less commonly, analysis of cerebrospinal fluid by way of a lumbar puncture. The most widely used diagnostic criteria are those of Poser et al. (1983; see Table 20.15).

Clinical Features

Any part of the CNS may be affected, so unsurprisingly symptoms vary tremendously according to which part of the CNS is affected. Some of the most common clinical features will be described here, but readers may need to refer to other texts for more detailed information (see also www.msif.org).

Vision

The optic nerve, cervical cord, brainstem and cerebellar peduncles are most commonly affected. Frequently at onset the first feature is of optic neuritis of varying severity. Pain is felt behind the affected eye with some element of visual disturbance occurring. In 58% of cases acuity is affected without pain. However, overall more than 90% of cases recover the majority of their visual acuity. Later on, other symptoms affecting eye movement are dysmetria, nystagmus, internuclear ophthalmoplegia (slowing of adduction) and occular flutter. Diplopia might be experienced.

Table 20.15 Diagnostic criteria in multiple sclerosis.

Category	Relapses	Minimum number of:		
		Deficits	Paraclinical evidence	Oligoclonal bands
Clinically definite	2	2		
	2 and	1		
Clinically probable	2	1		
	1	2		
	1	1 and	1*	+
Lab-supported definite	2	1 or		+
Lab-supported probable	1	1 and	1	+
	2		+	

* Progression of MRI abnormalities over time also constitutes paraclinical evidence for diagnosis of laboratory-supported definite MS.
From Poser CM, Paty DW, Scheinberg LC et al. 1983 New diagnostic criteria for multiple sclerosis: guidelines for research protocols. Ann Neurol 13:227–31.

Sensation

Sensory symptoms are common early on in the course of the condition. Numbness, pins and needles, tightness around a limb and other more unusual sensations, such as of water running down a limb, are the most frequently experienced. Later on joint proprioception is also commonly affected.

Motor function

Motor symptoms are more common than sensory symptoms and are usually more disabling in the long run. Changes in muscle tone, weakness, tremor, poor coordination and ataxia are all impairments that often result in difficulties with movement. Neurological conditions where the white matter is affected often result in considerable spasticity. Spasticity, most commonly in the legs, may be present with or without accompanying weakness. Other than cerebellar ataxia, spasticity is frequently the most disabling feature in people with MS. Individuals may report spasms, sometimes at night, which can be painful. Cerebellar ataxia can result in arm movements being uncoordinated (intention tremor), a wide-based gait pattern and speech disturbances.

Swallowing

Individuals entering the later stages of MS may experience swallowing difficulties (dysphagia). An underestimation of the degree of swallowing difficulties may result in bronchopneumonia and ultimately therefore can be potentially life-threatening. Swallowing is a highly complex motor skill that requires careful assessment by a speech and language therapist, dietician and radiographer. Videofluoroscopy using a modified barium swallow is an essential investigation if comprehensive assessment of dysphagia is to occur. Assessment of the individual's posture during swallowing should not be overlooked. Ultimately if severe difficulties persist with oral feeding then other alternatives such as a gastrostomy may need to be considered.

Bladder and bowel

Bladder disturbances in MS are very common and often take the form of either detrusor hyperreflexia or detruso-sphincter dyssernygia. Urgency, frequency, nocturnal disturbances and urge incontinence are the various types of bladder presentations. People often report that social trips have to be strategically planned around where the nearest toilet might be. The former type of bladder disturbance rarely occurs without the presence of spasticity in the legs. The second type of bladder disturbance (detruso-sphincter dyssernygia) presents as delay or inability to void, frequency, urgency and an inability to fully empty the bladder.

This may result in urinary retention and the susceptibility to urinary tract infections.

Treatment is often successful in the form of muscle relaxants, anticholinergic drugs and self-catheterisation.

Constipation is the main bowel problem and is relatively straightforward to treat.

Key point
One of the most common and usually most disabling symptoms is that of fatigue. Fatigue in its truest sense, for people with MS, is usually described as 'a deterioration in performance with continuing effort' (Barnes 2000).

Pain and fatigue

People with MS tend to be more susceptible to pain syndromes such as trigeminal neuralgia, myelopathies and musculoskeletal type pain. The latter is usually as a result of poor posture and poor alignment of joints – sometimes through soft tissue adaptations and over stressed joints.

As the day progresses, any activities involving physical effort are often increasingly difficult to carry out. This is an important consideration when it comes to planning physiotherapy treatment interventions.

Cognition

Cognitive difficulties such as disturbances in functional memory, reduced information processing speeds and impaired intellectual function are more common in people with MS than is widely recognised. Cognitive impairments in MS may contribute significantly to any reduction in functional capability. Although these types of impairments are more common in people with longstanding MS, they have also been shown to exist at a time when there are relatively few physical symptoms (Van den Burg et al. 1987).

Management

Medical management

Key point
Medical management can be divided into interventions that may influence the condition directly and those that help to manage the symptoms.

In acute relapses, rest and steroid therapy are the mainstay of medical management. In spite of the widespread use of steroids in MS there remains little consensus in the UK over the most appropriate dose and mode of administration. Steroid therapy is most commonly administered in the form of 1 g of intravenous methylprednisolone for 3–5 days with or without a reducing dose of steroids. The most common oral regimen is prednisolone 60 mg daily, reducing to zero over 1–3 weeks. Low-dose oral steroids are generally better tolerated, but evidence of efficacy is less robust.

Steroids have been shown to shorten the recovery time during relapses, although they do not seem to have an overall effect on the long-term progress of the condition. Longer-term use of steroids is less well supported in the literature and any potential benefits must be weighed against the potentially harmful side-effects of steroid therapy.

Interferone β has now unequivocally been proven to be of benefit to some people with MS, by reducing the number of relapses that occur in relapsing–remitting MS, thereby delaying progression of the condition.

Many other types of medical intervention are utilised to manage the consequences of the disease process, such as antispasmodic medication to reduce the effects of spasticity and referral for further investigations depending upon the presenting symptoms. For example an ultrasound scan of the bladder may be needed to establish incomplete voiding of the bladder.

Physiotherapy management

The key to any successful intervention is a comprehensive and ongoing assessment of the person's difficulties and needs. A coordinated interdisciplinary approach is also crucial if the condition is to be managed effectively (Ko Ko 1999). Rehabilitation programmes must be tailored to meet the needs of the individual and carers, who should be at the centre of the goal-setting approach.

Individuals with MS often feel their needs are best served by services that allow direct access to them at the time of need. They also often feel they benefit most from a consistent approach on an ongoing basis that allows continuity of management rather than episodes of care (Robinson et al. 1996).

The main aims of any physiotherapy intervention must be to keep the individual as functionally independent as possible. In order to do this, often in the face of increasing disability, it is vitally important that the physiotherapist works with the person on a psychological as well as physical level. Timing of interventions is crucial and is one of the main reasons for the need for ongoing monitoring of this group of patients.

Additional goals of a physiotherapy programme are to minimise abnormalities of muscle tone, preserve the integrity of the musculoskeletal system by preventing secondary problems (Thompson 1998), improve posture along with advice on postural management, facilitate the use of efficient functional movement patterns, re-educate gait, and encourage of self-management informed by an understanding of the condition.

Measurement

The most frequently used measurement tools to monitor outcomes of treatment for people with MS are:

- Functional Independence Measure (FIM)
- Barthel Index
- Rivermead Motor Assessment Scale
- SF-36
- Health Related Quality of Life (HRQoL) scale
- Multiple Sclerosis Quality of Life (MSQoL) scale
- Kurtzke Expanded Status Scale (Kurtzke 1981, 1983).

MOTOR NEURONE DISEASE

Introduction

Motor neurone disease (MND) is characterised by progressive degeneration of motor neurones:

- anterior horn cells in the spinal cord, resulting in lower motor neurone lesions (LMN)
- corticospinal tract cells, resulting in upper motor neurone lesions (UMN)
- motor nuclei in the brain stem, resulting in both upper and lower motor lesions.

Key point
'Motor neurone disease' is in fact a global term mainly used in the UK and Australia. In other parts of the world the condition is often referred to as 'amyotrophic lateral sclerosis'.

Although MND is primarily a disease of the motor neurones, there may be occasional involvement of other areas of the central nervous system. The autonomic nervous system, sensory nerves, lower sacral segments of the spinal cord and the three cranial nerves that control movement of the eyes are usually unaffected.

The aetiology of the condition is unknown, although 5% of people have a familial form (Figlewicz and Rouleau 1994). It is a condition that usually affects people in later life, starting at between 50 and 70 years, with a marginally higher occurrence in males.

Key point

Precise figures for incidence and prevalence are not known. The incidence is thought to be 2 per 100,000 per year, whilst the prevalence is estimated to be 7 per 100,000. The approximate number of people with MND in the UK is 5000 (MND Association 2000).

Clinical Features and Diagnosis

The onset of MND is usually insidious and the exact presentation depends upon the areas of the CNS affected. Where there is lower motor neurone degeneration, the main features are weakness, muscle wasting and fasciculation of the nerves undergoing degeneration. Degeneration of upper motor neurones usually results in spasticity with accompanying weakness and muscle wasting.

Forms of MND

The following is a broad categorisation of the forms of MND, but in reality there is often considerable overlap between the forms.

Amyotrophic lateral sclerosis (ALS)

This is the most common form of the condition (65%). It is more common in males and involves both upper and lower motor neurones. It is characterised by spasticity, muscle weakness, hyperactive reflexes, with possible bulbar signs of dysarthria, dysphagia and emotional lability. The hands tend to be affected initially with the person reporting clumsiness, with evidence of thenar eminence wasting with the shoulder also often being affected early on. With bulbar involvement, speech, swallowing and the tongue are affected. The average survival rate is 2–5 years.

Progressive bulbar palsy

This affects 25% of people with MND, with slightly older people and women being more commonly affected. Both upper and lower neurones may be involved. Dysphagia and dysarthria are characteristic of this form of the condition, owing to lower motor neurone damage causing nasal speech, regurgitation of fluids via the nose, tongue atrophy, pharyngeal weakness and fasciculation. Life expectancy is usually between 6 months and 3 years.

Progressive muscular atrophy

This affects approximately 7.5% of people with MND when there is predominantly lower motor neurone involvement. Males are more affected than females at a ratio of 5:1. Muscle wasting and weakness with weight loss and fasciculation are the main presenting features. Mental deterioration and dementia are found in fewer than 5% of people (Tandan 1994). Life expectancy is usually more than 5 years.

Primary lateral sclerosis

This is a rare form of the condition that affects mainly the upper motor neurones. It is characterised by spastic quadraperisis, pseudobulbar symptoms, spastic dysarthria and hyperreflexia. A survival rate of 20 years or more can be expected.

Diagnosis

As with many other progressive diseases, no one specific test exists for the diagnosis of MND. Investigations often include imaging (MRI), myelogram (EMG), blood tests, and clinical investigations to exclude the possibility of other conditions such as syringomyelia or cervical spondylosis (Swash and Schwartz 1995).

Management

Medical management

Medical and healthcare professionals have a significant role to play in the management of this condition owing to its complex and potentially rapidly deteriorating course. Owing to the high number of professionals involved in the person's care, it is vitally important that interventions be coordinated in some way. As in many cases where a high number of professionals from various agencies are involved, individuals with MND and their families often report that one of the most frustrating aspects of their management is the lack of coordination of service provision.

The family and their long-term needs must be considered. It is vitally important that the person with MND maintains as much control over his or her life as possible. Timely interventions, speedy responses,

Rilutek

In 1996 a drug called Rilutek, whose active ingredient is riluzole, became the first licensed drug treatment available for people with MND. It is not a cure for the condition but has been reported to extend life by several months (National Institute for Clinical Excellence 2001).

advice and support, ongoing assessment and access to equipment and services are the main needs for this group of people.

Physiotherapy management

Assessment of the person's needs on an ongoing basis is taken as a prerequisite before any treatment interventions. Again, a multidisciplinary team assessment and approach is necessary for this group of people.

In the early stages, information on MND and support agencies, advice on appropriate exercise programmes, support for the person with MND and the family, and providing a point of contact will be the main physiotherapy interventions.

As the condition progresses, and this will vary from person to person, physiotherapy interventions will take the form of advice on exercise programmes and how best to incorporate these into everyday activities. This will ensure that the movement is as functional as possible. Active assisted exercises may be required if the person needs assistance to move. The main aim at this stage is to keep the person as independent as possible for as long as possible. To this end, assistive devices may be needed and again the physiotherapist may need to liaise with the occupational therapist, orthotist and rehabilitation engineers in the case of environmental control systems.

As movement becomes more difficult through weakness or spasticity, passive movements are indicated to prevent secondary impairments of the musculoskeletal system. It is vital that carers be involved in this process, if they so wish, to assist in the process of maintenance. A large part of the physiotherapist's role will be teaching and advising carers and other members of the team. One aspect of advice from the physiotherapist might be how to move and position the client in the most appropriate manner. The client is likely to be increasingly reliant on other forms of mobility during this stage of the condition and as such will need advice on the type of wheelchair (often powered) required.

With individuals with dysphagia it is important that the physiotherapist works closely with the speech and language therapist and nursing staff to ensure optimum positioning for a safe swallow. Monitoring of respiratory function will also be necessary for this group of clients.

Terminal stage

In the terminal stage of the disease the person may be cared for at home or admitted to a hospice. Management of any prevailing symptoms and ensuring the person is as comfortable as possible are the main aims. It is of vital importance that both practical and emotional support is forthcoming for the family and carers. Deterioration is often rapid, with the most common cause of death being respiratory tract infection leading to respiratory failure.

TRAUMATIC BRAIN INJURY

Introduction

Traumatic brain injury (TBI) describes a wide range of conditions and has in the past been used interchangeably with the term 'head injury'. The prefix of traumatic differentiates this group of people from those who have sustained any disruption to the vascular supply of the brain.

TBI is often accompanied by other types of injury, particularly a fracture. Skull fractures may be simple or compound, undisplaced or depressed. The damage to the brain may be caused either at the time of injury (primary) or as a result of other injuries or complications (secondary).

Brain injury can be classified according to the Glasgow Coma Scale duration of coma, by the length of post-traumatic amnesia (PTA), or by results from a computerised tomography (CT) scan (Table 20.16; Jennet and Teasdale 1981). Post-traumatic amnesia is defined as 'the length of time between injury and the restoration of continuous day-to-day memory' (Russell and Smith 1961).

Key point

It is estimated that 270 people per 100,000 a year in England and Wales are admitted to hospital as a result of a TBI (Jennett and MacMillan 1981), although the number of people visiting accident and emergency departments with a head injury is much higher than this. The most frequently admitted groups are children and small babies. Men aged 15–24 have the most serious head injuries and account for more than 30% of all deaths in this age group; alcohol consumption has been found to be a contributing cause to many of these injuries. Road traffic accidents and sporting injuries are the other most common cause of TBI.

Pathology

Primary brain injury

Most commonly occurring mechanisms include direct blows to the head, deceleration and rotational forces. *Contrecoup lesions* can occur as a result of falls or direct

Table 20.16 Classification of brain injury.

Classification	Score on Glasgow Coma Scale (GCS)	Duration of coma	Length of PTA
Mild	13–15	<20 min	<1 hour
Moderate	9–12	<6 hours	1–24 hours
Severe	3–8	>6 hours	>24 hours

blows to the head where there may be contusions at the site of impact along with contusions at the opposite side to the impact. Often the frontal lobes are most prone to damage owing to their proximity to the orbital ridges. Vascular damage is the main form of damage in the form of subarachnoid bleeding with intracerebral and subdural haematomas appearing at the time of injury.

Secondary brain injury

This may be due to extracranial factors, such as chest or multiple injuries that lead to cardiac arrest, hypotension or hypoxia. If cerebral perfusion pressure reaches a critical low, regulatory mechanisms are lost and ischaemic damage occurs (Mendlow et al. 1983).

Alternatively, intracranial causes can be the result of damage, such as acute traumatic haematomas, raised intracranial pressure (ICP) and infection.

Potential Problems Following TBI

Post-traumatic epilepsy

This can be present in up to 40% of cases, depending on the severity of brain injury. The earlier practice of placing patients on prophylactic anticonvulsants for long periods has more recently been disputed (Temkin et al. 1990). Medication more commonly prescribed includes carbamazepine and valproic acid owing to their reduced side-effects in comparison to phenobarbital and phenytoin. Many anticonvulsants can produce significant side-effects.

Post-traumatic hydrocephalus

This refers to enlargement of the ventricular system and generally is nonobstructive. If hydrocephalus is diagnosed, ventricular shunting is the usual treatment.

Neuroendocrine and autonomic disorders

These types of problem include hypertension, hypothalamic–pituitary disorders, and hyperthermia. Hypertension can occur as a new condition in 10–15% of patients but is usually transient and can be managed effectively with beta-blockers.

Cranial neuropathies

These are a common occurrence following TBI, with cranial nerves I and III and less commonly IV, VI and VIII being affected.

Gastrointestinal and nutritional needs

Nutritional needs in the acute stages of TBI are reported to increase by an estimated 25%. Long-term outcomes have been more favourable owing to the nutritional needs of patients being met (Young et al. 1987). Alternative methods of feeding may need to be considered in the early stages to achieve this aim. Problems with dysphagia can occur in approximately 25% of patients and this might also be another reason why alternative methods of feeding may need to be adopted.

Orthopaedic and musculoskeletal complications

Fractures are a common feature in TBI, with occult fractures being amongst the most serious problems. Peripheral nerve injuries are frequently under-diagnosed, and heterotopic ossification occurs in 76% of cases.

Continence

Urinary incontinence following TBI is very common for a number of reasons but is primarily due to disinhibition.

Sexual dysfunction

The most common occurrence is oligomenorrhea. Other complications include impotence, altered libido along with difficulties created by any behavioural changes.

Motor function

Disturbances in the central nervous system can lead to hypertonicity, contractures and disordered movement. Hypertonicity can predispose patients to adaptive muscle shortening (contractures). Timely and effective management of hypertonicity can ultimately avoid the need for surgical intervention.

Movement disorders encountered might be rigidity, tremors, ataxia, akathisia and dystonias including chorea.

Sensation

Disturbances in sensory function can present in the form of diminished or absent cutaneous sensation (paraesthesia/anaesthesia), or various agnosias such as sensory neglect. Certain sensory disturbances can be addressed to some extent within the rehabilitation programme. However, long-standing sensory disturbances tend to persist.

Cognition

As mentioned earlier, altered behaviour can be the most troublesome aspect of a patient's rehabilitation and long-term social reintegration. Commonly occurring features include disturbances in level of arousal, speed of processing of information, memory, abstract reasoning and flexibility, self-awareness, distractability and limited attention span. Behavioural deficits and psychosocial adjustment after TBI include depression, poor social awareness, agitation, aggressive behaviour and difficulties initiating activities (Prigatano 1992; Wood 1990).

Management

Early medical management

The management immediately after trauma involves primarily life-support measures. It is important that levels of consciousness be recorded and measured using a scale such as the Glasgow Coma Scale. In conjunction with this, on transfer to an acute hospital setting, further investigations such as a skull X-ray, CT scan or MR imaging may be necessary. In some cases intracranial monitoring will be necessary to ensure further damage or deterioration in the patient's condition does not occur. Certain patients will require neurosurgical intervention, which cannot be covered in any detail within this text. Readers are referred to Black and Rossitch (1995) and Bullock and Teasdale (1990) for further information.

In summary, the overall goals in the acute setting are:

- medical stability
- clearing of post-traumatic amnesia
- reduction of behavioural and physical dependence.

If the patient does not require a high level of medical input, a less acute setting with intensive therapy services may be more appropriate.

Later stage medical management

As with many complex neurological conditions, patients are best managed by an experienced interdisciplinary rehabilitation team, using a patient-centred, goal-orientated approach. By this stage, patients should have been moved to an environment that is conducive to intensive rehabilitation. It is increasingly common for patients with complex disabilities to be managed using a key worker or case manager approach in order to provide more effective continuity of the services delivered.

Patients can present with a wide variety of impairments, depending on the site of the damage. Often even patients with severe physical impairments early on in their rehabilitation improve significantly. However, by far an overriding residual problem is one of cognitive impairment, including disruption of executive functions. These types of impairments, and the resultant psychosocial implications, can lead to significant limitations in social interactions and can be the main barriers to individuals returning to independent living (Lezak 1986; Brooks and McKinlay 1983; Oddy and Humphrey 1980; Oddy et al. 1978).

The effectiveness of rehabilitation is still under review. However, some evidence exists which suggests that rehabilitation is effective in improving patients' levels of independence (Malec and Basford 1996; Cope 1995; Hall and Cope 1995).

Physiotherapy management

Acute stage

The main priority at this stage is to ensure the patient is medically stable. However, it is also important not to lose sight of the fact that proactive management at this early stage, of potential secondary complications, can ultimately enhance patient outcomes. It is necessary to optimise the patient's respiratory function if secondary cerebral damage is to be avoided. All interventions during this stage need to be carefully balanced against the risk of raising the intracranial pressure (Ada et al. 1990).

The main goals of treatment are:

- to prevent build up of respiratory secretions and enhance oxygenation of the brain – by the use of bagging, suction and positioning
- to preserve the integrity of the neuromusculoskeletal system thereby preventing or minimising adaptive muscle shortening and contractures – by the use of passive movements, correct positioning, postural management, careful handling to avoid over-stimulation, prophylactic serial splinting in conjunction with antispasticity medication if necessary

- to provide an appropriate level of sensory stimulation – by careful handling, use of sensory stimulation regimes if appropriate
- to provide early family education and support – by means of involvement in aspects of the patient's care, providing time out to discuss the patient's progress and potential outcomes of interventions, advice on support groups and sources of information.

Later stage – after months or years

The cognitive abilities and behavioural presentation of individuals with TBI will have an impact upon their level of function. It is therefore vital that these elements be assessed and taken into account when agreeing goals for interventions. Historically, physiotherapists have failed to take sufficient account of these factors, and subsequent physiotherapy interventions have perhaps been less effective than they might have been. Access to a neuropsychologist, who can assess and advise on the most effective way to deal with these factors when planning treatment, is invaluable.

At this stage the main goals of physiotherapy interventions are to:

- encourage the return of active movement that carries over into function
- prevent secondary deformities
- prevent unnecessary and potentially damaging compensatory movement strategies
- maximise respiratory function
- encourage social and vocational reintegration
- provide advice to the family, carers and other members of the team on aspects of the patient's management.

Measurement

The most frequently used measurement tools to monitor outcomes of treatment for people with TBI are:

- Glasgow Outcome Scale (Jennet and Bond 1975)
- Disability Rating Scale (Rappaport et al. 1982)
- FIM and FAM
- Glasgow Coma Scale (Teasdale and Jennett 1974).

GLOSSARY OF TERMS

The following glossary is intended to provide a brief description of some of the terminology found in this chapter.

Agnosia   Loss of knowledge or inability to perceive objects
Anaesthesia   Absence of sensation

Ataxia   Loss of coordination affecting functional movement
Babinski sign   Abnormal response of the plantar reflex (great toe turns upwards on testing)
Bradykinesia   Slowness of movement
Clonus   Succession of intermittent muscular relaxation and contraction usually resulting from a sustained stretch
Diplopia   Double vision
Dysarthria   Incoordination of speech
Dysphagia   Difficulty in swallowing
Dysphasia   Disruption of expressive (produce) and or receptive (understand) speech
Dyspraxia   Inability to execute volitional purposeful movements
Dystonia   Involuntary movement characterised by twisting and repetitive movement
Flaccidity   Absence of muscle tone
Hemianopea   Loss of visual field in one half of each eye
Hemiplegia   Paralysis of one side of the body
Hypertonicity   Increased muscle tone
Hypotonicity   Decreased muscle tone
Nystagmus   Involuntary rhythmic oscillation of one or both eyes
Paraesthesia   Disruption of sensation causing abnormal sensation
Ptosis   Drooped eyelid
Rigidity   Stiffness of neurological origin, increased resistance to stretch throughout the range
Tone   The active resistance of muscle to stretch
Tremor   Fine type of involuntary movement (several types seen in neurological dysfunction)

FURTHER READING

General

Brincat CA 1999 Managed care and rehabilitation: adopting a true team approach. Top Stroke Rehabil 6(2): 62–5
Carr JH, Shepherd RB 1998 Neurological Rehabilitation: Optimizing Motor Performance. London: Butterworth–Heinemann
Edwards S 2002 Neurological Physiotherapy: a Problem-Solving Approach, 2nd edn. London: Churchill Livingstone
Greenwood R, Barnes MP, Mcmillan TM, Ward CD (ed.) 1993 Neurological Rehabilitation. Edinburgh: Churchill Livingstone
Partridge C (ed.) 2002 Neurological Physiotherapy: Bases of Evidence for Practice. London: Whurr
Reinkensmeyer D et al. 2002. Emerging technologies for improving access to movement therapy following neurological injury. In Emerging and Accessible Telecommunications: Information and Healthcare Technologies. New York: IEEE Press
Stokes M 1998 Neurological Physiotherapy. New York: Mosby International

Stroke

Alexander H, Bugge C, Hagen S 2001 What is the association between the different components of stroke rehabilitation and health outcomes? Clin Rehabil 15: 207–15

Ashburn A 1997 Physical recovery following stroke. Physiotherapy 83: 480–90

Bosworth H, Horner R, Edwards L, Matchar D 2000 Depression and other determinants of values placed on current health state by stroke patients: evidence from VAS Acute Stroke (VAS+) study. Stroke 31: 2603–9

Royal College of Physicians/Chartered Society of Physiotherapy intercollegiate working party 2000 National Clinical Guidelines for Stroke

Parkinson's disease

Deane KHO et al. 2001 Physiotherapy for patients with Parkinson's disease (Cochrane review). Cochrane Library, Oxford

Morris M 2000 Movement disorders in people with Parkinson's disease: a model for physical therapy. Phys Ther 80: 578–97

Plant R et al. 2000 Physiotherapy for People with Parkinson's Disease: UK Best Practice. Newcastle upon Tyne: Institute of Rehabilitation

Schenkman M et al. 1997 Reliability of impairment and physical performance measures for persons with Parkinson's disease. Phys Ther 77: 19–27

Suteeraiva Hananon M, Protas EJ 2000 Reliability of outcome measures in individuals with Parkinson's disease. Physiother Theory Pract 16: 211–18

Multiple sclerosis

Barnes D 2000 Multiple Sclerosis: Questions and Answers. Hampshire: Merit Publishing International

Motor neurone disease

Motor Neurone Disease Association 2000 A Patient and Carer Centred Approach for Health and Social Professionals: Motor Neurone Disease Resource File. Northampton: MND Association

Traumatic brain injury

Campbell M 2000 Rehabilitation for Traumatic Brain Injury: Physical Therapy Practice in Context. London: Churchill Livingstone

REFERENCES

Ada L, Canning C, Paratz J 1990 Care of the unconscious head-injured patient. In Ada L, Canning C (eds) Key Issues in Neurological Physiotherapy, p. 249. London: Butterworth–Heinemann

Ashburn A 1997 Physical recovery following stroke. Physiotherapy 83: 480–90

Banks MA, Caird FI 1982 Physiotherapy benefits patients with Parkinson's disease. Clin Rehabil 3: 11–16

Barnes D 2000 Multiple Sclerosis: Questions and Answers. Hampshire: Merit Publishing International

Black P, Rossitch E 1995 Neurosurgery: an Introductory Text. Oxford: Oxford University Press

Bohannon RW, Smith MB 1987 Interrater reliability of a modified Ashworth scale of muscle spasticity. Phys Ther 67: 206–7

Bohannon RW, Cassidy D, Walsh S 1995 Trunk muscle strength is impaired multidirectionally after stroke. Clin Rehabil 9: 47–51

Bonita R 1992 Epidemiology of stroke. Lancet 339: 342–43

Brooks DN, McKinlay WW 1983 Personality and behavioural change after severe blunt head injury: a relative's view. J Neurol Neurosurg Psychiat 46: 336–44

Caird FI (ed.) 1991 Rehabilitation in Parkinson's Disease. London: Chapman & Hall

Carr JH, Shepherd RB 1998 Neurological Rehabilitation: Optimizing Motor Performance. Butterworth–Heinemann

Carr JH, Shepherd RB, Nordholm L, Lynne D 1985 Investigation of a new motor assessment scale for stroke patients. Phys Ther 65: 175–80

Cella DF et al. 1996 Validation of the functioning assessment of multiple sclerosis quality of life instrument. Neurology 47: 129–39

Cope DN 1995 The effectiveness of traumatic brain injury rehabilitation: a review. Brain Inj 9: 649–70

Crow JL, Lincoln NB, Nouri FM, De Weerdt W 1989 The effectiveness of EMG feedback in the treatment of arm function after stroke. Int Disabil Studies 11: 155–60

Cutson TM et al. 1995 Pharmacological and non-pharmacological interventions in the treatment of Parkinson's disease. Phys Ther 75: 363–73

Dean G, Kurtzke JF 1971 On the risk of multiple sclerosis according to the age at immigration to South Africa. BMJ 3: 725–9

Duncan PW et al. 1990 Functional reach: a new clinical measure of balance. J Gerontol 45: 192–7

Department of Health (DoH) 2000 National Service Framework for Older People. London: DoH

Edwards S (ed.) 2002 Neurological Physiotherapy: a Problem-Solving Approach, 2nd edn. London: Churchill Livingstone

Elsworth JD, Marks JA, McGrath JR, Wade DT 1999 An audit of goal planning in rehabilitation. Top Stroke Rehabil 6(2): 51–61

Fawcus R (ed.) 2000 Stroke Rehabilitation: a Collaborative Approach. Oxford: Blackwell Scientific

Figlewicz DA, Rouleau GA 1994 Familial disease. In Williams AC (ed.) Motor Neurone Disease, pp. 427–50. London: Chapman & Hall

Freeman JA 2002 Assessment, outcome measurement and goal setting in physiotherapy practice. In Edwards S (ed.) Neurological Physiotherapy, 2nd edn, pp. 21–34. London: Churchill Livingstone

Granger CV, Cotter AC, Hamilton BB, Fiedler RC 1993 Functional assessment scales: a study of persons after stroke. Arch Phys Med Rehabil 74: 133–8

Hall KM, Cope DN 1995 The benefit of rehabilitation in traumatic brain injury: a literature review. J Head Trauma Rehabil 10(5): 1–13

Harwood RH, Gompertz P, Pound P, Ebrahim S 1997 Determinants of handicap 1 and 3 years after a stroke. Disabil Rehabil 19(5): 205–11

Hauser SL et al. 1983 Intensive immunosuppression in progressive multiple sclerosis: a randomised three-arm study of high-dose intravenous cyclophosphamide, plasma exchange and ACTH. N Engl J Med 308: 173–80

Hume-Adams J, Graham DI 1998 An Introduction to Neuropathology, 2nd edn. Edinburgh: Churchill Livingstone

Hunt SM, McKenna SP, Williams J 1981 Reliability of a population survey tool for measuring perceived health problems: a study of patients with osteoarthritis. J Epidemiol Commun Health 35: 297–300

Jennett B, MacMillan R 1981 Epidemiology of head injury. BMJ 282: 101–4

Jennett B, Teasdale G 1981 Management of Head Injuries. Philadelphia: FA Davis

Kamsma YPT et al. 1995 Training of compensational strategies for impaired gross motor skills in Parkinson's disease. Physiother Theory Pract 11: 209–29

Ko Ko C 1999 Effectiveness of rehabilitation for multiple sclerosis. Clin Rehabil 13 (suppl 1): 33–41

Kurtzke JF 1981 A proposal for a uniform minimal record of disability in multiple sclerosis. Acta Neurol Scand 64 (suppl 87): 110–29

Kurtzke JF 1983 Rating neurologic impairment in multiple sclerosis: an expanded disability status scale (EDSS). Neurology 33: 1444–52

Lezak MD 1986 Psychological implications of traumatic brain damage for the patient's family. Rehabil Psychol 31: 241–50

Lincon NB, Edmans JA 1989 A shortened version of the Rivermead Perceptual Assessment Battery. Clin Rehabil 3: 199–204

Lincoln NB, Leadbitter D 1979 Assessment of motor function in stroke patients. Physiotherapy 65: 48–51

Lundy-Ekman L 1998 Neuroscience: Fundamentals for Rehabilitation. London: WB Saunders

Mahoney FI, Barthel DW 1965 Functional evaluation: the Barthel Index. Maryland State Med J 14: 61–5

Malec JF, Basford JS 1996 Postacute brain injury rehabilitation. Arch Phys Med Rehabil 77: 198–207

Mathiowetz V, Weber K, Kashman N et al. 1985 Adult norms for the 9-hole peg test of finger dexterity. Occup Ther J Res 5: 24–37

McGrath JR, Adams L 1999 Patient-centered goal planning: a systematic psychological therapy? Top Stroke Rehabil 6(2): 43–50

Medical Research Council 1976 Aids to the Examination of the Peripheral Nervous System. London: HMSO

Mellerup E, Fog T, Raun N et al. 1981 The socio-economic scale. Acta Neurolog Scand 64: 130–8

Mendlow AD, Teasdale GM, Teasdale E et al. 1983 Cerebral blood flow and intracranial pressure in head injured patients. In Ishii S, Nagai H, Brock M (eds) Intracranial Pressure, pp. 495–500. Berlin: Springer-Verlag

Morris M 2000 Movement disorders in people with Parkinson's disease: a model for physical therapy. Phys Ther 80: 578–97

Motor Neurone Disease Association 2000 A Patient and Carer Centred Approach for Health and Social Professionals: Motor Neurone Disease Resource File. Northampton: MND Association

National Institute for Clinical Excellence 2001 Technology Appraisal: Guidance on the Use of Riluzole for the Treatment of Motor Neurone Disease. Appraisal no. 20

Norkin CC, White DJ 1975 Measurement of Joint Motion: a Guide to Goniometry. Philadelphia: FA Davies

Oddy M, Humphrey M 1980 Social recovery during the year following severe head injury. J Neurol Neurosurg Psychiat 43: 798–802

Oddy M, Humphrey M, Uttley D 1978 Subjective impairment and social recovery after closed head injury. J Neurol Neurosurg Psychiat 41: 611–16

Palastanga N, Field D, Soames R 2002 Anatomy and Human Movement, 4th edn. Butterworth–Heinemann: Oxford

Palmer SS et al. 1986 Exercise therapy for Parkinson's disease. Arch Phys Med Rehabil 67: 741–5

Partridge C (ed.) 2002 Neurological Physiotherapy: Bases of Evidence for Practice. London: Whurr

Petajan JH, Gappmaier E, White AT et al. 1996 Impact of aerobic training on fitness and quality of life in multiple sclerosis. Ann Neurol 39: 432–41

Peto V, Jenkinson C, Fitzpatrick R, Greenhall R 1995 The development and validation of a short measure of functioning and wellbeing for individuals with Parkinson's disease. Qual Life Res 4: 241–8

Plant R et al. 2000 Physiotherapy for People with Parkinson's Disease: UK Best Practice. Newcastle upon Tyne: Institute of Rehabilitation

Plum H, Morissey D 2002 Cross-speciality collaboration. Physiotherapy 88: 530–3

Podsialo D, Richardson S 1991 The timed 'up and go': a test of basic functional mobility for frail elderly persons. J Am Geriatr Soc 39: 142–8

Poser CM, Paty DW, Scheinberg LC et al. 1983 New diagnostic criteria for multiple sclerosis: guidelines for research protocols. Ann Neurol 13: 227–31

Prigatano GP 1992 Personality disturbances associated with traumatic brain injury. J Consult Clin Psychol 60: 360–8

Rappaport M, Hall KM, Hopkins K et al. 1982 Disability rating scale for severe head trauma: coma to community. Arch Phys Med Rehabil 63: 118–23

Robinson I et al. 1996 A Dispatch from the Front Line. The Views of People with Multiple Sclerosis about their Needs: a Qualitative Approach. London: Brunel MS Research Unit

Royal College of Physicians/Chartered Society of Physiotherapy intercollegiate working party 2000 National Clinical Guidelines for Stroke

Russell WR, Smith A 1981 Post-traumatic amnesia in closed head injury. Arch Neurol 5: 16–29

Sadovnick AD, Baird PA, Ward RH 1988 Multiple sclerosis: updated risks for relatives . Am J Med Genet 29: 533–41

Sadovnick AD, Ebers GC 1993 Epidemiology of multiple sclerosis: a critical review. Can J Neurol Sci 20: 17–29

Stokes M 1998 Neurological Physiotherapy. New York: Mosby International

Sunderland A, Tinson D, Bradley L, Langton Hewer R 1989 Arm function after stroke: an evaluation of grip strength as a measure of recovery and a prognostic indicator. J Neurol Neurosurg Psychiatr 52: 1267–72

Swash M, Schwartz MS 1995 Motor neurone disease: the clinical syndrome. In Leigh PN, Swash M (eds) Motor Neurone Disease: Biology and Management, pp. 1–17. London: Springer-Verlag

Tandan R 1994 Clinical features and differential diagnosis of classical motor neurone disease. In Williams AC (ed.) Motor Neurone Disease, pp. 3–27. London: Chapman & Hall

Teasdale G, Jennett B 1974 Assessment of coma and impaired consciousness: a practical scale. Lancet ii: 81–3

Temkin NR, Kikmen SS, Wilensky AJ et al. 1990 A randomized double-blind study of phenytoin for the prevention of post-traumatic seizures. N Engl J Med 323: 497–502

Thompson A 1998 Symptomatic treatment in multiple sclerosis. Curr Opin Neurol 11: 305–9

Turnbull GI (ed.) 1992 Physical Management of Parkinson's Disease. New York: Churchill Livingstone

Van den Burg W, Van Zomeren AH, Minderhoud JM et al. 1987 Cognitive impairment in patients with multiple sclerosis and mild physical disability. Arch Neurol 44: 494–501

Wade DT 1992 Measurement in Neurological Rehabilitation. Oxford: Oxford University Press

Wade DT 1999a Goal planning in stroke rehabilitation: how? Top Stroke Rehabil 6(2): 16–36

Wade DT 1999b Goal planning in stroke rehabilitation: what? Top Stroke Rehabil 6(2): 8–15

Wade DT 1999c Goal planning in stroke rehabilitation: evidence. Top Stroke Rehabil 6(2): 37–42

Ware JE et al. 1993 SF-36 Health Survey: Manual and Interpretation Guide. Boston, MA: Health Institute, New England Medical Center

Weiner WJ, Goetz CG 1994 Neurology for the Non-neurologist, 3rd edn. Philadelphia: Lippincott

Wichman T, DeLong MR 1993 Pathophysiology of parkinsonian motor abnormalities. Adv Neurol 60: 53–61

Wood RLI 1990 Neurobehavioural paradigm for brain injury rehabilitation. In Wood RL (ed.) Neurobehavioural sequelae of traumatic brain injury, pp. 3–17. New York: Taylor & Francis

Young B, Ott L, Twyman D et al. 1987 The effect of nutritional support on outcome from severe head injury. J Neurosurg 67: 668–76

APPENDIX – PHYSIOTHERAPY ASSESSMENT

For simplicity, the assessment outlined below is based on an initial contact with a patient sitting in a wheelchair. The assessment is by no means exhaustive and is intended to be used as a guide for students.

Database

Personal details
Name, address, DoB, consultant, GP

Medical diagnosis

Medication
Can impact on treatment effects e.g. antispasmodic medication

Investigations carried out
CT, MRI, blood tests …

Previous medical history
Operations, illnesses, conditions

Clinical Interview (with patient and carer where appropriate)

Patient's and carers' perception of their difficulties
What are they finding difficult including reason(s) why – personal activities of daily living, premorbid fitness, levels of fatigue …

History of present condition (HPC)
Onset of condition and how it has progressed to date. Might include previous physiotherapy treatment and how the patient responded to it

Social history/home circumstances
Occupation/lifestyle, family/partner support, general health of partner, input from support agencies, type of accommodation, toilet – upstairs/downstairs, bedroom – upstairs/downstairs, hand rail – which side, transport …

Equipment/adaptations
Stair lift, small equipment, wheelchair, walking aids …

Vision
Glasses, Hemianopia, diplopia, nystagmus …

Communication
Dysarthria, dysphasia, dysphonia, dyspraxia

Swallowing and nutritional status

Hearing aid

Cognition, perception, behaviour, emotional status
Attention or memory deficits, speed of processing information, neglect, spatial awareness, emotionally lability …

Continence
Bladder, bowel function

Pain
When, where, aggravating factors, methods of relief, irritability …

Expectations of intervention
What does the patient/carers expect to gain from this episode of treatment?

Clinical Examination (Supported sitting)

Posture
Alignment of body parts (e.g. head, shoulder girdles, pelvis, spinal curves, trunk creases, weight bearing aspects), symmetry vs asymmetry, acceptance of supporting surface, ability to move within base of support, dominated by flexion/extension/mixture of the two ...

Muscle tone (observe then handle) for upper limb, trunk and lower limb
Hypertonicity, hypotonicity, combination of tone, associated reactions (e.g. on preparation for movement, during movement – note movement precipitating them or present continuously)

Active movement
Observe all areas e.g. trunk, arms, head and legs, what can they do without assistance, with assistance ...

Passive range of movement
What is the available joint range, if limited what is it limited by, e.g. adaptive muscle shortening, joint stiffness, pain ... Use joint 'end-feel' to assist decision

At this point in the assessment, the person can be asked to move out of the chair and on to a plinth, if deemed appropriate. By now information needed to assess how much assistance the person requires to safely complete the transfer should be known. If assistance is required, the opportunity arises to evaluate the degree to which assistance is required and how effective that assistance might be. During the transfer, assessment of how effectively the patient moves from sitting to standing, transfers bodyweight and steps around can be carried out. Finally, analysis of how the person sits down can also be examined.

Transferring from Chair to Bed

Sit to stand sequence
What components of movement did they manage by themselves and what did they need assistance with? If assistance was required, what and why was this needed? Level type of associated reactions?

Once in standing (assess here or later)
Balance reactions, posture, awareness of midline, alignment of body parts, muscle tone ...

During moving from chair to bed
Does the patient effectively transfer bodyweight, awareness of midline, control of placing non-weight-bearing leg, control of stability on weight-bearing leg, were they independent or did they need assistance? Were they safe?

Standing to sitting
Is the person able to control all aspects of the movement sequence? Does the person sequence the movement correctly? Does the person compensate and if so how and why?

Unsupported sitting
Re-examine the patient's posture. Has it changed? If so why? Has the patient readily accepted the new base of support, and able to sit independently? Assess all aspects of sitting balance, use of arm support, level of muscle tone ...

Function whilst in unsupported sitting (if appropriate)
For example, getting undressed. Observe changes in muscle tone, balance reactions, weight transference, compensations, strategies employed to achieve the task, sequencing of task, ability to attend to multiple tasks ...

Sitting to Lying and Supine Lying

> **Sitting to lying**
> Can the patient lie down independently or do they need assistance? How was the task achieved? Did the patient compensate and if so why? Did the patient influence their level of tone?

> **In lying**
> Posture, acceptance of new base of support, testing of passive and active range of movement, sensory testing …

> **Moving within lying**
> Is the patient able to roll to either side? Compare analysis of movement with normal movement sequences. Does the patient compensate? Effort involved? Changes in level of tone? Functional?

> **Lying to sitting**
> Can the patient sit up independently onto the side of the bed or do they need assistance? Identify any assistance required and reasons why. Analysis of movement sequence and comparison with normal. Functional? Can they move into sitting to either side?

Sitting to Standing and Standing to Sitting

> **Sitting to standing**
> Which components of the movement could the person do independently and which needed assistance? What type and why? Did the person move using both sides equally? Comparison of movement sequences with normal. Did you observe any associated reaction? If so where and why? Functional and safe?

> **Standing to sitting**
> Which components of the movement could the person do independently and which needed assistance? What type and why? Did the person move using both sides equally? Comparison of movement sequences with normal. Did you observe any associated reaction? If so where and why? Functional and safe?

Standing and Moving in Standing

> **In standing**
> What can the person do independently? Is the patient symmetrical? Overall posture, alignment of limbs, level of muscle tone once in standing. Is the patient accepting the new base of support? Compensating in any way? If so how?

> **Standing balance**
> What balance mechanisms are used? How do these compare with normal balance strategies? Why does the patient choose those particular strategies? Compensations and if so how and why? Functional tasks in standing?

> **Moving in standing**
> Can the patient transfer weight laterally from one leg to another? Move weight in an A/P direction? Maintain own trunk, hip and knee extension? Do they compensate in any way?

> **Moving in standing**
> Able to step forward, backwards, across midline with either leg? Able to use saving reactions? If not why not? Level of muscle tone during tasks? Able to maintain stability on weight-bearing leg?

Walking

> **Walking**
> Is walking functional? Analyse the quality of the gait pattern. Use of a walking aid? If so is it being used correctly? Able to walk in different directions, on different surfaces, in different environments (with distractions)? Is walking an effort (energy expenditure)? Any associated reaction? If so when, where and why?

> **Walking pattern (stance phase on each leg)**
> Stability over stance leg, maintenance of hip extension and abduction, stability of hip and knee. Are all stages of stance phase (heel strike to toe off) equally as good? Muscle tone? Compensatory strategies?

> **Walking pattern (swing phase of each leg – from toe off to heel strike)**
> Able to alter tone from stance phase? Analyse movement sequences in comparison to normal. Able to clear the floor? If not why not? Recruitment of appropriate muscle groups? Timing of recruitment? Able to place either leg appropriately?

It is important during any assessment not to lose sight of the fact that many patients, following neurological damage, will have to compensate in some way. As long as the level of compensation is an appropriate one, that does not rob the patient of any further recovery, this is an acceptable, and often necessary compromise. Understandably, patients' main goal is to gain as much functional independence as possible.

List of Problems and Goals

Now the assessment is complete, a problem and goals list needs to be formulated. It is important to bring the problems identified as a physiotherapist together with the patient's/carers perceived problems. Problems and goals need to be agreed with the patient and family. At the end of the day it is important to remember that the goals should be the patient's, not the physiotherapist's.

Problem list (with date set in order of priority)	Reason for problems	Agreed goals (in order of priority)	Review date	Treatment plan	Date goal achieved, signature and job title. If not achieved state reason why

Concepts in Exercise Rehabilitation

21

Duncan Mason and Sean Kilmurray

MOBILISING EXERCISES: INTRODUCTION

Soft-tissue extensibility is a prerequisite for normal functioning. Unfortunately, following injury, inflammation, prolonged abnormal postures and other pathologies, this extensibility can be lost at an alarming rate.

Physiotherapists regularly encounter people who have well-established limitation of movement, and need to be able to recognise this phenomenon and act accordingly to restore the length of the soft tissues involved. It is also important that the physiotherapist is able to identify the muscles and soft tissues that are most prone to shorten and lose mobility. The initial sections of this chapter discuss the key concepts in the use of mobilising exercises in physiotherapy.

Mobilising exercises are a fundamental component of the rehabilitation process since they enhance normal tissue healing and are necessary to load the soft tissues progressively, thus enabling them to more effectively withstand the stresses and strains that they will encounter during normal functional use (Hunter 1998).

Mobilising exercises can be used to maintain or increase range of movement, for which the causes are numerous. These causes include:

- contractures of the joint capsule
- adhesions within the soft tissues
- muscle spasm or tightness
- neural sensitivity and inhibition due to pain.

Physiotherapists often use mobilising exercises in conjunction with other treatment modalities such as passive movements, heat, electrotherapy and soft-tissue techniques, depending on the presenting symptoms of the client.

For the purposes of this chapter, exercises are divided into the following classes:

1   passive
2   active assisted
3   auto assisted
4   active
5   stretching (including hold/relax).

CLASSES OF MOBILISING EXERCISE

Passive Exercises

With passive exercises, movement is produced entirely by an external force with the absence of voluntary muscle activity on behalf of the patient. This external force may be supplied by the physiotherapist (as is the case with passive movements), or by a machine. For exam-

---

Definitions of terms

- *Delayed-onset muscle soreness* (DOMS). A dull, aching sensation that follows unaccustomed muscular exertion. Soreness usually peaks 24–48 hours after exercise (Vickers 2001).
- *Kinematic chain*. Closed: an exercise performed where the distal part of the limb is fixed (e.g. squats with feet on the floor). Open: an exercise where the distal part of the limb is able to move freely in space (e.g. a biceps curl with a free weight).
- *Muscle contracture*. The adaptive shortening of muscle or other soft tissues that cross a joint, which results in limitation of range of motion (Kisner and Colby 1996).
- *Muscle spasm*. A persistent muscle contraction that cannot be voluntarily released.
- *Muscle spasticity*. A condition associated with hyperactivity of the stretch reflexes and tendon jerks, probably due to loss of inhibitory influences on the alphamotor neurones (Mense et al. 2001).
- *Muscle tension*. An increase in resistance to passive movement of a joint.
- *Muscle tone*. The resting tension of a muscle, clinically determined as resistance to passive movement or to deformation.
- *Myalgia*. Pain felt within a muscle.
- *Proprioception*. The specialised variation of the sensory modality of touch that encompasses the sensation of joint movement (kinaesthesia) and joint position (joint position sense) (Lephart et al. 1997).
- *Stretching*. Any therapeutic manoeuvre designed to lengthen pathologically shortened soft-tissue structures and thereby increase range of motion (Kisner and Colby 1996).

---

ple, continuous passive motion (CPM) units might be used following total knee arthroplasty or anterior cruciate ligament reconstruction.

Passive exercises are typically employed in the early stages of rehabilitation after the onset of trauma, provided that affected structures are stable enough to sustain movement without vulnerability to further injury. They may also be used to maintain range of movement during periods of joint inactivity, and in conjunction with stretching exercises to further increase the range achieved.

Active Assisted Exercises

These are exercises in which the movement is produced *in part* by an external force, but is completed by use of voluntary muscle contraction. These exercises are of obvious value when strengthening a weakened muscle;

but with the assistance given by the external force they can also be used to increase range of movement whilst allowing the individual to maintain control.

Equipment

All manner of equipment is used to facilitate active assisted exercises. Common examples are pulleys, slings and pole exercises for shoulders, re-education boards for knees and elbows, as well as many other external adjuncts. The physiotherapist can be as innovative as required.

Another important factor to be considered is *gravity*. If the exercise is performed with assistance from gravity, this may increase its effect on mobilising the targeted structure (Figure 21.1).

Auto assisted exercises

These exercises can be either passive or active assisted, as described above, and occur when the external force is applied by the individual rather than by the physiotherapist.

Active Exercises

Also known as *free active exercises*, these are activities in which the movement is produced solely by use of the individual's voluntary muscle action. They can be used as either strengthening for grade 2 and above on the Oxford scale (discussed later), or to mobilise structures – as is the case with dynamic stretching exercises.

Key point

With any exercise the correct choice of starting position is important. For example for a mobilising exercise aiming to increase range of movement, gravity will need to be counterbalanced. If an exercise is performed against gravity it will have more emphasis towards strengthening.

A clinically useful feature of active exercises is that they can be performed without the use of equipment, so they can be practised anywhere and can easily form the basis of a home exercise programme.

Stretching Exercises

Stretching exercises if performed appropriately may be a simple yet very effective form of treatment. For example, in the elderly a loss of hip extension during walking implies the presence of functionally significant hip flexor tightness (Kerrigan et al. 2001) and predisposes individuals to falls and subsequent femoral neck fractures. Overcoming hip tightness with specific stretching exercises is therefore worthy of investigation as a simple intervention to improve walking performance and fall prevention in the elderly.

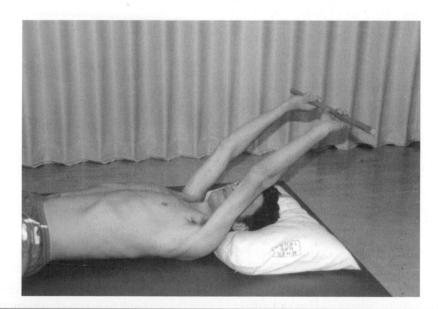

Figure 21.1   Active assisted shoulder elevation, demonstrating the use of gravity and the other arm (via a pole) to gain range of movement.

Key point
Stretching exercises are normally used to mobilise neural and muscle tissue to the limits of the available range. The issue of which stretching method is most effective is still not fully resolved (Etnyre and Lee 1987).

Stretching exercises are performed with the target structure towards a lengthened position. The stretching exercise will involve further movement in that direction, so as to further lengthen the structure. Collagen fibres realign rapidly as a result of stretching forces and become aligned (and therefore stronger) in the direction of the stretching force (Melis et al. 2002). The limiting factors to further movement, such as the degree of pain experienced, will govern the extent to which any further movement is possible. Stretches are commonly used to increase range of movement by mobilising restrictions within soft tissue (e.g. scar tissue), and are specifically used in the lengthening of tight muscles.

The time at which stretching is commenced after an injury needs careful consideration. After any soft-tissue injury the length of the immobilisation depends on the grade of injury and must be optimised so that the scar can bear the pulling forces operating on it without re-rupture. Mobilisation of soft tissues by stretching will aid resorption of the connective tissue scar and re-capillarisation of the damaged area (Kujala et al. 1997).

Stretching may also be used as a preventative measure, to prevent joint contractures for example. However, whilst the primary intervention for the treatment and prevention of contracture is to regularly stretch the soft tissues, and the rationale behind this intervention appears sound, the effectiveness of stretching has not been verified with well-designed clinical trials (Harvey and Herbert 2002).

Stretches may be applied in one of two ways: either dynamically or statically (Table 21.1).

Dynamic stretching

This involves gaining range by an active movement and should not be confused with ballistic stretching (see below) which involves the use of repetitive, bouncing, dynamic, rhythmic movements performed at higher velocities. Dynamic stretching involves progressively increasing the range through successive movements until the end of range is reached.

Dynamic stretching is especially useful when dealing with more advanced sports-related rehabilitation problems. The exercises enhance dynamic function and neuromuscular control through repetition and practice, thereby enhancing the movement memory. If the patient is suitable, this form of stretching can be highly effective to mobilise soft tissues and enhance motor control.

Note on ballistic stretching

Ballistic stretching uses repeated movement and *momentum* to gain range. The drawbacks to using this type of exercise with most individuals encountered in the hospital setting are that patients are typically not conditioned to use ballistic stretching effectively or *without sustaining further injury.*

During ballistic stretching, the stretch reflex is initiated to resist the change in muscle length and to protect the muscle from injury. This occurs due to stimulation of the non-contractile elements of muscle spindles, which send afferent information about the length of muscles to spinal cord level. This in turn causes stimulation of the extrafusal fibres via the alpha motor neurone, resulting in a muscle contraction (see Figure 21.15). Should this muscle contraction coincide with the next ballistic movement, a muscle unconditioned to cope with that stress may become injured.

Static stretching

As the name suggests, this involves maintaining a position for a sustained period to gain the desired effect – it is widely suggested that an effective time to hold a static stretch is 30 seconds (Bandy et al. 1997).

Table 21.1 Stretching exercises: a summary.

	Dynamic stretch	**Static stretch**
Feature of stretch technique	Faster, rhythmic, higher velocity, motor control, functional	Slow, controlled, emphasis on postural awareness, bodily alignment
Duration of stretch	Repetitive, progressive	Sustained 30-second hold
Stage employed	End-stage rehabilitation	Early and end-stage rehabilitation
Client types	Sportsmen, active persons	All

Static stretching is a controlled, slow movement with emphasis on correct bodily alignment. Static stretching protocols are commonly used and, for example, have been shown to be effective in terms of improving flexibility of muscle (Chan et al. 2001). An element of fine motor control and postural awareness is important during static stretching exercises and this can be enhanced by the use of feedback and correction from the physiotherapist, as well as mirrors. Exercise forms such as Pilates, Tai Chi and Yoga employ many of these principles and can be used effectively within a patient's exercise programme.

Key point
Correction of this type of exercise is frequently required to ensure an effective stretch is produced in the targeted tissue.

Therapeutic stretching or strengthening exercises are successful only if the target muscle is properly isolated (Gluck and Liebenson 1997), particularly when the tissue concerned crosses more than one body seg-

ment. Problems are often encountered when stretching two joint muscles. For example, when stretching the hamstrings, pelvic alignment needs to be controlled as well as considering hip flexion and knee extension components to stretch effectively.

The *order* in which the components are added can also influence the effect, depending on which area of the muscle's structure is to be targeted. In the case of a problem in the distal rectus femoris, one may wish to employ a stretch which extends the hip then flexes the knee, whilst proximally the components may be added alternatively (Figures 21.2 and 21.3).

It is also important to consider the functional anatomy of the area being targeted. Using the hamstrings as an example, the medial hamstrings (semimembranosus and semitendinosus) would require a component of lateral rotation to stretch them effectively. To effectively stretch biceps femoris would require an element of medial rotation, since it is a lateral rotator of the knee.

Spinal position
Many upper- and lower-limb muscles have their origins from the axial skeleton, so spinal position can

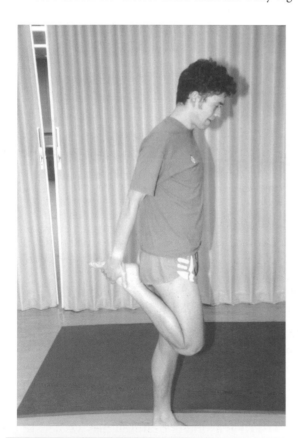

Figure 21.2   Demonstrating the order effect of adding components to a stretch of rectus femoris: knee flexion then hip extension.

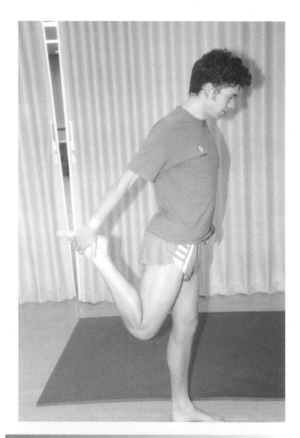

Figure 21.3   Hip extension then knee flexion. Note that the lumbar spine should remain in neutral throughout.

influence limb position. Consequently, throughout many stretching exercises it is important to consider any lumbo-pelvic or spinal movement to ensure that it is controlled throughout the exercise. Where possible there should be no spinal movement, ensuring a 'neutral' posture is maintained throughout.

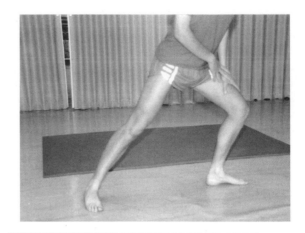

Figure 21.4   Static stretching of the right hip adductors.

Stretching exercises: a practical guide

Before performing the stretch

- Before commencing a stretching programme, ensure that your assessment has not identified any contraindications to stretching.
- Ensure that there is a logical, reasoned basis for your stretching programme. For example, if there is a bony block to movement caused by osteophytes, stretching is not appropriate (refer to Chapter 2 on end-feel).
- Consider how you will get the patient to assist in his or her own stretching programme at home.
- Explain how and why you are performing the stretch to ensure maximum compliance and minimal resistance.
- Consider how the stretch might be made more comfortable prior to stretching (e.g. use of a hot pack or hydrotherapy).

During the stretch

- Make your handling firm but maintain patient comfort. Reassure the patient that you will stop the stretch at his or her command.
- Stabilise the joints as necessary.
- Stretch across one joint at a time for two joint muscles.
- Make the stretch slow and sustained – do not bounce.
- The patient should experience a pulling sensation, not pain.
- Hold the position for 30 seconds.
- If tension releases, take the movement a little further.
- Release slowly.

After the stretch

- Warn the patient what feelings to expect following the stretch.
- Remember that once movement has been regained, active muscle control throughout that range will be needed as well as some form of maintaining the stretch in the long term.

Contraindications to stretching

These are some of the contraindications:

- bony block or end-feel to movement of the joint in question
- recent or unstable fractures
- the presence of infection or haematoma in the tissues
- after some surgical repairs and other procedures, such as skin grafting and tendon repair
- patient refusal.

> **Key point**
>
> Although static stretching is widely believed to cause an increase in a muscle's functional length, recent investigations suggest otherwise. It has been suggested by Magnusson et al. (1998) that the viscoelastic properties of muscles remain unaltered following stretching, and rather that it is the muscle's *tolerance* to stretch that is increased. Such details along with further developments in the area need to be considered when prescribing stretching exercises.

Hold/relax techniques

Hold/relax (or contract/relax) is a principle used when applying proprioceptive neuromuscular facilitation (PNF) and can be effective when trying to mobilise muscles. PNF stretching techniques may produce greater increases in range of motion than passive, ballistic or static stretching methods (Spernoga et al. 2001). PNF is a form of treatment that was devised to manually rehabilitate movement in specific patterns using a number of physiological principles to enhance its effectiveness.

A core principle of PNF is that after a muscle has contracted maximally it will then relax maximally. This principle can be used when using exercises to mobilise muscles which are in a shortened position. The patient is asked to contract the tight muscle strongly and hold the contraction isometrically for around 10 seconds, then relax. Following a short period of 2–3 seconds the physiotherapist then applies a stretch to the muscle, which is maintained for 20–30 seconds. Following a period of recovery this sequence is repeated.

Another useful principle used in PNF is that of *reciprocal inhibition*, which states that when a muscle (the agonist) contracts maximally, its opposite counterpart (antagonist) will relax maximally.

The two principles can also be combined with a hold/relax as described above followed by an active contraction of the antagonist of the muscle to be mobilised.

The principle of reciprocal inhibition can also prove useful and is worth considering during static stretching exercises where a contraction of the muscle's antagonist can act to relax and lengthen it.

PROGRESSION OF MOBILISING EXERCISES

An exercise plan without any progression will quickly become ineffective. It is essential to review the exercise programme regularly and revise it to match the patient's status. There are various ways to progress exercises, including:

1 changing the starting position
2 changing the length of the lever
3 changing the speed at which the exercise is performed
4 altering the range through which the movement is performed
5 applying resistance.

The starting position

Changing the starting position will change the base of support and may affect the difficulty of an exercise. Reducing the base of support will normally have the effect of advancing the difficulty of the exercise, and vice versa. For example, performing an exercise whilst standing on one leg will require more hip abductor control than when standing on two legs.

A change in starting position can also change a body segment's relationship to gravity, which will change the nature of an exercise. An exercise performed against gravity will require concentric muscle work and eccentric work to return to the starting position – it will therefore be a strengthening exercise.

With more grossly weakened muscles (Oxford scale 2 and below), exercises performed in a gravity counterbalanced position will be more effective. Exercises performed in this position will also be more effective in mobilising structures.

If an exercise is performed with the assistance of gravity it may have a strong mobilising effect upon reaching the end of the available range of movement. An example of this is performing squats from a standing starting position to increase the range of knee flexion, using the effects of gravity and bodyweight to increase knee flexion (Figure 21.7). Another example is shoulder flexion in lying and standing (Figure 21.5 and 21.6).

Length of the lever

Changing the length of the lever will affect the forces applied to the body during exercise (see Figures 21.8 and 21.9). A lengthened lever will result in a higher force being exerted at the fulcrum of the movement, so more muscle work will be needed to produce or control the movement. This will also result in a higher force applied to structures during mobilising exercises.

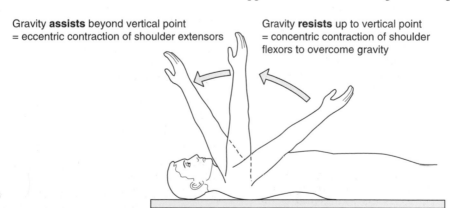

Gravity **assists** beyond vertical point = eccentric contraction of shoulder extensors

Gravity **resists** up to vertical point = concentric contraction of shoulder flexors to overcome gravity

Figure 21.5 Shoulder flexion in lying.

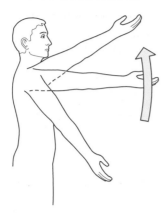

Figure 21.6   Shoulder flexion in standing. Gravity resists the movement throughout the range in standing even though the movement is the same as in Figure 21.5.

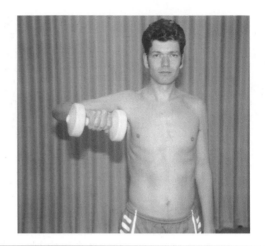

Figure 21.8   Shoulder abduction with a shortened lever.

Levers may be shortened or lengthened by flexing or extending joints, most commonly the elbow or knee joints. They may also be lengthened by holding or attaching an object to the end of a limb – such as holding a weight at arm's length.

The positioning of the application of resistance along the lever will also affect the muscle work required. Resistance applied distally will require more effort and will reduce when the same resistance is applied more proximally.

Speed of movement

A change in the speed at which a movement is performed will change the nature of an exercise. When altering the speed, the physiotherapist must be clear as to the desired effect. An exercise performed slowly

requires a great deal of precision and postural control. An exercise performed at higher velocities will produce a greater mobilising effect at the end of range, but the client will require adequate neuromuscular control to perform this without risking further injury.

Range of movement

A change in the range through which an exercise is performed will alter its difficulty. Muscles are at their strongest in middle range and weakest in outer range (a more lengthened position). This is discussed in more depth later in the context of muscle strengthening exercises.

Resistance to movement

The final way to progress an exercise is to apply resistance to strengthen a muscle (see Figure 21.10).

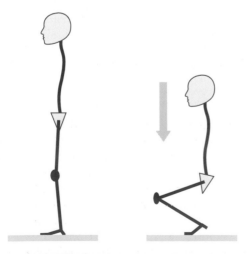

Figure 21.7   Squats in standing using gravity to mobilise knee flexion.

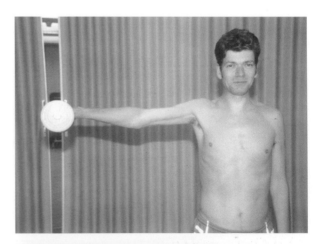

Figure 21.9   The muscle work of shoulder abduction is greatly increased by increasing the lever length.

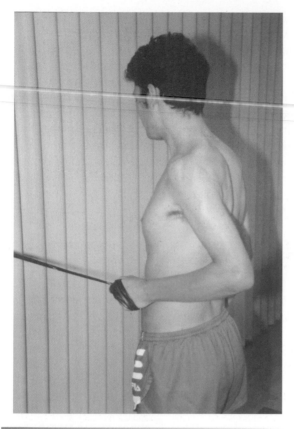

Figure 21.10 A resistance exercise to strengthen shoulder extensors.

Resistance can be applied in a number of ways. These are related to the desired effect – whether the aim is to produce a change in power or in endurance (this too will be discussed later).

MEASUREMENT OF MUSCLE STRENGTH

Key point

It is important for a physiotherapist to measure muscle strength objectively when assessing an individual, to obtain a baseline level from which future improvements (or lack of them) can be gauged. This allows the therapist to devise an individual exercise plan and to evaluate the effectiveness of a prescribed exercise regimen.

Muscle strength can be evaluated in a number of ways: manually, functionally, or mechanically.

The Oxford Scale

The Oxford scale has been devised to manually assess muscle strength and is widely used by physiotherapists.

Table 21.2 The Oxford scale.

Grade	Muscle contraction
0	No contraction
1	Flicker of a contraction
2	Full-range active movement with gravity eliminated (counterbalanced)
3	Full-range active movement against gravity
4	Full-range active movement against light resistance
5	Normal function/full-range against strong resistance

According to the Oxford scale, muscle strength is graded 0 to 5. Table 21.2 summarises the grades.

There are limitations to the usefulness of the Oxford scale. These include:

- a lack of functional relevance
- non-linearity (the difference between grades 3 and 4 is not necessarily the same as the difference between grades 4 and 5)
- a patient's variability with time (rarely falling into a fixed category)
- a degree of subjectivity between assessors
- assessment of muscles acting only concentrically
- the difficulty of applying the scale to all cases in clinical practice (so that strength is rarely evaluated throughout full range since many individuals seen by physiotherapists do not possess full range in the first place).

Functional Tools

Functional tools can be used to evaluate strength and can be related to a specific activity or to one of its components. These tools are commonly employed when rehabilitating sportsmen back to competition. Sport-specific activities can be monitored by a physiotherapist with knowledge of the demands of a particular sport.

Isokinetic Assessment

Isokinetic assessment has been used with increasing frequency since its inception in the 1970s. It involves the use of computerised evaluation of movement when exercising at a preset angular velocity on the isokinetic equipment (Figure 21.11). This means that the subject can push as hard or as little as desired and the machine will move only at the preset velocity. It is therefore the resistance provided by the machine that varies.

Use of isokinetics has functional relevance since it can evaluate both eccentric and concentric activity through range.

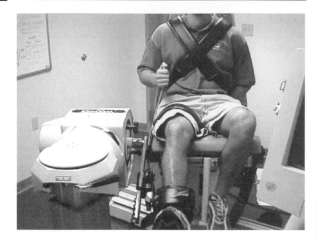

Figure 21.11   A typical isokinetic machine. (Photograph courtesy of Rehab World, Tennessee, USA.)

Key point

Isokinetic machines are used for treatment as well as assessment. They produce objective, reproducible and quantifiable data and therefore have obvious advantages over other methods of evaluating strength.

Drawbacks

The drawbacks of isokinetics relate to its function, as natural human movements rarely occur at fixed velocities. Also, the machine operates on a fixed axis of movement, which does not replicate the instantaneous axis of movement found in most normal joints. The equipment can also be time-consuming to set up and not all physiotherapists will have access to it.

Additional limitations have been acknowledged by Lieber (1992). These include the time required to recruit muscle fibres (50–200 milliseconds), making this period of data obtained unusable. Another drawback is the limb striking the testing bar at the end of the movement, although some isokinetic units employ a damping mechanism to prevent this.

Key point

While isokinetics can give the physiotherapist an idea of any underlying deficiencies in the musculoskeletal system, there is no single tool to evaluate strength that is both totally functional and quantifiable.

GROUP EXERCISE

Group exercise sessions are used widely, especially with more recent moves towards physiotherapists working in primary care as part of their educational or advisory role (Crook et al. 1998). Group work can take the form of exercise classes in a gym, in a hydrotherapy pool or as part of an educational programme, during which patients not only exercise but are also informed about the nature of their condition (Figure 21.12). Educational programmes are commonly employed

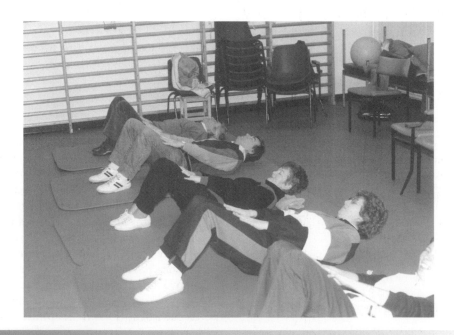

Figure 21.12   Group exercises in a chronic backpain management programme.

Table 21.3 Advantages and disadvantages of group exercises.

Advantages	Disadvantages
■ Competitive element can be useful in increasing a person's performance ■ A variety of exercises is possible ■ Group exercise can be fun if properly organised ■ Helps the individual to feel less isolated if meeting people with similar problems ■ Provides a good opportunity for the physiotherapist to educate and inform the group about the condition ■ Specialist groups such as ankylosing spondylitis or cardiac rehabilitation groups provide social support	■ Difficult to pitch the exercises at a level suitable for all group members ■ Temptation to put inappropriate individuals in the group to save time and relieve overburdened staff ■ Difficult to monitor all of the people all of the time ■ Difficult to progress all the members of the group appropriately ■ Competitive element may be counterproductive or dangerous ■ Some people do not respond well in a group situation

with the more longstanding pathologies and they encourage patients to take responsibility for the continued management of their condition (e.g. back education programmes or OA knee schools).

There are advantages and disadvantages to group work (Table 21.3).

Benefits and Drawbacks

Provided that members of a group are carefully selected there are several advantages to treating patients in groups. Exercising with patients who have experienced similar problems can provide peer support, encouragement, reassurance and camaraderie. It is also more economically effective with the therapist able to supervise several people at once.

The disadvantages of group work are that certain individuals may not respond to the group environment. In particular they may be embarrassed or dislike the interaction. Many clients will respond better to individual attention from their therapist, particularly in the early stages of rehabilitation; this is not possible in group work.

If groups are used solely as a way of treating large numbers of patients with diverse pathologies they will prove ineffective. This factor, along with a poorly organised treatment session, could lead to demotivation.

Finally, it is important that participants in the group do not become too competitive, thereby reducing the effectiveness of the exercise and also risking further injury.

Planning Group Work

Careful planning is necessary if group work is to be effective. The aims of the group session must be clearly

planned and stated so that selection criteria for participants can be agreed. This will ensure the session is both safe and effective. Factors such as age, gender, psychological status, the stage in rehabilitation, past medical history and general fitness need to be considered. The facilities and equipment that are available need to be appropriate for the activities planned. Important considerations are the space available and the layout and temperature of the room or gym – not only to provide a suitable environment but also a safe place to exercise.

Format of a Group Session

This should include:

1 patient assessment for suitability for group exercise (at an individual appointment)
2 warm-up session
3 main exercise session
4 cool-down period.

A warm-up is commonly used to start a session to improve circulation, and increase body tissue temperature, therefore physically as well as mentally preparing the participants for exercise. Warm-up exercise may also limit the build-up of metabolites and subsequent acidosis during intense exercise (Kato et al. 2000). It is also interesting to note that proprioception has been found to be significantly more sensitive after warm-up (Bartlett and Warren 2002).

Following the warm-up come the main exercises, and then it is important to also allow time for a cooling down, particularly following vigorous exercise, to assist with removal of lactic acid and waste products of metabolism.

Circuit training

Circuit training is often used in group work. Circuit training involves an exercise programme in which exercises are performed in successive stations with either a predetermined number of repetitions or for a set duration. Timed rest follows each exercise period prior to moving to the next station.

The exercises forming the circuit could be chosen from any of the aforementioned exercise types. The exercises included as part of the circuit must each form part of the client's overall rehabilitation goals. There will also usually be a cardiovascular element to circuit training, and it is commonly encountered in cardiac or pulmonary rehabilitation programmes.

The order of exercises in a circuit needs to be planned from a safety aspect so that group members do not endanger each other. Exercises also need to be ordered to achieve optimum effectiveness. For example two exercises targeted to achieve similar effects should not be placed adjacently on a circuit as that might cause excessive fatigue of the muscle groups involved.

Key point

During group work the physiotherapist facilitates the session by giving feedback and motivation to all participants to ensure that they benefit fully from the session. Also it is important that the participants have a home exercise programme to ensure their progress is continued at home.

HYDROTHERAPY

Hydrotherapy involves exercising in water. The same principles of exercise on dry land discussed in this chapter are generally true when exercising in water. It may be more appropriate to have clients performing individually devised exercises, concurrently, under supervision to gain the advantages of group activity, without the drawbacks of a class setting. This still, however, requires careful planning.

Hydrotherapy is used in the treatment of a wide range of conditions to enhance cardiovascular fitness, to mobilise, to strengthen, to coordinate movement, and to regain function of the neuromusculoskeletal system. Many hospital departments have purpose-built heated hydrotherapy pools. The warm environment may allow the muscles to work more effectively owing to a rise in temperature and of relaxation of any muscle spasm. It will also have a pain-relieving effect. Conditions commonly managed by hydrotherapy are wide ranging, from rheumatological conditions such as rheumatoid arthritis and ankylosing spondylitis to trauma cases and neurological conditions.

Contraindications and precautions are important when considering patients for any exercise programme, and more so with hydrotherapy. This is mainly due to the warm environment in which they are exercising and the dangers of slipping or drowning. Contraindications include the presence of certain medical conditions such as recent or severe neurological conditions (including uncontrolled epilepsy), certain cardiovascular problems and kidney failure. Hydrotherapy is also contraindicated with debilitating disease, and the presence of infections which may be exacerbated or risk transmission to other patients.

The most effective positions used to exercise in the pool will be different from those commonly used on dry land. Patients commonly exercise in standing or sitting in the pool or perform more dynamic exercises such as walking or swimming, but they can also be treated in lying with floats. Floats are placed around the neck and waist to support the patient, allowing the patient to exercise freely. Floats may also be placed around the limbs.

The factors that need to be considered, other than starting position, that change the nature of the exercise are those of buoyancy, turbulence and streamlining.

Buoyancy

This results from the relative density of the body or body part and the density of water. Buoyancy results in an apparent loss of weight of the object when placed in the water and it may be used to either assist or resist movement. Buoyancy will be of particular advantage in reducing the effect of gravity on the body, particularly on load-bearing joints. Buoyancy may increase the function or the range of movement that is possible – for example hip and knee flexion in standing. It may also be utilised to increase range of movement as a mobilising exercise, an effect that can be further enhanced by the use of a float or inflatable wrist or ankle bands – for example to mobilise shoulder flexion with a wrist float in sitting.

Buoyancy can also be used in strengthening exercises. *Buoyancy-resisted* exercise involves pushing against buoyancy. The effect can be graded by again adding floats – for example hip extension whilst floated in supine against an ankle float.

Key point

The greater the buoyancy of the float the greater the mobilising effect of the exercise. These types of exercise are classed as *buoyancy-assisted*.

As the exercises are progressed the inflatable bands can be further inflated or, alternatively, the position of the float on the lever can be adapted therefore changing the buoyancy effect on the limb. If buoyancy is to be counterbalanced the patient will need to exercise along the pool surface.

Turbulence

As limbs move through water they meet resistance – turbulence is created, resulting in the production of currents. Faster movements will produce more turbulence. These currents may act to make movement more difficult and so this principle is of value when progressing an exercise.

Streamlining

This refers to the surface area of the body part exposed to the water when moving through it. The simplest example is the orientation of the upper limb during exercise. If the hand moves with the palm facing the resistance of the water more effort is required than when the limb is rotated so that the ulnar border leads. This principle can be further used when progressing exercise by use of hand-held bats or by placing flippers on the feet.

Further study

For information on specific treatment techniques such as Bad Ragaz and Halliwick, further reading or study is required.

DEALING WITH MUSCLE IMBALANCE

This is an approach to rehabilitating patients who present with movement dysfunction and its associated problems. Several muscle imbalance classifications have been suggested relating to muscles' structure, function and response to injury. Movement dysfunction is said to occur at both a segmental or *local* or single-joint level (Bergmark 1989) and at a *global* level affecting many segments of a region. The cause of acute muscle strain injury in sport has been attributed in part to muscle imbalance (Emery 1999).

Muscles can be classified as either stabilisers or mobilisers depending on their structure and function (Table 21.4).

- *Stabiliser muscles* characteristically are deep, have broad, aponeurotic attachments and their primary function is one of postural and dynamic control.
- *Mobiliser muscles* have features which enable them to fulfil their role as the main producers of force to generate a particular movement. They tend to be

Table 21.4 The muscle groups commonly affected by muscle imbalance.

Muscles prone to tightness (mobilisers)
- Sternocleidomastoid
- Scalene muscles
- Levator scapulae
- Pectoralis minor
- Upper trapezius
- Rhomboids
- Erector spinae
- Rectus abdominis
- Hamstrings
- Gracilis
- Vastus lateralis
- Tensor fascia latae
- Rectus femoris
- Quadratus lumborum
- Piriformis
- Gasrocnemius

Muscles prone to weakness (stabilisers)
- Deep cervical flexors
- Serratus anterior
- Lower fibres trapezius
- Subscapularis
- Transversus abdominis
- Gluteus medius and minimus
- Vastus medialis
- Psoas major
- Multifidus

From Jull GA, Janda V 1987 Muscles and motor control in low back pain. In Twomey LT, Taylor JR (eds) Physical Therapy of the Low Back, pp. 253–78. Edinburgh: Churchill Livingstone.

more superficially situated and have long, cylindrical muscle bellies.

In certain pathological states these two classes of muscles will change their recruitment patterns, and typically this results in an alteration in function. This can happen at a local level resulting in a loss of control of a segment (Hodges and Richardson 1996). It can also occur at a global level whereby the stabilisers become inhibited, weakened and have increased functional length whereas the mobilisers become increasingly facilitated, overactive, and have shortened functional length.

These changes in muscle function may eventually cause muscle imbalance problems such as damage to the muscles involved along with the soft tissues implicated by changes in movement patterns. A shortened muscle in a region shows a lowered irritability threshold and is recruited first in a movement, causing changes in motor programming (Norris 1995).

When a movement dysfunction has been identified, changes in movement patterns are influenced by structures producing either a 'give' or a 'restriction' (Comerford and Mottram 2001). These structures may not just be muscular; they may be bony, such as joint surfaces or osteophytes, and they could be articular such as changes in ligaments or capsular laxity and tightness. The factors influencing movement could also be neurological, as is the case with neural irritability. Pain is often clinically associated with movement dysfunction, as it is usually pain that causes the patient to initially seek treatment. The give and the restriction may be occurring at a segmental, global level or both levels concurrently.

Treatment

Treatment of this type of pathology involves re-education of stability function. To allow the patient to control the position of the affected joint may involve controlling the segmental 'give'. For example, in the case of scapulothoracic instability this would involve positioning of the scapula in its correct alignment progressing through a variety of starting positions.

The next stage in treatment involves progressively challenging the stability with movement. This may involve moving into a restriction. Using the same example as above, this would involve 'setting' the scapula in neutral, then (whilst maintaining this position) moving the glenohumeral joint into flexion or abduction.

As the stability is recruited more readily, exercises are then progressed to gain through-range control of the stabilisers, into first inner then outer range, involving concentric then eccentric work respectively. As the stabiliser function improves through exercise, it is perceived that they are more readily recruited during normal functional activity and the normal recruitment patterns return.

The final treatment priority is to lengthen the mobilisers. This will often occur as a result of increased stability.

Rehabilitation using this approach can be lengthy, as the problems of movement dysfunction are likely to have built up over a considerable time.

Further study
The topic of muscle imbalance has been outlined briefly here. Further reading should be undertaken prior to practising the techniques suggested.

PROPRIOCEPTIVE REHABILITATION: BASIC ISSUES

Introduction

Normal proprioception is essential to everyday functioning, whether it involves simply placing a cup on a table or running around a football field. Definitions of proprioception have been the cause of some debate within the literature. Some authors include the motor response as well as the initial sensory input within their definition.

Definition
Proprioception is 'specialised variation of the sensory modality of touch and encompasses the sensations of joint movement (kinaesthesia) and joint position (joint position sense)' (Lephart and Henry 1995).

The above definition implies that proprioception is very much an *afferent* (sensory) response. However, sense of force has also been incorporated into definitions of proprioception (Jerosch and Prymka 1996), and is another example of the amount of afferent input entering the central nervous system (CNS).

Physiotherapists are concerned with the normal functioning of this afferent response, but more importantly it is the efferent (motor) response to this sensory input that physiotherapists are most involved with from a rehabilitation point of view.

Loss of proprioception is a commonly encountered clinical problem. The key areas where proprioceptive deficits have been identified through research are presented in Table 21.5. The first column in the table illustrates the importance of being aware of the potential scope of proprioceptive loss, and how important appropriate sensorimotor rehabilitation is with a large percentage of patients. It has also been hypothesised that proprioceptive deficiency could in fact precipitate degenerative joint changes (Barrett et al. 1991).

Key point
Proprioception could also play a vital role in prevention of injury as well as in reducing symptoms of pathology. Caraffa et al. (1996) found a seven-fold reduction in anterior cruciate ligament injuries in a group of 300 semi-professional and amateur footballers when compared to a matched control group.

Table 21.5 Conditions commonly exhibiting reduced proprioception.

Proprioceptive deficits identified in:	Clinical example
Osteoarthritis	Particularly joint degeneration in the lower limb, the knee encountered most commonly
Ageing	Any elderly patient
Immobility	Patients on bedrest due to illness or trauma
Trauma	Anterior cruciate ligament (ACL) injuries, glenohumeral dislocation and instabilities, lateral ligament injuries of the ankle

The Mechanism of Proprioception

There are many *receptors* within joints, muscles and skin that continually convey information to the central nervous system (CNS). Using this information we continually make subconscious and conscious modifications to how we move, allowing us to carry out normal functional activities. Each receptor supplies a different type of information – for example joint pressure, joint acceleration/deceleration and joint velocity. When the receptors are stimulated through movement or other forces, they act as transducers and convert this mechanical deformation into an electrical sensory impulse (Barrack et al. 1994). This sensory impulse then passes on to the CNS, triggering the appropriate motor response (Figure 21.13).

A practical illustration of this can be seen in Figure 21.14. When walking on uneven ground the muscles of the foot and ankle continually have to adjust in order to keep the body upright and prevent a fall. The peronei and anterior tibials, for example, will be continually controlling the movement of the foot and ankle, responding to constant positional changes. This example illustrates the nature of proprioception, as a continuous process occurring at different levels of the CNS at the same time.

Consider all the potential tasks that you might undertake whilst walking, such as carrying a rucksack, using a walking pole, or exercising a dog. All of these tasks will be bombarding the CNS with all sorts of afferent information. If the responses to this information were all at the conscious level it would be a slow walk. This is a key point to understand when rehabilitating a patient with a proprioceptive deficit – many actions need to function at a subconscious level.

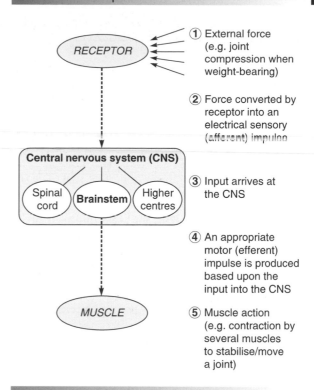

① External force (e.g. joint compression when weight-bearing)

② Force converted by receptor into an electrical sensory (afferent) impulse

③ Input arrives at the CNS

④ An appropriate motor (efferent) impulse is produced based upon the input into the CNS

⑤ Muscle action (e.g. contraction by several muscles to stabilise/move a joint)

Figure 21.13   Diagrammatic representation of the mechanism of proprioception.

Receptors, as well as having different functions, also have different properties. For example they may react at different speeds, and can be rapidly or slowly adapting (Barrack et al. 1994; Borsa et al. 1994). The impulse from a rapidly adapting receptor drops off quickly, whereas that from a slowly adapting receptor fires for longer periods. Some examples are presented in Table 21.6.

Importantly, many joint receptors are also only active at the beginning and ends of range. Therefore as

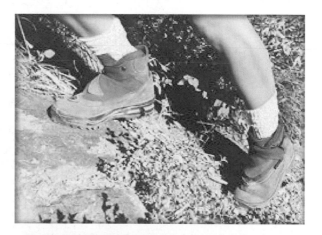

Figure 21.14   Subconscious muscular action to control the ankle when walking on uneven ground.

Table 21.6 Examples of receptors and their functions.

Receptor	Type	Function
Ruffini end organs	Slowly adapting	Monitoring position of the limb in space
Pacinian corpuscles	Slowly adapting	Detection of acceleration and deceleration or sudden mechanoreceptor deformation
Muscle spindles	Rapidly adapting	Changes in muscle length
Golgi tendon organs	Slowly adapting	Changes in muscle tension

a joint moves through a range of movement it is reliant on other receptors to keep the CNS informed of its activity. Particularly important in maintaining this function are the muscle spindles (Figure 21.15).

The large volume of proprioceptive information entering the CNS is utilised at three different levels:

- *Spinal level.* Reflex contractions occurring at this level contribute to reflex stability within a joint, helping to reduce the risk of injury from sudden forces acting on the joint.
- *Brainstem.* This is the part of the brain which receives input from the vestibular centres in the eyes and ears and helps to control balance.

- *Motor cortex, cerebellum and basal ganglia.* Responsible for control of complex movement patterns.

Instability

The word 'instability' is frequently encountered when dealing with patients who display reduced proprioception. Instability can effectively be divided into two types:

- *Mechanical (true) instability.* Disruption of the ligamentous structure of the joint produces instability.

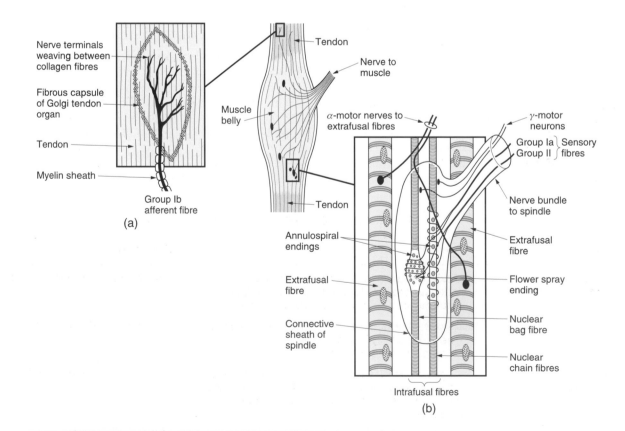

Figure 21.15   (a) The Golgi tendon organ and (b) the muscle spindle.

This is the type of instability detected by manual testing – for example valgus stress testing at the knee to test the medial collateral ligament.

- *Functional instability.* Ligamentous structures are intact with no laxity detected through manual testing. The patient will, however, complain of symptoms such as 'giving way' (lower limb) or 'pain' and 'heaviness' (upper limb). The problem is one of poor neuromuscular control and was initially described by Freeman et al. (1965) with reference to ankle inversion injuries.

The above definitions illustrate the fact that joint stability is multifactoral and relies significantly on dynamic as well as passive control (Waddington and Shepherd 1996). This is a key point and has major implications for the rehabilitation process. Functional instability is, however, the type of instability most commonly encountered by physiotherapists. Recent work on ankle injuries has shown that the majority of patients suffer from functional instability only (Richie 2001). The potential courses of functional instability are presented in Table 21.7.

Correcting functional instability is the primary aim during functional rehabilitation (Lephart et al. 1997) and it is particularly important before undertaking rapid dynamic activities, such as sudden deceleration, which are seen in many sports, but just as importantly, may also be seen in many occupations.

> **Key point**
>
> Individuals suffering from mechanical instability are also likely to have functional instability – a breakdown in the afferent efferent loop resulting in lack of muscular control around the joint.

It is possible in some situations to reduce or even alleviate the symptoms of mechanical instability through appropriate neuromuscular training. If functional instability is not addressed, chronic injury syndromes can develop (Figure 21.16).

ASSESSING PROPRIOCEPTION

Assessment of proprioception takes several forms, many of which rely on complex equipment. There is currently a lack of validated tests that can be used easily within the clinical setting. The key measurements of proprioception often quoted in a research context are discussed below.

Threshold to detection of passive movement (TTDPM)

Isokinetic dynamometers are usually used to assess this component of proprioception. Using the ankle as an example, the blindfolded subject sits on the machine and the dynamometer starts to move the ankle passively. The subject then indicates the point at which movement has been sensed (normally by pressing a button). This result is compared to the unaffected side.

Reproduction of positioning
Reproduction of passive positioning (RPP)

In this instance the joint is moved passively to a position and back (usually by an isokinetic dynamometer or similar device). The patient then presses a button, which takes the joint back towards the position and stops the machine when the subject feels the identical position has been reached.

Table 21.7 Potential causes of functional instability within a joint.

Cause	Rationale	Reference
Articular deafferentation	Articular mechanoreceptors are damaged, reducing the afferent impulse to the CNS, resulting in a decreased motor response	Freeman et al. (1965)
Differentiation	Trauma can result in direct damage to the motor supply, resulting in a decreased muscular response to perturbation	Wilkerson and Nitz (1994)
Neurogenic Inflammation	Thought to be related to joint inflammation and inflammatory mediators directly affecting the motor endplate and therefore the motor response	Wilkerson and Nitz (1994)
Capsular distension	Joint effusion following trauma can cause muscle inhibition, leading to instability	Wilkerson and Nitz (1994)

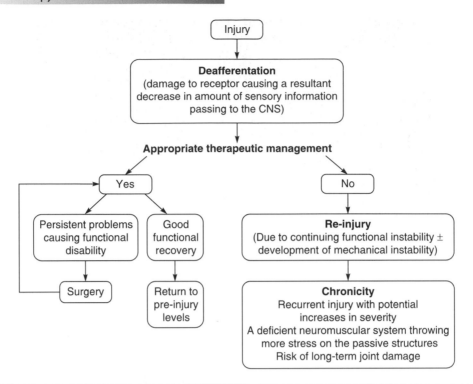

Figure 21.16   Illustration of the importance of early effective rehabilitation in preventing chronic injury.

Reproduction of active positioning (RAP)

This is less frequently used, and involves the subject actively moving a joint to a given position.

Measurement of reflex latency

Beard et al. (1994) tested anterior cruciate deficient knees, and suggested that a latent or slow muscle contraction in response to sudden movement could be used as an assessment method. In terms of functional significance this is a very useful test but it requires electromyographic equipment to produce quantifiable data.

An appreciation of the presence of latency of contraction can, however, be gauged manually when comparing affected and non-affected limbs, particularly at the ankle. For example the patient can be instructed to evert the foot as soon as it is tapped into inversion by the therapist. The two sides are then compared.

PROPRIOCEPTIVE REHABILITATION OF THE LIMBS

Issues

The key aims of proprioceptive rehabilitation are:

- to provide early afferent input to a joint
- to restore reflex stability
- restore normal neuromuscular coordination
- to enhance the neuromuscular response.

Early commencement of proprioception can sometimes be neglected. This can be particularly so in the lower limb, when partial weight-bearing at least is seen as a prerequisite of proprioceptive training. Wobbleboard work in sitting is an excellent early exercise that can be made as easy or difficult an exercise as is required (Figure 21.17).

There is a wide variety of equipment available to facilitate rehabilitation of the sensorimotor system. There are numerous types of balance boards, starting with simple unidirectional wobbleboards to [the more novel] core stability boards. Wobbleboards are an excellent way of bombarding a joint with afferent input in the early stages of rehabilitation, but they are not a functional piece of equipment and it is important to progress from these types of apparatus if required. Other equipment such as slide boards can be useful acquisitions to enhancing dynamic functional stability. Coloured floor markers and even treadmills can also be used. The only limit to devising proprioceptive exercises should be your imagination.

There are several means open to the physiotherapist to progress proprioceptive exercises. These include:

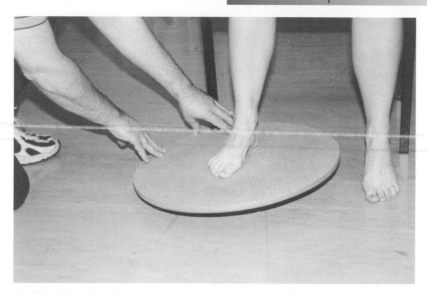

Figure 21.17 Wobbleboard work in sitting.

- removing visual stimulus
- altering the base of support
- increasing weight-bearing
- increasing speed of an activity
- making an exercise more complex.

Visual input provides additional afferent input to the CNS. Without it any given exercise becomes more difficult to perform, even with wobbleboard activities in sitting.

An example of altering the base of support is illustrated in Figures 21.18 and 21.19. This activity progressively requires greater neuromuscular control and strength to maintain a given position.

Key point

It is important during rehabilitation to place the joint(s) in situations that encourage the necessary reflex stability required to meet the functional demands of the individual. Stability work should therefore be progressed to place joints in vulnerable yet functional positions.

The Lower Limb

Proprioceptive exercises in the lower limb are progressions towards full weight-bearing, with the addition (if

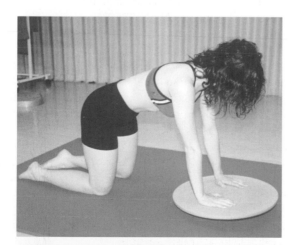

Figure 21.18 Altering the base of support with proprioceptive exercises.

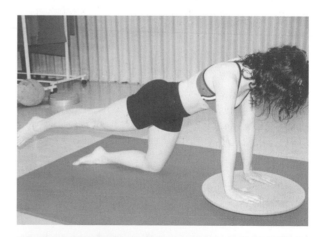

Figure 21.19 Altering the base of support with proprioceptive exercises.

required) of more dynamic stop–start activities that require aspects of acceleration deceleration and strong reflex stability around the ankle and knee.

Figures 21.20 and 21.21 illustrates a typical exercise for the lower limb. It is important to remember that this is not a particularly functional exercise as the limb remains static, yet this often becomes the end-point of rehabilitation. The more dynamic activities outlined above can be described as proprioceptive as they stress the joints in vulnerable positions and encourage the reflex actions that are required.

The Upper Limb

> **Key point**
> The objective of proprioceptive reha-bilitation is to 'enhance cognitive appreciation of the respective joint rel-ative to position and motion, and to enhance muscular stabilization of the joint in the absence of structural restraints' (Borsa *et al.* 1994).

The above quotation refers to rehabilitation of unstable shoulders and perhaps highlights the potential differences in the nature of pathologies between the upper and lower limb. The shoulder is inherently more unstable than the joints of the lower limb, and is therefore much more vulnerable to mechanical as well as functional instability. Consequently a degree of caution should be exercised and a comprehensive assessment undertaken when rehabilitating these types of injury.

Owing to this potential level of instability, close chain exercises are often a useful starting point as they help to encourage joint stability through co-contraction of the surrounding muscles induced by the axial compression (Davies and Dickoff-Hoffman 1993). Variations of the four-point kneeling position are commonly used to achieve this (Figures 21.18 and 21.19). These positions are also useful in rehabilitating scapula stability, which will also be affected (or be a cause) with shoulder instability problems.

When rehabilitating older patients or those with poorer physical condition, four-point kneeling may not be an appropriate position and variations of closed chain exercises can be used. These can include

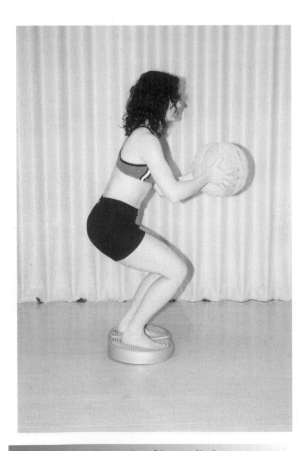

Figure 21.20   Example of lower limb proprioceptive exercises.

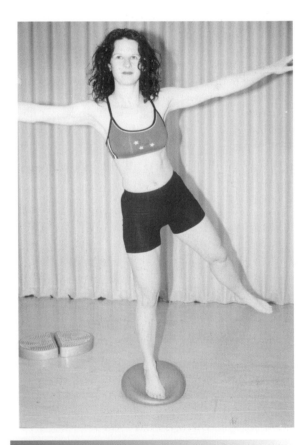

Figure 21.21   Example of lower limb proprioceptive exercises.

resting the hand on a wobbleboard in sitting, or pressing the hand against a wall or table and moving the shoulder.

Once a degree of control has been restored, more functional exercises can be taught. The reflex stabilisations illustrated in Figures 21.22 and 21.23 are aimed at eliciting the correct motor response at the appropriate speed and in the most functional position. This particular exercise and variations of it could be used with a rugby player who would require stability in this vulnerable position when making a tackle.

The weighted-pan exercise is another example of devising an exercise based upon function. The patient is asked initially to observe weights being dropped into the pan he or she is holding. The arm is placed progressively in more vulnerable positions, and the patient is instructed not to let the arm drop. The patient then closes his or her eyes and the exercise is repeated. This helps restore reflex stability in the upper limb.

Rehabilitating the sensorimotor system requires adequate strength and endurance within the muscle. Many of the exercises illustrated can also be viewed as strengthening exercises; and although much of the preceding discussion has emphasised sensorimotor rehabilitation in isolation, the need for an accompanying strength and endurance programme is paramount. Indeed muscular fatigue has been shown to induce proprioceptive deficits (Voight et al. 1996).

There is no definitive way to rehabilitate the sensorimotor system, and issues of progression depend on functional need, pain, swelling and an appropriate strength base. Table 21.8 provides an example of a potential rehabilitation programme for a footballer

recovering from a lateral ligament injury of the ankle. The stages illustrated are intended as a guide only.

PROPRIOCEPTIVE REHABILITATION OF THE SPINE

The spine needs an effective neuromuscular control system and so may benefit from proprioceptive rehabilitation. Means of assessing proprioceptive deficits within the spine are, however, less clearly defined than for the upper and lower limbs. Dynamic postural control requires reflex stabilisation of the trunk musculature. Swiss-ball exercises are useful to help restore this dynamic control (Figure 21.24).

Key point
Panjabi (1992) uses the phrase 'clinical instability' when referring to a decrease in the effectiveness of the passive and dynamic stabilisers within the spine.

The mechanisms of proprioception within the spine are less clearly defined, as are the means of assessing it. Research into the rehabilitation of such problems is also limited (Richardson et al. 1999). However, one can assume that the different levels at which proprioception works are the same for spinal as for the peripheral joints. There is a need for reflex muscular stabilisation as well as an initial conscious appreciation of muscle activity to control the multisegmental spine in both

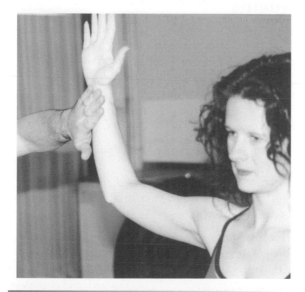

Figure 21.22 Reflex stability exercises applied to the shoulder.

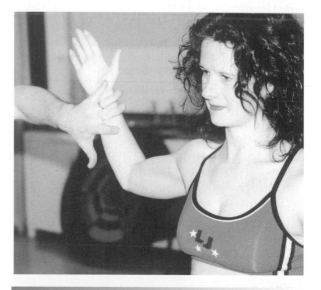

Figure 21.23 Reflex stability exercises applied to the shoulder.

Table 21.8 Example of a proprioceptive training programme for a footballer who has suffered a lateral ligament sprain of the ankle.

Stage	Examples of exercises	Rationale
Stage 1 (early, acute injury, pain on weight-bearing of varying degree)	(a) Wobbleboard exercises in sitting; basic controlled uniplanar movements progressing to multiplanar with physiotherapist input (see Figure 2.17) (b) As (a) but partial weight-bearing in standing progressing as able (c) Walking on a trampette	Provision of early afferent bombardment to the area Low-load reflex stabilisation Conscious appreciation of movement and position
Stage 2 (pain and swelling resolving, minimal if any discomfort with normal gait)	(a) Dynamic balance board activities: throwing and catching a ball (b) Use of other equipment such as the fitter and slide board (c) Variations on the above incorporating functional activities (d) Trampette work with football	Encouraging reflex stabilisation, functional movement patterns Subconscious activity
Stage 3 (mid/late, pain-free with all ADLs, may be mild discomfort with dynamic functional activities, e.g. running and twisting)	(a) Dynamic multidirectional functional activities at less than full pace: 'W' runs, sidestepping activities (b) Bilateral jumping activities (c) Running activities incorporating ball work	Increasing dynamic functional stability, increasing specificity
Stage 4 (late stage, full function)	(a) Full speed activities/ball work (b) Single leg drills, e.g. zig-zag hopping (c) Advanced plyometric drills (d) Return to full training	Preparation for return to full training/competition

static and dynamic postures. The emphasis is on maintaining a neutral spinal position (Panjabi 1992), thus reducing shear and compressive forces around the spinal joints.

Conscious appreciation of spinal position and associated muscle activity has been aided by the use of equipment such as the Stabilizer pressure biofeedback device (Chattanooga, Australia). This is a simple device consisting of an air-filled chamber and an attached dial that monitors pressure changes. Patients are instructed to perform exercises while maintaining a constant pressure reading or altering the pressure through exercise.

Exercises may be commenced in lying initially and progressed into more functional upright positions. Pain is often the major concern in these patients and a neuromuscular training programme will aim to decrease or alleviate pain. The mechanisms of spinal pain are, however, varied and often poorly understood.

The term 'core stability' is used also with reference to back rehabilitation – 'core' referring to the trunk as the central control point of all movement.

RESISTANCE TRAINING

Benefits

Resistance training can include strength training, which is described as the maximum force or tension generated by a muscle. It can also refer to sub-maximal and endurance work. All aspects of resistance training can be incorporated into various rehabilitation programmes. Some of the reported physiological benefits of resistance training are:

- increased cross-sectional area of muscle
- increased muscle fibre size
- increased or maintained bone density
- increased tensile strength of tendons and ligaments
- decreased heart rate.

In order for a muscle or muscle group to develop sufficient strength gains it must be loaded progressively, otherwise strength improvements will be limited. This factor can often be overlooked, and countless repetitions of straight leg raises, for example, can be given without producing the desired effect.

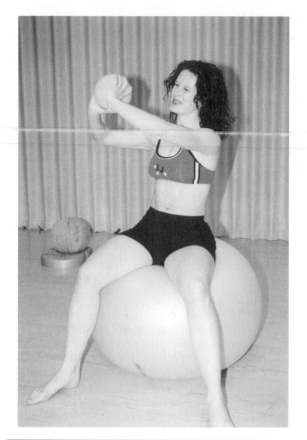

Figure 21.24   Swiss-ball exercise designed to develop neuromuscular control around the trunk.

Initial improvement in strength, when measured objectively, may be rapid without noticeable changes in physical characteristics. This is due to enhanced neuromuscular coordination. More motor units are recruited within a given muscle and a stronger contraction of the muscle is therefore produced. This neural adaptation occurs before other physical and physiological changes that result from resistance training.

Muscle Contractions

Muscles can contract in three different ways: concentrically, eccentrically and isometrically. The characteristics of these different types of contractions are summarised in Table 21.9.

Key point

Sometimes the terminology *isotonic shortening* and *isotonic lengthening* may be seen instead of concentric and eccentric contraction. These terms are best avoided as they imply one contraction is an opposite of the other, whereas physiologically their characteristics vary greatly.

Table 21.9 Types of muscle contraction.

Type of contraction	Characteristics
Isometric	Muscle maintains same length throughout the contraction
Concentric	Muscle shortens during contraction
Eccentric	Muscle lengthens during contraction

Individual muscles may exhibit more than one type of contraction at a time. Consider the muscle work occurring at the hamstrings in Figure 21.25. The proximal part of the muscle is lengthening (controlling hip flexion), and the distal part is shortening, controlling tibial movement.

Types of Muscle Fibre

There are three main types of muscle fibre, usually called I, IIa and IIb. Newer subdivisions are now being described, such as Ic, IIc and IIab (Scott *et al.* 2001). Individual muscles have different percentages of each

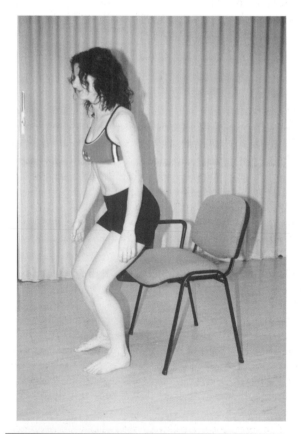

Figure 21.25   Moving towards sitting from a standing position.

of the fibre types. Some of the differences in the physiological make-up of these muscle fibres are illustrated in Table 21.10.

The proportion of different fibre types is not consistent between muscles or between individuals. These characteristics are generally thought to be genetically determined and are part of the reason for the natural selection that sees individuals excel in different sports or play in different positions within a team. Some general points can be made, however.

- Postural muscles such as soleus are involved in maintaining position rather than dynamic activity and therefore have a higher number of type I fibres.
- Muscles that may be involved in more dynamic activity, such as the gastrocnemius, will have proportionately greater numbers of fast twitch fibres – types IIa and IIb.
- With age the number and size of type II fibres decreases (Rogers and Evans 1993), making tasks that require a quick burst of strength more difficult. This should be an important consideration when rehabilitating elderly patients.
- There is evidence that muscle fibres can convert from one fibre type to another. This occurs particularly between types IIa and IIb (Scott et al. 2001). This is known as *plasticity*.

Number of Repetitions

The number of repetitions performed of a particular exercise determines the type of muscle work. Resistance training includes pure strength work as well as endurance work and as a consequence the number of repetitions will be based on the required outcome.

There is little clear evidence on the number of repetitions that should be used, but there are many protocols that can be used or adapted. A group of repetitions is known as a *set*, with three or four sets of an exercise usually being performed.

Instructing a patient to perform 10 repetitions may be the most appropriate number to prescribe for the particular weight and exercise, but there needs to be a method of determining the weight required for these repetitions. It is important not to lose sight of the purpose of resistance training, particularly strength training – one of progressive overload to increase muscle strength and improve function. Progressive overload will not occur with repetitions of a weight that is too light and as a consequence recovery will be slower.

The majority of protocols that are in existence for strength training are based upon what are known as the 'one repetition maximum' (1RM) and the '10 repetition maximum' (10RM). The 1RM is when only one repetition of an exercise is possible, further completed effort being prevented by fatigue (Cahill et al. 1997). Determining the 1RM therefore prevents a challenge in the clinical environment and perhaps explains the sometimes arbitrary nature of repetitions given.

Key point

Sets consisting of 10 repetitions are commonplace within exercise prescription. However, this is often just an arbitrary number. Avoid giving 'sets of 10' without any underlying rationale.

As their names suggest, 1RM and 10RM relate to the maximum amount of weight that can be lifted by a muscle or muscle group, for 1 and 10 repetitions respectively. Examples of some of these protocols are illustrated in Table 21.11. The numbers of repetitions that should be used during sub-maximal and endurance exercises are less clearly defined.

Open-Chain and Closed-Chain Kinetic Strengthening

The emphasis on closed kinetic chain exercises has developed since the onset of accelerated protocols for anterior cruciate ligament rehabilitation. A closed kinetic chain exercise occurs when the distal part of the limb (upper or lower) is firmly in contact with a firm

Table 21.10 Some characteristics of the muscle fibre types.

	Type I	Type IIa	Type IIb
Fitness component	Cardiorespiratory fitness	Muscular endurance	Strength/power
Energy system utilised	Aerobic	Anaerobic	Anaerobic
Contraction speed	Slow	Fast	Fast
Numbers of mitochondria	Many	Moderate	Low
Resistance to fatigue	High	Moderate	Low

Table 21.11 Sample of strength training protocols.

Programme	Protocol	
DeLorme	1 set of 50%	10RM × 10
	1 set of 75%	10RM × 10
	1 set of 100%	10RM × 10
Oxford	1 set of 100%	10RM × 10
	1 set of 75%	10RM × 10
	1 set of 50%	10RM × 10
DAPRE	1 set of 50%	6RM × 10
(daily adjusted	1 set of 75%	6RM × 10
progressive resistance	1 set of 100%	6RM × as many as possible
exercise)	Next set: on a sliding scale depending on performance in the third set	

surface. Squatting is a commonly quoted example of a closed chain kinetic exercise, but performing a leg press exercise with the feet in contact with a metal footplate is also an example.

The following are some of the proposed benefits of closed chain exercises in the lower limb:

- The shear force acting at the knee joint is reduced compared with the last 30 degrees of open chain extension.
- They encourage more functional movement patterns.
- They stimulate co-contraction of the hamstrings, helping to reduce anterior tibial translation (important in ACL rehabilitation).
- They increase shoulder stability in the upper limb by stimulating co-contraction of surrounding muscles.

Eccentric Muscle Work

Eccentric muscle work has different physiological properties compared with concentric muscle work and may be described as a controlled lengthening of a muscle under tension (Table 21.12).

Reported physiological differences in eccentric muscle work when compared to concentric are:

- greater mechanical efficiency
- greater metabolic efficiency
- less resistant to fatigue
- delayed-onset muscle soreness experienced.

Delayed-onset muscle soreness (DOMS) is a dull aching sensation that follows unaccustomed muscular exertion. It is a key characteristic occurring only in eccentric muscle soreness. DOMS should be differentiated from other types of muscle soreness that occur during or soon after exercise owing to metabolic deficiencies.

DOMS is typically felt most acutely 48 hours after eccentric exercise has been completed (Leger and Milner 2001; Howell et al. 1993; Rodenberg et al. 1993). This commonly occurs in certain muscles of individuals infrequently undertaking a particular activity that has quite a high eccentric component. Examples include hill walking (quadriceps in the downhill component) or playing squash (gluteus maximus when reaching for a low shot).

DOMS is effectively the occurrence of local microtrauma within the muscle. A key site for this inflammation is between adjacent sarcomeres, or within the Z bands. Evidence for this inflammatory reaction can be found in increased levels of creatine kinase (CK) in the blood following exercise. This enzyme is released into the bloodstream following a muscular injury. Occasionally the high creatine kinase levels found following eccentric exercise can confuse the clinical picture of a patient in whom CK levels may be used as a means of informing clinical diagnosis (Gralton et al.

Table 21.12 The functions of eccentric muscle work.

Function	Example
Deceleration of a limb part	Kicking a football; the hamstrings act to decelerate hip flexion and knee extension
Force absorption	Landing from a jump; the quadriceps contract absorbing some of the ground reaction force thus reducing the joint reaction forces
Controlling a movement against gravity	Sitting down in a chair; gluteus maximus and the upper part of the hamstrings are controlling hip flexion

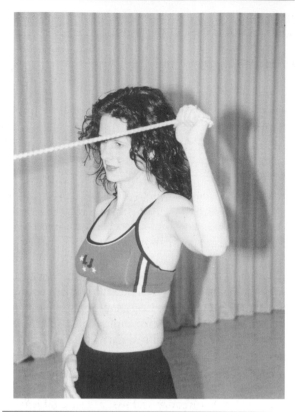

Figure 21.26   Eccentric training of the lateral rotators for throwing activities.

1998). Saxton et al. (1995) have also reported a decrease in proprioceptive function with high-level eccentric exercise.

Undertaking low-level bouts of eccentric exercise has been found to enhance recovery from DOMS following previous eccentric exercise and has also been found to reduce the effects of DOMS when undertaken prior to bouts of heavy eccentric exercise.

Treatment with eccentric exercise

Eccentric exercise has been identified as a key treatment technique when rehabilitating tendon injuries. Stanish *et al.* (1985) proposed treatment protocols with eccentric exercise involving alteration in both load and speed. An example of an eccentric training programme for the lateral rotators of the glenohumeral joint is presented in Table 21.13.

The benefits of using eccentric exercise programmes for tendon injuries are thought to include:

- increasing the tensile strength of the tendon
- stressing healing tissue in a functional manner
- utilising a rehabilitation programme that mimics the functional role of the appropriate musculo-tendinous unit.

Resistance Training in Different Populations

The elderly

Physical strength is known to decrease with age. Some of the reported reasons for this decline are the following:

- a decrease in the number of actual muscle fibres
- muscle fibre atrophy
- impaired excitation–contraction coupling
- an inability or decreased ability to recruit type II motor units (Rogers and Evans 1993).

Table 21.13 Example of eccentric exercises that could be used as part of a rehabilitation programme for a throwing injury involving the posterior rotator cuff (infraspinatus and teres minor).

Timescale	Exercise	Load
Early (still pain and dysfunction)	Low load, low speed controlling the arm into medial rotation (in prone)	Light dumbbell, low strength bungee cord anchored to floor
	Increase load ± speed	Heavier dumbbell increases strength of bungee cord
Mid stage	Low/moderate load in standing incorporating some diagonal movement patterns	Moderate-resistance bungee cord
	As above increasing load ± speed in standing towards functional level	
Late stage (symptom free)	Functional activities – various throwing drills progressing to functional speeds	Different size/weight of balls

It is important to appreciate these long-term declines when addressing rehabilitation programmes with this section of the population. The issues outlined above related to progressive overload are just as significant but can be forgotten. An increase in basic strength may mean improved performance in functional tasks.

Children and adolescents

There is currently no evidence to suggest that resistance training in children is harmful, provided it is well supervised. The vast majority of adverse incidents have been related to poor technique and/or unsupervised activity. There have been no reports of growth plate fractures in studies related to youth strength training programmes.

The American Academy of Pediatrics has produced a series of recommendations in this area that stress supervision and numbers of repetitions of between 8 and 15. Practising technique with no load is also highlighted.

From a clinical viewpoint it is important to consider appropriate resistance training programmes when rehabilitating children and adolescents, adhering to the same principles of progressive overload.

FUNCTIONAL TESTING AND REHABILITATION

All rehabilitation should be geared towards a return to normal functional activity. Towards the later stages of rehabilitation the functional aspects are perhaps of greatest importance.

Rehabilitation should not be measured as complete solely by outcomes such as bilateral symmetry of strength and range of movement, or an individual's ability to balance on a wobbleboard on the injured leg for 60 seconds. The physiotherapist needs to have a clear insight into the specific occupational and functional requirements of an individual to make sure the person is rehabilitated to the correct level. Such demands may involve carrying heavy weights, working on a building site or playing professional sport.

Figures 21.27 and 21.28 illustrates a fireman undergoing specific functional rehabilitation whilst wearing full kit, thus mimicking the working environment. This provides psychological as well as physical benefits. Functional rehabilitation allows a more objective measure of fitness to return to work. However, unless working in a specialist centre, being able to completely replicate a particular working environment as described above may not always be possible. In this situation the physiotherapist needs to be inventive and

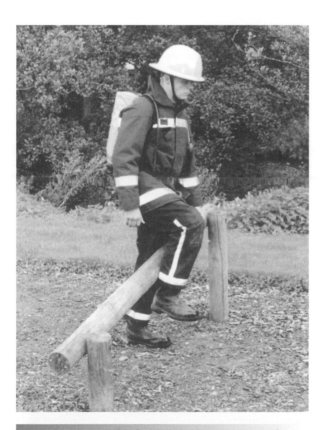

Figure 21.27   A firefighter undergoing specific functional rehabilitation.

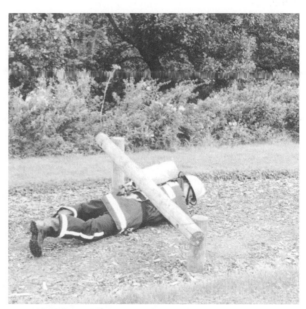

Figure 21.28   A firefighter undergoing specific functional rehabilitation.

(Photos courtesy of Firebrigade Rehabilitation Centre Penrith UK.)

reproduce the tasks to be undertaken in the working environment as closely as possible, using any equipment or apparatus that may be available. This can include benches, wall bars, bungee cord, rucksacks, and sports-specific equipment such as tennis racquets.

Functional testing is an extension of functional rehabilitation and plays a major role in determining an individual's ability to return to pre-injury levels. This can take the form of one particular drill that encompasses several of the most difficult aspects of the individual's occupation or sport. For example, a soccer player needs to be able to run quickly, accelerate and decelerate, change direction, and jump. A circuit could be set up similar to the one illustrated in Figure 21.29 to test any number of skills. This circuit could be timed over a number of sessions to determine improvement, or may simply be used as a one-off test to determine a return to full training.

Key point

When devising functional tests it is useful to apply the SMART principle: specific, measurable, achievable, realistic, timed. In this way they can be developed as a valuable objective measure. There is a large scope for development of such tests, but it is also important that once such tests are devised they are seen to be reliable and valid. This therefore requires ongoing data collection.

Further occupational tests are presented in Figures 21.30 and 21.31. In these situations the fireman has to perform timed functional tests, based upon set criteria.

Functional testing does not always need to be used as a measure for determining return to full function; it may instead be used as a baseline measure of functional

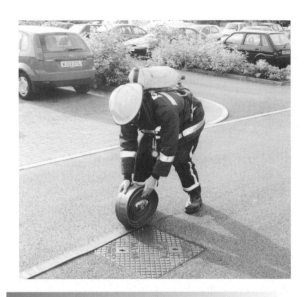

Figure 21.30   Timed functional occupational tasks.

ability. Examples of this include the various timed and distance hop tests which are used to test ACL deficient knees. Tippet and Voight (1995) suggest the following times when functional testing is undertaken within a sports environment:

- preseason training
- during rehabilitation
- immediately after injury.

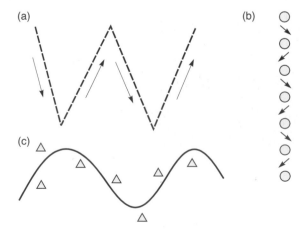

Figure 21.29   Example of a timed circuit.

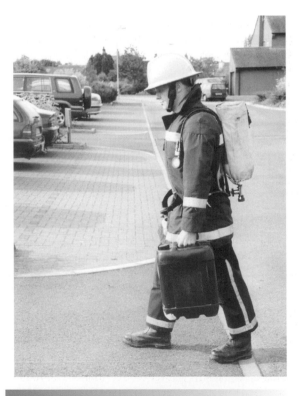

Figure 21.31   Timed functional occupational tasks.

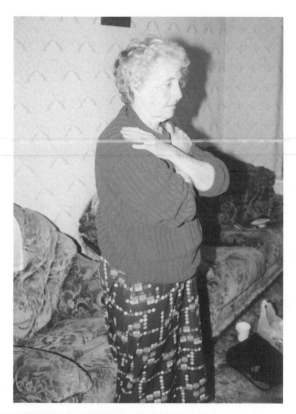

Figure 21.32   The sit to stand functional test. An example of a simple functional test requiring no equipment.

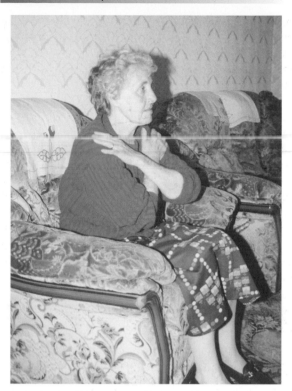

Figure 21.33   The sit to stand functional test.

Although the examples highlighted above involve quite dynamic activities, functional testing and rehabilitation can be applied to all populations. An example of functional testing in the elderly population is the sit-to-stand test (Figures 21.32 and 21.33). This can be either be timed or judged on the number of repetitions.

Task

There should be no limit other than your imagination on the exercises and tests you can devise as long as you follow the guidelines above. For practice, devise some specific exercises and tests for the following individuals: (a) a scaffolder working on a building site; (b) a professional tennis player.

PLYOMETRIC EXERCISES

Plyometric exercises are normally incorporated in the later stages of a rehabilitation programme and are aimed predominantly at those individuals who require more dynamic neuromuscular control as part of their normal functional activities. Plyometric exercises utilise the stretch shortening cycle to produce an enhanced concentric contraction.

A plyometric activity consists of a rapid eccentric contraction followed by an immediate concentric contraction. Typically these exercises are performed in the lower limb and involve various jumping-type activities (Figure 21.34). Successful performance involves a rapid

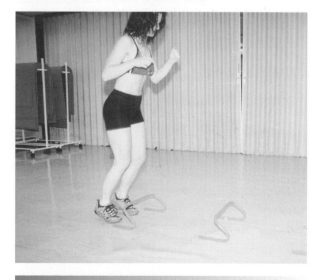

Figure 21.34   A plyometric drill for the lower limb.

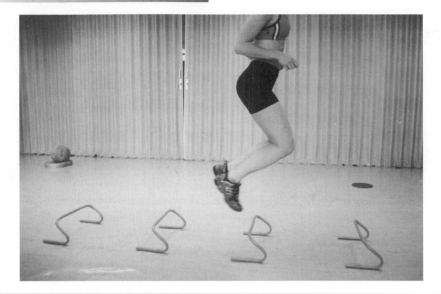

Figure 21.35   A plyometric drill for the lower limb.

change from the eccentric to the concentric contraction. The time between the eccentric and concentric contractions is known as the *amortisation phase* – the quicker this phase the more powerful the muscular concentric contraction.

Consider the jumping activity in Figure 21.35. As the feet hit the floor the knees flex and stretch in what is known as the series elastic component. The series elastic component consists of three structures:

- Z lines
- myosin hinges
- Sharpey's fibres.

Sharpey's fibres are located at the site of tendon insertion into bone. Acting together these structures behave like an elastic band that is stretched quickly – it stores up energy that can be suddenly released. This energy is added to the stretch reflex that occurs in the quadriceps on landing and, together with the following concentric contraction, combines to provide a more powerful contraction.

Plyometrics are used in the upper limb and certainly have functional applications. Medicine-ball drills are often incorporated into upper-limb exercises. Figure 21.36 illustrates one such drill using a trampette. The aim of the exercise is to throw a ball towards the tram-

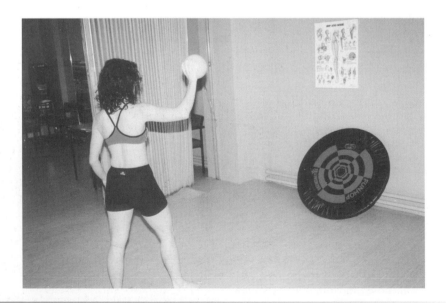

Figure 21.36   Pylometric drill using a trampette.

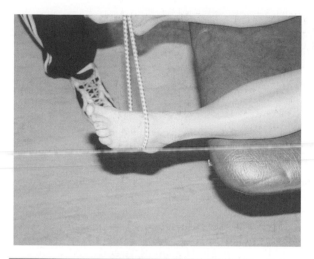

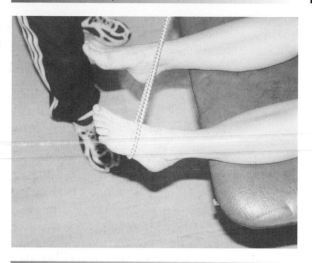

Figure 21.37   Plyometrics improve muscular response following injury.

Figure 21.38   Plyometrics can help improve muscular response following injury.

pette; it is then caught on the rebound and immediately thrown again. This exercise utilises the same components as the lower-limb exercise illustrated in Figure 21.35. There is a rapid eccentric contraction and sudden stretch of the lateral rotators, followed by an immediate concentric contraction of the medial rotators as the ball is thrown back.

The stated benefits of plyometric exercise are:

• increased power of muscular contraction
• enhanced neuromuscular coordination.

Before deciding to use plyometric exercises in the clinical situation, this checklist should be considered:

1   Is the person free of pain?
2   Is there an absence of recurrent swelling?
3   Does the person demonstrate a sufficient level of stability?

There are a number of tests reported in the literature to determine whether or not an individual has sufficient stability to be able to undertake plyometric exercises.

Despite the emphasis of plyometrics being on advanced rehabilitation, it can also play a role in improving the neuromuscular response following injury. An example of this is illustrated in Figure 21.37.

Latency of contraction is commonly seen in the peronei following an inversion injury to the ankle. The

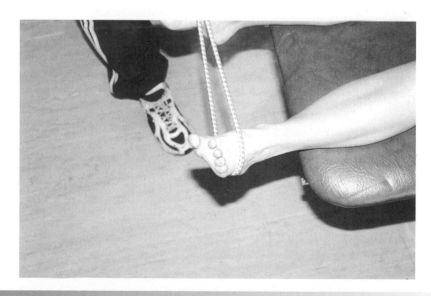

Figure 21.39   Plyometrics can help improve muscular response following injury.

principles of plyometrics can be used, using bungee cord, to work on improving the neuromuscular response and strengthening the peronei at the same time. The patient takes the strain on the bungee cord, holding the foot in an everted position. The patient is then instructed to release the tension on the bungee cord and then immediately evert the foot again. The condition of the ankle needs to be carefully assessed before commencing this type of exercise, in the same way as the inclusion criteria are checked for weight-bearing exercises.

There is little information on the number of repetitions that should be completed with plyometric exercises. Foot contacts have been suggested as an effective way of measuring the intensity of activity (Tippet and Voight 1995) in lower limb exercise, with a beginner counting 75–100 foot contacts and progressing up to 200–250 of low to moderate intensity. No values have been stated for the upper limb. Common sense should also prevail in monitoring performance, looking out for loss of quality of performance, obvious fatigue, and increase in the amortisation phase, etc.

Plyometric exercises should be performed no more than two or three times per week. The eccentric component is likely to cause a degree of DOMS and the muscle will need adequate time to recover.

FURTHER READING

Barrack RL, Lund PJ, Skinner HB 1994 Knee joint proprioception revisited. J Sport Rehabil 3: 18–42

Barrett DS, Cobb AG, Bentley G 1991 Joint proprioception in normal, osteoarthritic and replaced knees. J Bone Joint Surg 73B(1): 53–0

Crook P, Stott R, Rose M et al. 1998 Adherence to group exercise: physiotherapist-led experimental programmes. Physiotherapy 84: 366–72

Janda V 1983 Muscle Function Testing. London: Butterworth

Jerosch J, Prymka M 1996 Proprioception and joint stability. Knee Surg Sports Traum Arthrosc 4: 171–9

Kato Y, Ikata T et al. 2000 Effects of specific warm-up at various intensities on energy metabolism during subsequent exercise. J Sports Med Phys Fitness 40(2): 126–30

Kisner C, Colby LA 1996 Therapeutic Exercise: Foundations and Techniques, 3rd edn. Philadelphia: FA Davies

Lieber 1992 Skeletal Muscle Structure and Function: Implications for Rehabilitation and Sports Medicine. Baltimore: Williams & Wilkins

Mense S, Simons DG, Russell J (eds) 2001 Muscle pain: understanding its nature, diagnosis and treatment. Philadelphia: Lippincott Williams & Wilkins

Richie DH 2001 Functional instability of the ankle and the role of neuromuscular control: a comprehensive review. J Foot Ankle Surg 40: 240–51

Tippet SR, Voight ML 1995 Functional Testing in Functional Progressions for Sport Rehabilitation. Champaign, IL: Human Kinetics

Vickers AJ 2001 Time course of muscle soreness following different types of exercise. BMC Musculoskelet Disord 2(1): 5

REFERENCES

Bandy WD, Irion JM, Briggler M 1997 The effect of time and frequency of static stretching on flexibility of the hamstring muscles. Phys Ther 77: 1090–6

Barrack RL, Lund PJ, Skinner HB 1994 Knee joint proprioception revisited. J Sport Rehabil 3: 18–42

Barrett DS, Cobb AG, Bentley G 1991 Joint proprioception in normal, osteoarthritic and replaced knees. J Bone Joint Surg 73B(1): 53

Bartlett MJ, Warren PJ 2002 Effect of warming up on knee proprioception before sporting activity. Br J Sports Med 36(2): 132–4

Beard DJ, Kyberd PJ, O,Connor JJ, Ferguson CM, Dodd CAF 1994 Reflex hamstring contraction latency in anterior cruciate ligament deficiency. J Orthopaed Res 12: 219–28

Bergmark A 1989 Stability of the lumbar spine: a study in mechanical engineering. Acta Orthopaed Scand Suppl 230: 1–54

Borsa PA, Lephart SM, Kocher MS, Lephart SP 1994 Functional assessment and rehabilitation of shoulder proprioception for glenohumeral instability. J Sport Rehabil 3: 84–104

Cahill BR, Misner JE, Boileau RA 1997 The clinical importance of the anaerobic energy system and its importance in human performance. Am J Sports Med 25: 863–72

Caraffa A, Cerulli G, Projetti M, Aisa G, Rizzo A 1996 Prevention of anterior cruciate ligament injuries in soccer: a prospective controlled study of proprioceptive training. Knee Surg Sports Traum Arthrosc 4: 19–21

Chan SP, Hong Y, Robinson PD 2001 Flexibility and passive resistance of the hamstrings of young adults using two different static stretching protocols. Scand J Med Sci Sports 11(2): 81–6

Comerford MJ, Mottram SL 2001 Masterclass. Functional stability re-training: principles and strategies for managing mechanical dysfunction. Manual Ther 6(1): 3–14

Crook P, Stott R, Rose M et al. 1998 Adherence to group exercise: physiotherapist-led experimental programmes. Physiotherapy 84: 366–72

Davies GJ, Dickoff-Hoffman S 1993 Neuromuscular testing and rehabilitation of the shoulder complex. J Orthopaed Sports Phys Ther 18: 449–58

Emery CA 1999 Does decreased muscle strength cause acute muscle strain injury in sport? A systematic review of the evidence. Phys Ther Rev 4(3): 141–51

Etnyre BR, Lee EJ 1987 Comments on proprioceptive neuromuscular facilitation stretching techniques. Res Quart Exer Sport 58(2): 184–8

Freeman MAR, Dean MRE, Hanhan IWF 1965 The aetiology and prevention of functional instability of the foot. J Bone Joint Surg 47B: 678–85

Gluck NI, Liebenson CS 1997 Clinical implications of paradoxical muscle function in muscle stretching or strengthening. J Bodywork Mov Ther 1: 219–22

Gralton E, Wildgoose J, Donovan WM, Wilkie J 1998 Eccentric exercise and neuroleptic malignment syndrome. Lancet 352: 1114

Harvey LA, Herbert RD 2002 Muscle stretching for treatment and prevention of contracture in people with spinal cord injury. Spinal Cord 40(1): 1–9

Hodges PW, Richardson CA 1996 Inefficient muscular stabilization of the lumbar spine associated with low back pain: a motor control evaluation of transversus abdominis. Spine 21:2640–50

Howell JN, Chlebourn G, Conaster R 1993 Muscle stiffness, strength loss, swelling and soreness following eccentric induced exercise in humans. J Physiology 464: 183–96

Hunter G 1998 Specific soft tissue mobilization in the management of soft tissue dysfunction. Manual Ther 3(1): 2–11

Janda V 1983 Muscle Function Testing. London: Butterworth

Jerosch J, Prymka M 1996 Proprioception and joint stability. Knee Surg Sports Traum Arthrosc 4: 171–9

Jull GA, Janda V 1987 Muscles and motor control in low back pain. In Twomey LT, Taylor JR (eds) Physical Therapy of the Low Back, pp. 253–78. Edinburgh: Churchill Livingstone

Kato Y, Ikata T et al. 2000 Effects of specific warm-up at various intensities on energy metabolism during subsequent exercise. J Sports Med Phys Fitness 40(2): 126–30

Kerrigan DC, Lee LW, Collins JJ, Riley PO, Lipsitz LA 2001 Reduced hip extension during walking: healthy elderly and fallers versus young adults. Arch Phys Med Rehabil 82: 26–30

Kisner C, Colby LA 1996 Therapeutic Exercise: Foundations and Techniques, 3rd edn. Philadelphia: FA Davies

Kujala UM, Orava S et al. 1997 Hamstring injuries: current trends in treatment and prevention. Sports Med 23: 397–404

Leger AB, Milner TE 2001 Muscle function at the wrist after eccentric exercise. Med Sci Sports Exer 33: 612–20

Lephart SM, Henry TJ 1995 Functional rehabilitation for the upper and lower extremity. Orthoped Clin N Am 26: 579–92

Lephart SM, Pincivero DM et al. 1997 The role of proprioception in the management and rehabilitation of athletic injuries. Am J Sports Med 25: 130–7

Lieber 1992 Skeletal Muscle Structure and Function: Implications for Rehabilitation and Sports Medicine. Baltimore: Williams & Wilkins

Magnusson SP 1998 Passive properties of human skeletal muscle during stretch manoeuvres. Scand J Med Sci Sports 8(2): 65–77

Melis P, Noorlander ML et al. 2002 Rapid alignment of collagen fibres in the dermis of undermined and not undermined skin stretched with a skin-stretching device. Plast Reconstr Surg 109: 674–80

Mense S, Simons DG, Russell J (eds) 2001 Muscle pain: understanding its nature, diagnosis and treatment. Philadelphia: Lippincott Williams & Wilkins

Norris CM 1995 Spinal stabilisation. 4: Muscle imbalance and the low back. Physiotherapy 81(3): 127–38

Panjabi MM (1992) The stabilising system of the spine. Part II Neutral zone and stability hypothesis. J Spinal Dis 5: 390–7

Richardson C, Jull G, Hodges P, Hides J 1999 General considerations in motor control and joint stabilization: the basis of assessment and exercise techniques. In Therapeutic Exercise for Spinal Segmental Stabilisation in Low Back Pain: Scientific Basis and Clinical Approach. London: Churchill Livingstone

Richie DH 2001 Functional instability of the ankle and the role of neuromuscular control: a comprehensive review. J Foot Ankle Surg 40: 240–51

Rodenberg JB, Bär PR, De Boer RW 1993 Relations between muscle soreness and biochemical and functional outcomes of eccentric exercise. J Appl Physiol 74: 2976–83

Rogers, MA, Evans WJ 1993 Changes in skeletal muscle with aging: effects of exercise training. Exer Sports Sci Rev 21: 65–102

Saxton JM, Clarkson PM, James R et al. 1995 Neuromuscular dysfunction following eccentric exercise. Med Sci Sports Exer 27: 1185–93

Scott W, Stevens J, Binder-Macleod SA (2001) Human skeletal muscle fibre type classifications. Phys Ther 81(11): 1810–16.

Spernoga SG, Uhl TL, Arnold BL, Gansneder BM 2001 Duration of maintained hamstring flexibility after a one-time, modified hold–relax stretching protocol. J Athlet Train 36(1): 44–8

Stanish WD, Curwin S, Rubinovich M (1985) Tendinitis: the analysis and treatment for running. Clin Sports Med 4(44): 593–609

Tippet SR, Voight ML 1995 Functional Testing in Functional Progressions for Sport Rehabilitation. Champaign, IL: Human Kinetics

Vickers AJ 2001 Time course of muscle soreness following different types of exercise. BMC Musculoskelet Disord 2(1): 5

Voight ML, Hardin JA, Blackburn TA, Tippet S, Canner GC 1996 The effects of muscle fatigue on and the relationship of arm dominance to shoulder proprioception. J Orthop Sports Phys Ther 23: 348–52

Waddington GS, Shepherd RB 1996 Ankle injury in sports: role of motor control systems and implications for prevention and rehabilitation. Phys Ther Rev 1: 79–87

Wilkerson GB, Nitz AJ 1994 Dynamic ankle instability: mechanical and neuromuscular interrelationships. J Sport Rehabil 3: 43–57

Physiotherapy for Amputees

Alison Chambers

22

INTRODUCTION

Amputation is a devastating and traumatic experience. The decision to amputate is often a last resort irrespective of the underlying pathology or problem. Patients facing amputation have usually already been through a series of other medical and surgical interventions in an attempt to save the affected limb, so the decision to amputate comes at the end of what for many patients has been an emotional and taxing period.

The psychological impact of the realisation of the necessity to amputate is immense. The adaptation and adjustment required by the patient and family facing such invasive surgery is challenging and can take place over many months. Its success depends on the person's ability to cope with amputation and also on the acceptance of those around the person of the change amputation inevitably imposes on physical and psychological health. Societal responses to disability and impairment also impact upon the rehabilitation process (Seymour 1998).

A team approach to management is the only way in which healthcare professionals can meet the needs of the patient to promote maximum recovery and function. Many of the amputee population are elderly and suffering from concurrent illness and disease, adding to the challenge faced by physiotherapists working within this clinical area.

Key point

Physiotherapists have been involved in the management of amputees for many years and are an integral part of the multidisciplinary team (MDT). The MDT comprises physiotherapists, occupational therapists, prosthetists, nurses, doctors, surgeons, psychologists, social workers – and last but not least the patient and significant others. The MDT approach enables a holistic approach to be adopted.

Patients are managed by a multidisciplinary team in primary, secondary and tertiary health and social care environments. This care is often provided in specialist units such has disabled services centres (DSCs) (Engstrom and Van de Ven 1999).

This chapter provides an overview of the management of amputees and an outline of the role of the physiotherapist (the examples given here focus on the lower-limb amputee patient). Readers are reminded that it will be necessary to refer to appropriate texts for details of the specifics of physiotherapy treatment, and of the causative factors and pathophysiology associated with amputation. In particular, readers will need to understand the pathology of:

- peripheral vascular disease (PVD)
- diabetes mellitus (DM)
- congenital abnormalities and the trauma associated with limb amputation.

Peripheral vascular disease is the most common indication for amputation in the UK – 85% of lower-limb amputees have PVD as the causative factor, and many of these individuals also have DM (Engstrom and Van de Ven 1999).

Further reading

General management principles apply equally to all levels of amputation. For detail relating to other specific levels of amputation, readers are directed to the texts listed in the further reading and reference lists.

LEVELS OF AMPUTATION

The decision to amputate a limb involves four principal considerations:

- preservation of life
- improvement of general health
- restoration of function
- reduction of pain.

Key point

Of course, people with congenital abnormalities may *elect* for amputation in order to improve function, so in those cases it is not associated with the preservation of life.

The underlying causative factors that result in amputation are (Engstrom and Van de Ven 1999):

- peripheral vascular disease (arteriosclerosis, gangrene)
- diabetes mellitus
- renal disease
- trauma
- tumour
- congenital limb deficiency
- infection.

The level of amputation is decided by tissue viability. A limb needs to be amputated to a level which ensures that all necrotic tissue has been excised and that the residual portion of limb will heal and be viable. The decision must also take account of the length of the residual limb and its suitability for prosthetic fitting, function and cosmesis. Table 22.1 lists the levels of amputation seen in clinical practice.

The proprioceptive feedback from the joint receptors in joints is extremely important to gait re-education, so joints will be preserved if possible.

GENERAL APPROACH TO MANAGEMENT

The overall management of an amputee patient is aimed at improving general health, reducing pain and restoring function. A team approach with clinical reasoning, clinical effectiveness, evidenced-based healthcare and problem-solving at its centre is advocated. Management spans all spheres of health and social care, from initial contact in a primary care setting through to tertiary care in a specialist centre. The partnership between health and social care is paramount to a successful outcome.

Because amputation is the last resort when all other possible treatments have been exhausted, patients have often had other interventions such as angioplasty, endarterectomy and pharmacological therapy (Pell et al. 1997; Robicsek 1997; Redhead 1984).

Not all amputees are suitable for a prosthetic limb. Assessment of suitability is made by the multidisciplinary team and is based (for a lower-limb amputee) on the following criteria:

1 Does the patient *want* to walk?
2 Does the patient have the *potential* to walk?
3 Who will help the patient in the home setting?

PHYSIOTHERAPY MANAGEMENT

Basic Issues

Physiotherapy management includes assessment and management of all aspects of the patient's well-being. The physiotherapist needs to take into account the physical, psychological and social aspects of the patient's life. Rehabilitation is an inclusive process giving due regard to the whole patient and not just his or her physical status (Buttenshaw and Dolman 1992).

The overall aim of physiotherapy is to promote *optimal independence in the use of a specific limb*. The goals can be summarised as:

- recovery of good general health
- maximisation of functional outcome
- prevention of complications
- reduction of pain.

Accurate and ongoing assessment of the patient throughout the four stages of amputee management is an essential component of physiotherapy.

Table 22.1 Principal amputation levels.

Upper limb	Lower limb
Forequarter	Hindquarter
Shoulder disarticulation	Hip disarticulation
Transhumeral	Transfemoral*
Elbow disarticulation	Supracondylar
Wrist disarticulation	Transtibial
Transmetacarpal	Gritti–Stokes
	Knee disarticulation
	Transtibial*
	Symes
	Choppat/Lisfranc
	Transmetatarsal

* The most common levels seen in clinical practice (Fyfe 1990).

Initial assessment at the preoperative stage should be followed by regular reassessment and evaluation of the outcomes of the treatment process. A problem-solving approach to assessment is required. This type of approach allows the physiotherapist to 'tailor' a treatment programme that best suits an individual patient at any given time. The physiotherapist's knowledge of normal human movement is essential to provide effective limb re-education.

The physiotherapist is involved in the management of a patient from the preoperative stage to the rehabilitation stage. Contact with the physiotherapist is often frequent and takes place over many months. The physiotherapist is instrumental to the decision regarding prosthetic prescription and works closely with the prosthetist to facilitate the best mobility outcome. It is often the physiotherapist who discovers problems with the prosthesis during the rehabilitation stage.

Physiotherapy intervention can be divided into four distinct stages: *preoperative*, *postoperative*, *preprosthetic* and *prosthetic* (the preprosthetic and prosthetic stages collectively make up the rehabilitation stage). Table 22.2 summarises these four stages of physiotherapy intervention, with lower-limb amputation used for illustrative purposes. Assessment is an integral part of all stages.

The Preoperative Stage

The physiotherapist's full preoperative assessment should include the respiratory status of the patient, because the effects of anaesthesia can mean that this status is compromised following surgery.

This preoperative stage is very important to the overall outcome as it is a time when the physiotherapist can explain to the patient what will occur postoperatively and prepare the person for the rehabilitation pro-

Table 22.2 Lower-limb amputation used to illustrate the four stages of physiotherapy management.

Stage of management	Components
Preoperative	Respiratory and musculoskeletal status Physical, psychological and social status Past medical, drug and social history Premorbid mobility Explanation of postoperative regimen
Postoperative	Respiratory status Bed mobility exercises Mobility and strength exercises for the residual limbs and trunk Assessment for walking aid, transfers Wheelchair assessment Balance and posture re-education Stump care and pain relief
Preprosthetic rehabilitation stage (patient assessed for suitability for prosthesis)	As above, plus: Use of pneumatic postamputation mobility (PPAM) aid 7–10 days postoperatively Gait, posture and balance re-education Activities of daily living (ADLs).
Prosthetic rehabilitation stage	As above, plus: Prosthetic management Continuing gait re-education Promotion of functional independence Stump care

gramme. The physiotherapist is involved in the preparation of the patient for surgery (Cutson and Bougiorni 1996).

Ideally the preoperative stage involves assessing the patient several days prior to surgery. However, the decision to amputate may occur as an emergency, in which case the physiotherapist possibly has only a few hours to complete the assessment.

The Postoperative Stage

During the postoperative stage the physiotherapist is involved in the assessment of suitability for walking aids and wheelchair prescription. Early on, prior to the use of a temporary prosthesis, the walking aid of choice is a walking frame – except for the younger patient when crutches may be possible.

Whilst there is no fixed protocol following surgery, Table 22.3 provides a guide to the type of programme used in clinical practice. The physiotherapist must work in line with the protocol stipulated by the operating surgeon, which may vary.

An important role of physiotherapy during the postoperative stage is the prevention of contractures. This is vital to ensure the success of the prosthetic

stage. Contractures will severely hamper the rehabilitation process and could result in the inability to use a prosthesis. The physiotherapist educates the patient in the prevention of contractures through a range of exercises and posture management. The typical contractures associated with lower-limb amputation are *transtibial* and *transfemoral*:

- Transtibial contracture can be described as knee flexion. It is positional as patients may spend a lot of time sitting. The use of a stump board and regular supine lying will help to prevent this.
- Transfemoral contracture can be described as hip flexion. There may be abduction due to unopposed hip flexors and abductors. Adduction may be a problem with a long residual stump owing to unopposed adductor longus.

Key point
Stump shape is to some extent determined by the use of a *juzo sock*, which controls oedema. The size and shape of the residual stump are important for ensuring a good prosthetic fit (Lambert et al. 1995).

Table 22.3 Example of post-operative physiotherapy management.

Day 1 – in bed
- Respiratory maintenance
- Exercises to include strengthening, mobility, balance
- Pain control

Day 2 – In chair
- Strengthening exercises (e.g. static quadriceps, upper limb exercise, knee flexion, bridging)
- Balance work
- Transfer practice
- Contracture prevention
- Assessment for wheelchair

Day 2–3 – Standing with walking frame
- Balance work
- Posture management

Day 3–4 – Walking with walking frame
- Transfer practice
- Stump maintenance
- Balance work

Day 7–10
- Begin early walking (PPAM) aid
- Re-education in the gym: posture, balance work
- Continue contracture prevention and stump care

Day 10
- Discharge, or transfer to rehabilitation unit
- Refer to DSC for prosthetic assessment

The Preprosthetic Stage

Early mobility is an important element in the rehabilitation of the patient. Not only does it provide early ambulatory practice for the patient, it also provides a psychological boost. It helps to prevent the onset of contractures and to re-educate posture and balance, two essential components of gait.

The pneumatic postamputation mobility (PPAM) aid

This mobility aid is advocated in the literature (Engstrom and Van de Ven 1999). It is introduced approximately 7–10 days after the operation, provided the residual limb is healing and there are no complications. It provides the patient with the opportunity to bear weight through the residual limb. Care must be taken when using the PPAM aid to ensure no damage to the stump.

The PPAM aid uses inflatable bags inside a metal frame. The inflatable bags are placed over the stump and support the residual limb inside the frame. Owing to the vulnerability of the stump the bags should not be inflated beyond 40 mmHg. It is essential that a pump be used that is capable of measuring exactly the amount of pressure in the bags. Over-inflation may compromise tissue viability.

The decision whether or not to proceed to a prosthesis is usually taken at this stage. Not all patients are suitable for prosthetic use. There is also little point providing a prosthesis if it will gather dust in a cupboard!

Some people are unable to cope with a prosthesis, for a variety of reasons. However, all patients should be assessed for prosthetic use on an equal basis. For those patients not going on to the prosthetic stage, an important part of the physiotherapist's role is to promote wheelchair independence.

The Prosthetic Stage

The majority of amputees go on to successful prosthetic independence and often enjoy a greater degree of quality of life than they had prior to the amputation. The improvement in function after possibly years of pain, discomfort and poor function can mean that the amputation has an eventual positive outcome. This does take time. Often it is the *psychological* impact of the change in body image that has a more significant effect on the patient (Henker 1979).

For the lower-limb amputee this stage involves intensive re-education of gait, along with detailed education of stump maintenance. The ultimate outcome of physiotherapy at this stage is to ensure the functional independence of the patient with a definitive limb. Ideally the outcomes of this final stage should be:

- understanding of the components of the prosthesis
- independent fitting and removal of the prosthesis, and checking its fit
- care of the prosthesis
- independent mobility with or without a walking aid, inside and outside, and the ability to cope with obstacles
- functional tasks with the prosthesis
- ability to perform occupational and/or leisure activities
- ability to cope with falls.

Prosthetic training
Prosthetic training is essential to the success of the rehabilitation process. Readers are directed to the numerous texts, which include Buttenshaw (1992), Jaegers et al. (1995) and Lemaire et al. (1993).

Common gait abnormalities

The following lists are extracted from Engstrom and Van deVen (1999).

Transtibial

- Excessive knee flexion.
- Insufficient knee flexion.
- Delayed knee flexion during the swing phase.
- Early knee flexion ('drop off').
- Lateral shift of the trunk.
- Lateral shift of the prosthesis.
- Rotation of the foot.

Transfemoral

- An abducted pattern.
- Rotation of the foot.
- Circumduction.
- Uneven step length.
- Uneven timing.
- 'Drop off'.

- 'Foot slap'.
- Uneven heel rise.
- Rising up on the toes of the opposite limb ('vaulting').
- Medial or lateral heel travel in swing phase ('medial whip'/'lateral whip').
- Terminal swing impact.
- Uneven arm swing.
- Lateral side bend of the trunk.
- Forward trunk flexion.
- Lumbar lordosis.

PSYCHOLOGICAL IMPLICATIONS OF AMPUTATION

All members of the healthcare team must understand the psychological implications associated with amputation. In some patients the reaction is transient and minor, for others it is more profound and longer lasting (Bridway et al. 1984; Butler et al. 1992). The normal reactions to grief and bereavement are well documented (e.g. Kubler-Ross 1969; Parkes 1972, 1975; Campling 1981), and the loss of a limb and the associated alteration in body image can be likened to other grieving processes.

Henker (1979) found that patients who had an amputation were likely to suffer from the alteration in body image and this had more of a detrimental effect than the resultant functional loss. The psychological adjustments required by people who have, as a result of illness and disease, a body which falls outside the accepted definition of 'normal' are enormous and well documented (Seymour 1998; Campling 1981; Jones and Davidson 1988).

Psychological well-being is important to the whole process of rehabilitation. It is essential that the management of amputation be explained to the patient. Physiotherapists need to acknowledge the enormous challenges patients face and use their knowledge of the normal grieving process to inform their approach to therapy. The Zigmond 'difference and adjustment' model (Engstrom and Van de Ven 1999) is seen to be particularly applicable to the grief and bereavement effects of amputation.

Key point
Models of grief and bereavement offer *frameworks* for understanding the grief associated with loss, but it must be acknowledged that grief manifests itself in many different ways and does not follow a linear pattern often outlined in such models.

PAIN IN AMPUTATION

There are essentially two types of pain, *residual limb pain* and *phantom pain*.

Residual limb pain

Residual limb pain can be attributed to a variety of causes, including the formation of a neuroma – a nodule formed at the end of a cut peripheral nerve, which folds back on itself and creates an enlargement. Pain caused by an ill-fitting prosthesis is referred to as 'prosthetic pain' and has a number of causes. In addition, postoperative pain is likely.

Phantom limb pain

Phantom limb pain can be described as distressing pain sensation felt by patients in the limb that is no longer there. It is well documented and is a feature that can impact significantly on the life of a patient (Weiss and Lindell 1996; Williams and Deaton 1997; Hill et al. 1995). It is a pain that seems to be an increasing factor with increasing age (Houghton et al. 1994). The psychological status of the patient also has an impact on phantom limb pain.

Phantom limb pain is described variously as cramping, squeezing, burning, sharp and shooting. Table 22.4 lists typical descriptions patients use to describe it.

OUTCOME MEASURES

The responsibility of healthcare professionals to provide evidence of the effectiveness of their treatments and management is of increasing importance. The introduction of the clinical governance framework within the National Health Service and the implications this has for accountability and clinical effectiveness has resulted in the growth of outcome measurement.

Outcome measures are designed to take the guesswork out of evaluation. They provide physiotherapists with a universal system of evaluation. This can then be utilised to identify best practice, ultimately leading to the improved health outcomes of patients. The field of amputee management is no exception. Many outcome measures offer a universal utility, whilst others provide specificity to a clinical area. Outcome measures measure function, treatment techniques and quality of life.

Outcome measures are essential to physiotherapists (Wade 1992). The range available is comprehensive, so the following examples of outcome measures used within the specialism of amputee management are not intended to be exhaustive:

- Rivermead Mobility Scale
- Functional Measures for Amputees
- Prosthetic Profile of Amputee (PPA)
- Houghton scale.

USEFUL SOURCES

- British Association of Chartered Physiotherapists in Amputee Rehabilitation (BACPAR)
- Scottish Physiotherapy Amputee Research Group (SPARG)
- CSP: www.csp.org.uk

FURTHER READING

Campling J 1981 Images of Ourselves: Women with Disabilities Talking. London: Routledge
Engstrom B, Van de Ven C (eds) 1999 Therapy for Amputees, 3rd edn. Edinburgh: Churchill Livingstone
Ham R, Bardsley P (eds) 1995 Amputee Rehabilitation: a Handbook. York: Lumley Associates
Ham R, McCreadie M 1992 Rehabilitation of elderly patients in the UK following lower limb amputation. Topics Geriatr Rehabil 8(1): 64–71
Houghton AD, Nicholls G, Houghton AL, Saadah E, McColl I 1994 Phantom pain: a natural history and association with rehabilitation. Ann R Coll Surg 76: 22–5
Jeffries GE 1998 Pain management. In Motion 22–36

Table 22.4 Patient descriptions of phantom limb pain.

Upper limb	Lower limb
Thumbnail being pulled out at the roots	Feeling that the tibia and fibula are being broken
Fist clenched so tightly that the fingernails are digging into the flesh	Rope-burn sensation between the great and second toe
Bones in the non existent arm being crushed	Steamroller running over the front part of the foot
Hand being crushed in a vice	Hammer smashing the great toe
	Five toes being stretched

Thompson DM, Haran D 1985 Living with an amputation. Soc Sci Med 20: 319–23

Williams AM, Deaton SB 1997 Phantom pain, elusive yet real. Rehabil Nurs 22(2): 73–7

REFERENCES

Bridway JK, Malone JM, Racy J, Leal J, Poole M 1984 Psychological adaptation to amputation an overview. Orthot Prosthet 38: 46–50

Butler DJ, Turkal NW, Seidl JJ 1992 Amputation: preoperative psychological preparation. J Am Board Fam Pract 5: 69–73

Buttenshaw P, Dolman J 1992 The Roehampton approach to rehabilitation: a retrospective survey of prosthetic use in patients with primary unilateral lower limb amputation Topics Geriatr Rehabil 8(1): 72–8

Campling J 1981 Images of Ourselves: Women with Disabilities Talking. London: Routledge

Cutson TM, Bougiorni DR 1996 Rehabilitation of the older lower limb amputee: a brief review. J Am Geriatr Soc 44: 1388–93

Engstrom B, Van de Ven C (eds) 1999 Therapy for Amputees, 3rd edn. Edinburgh: Churchill Livingstone

Fyfe NCM 1990 An audit of amputee levels in patients referred for prosthetic rehabilitation. Prosthet Orthot Int 14: 67–70

Henker FO 1979 Body Image conflict following trauma and surgery. Psychsomatics 20: 812–20

Hill A, Niven CA, Knussen C 1995 The role of coping in adjustment to phantom limb pain. Pain 62: 79–86

Houghton AD, Nicholls G, Houghton AL, Saadah E, McColl I 1994 Phantom pain: a natural history and association with rehabilitation. Ann R Coll Surg 76: 22–5

Jaegers SMHJ, Arenden JH, deJough HJ 1995 Prosthetic gait of unilateral transfemoral amputees a kinematic study. Arch Phys Med Rehabil 76: 736–43

Jones G, Davidson J 1988 How spinal cord paralysis alters body image. In Salter M (ed.) Altered Body Image: the Nurse's Role. Chichester: John Wiley

Kubler-Ross 1969 On Death and Dying. London: Macmillan

Lambert A, Johnson J 1995 Stump shrinkers: a survey of their use. Physiotherapy 81: 234–6

Lemaire ED, Fisher FR, Robertson DGE 1993 Gait patterns of elderly men with transtibial amputation. Prosthet Orthot Int 17: 27–37

Parkes CM 1972 Bereavement studies of grief in adult life. London: Tavistock

Parkes CM 1975 Psychosocial transition comparison between reactions of loss of limb and loss of spouse. Br. J Psychol 127: 204–10

Pell JP, Fowkes FGR, Lee AJ 1997 Indications for the arterial reconstruction and major amputation in the management of chronic critical lower limb ischaemia. Eur J Vasc Endvasc Surg 13: 315–21

Redhead RG 1984 The place of amputation in the management of ischaemic lower limb in the dysvascular geriatric patient. Int Rehabil Med 6: 68–71

Robicsek F 1997 Impact of arterial surgery and balloon angiography on amputation: a population based study. J Vasc Surg 26: 353

Seymour W 1998 Remaking the Body: Rehabilitation and Change. London: Routledge

Wade D 1992 Measurement in Neurological Rehabilitation. Oxford: Oxford University Press

Weiss SA, Lindell B 1996 Phantom limb pain and etiology of amputation in unilateral lower extremity amputees. J Pain Sympt Mgmt 11(11): 3–17

Williams AM, Deaton SB 1997 Phantom pain, elusive yet real. Rehabil Nurs 22(2); 73–7

Appendices

Glossary of Common Research Terms

Abstract A succinct summary of a research paper.

Action research The researcher uses some form of intervention in a situation and evaluates the impact of the intervention.

Bias Deviation of the results from their true values. This list contains several examples.

Central tendency The middle of a distribution.

Chance Random variation. Statistical methods are used to estimate the probability that chance alone has accounted for the difference in outcome.

Coding A qualitative research term, it refers to the task of ascribing codes to concepts and themes that occur in an interview transcript.

Cohort study Longitudinal study that begins with the gathering of two groups of patients (the cohorts), one which received the exposure of interest, and one which did not, and then following this group over time (prospective) to measure the development of different outcomes.

Confidence interval Often expressed as 95% confidence interval. The confidence interval (CI) quantifies uncertainty. It is derived from the sample mean and the standard error.

Confounding bias Occurs when two factors are closely associated and the effects of one confuses or distorts the effects of the other factor. The distorting factor is called a confounding variable.

Control group The study patients that have not received the experimental manoeuvre or test.

Correlational designs These look for a relationship between two variables. They do not involve the manipulation of variables, and they do not look for

cause and effect. A correlation is expressed as a number between −1 and +1 (see figures). Minus one signifies a negative correlation. Plus one signifies a positive correlation.

Crossover study design The administration of two or more experimental therapies one after the other.

Cross-sectional study Survey of an entire population for the presence or absence of a disease and/or other variable in every member (or a representative sample) and the potential risk factors at a particular point in time or time interval.

Data (singular = datum) The pieces of information, facts and figures that have resulted from the study. Data can be one of four types: nominal (naming data, e.g. male or female, yes or no); ordinal (slightly more detailed, puts data into an order, e.g. strongly agree, agree, neither agree nor disagree, disagree, disagree strongly); interval (as ordinal but assumes equal intervals between the categories); ratio (as interval but also possesses a zero point).

Dependent variable The variable which alters as a result of manipulation of the independent variable.

Double-blind Experimental method in which both the patients and the research staff do not know which patients are receiving treatment and which are receiving placebo.

Epistemology The theory of knowledge.

Ethnography The description or study of a culture.

Exclusion criteria The criteria by which members of the population of the sample will be excluded. For example in a study of heart rate, people with a history of cardiac problems would be excluded.

External validity Whether or not the results are valid outside the population that has been studied. For example, are results from studies done on dogs valid for cats?

Field notes Records or reflections kept by the researcher which act to enrich the data obtained or put them into some sort of context. Commonly used in qualitative research.

Focus group A group of people who have been gathered together in order to gain some insight into their ideas and attitudes towards a particular subject.

Generalisability Given the validity of the results, the similarity of the study population to the population in general.

Grounded theory Research approach which attempts to generate theory from the data.

Hawthorne effect When subjects systematically alter their behaviour when they are being watched.

Positive correlation:
As one gets larger, so does the other (e.g. the relationship between length of a person's foot and their shoe size)

Correlation of +1

Negative correlation:
As one gets larger, the other gets smaller (e.g. as age increases, height tends to decrease)

Correlation of −1

No correlation:
For example, there is no relationship between the colour of your socks and what you had for breakfast

Correlation of 0

Hypothesis (pleural = hypotheses)   A proposition that may be either supported or rejected.

Independent variable   The variable which is actually changed (manipulated) so that its effects on the dependant variable can be seen.

Inferential statistics   Determines how likely a given result occurred by chance alone. Since we can rarely study an entire population, we study a sample of the population and by inference apply that result to the entire population.

Intention-to-treat analysis   In a randomised control trial patients can be randomly assigned to different treatments After randomisation, patients who have been assigned conservative therapy may decide to have surgery instead. Conversely, patients assigned to the surgical treatment may decide not to undergo surgery. In an intent-to-treat analysis patients would be analysed for mortality according to the groups for which they were originally assigned.

Internal validity   Are the results of the study valid for the patient population studied?

Interobserver variability   Variability between different observers. For example, do two or more senior clinicians give the same reading from the same knee joint?

Intraobserver variability   Variability between the same observer on repeated occasions. For example, does a senior clinician give the same reading of knee flexion when goniometry is performed on more than one occasion?

Investigator bias   Occurs when the interviewer is aware (not blinded) of the outcome variable. An unblinded interviewer may be more vigorous in searching for the exposure of interest.

Mean   The average number in a set of values.

Measurement bias   The act of being studied or measured can affect the outcome.

Median   When values are arranged in order of magnitude, the median is the middle value for odd number of values and the average of the two middle values in the case of an even number of values.

Mode   The mode is the value that occurs most often.

Multivariate analysis   An analysis where the effects of many variables are considered.

Non-parametric test   Statistical test which is less sensitive than a parametric test but which can be used on nominal and ordinal data.

Normal distribution   Data which are spread out in a bell-shaped curve (see figure).

Null hypothesis   The proposal that there is no difference between groups. If the null hypothesis is true then the study findings are the result of chance or other random factors. A typical study aims to 'reject the null hypothesis'.

***p*-value**   The probability of a finding occurring by chance alone given that the null hypothesis is actually true. A *p*-value <0.05 is often considered significant.

Parametric test   Type of statistical test which is more sensitive and robust than a non-parametric test. In order to be able to carry out a parametric test on your data, the data must be interval/ratio, and should ideally be Normally distributed.

Phenomenology   The study of the lived experiences of people.

Pilot study   A small-scale 'test' run of the proposed larger research study under the same conditions. Useful as a means of ironing out problems before the study starts.

Placebo   An intervention that is actually a 'mock' intervention (e.g. giving a person a tablet which has no active ingredients but resembles the active drug in outward appearance).

Population   Every person who satisfies inclusion criteria for the study about to be performed.

Qualitative research   Research not based on numbers. Useful for assessing opinions, attitudes, feelings and so on.

Quantitative research   Research which is based on numbers.

Randomisation   The process by which every member of a population has an equal chance to be included in the sample.

Randomised controlled trial (RCT)   An experiment in which the researcher randomly assigns some patients to at least one manoeuvre and other patients to a placebo. When properly done, an RCT can be used to determine cause and effect.

Recall bias   The recall of events may differ in cases and controls. Questions may be asked more times and more intensively in cases compared to controls.

Referral bias   Healthcare referrers may attract individuals with specific disorders or exposures.

Reliability   The repeatability of a study.

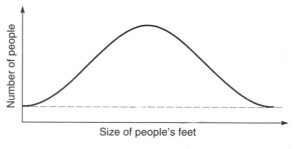

Normal distribution.

Research question   The question contains the population, the manoeuvre, the study population, and the outcomes. The research question should specify one measurable outcome, in addition to all conditions and any other important variables.

Sample   The individuals who satisfied the inclusion criteria and who actually entered the research study.

Sensitising concept   Term used to describe how certain concepts may guide the researched towards a certain behaviour.

Significance level   Probability of incorrectly rejecting the null hypothesis; i.e. saying that there is a difference between two groups when actually there is no difference. Otherwise known as the probability of a type I error. By convention, the level of significance is often set to a *p*-value of 0.01 (99% significance level) or 0.05 (95% significance level).

Spectrum bias   The sample population chosen is not representative of the population. For example, an appropriate spectrum of students were not included in the study of their exam results.

Standard deviation (SD)   Measure of variability or spread of data. The standard deviation quantifies how much the values vary from each other. It is a measure of the spread of individual observations around the mean value of the sample. A normal, unskewed curve will have 34% of the cases between the mean and 1SD above or below the mean; 68% of cases between 1SD above and 1 below the mean; and 95.5% of cases will be within 2SDs of the mean.

Standard error of the mean (SE)   Measure of variability. The standard error of the mean quantifies how accurately the true population mean is known.

Thematic analysis   In qualitative research the researcher attempts to categorise and analyse the themes that are produced from interviews.

Theoretical saturation   (data saturation) Used in qualitative research, the point where no new themes of concepts emerge from the data being collected.

Triangulation   Process whereby the same data are obtained from various means as an attempt to improve their validity.

Type I error   Rejecting the null hypothesis when it is actually true.

Type II error   Accepting the null hypothesis when it is actually false.

Volunteer bias   Volunteers may exhibit outcomes that may differ from non-volunteers (e.g. volunteers tend to be healthier).

Withdrawal bias   Patients who withdraw from studies may differ systematically from those who remain.

Common Medical Abbreviations

Check before using abbreviations in any legal documentation. The use of abbreviations might not be permitted in certain circumstances. Note that some common abbreviations have more than one meaning.

ACBT	Active cycle breathing technique
ACL	Anterior cruciate ligament
ADL	Activities of daily living
AE	Air entry
AFO	Ankle foot orthosis
AP	Antero-posterior
AF	Atrial fibrillation
AS	Ankylosing spondylitis
BCG	Bacille Calmette–Guérin
b.i.d.	Twice a day (medication)
BP	Blood pressure
BS	Breath [or bowel] sounds
B/slab	Back slab
CBC	Complete blood cell count
CDH	Congenital dislocation of hip
CK	Creatine kinase
CNS	Central nervous system
CPK	Creatine phosphokinase
CT	Computerised tomography
CoP	Completion [or change] of plaster
COPD	Chronic obstructive pulmonary disease
CPAP	Continuous positive airway pressure
CPM	Continuous passive motion
CRP	C-reactive protein
Crash team	Cardiac arrest team
C-section	Caesarean section
CVI	Cerebrovascular incident
CVS	Cardiovascular system
c/w	Consistent with
CXR	Chest X-ray
D&C	Dilation and curettage
DDD	Degenerative disc disease
DISH	Diffuse idiopathic skeletal hyperostosis
DOA	Dead on arrival [or date of admission]
DMARD	Disease-modifying anti-rheumatic drug
DNA	Deoxyribonucleic acid [or 'did not attend']
DM	Diabetes mellitus
DTs	Delirium tremens
DU	Duodenal ulcer
DVT	Deep-vein thrombosis
ECG	Electrocardiogram
EMG	Electromyogram

ESR	Erythrocyte sedimentation rate
ET	Endotracheal tube
EUA	Examination under anaesthesia
FH	Family history
F(A)RoM	Full (active) range of motion
GH	Glenohumeral
GI	Gastrointestinal
Hb	Haemoglobin
HDL	High-density lipoprotein
HIV	Human immunodeficiency virus
HPC	History of present condition
IBS	Irritable bowel syndrome
ICP	Intracranial pressure
IF	Interferential therapy
IgG	Immunoglobulin G
IM	Intramedullary
i.m.	Intramuscular (injection)
INH	Inhalation
INR	International Normalised Ratio
IRQ	Inner-range quadriceps
IPPV	Intermittent positive-pressure ventilation
i.v.	Intravenous
°JACCOL	No jaundice, anaemia, clubbing, cyanosis, oedema, lymphadenopathy
°LKKS	No liver, kidney, kidney, spleen
LBP	Low back pain
LCL	Lateral collateral ligament
LDL	Low-density lipoprotein
LFA	Low-friction arthroplasty
LFT×2	Lung or liver function tests
MAOI	Monoamine oxidase inhibitor
MCL	Medial collateral ligament
MDT	Multidisciplinary team
ME	Myalgic encephalomyopathy
MI	Myocardial infarction
MMR	Measles–mumps–rubella (vaccine)
MUA	Manipulation under anaesthesia
MRI	Magnetic resonance imaging
MWM	Mobilisations with movement
NAD	No abnormality detected
NAG	Natural apophyseal glide
NAI	Non-accidental injury
NBI	No bony injury
NBM	Nil by mouth
NoF	Neck of femur
NSAID	Non-steroidal-anti inflammatory drug

NIDDM	Non-insulin-dependent diabetes mellitus
NWB	Non-weight-bearing
OA	Osteoarthritis
Occ	Occasional
OE	Objective examination [or on examination]
ORIF	Open reduction internal fixation
PA	Postero-anterior
PCL	Posterior cruciate ligament
PE	Pulmonary embolism
PERLA	Pupils equal reacting to light and accommodating
PEME	Pulsed electromagnetic energy
PFT	Pulmonary function test
PFJ	Patellofemoral joint
PMH	Past medical history
PMR	Polymyalgia rheumatica
PID	Pelvic inflammatory disease [or prolapsed intervertebral disc]
PAIVM	Passive accessory intervertebral movement
PPIVM	Passive physiological intervertebral movement
POMR	Problem-oriented medical records
PoP	Plaster of Paris
PU	Passed urine
p.r.	*Per rectum*
p.r.n.	As needed (pro re nata)
PWB	Partial weight-bearing
Px	Prescribing
q.d.	Every day
q.i.d.	Four times per day
q.o.d.	Every other day
RA	Rheumatoid arthritis
RBC	Red blood cell
RS	Respiratory system
RSD	Reflex sympathetic dystrophy
RSI	Repetitive strain injury
RTA	Road traffic accident
Rx	Treatment
SAB	Subacromial bursa
SC	Subcuticular
SFL/SFR	Side flex left/right

SH	Social history
SIJ	Sacro iliac joint
SL	Sublingual
SLE	Systemic lupus erythematosus
SLR	Straight leg raise
SUF(c)E	Slipped upper femoral (capital) epiphysis
SNAG	Sustained natural apophyseal glide
SOB(OE)	Short of breath (on exertion)
SVT	Supraventricular tachycardia
TA	Tendo-achilles
TATT	Tired all the time
TAR	Total ankle replacement
t.d.s.	Three times a day
TFCC	Triangular fibrocartilaginous complex (at the wrist)
TFT	Thyroid function tests
THR	Total hip replacement
TIA	Transient ischaemic attack
TKR	Total knee replacement
TTO	To take out (medication)
TURP	Transurethral resection of prostate
U&E	Urea and electrolytes
URTI	Upper respiratory tract infection
US	Ultrasound
UTI	Urinary tract infection
VAS	Visual analogue scale
VF	Ventricular fibrillation
VMO	Vastus medialis obliquus
WBC	White blood cell
X-ray	X-ray

Other Symbols Seen in Medicine

< Less than
> More than
° No (absence of)
Fracture
Δ Diagnosis

Diagram of abdomen

Points on Critical Evaluation of a Research Paper

Physiotherapists need to be able to read and critically evaluate research reports and papers if they are to successfully incorporate them into their clinical practice. The following basic steps may help you when reading research articles and papers.

START

Read the article carefully.
Does the title give a clear guide as to what is to follow?
The title should be concise and precise

What is the theme or the broad aims of the piece of work in front of you?
What is your opinion of the general layout of the research paper?

Has the writer(s) explained or justified why they have done this study?
Have they explained and summarised the previous literature in the subject area?
(i.e. What is the context of this study?)

Why did the author(s) decide to do this study?

What is the research question?
Is there a research question?

What is the study design?
Is it qualitative, quantitative, case
study, systematic review or other format

More importantly, does the design fit the question?

Have the researchers used 'the right tool
for the right job?'

How did the researchers collect their data?
Have they acknowledged any limitations of the study?

Did they perform a pilot study?

Have they discussed validity and reliability?

What was their sample size, and do they note inclusion and
exclusion criteria if relevant?

How was sampling achieved?

Ethics: Were there any ethical issues? Did they obtain consent?

Presentation of the paper:
How is the information presented?
Are the statistical tests appropriate?
Are any graphs clearly presented?
Has any level of statistical significance been used?

What are the findings of the paper?
Did they answer their own research question?
Does it add to the body of existing knowledge?

Conclusion
How has the author(s) interpreted the result?
Have they made unsupported claims or missed the important points?

The 'so what' question:
Was it all worthwhile? Will it change anything about your work as a physiotherapist,
or could it be used in your own future clinical practice?
How can you integrate the paper into your work as a physiotherapist?

END

Ranges of Joint Motion (typical normal values)

Shoulder

Flexion	0–165°
Extension	60°
Abduction	0–180°
Internal rotation	70°
External rotation	90°

Elbow

Flexion	150°
Pronation	75°
Supination	80°

Wrist

Flexion	80°
Extension	70°
Ulnar deviation	30°
Radial deviation	20°

Thumb

CMC flexion	15°
CMC extension	20°
CMC abduction	70°

Finger

MCP flexion	90°
PIP flexion	100°
DIP flexion	80–90°

Hip

Flexion	120°
Extension	10–20°
Abduction	45°
Adduction	25°
Internal rotation	45°
External rotation	45°

Knee

Flexion	135°
Extension	0–5° (hyperextension)
Internal rotation	30°
External rotation	40°

Ankle

Dorsiflexion	20–30°
Plantarflexion	50°

Subtalar

Inversion	35°
Eversion	15°

Clinical Interest Groups: Worldwide Web Addresses

- For revisions, updates and further information, please see the website of the Chartered Society of Physiotherapy at www.csp.org.uk.
- In all the following, enter

  www.csp.org.uk/membergroups/clinicalinterestgroups/microsites

  into your browser address line, followed by the link **/*.cfm** (e.g. /aacp.cfm).

Area	Group	Website
Acupuncture	AACP	/aacp.cfm
Amputee rehabilitation	BACPAR	/bacpar.cfm
Animal therapy	ACPAT	/acpat.cfm
Bobath trained	BABTT	/babtt.cfm
Bobath tutors	BBTA	/bbta.cfm
Burns care	BBATG	/bbatg.cfm
Cardiac rehabilitation	ACPICR	/acpicr.cfm
Community	ACPC	/acpc.cfm
Continence treatment	CPPC	/cppc.cfm
Craniosacral therapy	CTACP	/ctacp.cfm
Cystic fibrosis	ACPCF	/acpcf.cfm
Electrotherapy	ACPIE	/acpie.cfm
Energy medicine	ACPEM	/acpem.cfm
Haemophilia	HCPA	/hcpa.cfm
Hand therapy	BAHT	/baht.cfm
HIV	CPIHIV	/cphiv.cfm
Hydrotherapy	HACP	/hacp.cfm
Hyperventilation	PFH	/pfh.cfm
Learning disabilities	ACPPLD	/acppld.cfm
Manipulation	MACP	/macp.cfm
Massage	ACPIM	/acpim.cfm
Mechanical diagnosis	MIMDT	/mimdt.cfm
Mental health	CPMH	/cpmh.cfm
Neurology	ACPIN	/acpin.cfm
Older people	AGILE	/agile.cfm
Oncology & palliative care	ACPOPC	/acpopc.cfm
Orthopaedic	AOCP	/aocp.cfm
Orthopaedic medicine	ACPOM	/acpom.cfm
Paediatrics	APCP	/apcp.cfm
Reflex therapy	PPA	/ppa.cfm
Respiratory care	ACPIRT	/acpirt.cfm
Rheumatic care	ACPRC	/acprc.cfm
Pain	RCACP	/rcacp.cfm
Sensory integration	SINetwork	/sine.cfm
Spinal injuries	SIUPLC	/siuplc.cfm
Sports medicine	ACPSM	/acpsm.cfm
Therapeutic riding	ACPTR	/acptr.cfm
Vestibular rehabilitation	ACPVR	/acpvr.cfm
Women's health	ACPWH	/acpwh.cfm

Dermatomes
(of the upper and lower limbs)

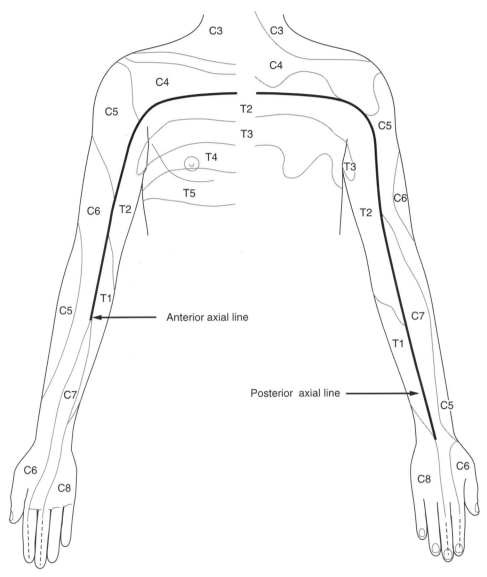

(Reproduced from Palastanga N, Field D, Soames R 2002 Anatomy and Human Movement, 4th edn. Butterworth–Heinemann: Oxford.)

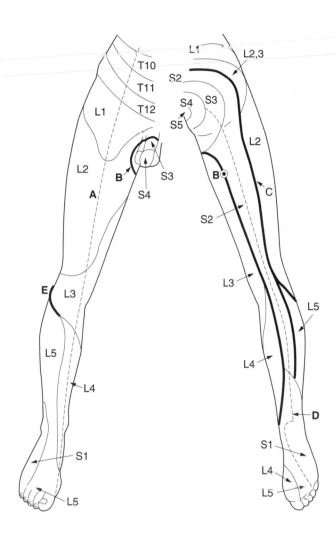

(Reproduced from Palastanga N, Field D, Soames R 2002 Anatomy and Human Movement, 4th edn.
Butterworth–Heinemann: Oxford.)

Myotomes

C4	Shoulder shrug
C5	Shoulder abduction, external rotation
C6	Elbow flexion, wrist extension
C7	Elbow extension, wrist flexion
C8	Ulnar deviation, thumb abduction, finger abduction
T1	Finger adduction
L2	Hip flexion
L3	Hip flexion, knee extension
L4	Knee extension, ankle dorsiflexion
L5	Great toe dorsiflexion (extension) eversion
S1/S2	Ankle plantarflexion, knee flexion
S3/S4	Rectal sphincter

Biomechanics: background maths and questions

TRIGONOMETRY

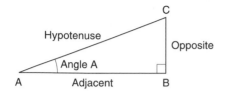

The tangent of an angle

> Tangent of angle A (tan A) = $\dfrac{\text{opposite}}{\text{side/adjacent side}}$

In this way, if we know the lengths of the opposite side and the adjacent side we can find the angle A. Likewise, if we know the angle at A and the length of the opposite side we can find the length of the adjacent side.

The sine and cosine of an angle

Two other ratios exist between the sides of a right-angled triangle and the angles of the triangle. These are sine and cosine, which are commonly written sin and cos.

> Sine of angle A (sin A) = $\dfrac{\text{opposite}}{\text{side/hypotenuse}}$
>
> Cosine of angle A (cos A) = $\dfrac{\text{adjacent}}{\text{side/hypotenuse}}$

With this information, if we know the length of one side and one angle of a right-angled triangle we can find the length of all the other sides and their angles. Within biomechanics it is possible to use only right-angled triangles. With the tools above it is possible to solve all the trigonometry necessary for biomechanical assessment.

Pythagoras' theorem

Pythagoras' theorem states that, *in a right-angled triangle*, the square of the hypotenuse is equal to the sum of the squares of the other two sides:

$$AC^2 = AB^2 + BC^2$$

So, if any two sides of a right-angled triangle are given, the third side can be found.

In a right-angled triangle the ratios of the sides of the triangle determine the angles within the triangle, and vice versa.

Self-assessed Questions: Trigonometry

Find all the sides and angles for the following triangles.

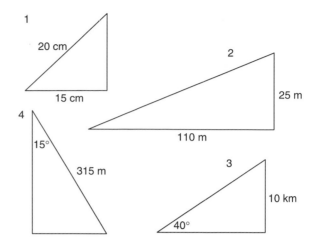

Solutions

1   Missing side = 13.2, missing angles = 41.4, 48.6 degrees
2   Missing side = 112.8, missing angles = 12.8, 77.2 degrees
3   Missing sides = 11.9, 15.6, missing angle = 50 degrees
4   Missing sides = 304.3, 81.5, missing angle = 75 degrees.

VECTORS

What is a vector?

Vectors have both *magnitude* (i.e. size) and *direction*. All vectors can be described in terms of components in the vertical and horizontal directions. Vectors may also be described by a *resultant* acting at a particular angle.

Displacement is a vector, i.e. a change in position in a particular direction. Other examples of vectors include force, velocity and acceleration.

The resultant

This is the combination effect of all the vectors. In this example the resultant is the distance travelled in a straight line. This can be found using Pythagoras' theorem.

The components

The components of a resultant act at 90 degrees to each other. This creates a right-angled triangle, which may be solved using the methods above.

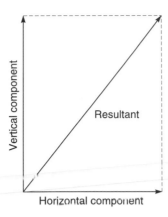

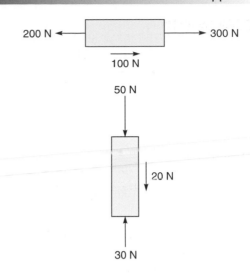

Rules to use when working out vector problems

First decide on a frame of reference (this may be compass points or planes of the human body; e.g. sagittal, coronal or transverse). If given the resultant and an angle find the component vectors acting in each of the directions of your reference system. If given the components of the resultant then use Pythagoras' theorem to find the magnitude of the resultant. Then use sine or cosine to find the angle at which it acts.

Adding and resolving forces

In practical biomechanical problems, the limbs or orthoses which are analysed will usually be subjected to a number of forces acting in various directions. Often, we will wish to 'add' (combine) these forces together to determine their overall or resultant effect. However, as forces are vectors – that is, they have direction as well as magnitude – they cannot simply be added numerically. If all the forces involved act along the same line they can be added algebraically – that is forces acting in one direction are regarded as positive, whilst those acting in the opposite direction are regarded as negative.

How to cope with problems that require resolving

Resolving is the term used for finding the component vectors from a resultant vector, or vice versa. This may be required if a force and its direction are known, but the magnitudes of the components in the different directions are not.

The component vector may be found by using trigonometry, but first we need to decide on a sensible frame of reference. When dealing with the human body this can either be:

- in the vertical and horizontal directions relative to the ground, or
- along a body segment, or object, and at 90 degrees to it.

Worked Example: Resolving

Find the horizontal and vertical components of the vector shown.

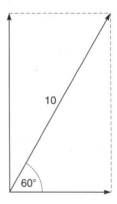

Horizontal force = 10 × cos 60
Horizontal force = 5
Vertical force = 10 × sin 60
Vertical force = 8.66

Self-assessed Questions: Resolving

Resolve the following to find either the resultant or the component vectors:

1 If the resultant of two vectors is 453 N (newtons) acting at 30 degrees from the horizontal, find the horizontal and vertical components of resultant.

2 If a plane moves along horizontally at 500 km/h and down at 25 km/h, find the resultant speed and the angle the plane is flying at.

3 A force acts on a mass in the direction shown. Find the components of the force acting in the x and y directions.

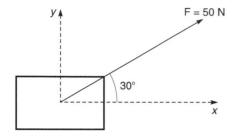

4 What is the resultant velocity of the boat shown?

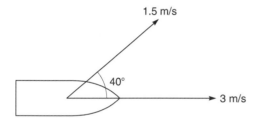

5 Find the resultant of all the forces acting on the mass shown.

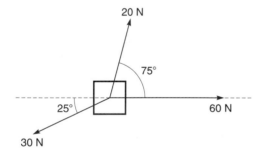

Solutions

1 Horizontal = 392 N, vertical = 226.5 N
2 Resultant speed = 500.6 km/h, angle = 2.86 degrees down
3 x = 43.3 N, y = 25 N
4 Up 0.96 m/s, right 1.15 m/s and 3 m/s (total right = 4.15), resultant = 4.25 m/s
5 Up 19.3 N, down 12.7 N, right 5.2 N and 60 N, left 27.2 N; total up = 6.6, total right = 38, resultant = 38.56.

NEWTON'S LAWS, MASS AND WEIGHT

Self-assessed Questions

1 A person has a mass of 60 kg. What is the weight of the person?

2 An apple has a weight of 5 N. What is its mass?

3 The diagram shows a plan view of a block on a smooth surface. Calculate the magnitude and direction of the resultant force on the block. At what rate will the block accelerate and in what direction? The mass of the block is 10 kg.

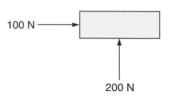

4 From the sketch of a person pulling a block, draw a free body diagram of the block. Calculate the acceleration of the block in the horizontal direction, ignoring friction, and calculate the reaction force at the ground on the block. The mass of the block is 25 kg, and the force which the rope exerts on the block is 100 N at an angle of 15 degrees to the horizontal.

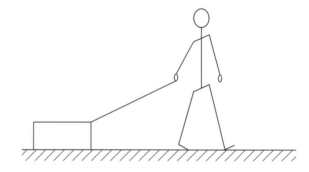

Solutions

1 588.6 N
2 0.51 kg
3 Force = 223.6 N, angle = 26.6 degrees, acceleration = 22.4 m/s²
4 Acceleration = 3.86 m/s², ground reaction force = 224 N.

GROUND REACTION FORCES

Self-assessed Questions

1 Draw the ground reaction forces in the three directions during normal gait.

2 Explain the functional implications of the following: (a) a low first peak on the vertical force trace; (b) a trough that does not fall below 0.9 times bodyweight; (c) a low second peak on the vertical force trace; (d) low anterior and posterior forces.

3 Describe the functional deficits of the force pattern shown below. How does it compare with that of normal? The subject's weight is 450N.

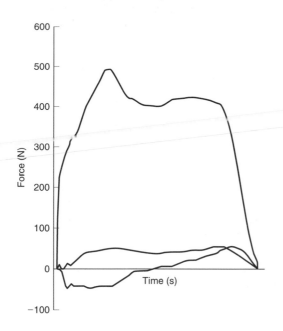

Solutions

1 See the main text in Chapter 6 on ground reaction forces during the gait cycle.
2 (a) Poor loading response. (b) Poor movement of the body over the stance limb. (c) Poor vertical propulsion. (d) Low anterior forces indicate poor propulsion forwards; low posterior forces indicate poor loading response.
3 Calculate how big the peaks and troughs are in relation to the bodyweight given. Then compare this information with the normal values given in Chapter 6. Describe the difference seen in the vertical peaks and troughs and the anterior/posterior peaks.

MOMENTS

Self-assessed Questions

1 Find the force F that will balance the seesaw shown below.

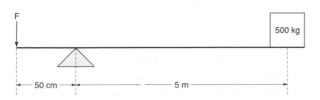

2 Find the force F that will balance the seesaw shown below.

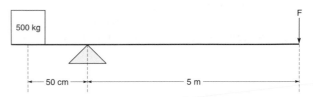

3 The weight of the beam shown below acts 1 m away from the pivot P. If a force acts at 30 degrees from the horizontal at a distance 3 m from the pivot, calculate the force F needed to support the beam. The mass of the beam is 10 kg.

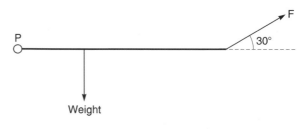

Solutions

1 50,000 N
2 500 N
3 66.7 N.

MUSCLE FORCE AND JOINT MOMENTS

Self-assessed Questions

1 The diagram below shows an arm flexed at the elbow with the hand holding a mass of 5 kg. The

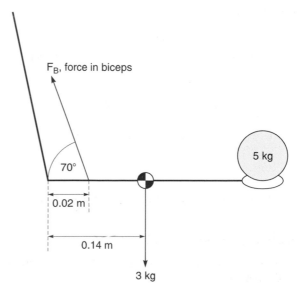

mass of the forearm is 3 kg and its length is 0.32 m. Calculate the muscle force in the biceps, F_B

2   If the forearm is now inclined to 20 degrees from the horizontal, as below, calculate the new muscle force in the biceps, F_B.

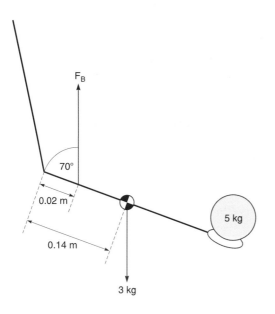

3   The diagram below represents a leg and foot in contact with the ground. If the point of application of the ground reaction force and the positions of the ankle, knee and hip are as shown, calculate the turning moments produced by the ground reaction force about (a) the ankle joint; (b) the knee joint; (c) the hip joint.

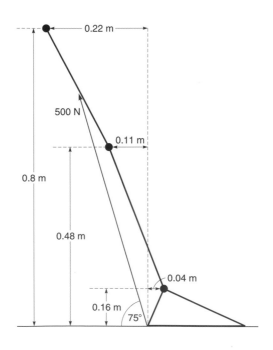

Solutions

1   weight of ball × 0.32 + weight of forearm × 0.14 − F_B sin 70 × 0.02 = 0
$5 \times 9.81 \times 0.32 + 3 \times 9.81 \times 0.14 − F_B \sin 70 \times 0.02 = 0$
$15.69 + 4.12 − F_B \sin 70 \times 0.02 = 0$
$19.81 − F_B \sin 70 \times 0.02 = 0$
$19.81 − F_B \sin 70 \times 0.02$
$19.81 / \sin 70 \times 0.02 = F_B$
$\underline{1054\,N = F_B}$

2   weight of ball × cos 20 × 0.32 + weight of forearm × cos 20 × 0.14 − F_B sin 70 × 0.02 = 0
$5 \times 9.81 \times \cos 20 \times 0.32 + 3 \times 9.81 \times \cos 20 \times 0.14 − F_B \sin 70 \times 0.02 = 0$
$14.75 + 3.87 − F_B \sin 70 \times 0.02 = 0$

$18.62 − F_B \sin 70 \times 0.02 = 0$
$18.62 = F_B \sin 70 \times 0.02$
$18.62 / \sin 70 \times 0.02 = F_B$
$\underline{990.7\,N = F_B}$

3   500 × cos 75 = Horizontal force
500 × sin 75 = Vertical force

Horizontal force = 129.4 N
Vertical force = 483 N

$M_{ankle} = 483 \times 0.04 + 129.4 \times 0.16$
$M_{ankle} = 19.32 + 20.7 = 40.02\ Nm$

$M_{knee} = −483 \times 0.11 + 129.4 \times 0.48$
$M_{knee} = 53.13 + 62.11 = 8.98\ Nm$

$M_{hip} = −483 \times 0.22 + 129.4 \times 0.80$
$M_{hip} = −106.26 + 103.52 = −2.74\ Nm$

ANGULAR WORK, ENERGY AND POWER

Self-assessed Questions

1   If a man, mass 90 kg, climbs a ladder to a height of 3 m, how much work has he done?
2   From (1), if the man climbs in 10 s, how much power has he produced?
3   On an isokinetics machine an individual produces a moment of 40 Nm over an angle of 45 degrees. (a) How much work was done? (b) If this were carried out over 0.25 s, how much power was produced?
4   An individual with a leg length of 0.9m produces a force at his toes of 46 N over an angle of 25 degrees in 0.2 s. How much power has been produced?
5   The diagram below shows an individual walking. During loading response the ground reaction force is 800 N acting at 80 degrees to the horizontal. If the knee joint flexes at a constant angular velocity of 150 degrees/s, find the knee joint power.

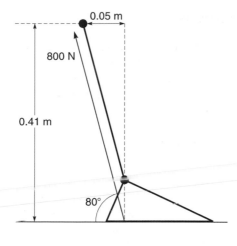

Solutions

1   Work done = mgh
Work done = $90 \times 9.81 \times 3$
Work done = 2649 J

2   P = work done / time = 2649 / 10 = 264.9 W

3   Work done = MΘ (rad)
Work done = $40 \times (45/57.3)$
Work done = 31.4J

P = work done / time
P = 31.4 / 0.25
P = 125.6 W

4   P = (Γ × d × Θ (rad)) / t
P = $(46 \times 0.9 \times (25 / 57.3)) / 0.2$
P = 90.3 W

5   Mk = $-800 \sin 80 \times 0.05 + 800 \cos 80 \times 0.41$
Mk = $-39.4 + 56.9$
Mk = 17.6 Nm

P = M × ω (rad/s)
P = $17.6 \times (150 / 57.3)$
P = 46 W

Respiratory Anatomy and Physiology

Surface Marking of the Lungs

It is important for a physiotherapist to understand how the lungs and lobes relate to the surface of the thorax. The lung borders may be traced as follows.

Right lung anterior border

Start at the level of the apex 2–3 cm above the medial third of the clavicle. Trace a line behind the right sternoclavicular joint vertically down behind the right side of the sternum to the 6th chondrosternal junction

Right lung inferior border

Trace from the 6th chondrosternal junction laterally on a line which crosses the 6th costal cartilage in midclavicular line and the 8th rib in midaxillary line, then medially to the 10th rib in line with the inferior angle of the scapula to the 10th thoracic spine.

Right lung posterior border

Trace from a point 2 cm right of 10th thoracic spine, vertically up the back to the level of the neck of the first rib, and thence to the apex.

Left lung anterior border

Trace the same as for the right lung on the left side down to the 4th chondrosternal junction. Then trace laterally along the lower border of the 4th costal cartilage for 3.5 cm, turn down and curve slightly medially to the 6th costal cartilage 4 cm from midline of sternum (this curve is the cardiac notch).

Left lung inferior and posterior borders

These are like those of the right lung.

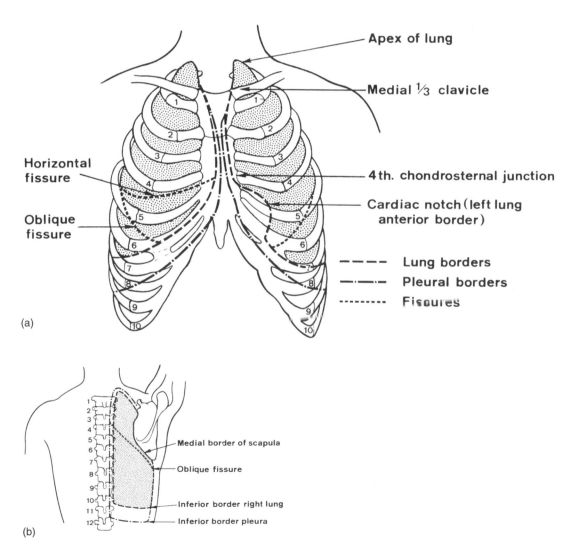

(a) anterior aspect of thorax showing surface marking of lungs and pleural borders
(b) posterior aspect of thorax showing right lung

Fissures

Oblique

This is traced from the posterior border of the right lung level with the spine of the 3rd thoracic vertebra to the 5th interspace in midaxillary line and ends anteriorly near the 6th costochondral junction at the inferior border, 7.5 cm from the midline of the sternum. The oblique fissure of the left lung is equivalent on the left side.

Horizontal

This is traced from the oblique fissure of the right lung in midaxillary line horizontally forwards and medially to the sternal end of the 4th costal cartilage. There is no horizontal fissure in the left lung.

Pleura

The right pleura starts 3 cm above the medial third of the clavicle, passes down behind the sternoclavicular joint and meets the left pleura at the sternal angle just left of midline. It passes vertically down to the level of the 4th chondrosternal junction and then obliquely to the 6th chondrosternal junction. It may then be traced laterally to the 8th costal cartilage in mid-clavicular line, the 10th rib in mid-axillary line, and the 11th rib in line with the inferior angle of the scapula to the level of the 12th thoracic spine, just lateral to midline.

The left pleura is traced in the same way as the right except that from the 4th chondrosternal junction it is traced obliquely laterally to the 8th costal cartilage in midclavicular line. Thereafter it is traced like the right pleura.

Mechanics of Respiration

The principal effect of movements of the thorax is to alter the capacity of the thoracic cavity to enable air to be drawn in (inspiration) or expelled (expiration) and thus produce ventilation of the lungs. This capacity may be increased in three dimensions anteroposteriorly, laterally and vertically by the muscles of respiration which are the diaphragm and the intercostals. The amount of movement depends on the depth of respiration (ventilation).

Inspiration

The muscular fibres of the diaphragm contract and pull down the central tendon thus increasing the vertical dimension. The excursion of the tendon is limited by the abdominal organs. As the muscle fibres continue to contract the tendon becomes the fixed point and the lower ribs are pulled upwards and outwards. As inspi-

ration continues the intercostal muscles also contract to produce these lower rib movements, and in addition the upper ribs move forwards and upwards and then outwards. Thus the capacity of the thoracic cavity is increased in all three dimensions.

Since the parietal pleura is attached to the upper surface of the diaphragm and inner surface of the thorax, the negative intrapleural pressure is made more negative, thus stretching the elastic tissue of the lungs and increasing the volume of the air spaces. Air rushes in because the pressure inside the lungs is subatmospheric. The deeper the inspiration the greater is the pressure difference and therefore the greater is the volume of air entering the lungs.

Expiration

This is a passive movement produced by the elastic recoil of the chest wall and the lung tissue which forces air out of the lungs. Momentarily, the pressure inside the lungs (alveolar pressure) is greater than atmospheric pressure. Then when the two pressures are equal expiration stops. In forced expiration the abdominal muscles contract to aid expulsion of air by increasing intra-abdominal pressure.

The volume of air that passes in and out of the lungs and the total lung capacity varies according to age, sex and height. Deviations from the normal predicted values indicate a functional disorder.

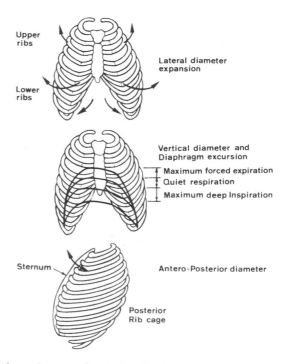

Thoracic excursion in inspiration

Lung Volumes and Capacities

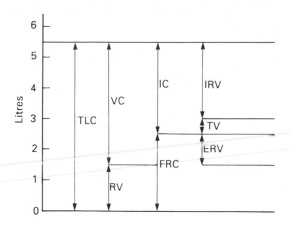

Lung volumes

The total lung capacity can be divided into various volumes:

- Tidal volume (TV) is the volume of air moved into or out of the lungs during quiet breathing at rest.
- Inspiratory reserve volume (IRV) is the volume of air additional to TV that can be inspired during a maximum inspiration.
- Expiratory reserve volume (ERV) is the volume of air additional to TV that can be expired during a maximum expiration.
- Residual volume (RV) is the volume of air remaining in the lungs after a maximum expiration.

Lung capacities

- Total lung capacity (TLC) is the total volume of air in the lungs after a maximum inspiration.
- Vital capacity (VC) is the maximum volume of air that can be expired after a maximum inspiration.
- Inspiratory capacity (IC) is the maximum volume of air that can be inspired from the endpoint of quiet expiration at rest.
- Functional residual capacity (FRC) is the volume of air remaining in the lungs at the end of quiet expiration at rest.

Tidal volume, inspiratory reserve volume, expiratory reserve volume, vital capacity and inspiratory capacity can be measured with a spirometer. Functional residual capacity can be measured indirectly using helium or nitrogen in a closed-circuit spirometer, a whole-body plethysmograph or radiographs. Residual volume and total lung capacity are calculated arithmetically from the measurements mentioned above.

Values for the average male adult are: TLC 5500 mL, RV 1500 mL, VC 4000 mL, IRV 2500 mL, IC 3000 mL, TV 500 mL, FRC 2500 mL, ERV 1000 mL. Values for the average female adult are 25% less.

In exercise the tidal volume gradually increases while both the inspiratory and expiratory reserve volumes decrease.

Respiratory rate

At rest a normal adult breathes in and out between 12 and 16 times per minute. During exercise this may increase to over 30 times per minute.

Respiratory minute volume is the tidal volume multiplied by the respiratory rate; e.g. 500 mL × 14 = 7000 mL.

Anatomical dead space is the volume of air in the conducting airways from the nose and mouth to the alveoli and is 150 mL.

Forced vital capacity (FVC) is the maximum volume of air forcibly expired after a maximum inspiration. Forced expiratory volume in one second (FEV_1) is the volume of air forcibly expired after a maximum inspiration in one second and this is usually 80% FVC. Thus the ratio FEV_1/FVC in healthy people is 80%.

Peak expiratory flow rate (PEFR) is the maximum flow rate of air from full inspiration during a forced expiration and is measured with a Wright peak flow meter. In the normal adult PEFR is over 400 L per minute.

Disease states

Lung measurements are altered in respiratory diseases which have characteristic patterns.

In obstructive airways disease such as asthma, emphysema and chronic bronchitis, there is a greater reduction in FEV_1 than FVC, so that the ratio FEV_1/FVC may be as low as 30%. These diseases result in hyperinflation of the lungs and the TLC, FRC and RV are increased. PEFR can be reduced to less than 100 L per minute. In reversible airways obstruction the FEV_1/FVC and PEFR are improved after the administration of bronchodilators or corticosteroids and other measurements are nearer normal values.

In restrictive airways disease such as fibrosing alveolitis pneumonia, pleural and neuromuscular diseases and pulmonary collapse, the FEV and FVC are both reduced in the same proportion resulting in the FEV_1/FVC ratio remaining about 80%. The TLC, VC and RV are all decreased but PEFR is normal. Ankylosing spondylitis can produce results similar to restrictive airways disease.

Lung measurements obtained with a vitalograph spirometer

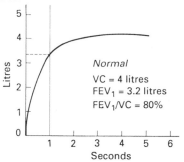

Normal
VC = 4 litres
FEV$_1$ = 3.2 litres
FEV$_1$/VC = 80%

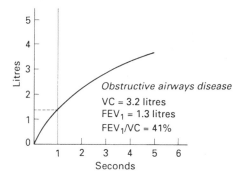

Obstructive airways disease
VC = 3.2 litres
FEV$_1$ = 1.3 litres
FEV$_1$/VC = 41%

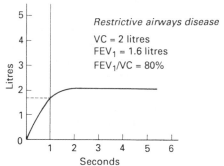

Restrictive airways disease
VC = 2 litres
FEV$_1$ = 1.6 litres
FEV$_1$/VC = 80%

Composition of air (%)

	Inspired air	Expired air	Alveolar air
Oxygen	20.95	16.40	13.80
Carbon dioxide	0.04	4.00	5.50
Nitrogen	79.01	79.60	80.70

Alveolar air has the least amount of O2 because it is from the alveoli that O2 diffuses out into the blood. Similarly alveolar air has most CO2 because CO2 diffuses from the blood into the alveoli.

Expired air is a mixture of alveolar air and dead space air which has the composition of inspired air.

Chest Radiographs

Radiograph films are generally posteroanterior (PA) or lateral (L) views taken at total lung capacity (i.e. at maximum inspiration). Prior to reading a radiograph it is important to check the patient's name, whether it is posteroanterior or anteroposterior (AP) and to identify left from right.

- Clavicles – check level and position.
- Scapulae – identify medial border, which is well round the chest wall due to the protracted position of the shoulder girdles.
- Trachea central and vertical.
- Upper border of right hemi diaphragm is level with 10th rib at the back and 6th rib at the front. The left side is 1–3 cm lower.
- The heart shadow. The width at its broadest part should not exceed 50% of the total width of the chest.
- The right border of the heart shadow represents the border of the right atrium.
- The left border of the heart shadow comprises from above down, the aorta, pulmonary artery and left ventricle.
- Lung markings. Identify level of vascularity. This should decrease towards the periphery.

NB. Air shows as a dark area while bone and soft tissues which absorb X-rays appear light. Abnormal lesions that absorb X-rays show as grey/white areas and may be referred to as *shadows* or *opacities*.

Common abnormalities on chest radiographs

- *Lobar collapse.* Identify shift of trachea, raised hemi-diaphragm and fissures which may be obviously displaced. A collapsed area looks like a homogenous opacity.
- *Consolidation.* Characterized by patchy opacity usually localized to a lobe or segment.
- *Pleural effusion.* Always associated with loss of the costophrenic angles, and is seen as a dense opacity.
- *Coin lesion.* Round dense areas anywhere in the lung fields may indicate carcinoma, tuberculosis or rheumatoid nodule.
- *Pneumothorax.* No lung markings are seen, and the edge of the collapsed lung may be identified.
- *Lung abscess.* Appears as a rounded opacity with concave meniscus at edges showing fluid level.

Other radiographic tests

- *Bronchograms.* Radiographs are taken after a radio-opaque fluid has been introduced to the lung fields.

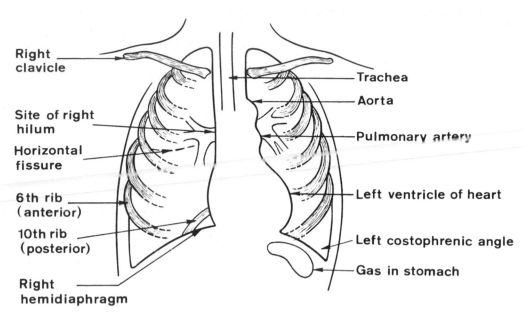

Main features on an antero-posterior chest radiograph.

- *Tomography.* Radiographs are taken with a specific area of the lung in focus and surrounding structures are blurred.
- *CAT scans.* Computerized axial tomograph provides views of horizontal 'slices' through the chest wall.

Breath Sounds

A stethoscope is used to determine the quality, character and intensity of breath sounds, vocal resonance and adventitious sounds.

Normal breath sounds

Normal breath sounds are of two types: (1) over the trachea, and (2) over lung tissue. Two tracheal sounds are heard: (1) on inspiration of low pitch, and (2) on expiration – at a higher pitch and for longer. The two are separated by a pause, and are blowing in quality.

The stethoscope diaphragm is placed near the root of the neck. Two lung tissue sounds are heard:

1 On inspiration – A 'wind through trees' sound heard throughout inspiration.
2 On expiration – A very short low pitched sound or no sound at all.

There is no pause between the two and they are rustling in quality. They are often referred to as vesicular breath sounds.

The stethoscope diaphragm is placed on various parts of the chest wall, covering each side equally

Abnormal breath sounds

- Tracheal breath sounds heard over lung tissue areas (often referred to as bronchial breathing). This is due to transmission of these sounds by fluid or consolidation (e.g. in pneumonia). The sound is muffled by pleural effusion.
- Absence of lung tissue sounds occurs when transmission of sound is impeded (e.g. in pneumothorax, lung tissue collapse or pleural effusion). In severe asthma airflow obstruction may be so extensive as to prevent transmission of breath sounds and this is known as 'silent chest'.

Stethoscope positional sounds

Vocal resonance are the sounds heard through the stethoscope when the patient is asked to say 'Aaa' or '99'.

Normal

The sounds can be heard clearly over the trachea and are muffled and softer over lung tissue. If the patient is asked to whisper, the sound can be heard over the trachea but not at all over lung tissue.

Abnormal: increased sounds

- Broncophony – The number '99' can be clearly heard over lung tissue.
- Whispering pectoriloquy – The whispered '99' can be heard over lung tissue.

Both of these are due to consolidation.

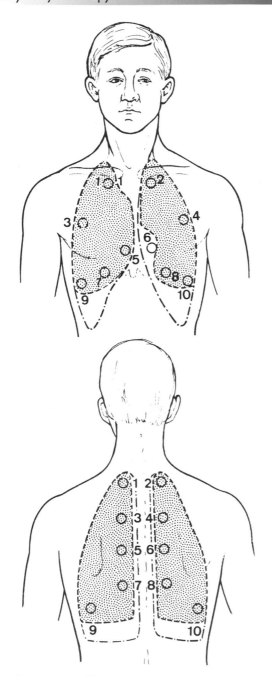

Stethoscope positions.

Abnormal: adventitious sounds

These are always a sign of abnormality. There are three types:

- rhonchi or wheezes
- crepitations or crackles
- pleural rub.

Rhonchi or wheezes indicate obstruction or narrowing of airways. They may be low-pitched and sonorous or high-pitched and whistling. The greater the narrowing, the higher the pitch of the sound.

Abnormal: crepitations or crackles

These are short, interrupted sounds possibly due to the opening of previously closed airways. They are heard on inspiration and can help determine the site of abnormality as follows:

- Start of inspiration – large airways.
- Mid-inspiration – medium/smaller airways.
- End of inspiration – small airways and lung tissue.

They may be coarse as in bronchiectasis or fine as in pulmonary oedema.

Abnormal: pleural rub

This is a squeaky sound present on both inspiration and expiration. It is due to roughening of the pleural surfaces as in pleurisy.

Percussion

This is performed by placing one hand flat on the patient's chest and the middle phalanx of that hand is then tapped with the middle finger of the other hand. The resonance of the percussion note and resistance to percussion are identified.

The note is affected by the nature of the underlying tissues, being duller over the heart and liver and more resonant over air-filled lung tissue. Abnormal dullness may be caused by pleural effusion, lung collapse or consolidation or localised fibrosis. Increased resonance is indicative of pneumothorax or emphysema.

Index

Note: Page numbers in italics refer to figures and/or tables. Abbreviations used as sub entries include: ACBT, active cycle of breathing technique; COPD, chronic obstructive pulmonary disease; DMARDs disease-modifying antirheumatic drugs; ECG, electrocardiography, NSAIDs, non-steroidal anti-inflammatory drugs and TBI, traumatic brain injury, other common abbreviations are listed on pages 517–518.